Annual Update in Intensive Care and Emergency Medicine 2016

GW00602725

The series *Annual Update in Intensive Care and Emergency Medicine* is the continuation of the series entitled *Yearbook of Intensive Care Medicine* in Europe and *Intensive Care Medicine: Annual Update* in the United States.

Jean-Louis Vincent
Editor

Annual Update in Intensive Care and Emergency Medicine 2016

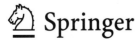 Springer

Editor
Prof. Jean-Louis Vincent
Université libre de Bruxelles
Dept. of Intensive Care
Erasme Hospital
Brussels, Belgium
jlvincen@ulb.ac.be

ISSN 2191-5709   ISSN 2191-5717 (electronic)
Annual Update in Intensive Care and Emergency Medicine
ISBN 978-3-319-27348-8   ISBN 978-3-319-27349-5 (eBook)
DOI 10.1007/978-3-319-27349-5

Cover design: WMXDesign GmbH, Heidelberg

Printed on acid-free paper

This Springer imprint is published by Springer Nature
The registered company is Springer International Publishing AG Switzerland.

Contents

Part III   Renal Issues

Part IV   Fluid Therapy

Part V   Bleeding

Part VI   Cardiovascular System

Part X   Metabolic Support

Part XI   Ethical Issues

Part XII   Applying New Technology

Part XIII   Intensive Care Unit Trajectories: The Bigger Picture

Common Abbreviations

AKI — Acute kidney injury
ARDS — Acute respiratory distress syndrome
BMI — Body mass index
CAP — Community-acquired pneumonia
CI — Confidence interval/cardiac index
COPD — Chronic obstructive pulmonary disease
CPB — Cardiopulmonary bypass
CPR — Cardiopulmonary resuscitation
CRP — C-reactive protein
CRRT — Continuous renal replacement therapy
CT — Computed tomography
CVP — Central venous pressure
ECMO — Extracorporeal membrane oxygenation
EKG — Electrocardiogram
ICU — Intensive care unit
IL — Interleukin
LPS — Lipopolysaccharide
LV — Left ventricular
MAP — Mean arterial pressure
MRI — Magnetic resonance imaging
OR — Odds ratio
PEEP — Positive end-expiratory pressure
PCR — Polymerase chain reaction
RCT — Randomized controlled trial
RRT — Renal replacement therapy
RV — Right ventricular
SvO_2 — Mixed venous oxygen saturation
SOFA — Sequential organ failure assessment
TNF — Tumor necrosis factor
VILI — Ventilator-induced lung injury

Part I
Infections and Antibiotics

Interpreting Procalcitonin at the Bedside

J. Fazakas, D. Trásy, and Z. Molnár

Introduction

One of the most challenging tasks in critical care medicine is the treatment of serious infection-related multiple organ dysfunction. Early detection of infection and the immediate start of resuscitation paralleled with adequate antimicrobial therapy undoubtedly give the best possible chance for survival and are strongly recommended in the Surviving Sepsis Campaign guidelines [1]. However, although recognizing organ failure via objective signs is relatively easy, diagnosing infection as a possible underlying cause remains a challenge. Because of the non-specific properties of conventional signs of infection, such as body temperature and white blood cell (WBC) count, biomarkers to aid diagnosis have been looked for for decades. One of the most studied biomarkers is procalcitonin (PCT) [2]. Its role in assisting antibiotic therapy has been studied extensively, with contradicting results. There are positive studies [3, 4] showing that PCT-guided patient management reduced antibiotic exposure and length of antibiotic therapy without affecting patient outcomes. There are also negative studies, which did not show this benefit [5–7]. However, to understand the values and limitations of inflammatory biomarkers it is necessary to understand the immunological background of critical illness determined mainly by the host response. Putting the results of these studies into context, based on new insights of the pathomechanisms of sepsis and systemic inflammation generated mainly by the individual's host response, may help explain the differences between the reported results and help the clinician to interpret PCT data with more confidence at the bedside.

J. Fazakas
Department of Transplantation and Surgery, Semmelweis University
Budapest, Hungary

D. Trásy · Z. Molnár (✉)
Department of Anesthesiology and Intensive Therapy, University of Szeged
Budapest, Hungary
email: zsoltmolna@gmail.com

© Springer International Publishing Switzerland 2016
J.-L. Vincent (ed.), *Annual Update in Intensive Care and Emergency Medicine 2016*,
DOI 10.1007/978-3-319-27349-5_1

Sepsis Is not a 'Definitive' Disease

In classical medicine, for example, in most fields of surgery and internal medicine, after taking a medical history, performing physical examination and diagnostic tests, the diagnosis is often straightforward, and patients can receive treatment, which is by-and-large well defined around the world. As examples, in stroke, myocardial infarction, bone fractures, intracranial hemorrhage, etc., we have diagnostic tests with very high sensitivity and specificity. However, defining sepsis is not that simple.

The term "sepsis syndrome" was conceived in a hotel in Las Vegas in 1980, during the designing of the protocol of one of the first prospective randomized trials in sepsis, performed by a group of scientists led by the late Roger Bone [8]. The study ended with non-significant results, but a statement paper was later published by the same authors entitled "Sepsis syndrome: a valid clinical entity" [9], after which medical society started to deal with sepsis as a definitive disease. As a definitive disease, physicians wanted a single test with high sensitivity and specificity to diagnose sepsis, and there was an urge to find an 'anti-sepsis magic bullet'. Neither of these wishes has or will ever come true.

Regarding the definition and diagnosis of sepsis, the classical signs of the "sepsis syndrome", such as fever/hypothermia, leukocytosis/leukopenia, tachycardia and hypotension, were met by a very large and non-specific cohort of patients. For this reason, a consensus conference was convened and defined 'consensus criteria' of sepsis, which have been used for decades in research and clinical practice [10]. In the most recent Surviving Sepsis Campaign guidelines more robust, more detailed criteria were used as definition [1], but these were almost immediately questioned by experts who had also taken part in the Surviving Sepsis Campaign process [11].

These efforts clearly show that finding the appropriate definition of sepsis has been a continuous challenge for more than 30 years. The difficulty in defining sepsis originates from its complex pathophysiology, which is affected by numerous individual variations of the host response. Furthermore, in most specialties, diagnostic laboratory or radiological tests have very high sensitivity and specificity, often reaching almost 95–100% [12]. However, in the case of sepsis, as we will see in the subsequent paragraphs, the situation is different, which makes not just diagnosis, but also interpretation of the results of clinical trials and epidemiological data very difficult.

From Localized Insult to Cytokine Storm

The immune system is a complex network and the immune response to pathogens relies on both innate and adaptive components, dynamically defined as the pro- and anti-inflammatory forces. The innate immune system (including the complement system, sentinel phagocytic and natural killer cells), is responsible for the eradication of the invaders, whereas the adaptive immune system's role is to control the process and keep it localized to the site of the insult [13]. Under normal circumstances, these mechanisms remain in balance. The innate system acts by broad recognition of antigens, mainly by triggering pathogen-associated molecular patterns (PAMPs) of lipopolysaccharide (LPS) elements of the surfaces of invading pathogens. When there is an imbalance due to dysregulation of the pro- and anti-inflammatory forces, the local response escalates into a systemic host response also termed a "cytokine storm" [14]. It was a surprising finding that after trauma, burns, ischemia-reperfusion, pancreatitis, major surgery, etc., the same or similar molecules that are found in PAMPs are released, mainly from the mitochondria of the injured or stressed cells, and can also cause a cytokine storm. This process accompanying tissue injury is called damage-associated molecular patterns (DAMPs). This similarity is due to the fact that the bacteria and the mitochondria (which are more-or-less encapsulated bacteria) share very similar genetic backgrounds, and explains why tissue injury-induced DAMPs and bacterial infection-induced PAMPs manifest as similar host responses and clinical manifestations [15].

The Role of PCT in Diagnosing Infection

The question "Is this patient septic?" is frequently asked on intensive care unit (ICU) rounds. However, this may be an irrelevant issue. Why? Because, first, we should recognize a critically ill patient via objective signs of organ dysfunction, which determines the immediate start of basic and organ-specific resuscitation, regardless of the actual diagnosis. And, second, what is of pivotal importance is not that the patient is septic or not, but whether the onset of critical illness is due to infection or not? Because, if it is due to infection, then we should start antibiotics or perform another form of source control. But if there is no infection, then antibiotic therapy should not be commenced, because of its undesired effects. Therefore, it is not 'sepsis' that we treat, but organ dysfunction and infection.

Diagnosing infection on the ICU is not easy and requires a multimodal approach. Clinical signs are obviously the most important in recognizing critical illness and suspecting infection and even the source of infection, but they cannot prove it on their own. Conventional indicators, such as fever/hypothermia, leukocytosis/leukopenia, tachypnea, tachycardia, hypotension, taken from the classical sepsis-syndrome criteria are non-specific, and in fact poor indicators of infection. To fill this gap, inflammatory biomarker measurements have been developed [2]. Every biomarker has its own merits and limitations, but there is no 'ideal' biomarker, and there may never be one. Biomarkers can support decision-making but they will never be able to differentiate between the inflammatory response to infection and the host response to non-infectious insults with 100% sensitivity and specificity because of the complex, overlapping pathomechanism of PAMPs and DAMPs. This situation is in sharp contrast with the diagnostic power of certain biomarkers used in the world of 'definitive' diseases, where several laboratory parameters have this ability. Furthermore, learning how to use biomarkers is not easy either.

The two markers most commonly used in infection/sepsis diagnostics and for guiding therapeutic interventions are PCT and C-reactive protein (CRP) [2]. One of the main limitations of CRP is that it moves 'slowly', and after a certain insult reaches its maximum value usually 48 h later. This is in general unacceptable on the ICU, as every hour delay in starting, for example, appropriate antibiotic treatment can affect mortality as indicated in the study of Kumar et al. [16]. Furthermore, levels are generally elevated in most ICU patients, making interpretation of CRP very difficult [17].

PCT is detectable in the serum within a few (4–6) h after its induction, which is most often by bacterial infection. During the 'normal' course of an infection it reaches its peak within 24 h and then starts to decline, if treatment is adequate, with levels reducing by roughly 50% daily according to its half-life [18]. PCT differentiates bacterial infections from a systemic inflammatory response of other etiologies with higher sensitivity and specificity than CRP [19], and also has good prognostic value [20]. However, interpreting PCT concentrations on admission or after the onset of an acute insult, whether infectious or not, is not simple. There are many studies reporting that PCT concentrations correlate with severity and differ significantly in patients with SIRS, sepsis, severe sepsis and septic shock [21]. Clec'h et al. found that patients with septic shock had more than 10 times higher median PCT concentrations as compared to those admitted with shock of non-septic origin [22]. However, looking at the data carefully reveals that although there was a remarkable and statistically significant difference, there was also a huge scatter and overlap of the PCT data between the groups (septic shock: 14 (0.3–767) vs. non-septic shock: 1 (0.15–36) ng/ml), which makes individual interpretation of a single measurement very difficult – a finding, which is generally true for every biomarker of inflammation. This observation was reinforced by the same group in a subsequent study, in which they found that the median PCT concentrations in medical vs. surgical patients differed in SIRS (0.3 (0.1–1.0) vs. 5.7 (2.7–8.3)) and in septic shock (8.4 (3.6–76.0) vs. 34.0 (7.1–76.0) ng/ml) [23]. These differences and the large overlap can be explained by the PAMP- and DAMP-based host response. In certain cases, there is a single PAMP or DAMP, but they can also occur in combination as PAMP + DAMP. The latter is bound to have a pronounced inflammatory response reflected in higher PCT concentrations. Therefore, it has become clear that the same PCT concentration, in other words a given 'normal' concentration, cannot be used in every condition. Medical patients with infection should, in general, have lower PCT concentrations (single PAMP insult) as compared to surgical patients with infection, in which DAMP and PAMP are present at the same time. Moreover, it is also important to acknowledge that any cellular injury, whether direct tissue or ischemia-reperfusion injury without infection, can result in elevation of PCT induced by a single DAMP type insult.

In recent large multicenter trials some authors did not show benefit of a PCT-based approach to antibiotic management in ICU patients [5–7]. However, in these studies, fixed PCT values were applied in the protocols with a low (1 ng/ml) cut-off value for intervention. In the studies by Jensen et al. [6] and Layios et al. [5], 40% of the patients were surgical, in whom, as we have shown before, this threshold of PCT is too low; hence these patients may have received antibiotics unnecessarily, which may in part explain the negative results.

Although PCT absolute values have the above mentioned limitations, there is overwhelming evidence that in most cases, high PCT concentrations indicate bacterial infection. The shortcomings of absolute PCT values may be compensated when the kinetics of PCT are taken into account to indicate infection. In a recent study by Tsangaris et al., daily measurements of PCT were performed and kinetics were evaluated in patients who had already been treated on the ICU for > 10 days and had a sudden onset of fever [24]. These authors found a two-fold increase in PCT levels from the day before to the day when there was a sudden onset of fever in patients with proven infection, but there was no change in PCT concentrations in patients with fever but no infection. They concluded that in patients treated longer-term on the ICU, PCT values on the day of fever onset must be compared to values measured on the previous day in order to define whether this rise in temperature is due to infection or not. It is also important to note that these were medical patients, in whom median PCT concentrations varied between 0.1–0.75 ng/ml. Nevertheless, despite the low absolute values, a two-fold increase was able to detect those with proven infection.

In a recent observational study, we also found that an increase in PCT from the day before (t_{-1}) to the day when infection was suspected (t_0) predicted infection. The best cut-off for the absolute PCT concentration was 0.84 ng/ml, with a sensitivity of 61% (95% CI 50–72) and specificity 72% (95% CI 53–87), which shows that the absolute value was a poor indicator. However, the percentage change in PCT concentration, with an increase of > 88% from t_{-1} to t_0, had a sensitivity of 75% (95% CI 65–84) and specificity of 79% (95% CI 60–92) and a PCT delta change of > 0.76 ng/ml had a sensitivity of 80% (95% CI 70–88) and specificity of 86% (95% CI 68–96) to indicate infection. Furthermore, neither the absolute values of conventional indicators of infection, such as WBC, body temperature and CRP, nor their change from t_{-1} to t_0, could predict infection [25].

Despite the discussed limitations, elevated PCT concentration has so far been shown to have the best sensitivity and specificity to indicate infection compared to other markers, and in the case of high levels one must at least suspect infection, whereas low PCT concentrations may help to exclude infection and suggest that antibiotics not be started. However, careful multimodal evaluation of the clinical picture together with PCT results and consideration of all the issues discussed earlier is necessary to correctly interpret PCT results and make the best decisions for our ICU patients.

PCT-assisted Antibiotic Therapy

There are three fundamental questions to be answered during our ward rounds when treating patients with suspected or proven infections on the ICU: 1) is there infection, in other words should we start empirical antibiotic therapy?; 2) is the commenced antibiotic effective?; and finally, 3) when should we stop antibiotic treatment?

Fig. 1 Starting antibiotic (AB) therapy. PCT: procalcitonin; *: patient requires clinically significant dose of vasopressors after initial resuscitation. For explanation see text

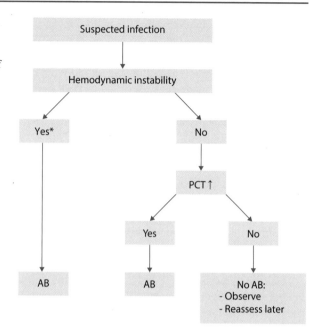

Diagnosing Infection and Starting Antibiotics

The role of PCT in diagnosing infection has been discussed in detail earlier. Several studies have investigated the effects of PCT-guided antibiotic therapy on patient outcomes. In a landmark study by Christ-Crain et al., antibiotic exposure was reduced by 50% (44% versus 83%) in patients admitted to emergency wards with acute respiratory complaints when antibiotic therapy was guided by admission PCT levels as compared to using conventional signs of infection only [3]. Two subsequent multicenter trials also found a decrease in antibiotic exposure in patients treated on the ICU with infections [4, 26]. The possible reasons why other studies [5, 7], could not find positive results were discussed earlier.

Patients treated on the ICU for a longer period of time may develop an imbalance between pro- and anti-inflammatory forces such that the latter become prominent. These patients will become immunoparalyzed, making them prone to a series of recurrent infections. Detecting infection in these patients may prove even more difficult. Rau et al. [27] found that in patients with secondary peritonitis, PCT levels increased and indicated infection, but the peak values decreased significantly with each new insult. This observation was also supported by Charles et al. [28]. They found that during the first infectious insult, the mean PCT concentration was 55 ng/ml, but during the second infectious insult, despite the same clinical gravity, it was several fold less at 6.4 ng/ml. These data indicate that with time, patients become immunoparalyzed and lower PCT concentrations should then be taken just as seriously as higher levels in the early course of the disease. Furthermore, this

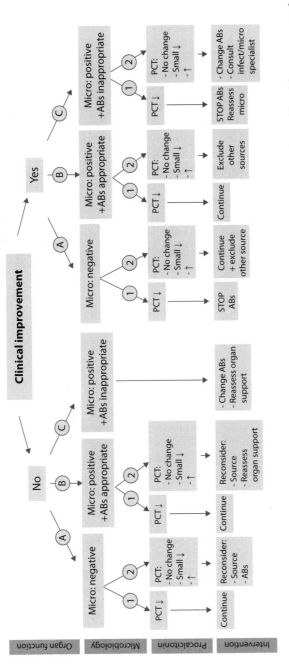

Fig. 2 Multimodal reassessment of antibiotic (AB) therapy on day 2–3. After empirical antibiotics have been commenced, a multimodal reassessment of the situation when microbiological data are available, usually on day 2 or 3, is strongly recommended. *No clinical improvement:* Despite no clinical improvement, a decrease in procalcitonin (PCT) (A-1) may still indicate that the infection is under control, but the patient needs more time to benefit from treatment; therefore, antibiotics should be continued. By contrast (A-2), if PCT is not decreasing or even increasing, these can be important signs that infection is not under control, hence source of infection and antibiotics (type, dose) should be reassessed. If antibiotics are appropriate, depending on PCT changes, antibiotics should either be continued (B-1) or other sources of infection should be looked for (B-2). In case of inappropriate antibiotics and no clinical improvement, regardless of the PCT concentration, therapy should be changed (C). *Clinical improvement:* If there is no proof of infection (micro: negative), based on PCT changes (↓ or ↑) infection may be excluded and antibiotics stopped (A-1) or continued (A-2). Similar algorithms can be applied if antibiotics are appropriate (B-1, 2). If antibiotics are inappropriate and PCT decreases, then one may consider the microbiology as a false positive and stop antibiotics (C-1), because it is highly unlikely that there is clinical improvement and decreasing PCT if an infection is not under control due to inappropriate antibiotics. This scenario happens when there are pathogens (colonization for example), but no infection. Finally, if antibiotics are inappropriate and PCT changes unfavorable (C-2), consultation with infectious disease specialists/microbiologists is recommended. Micro: microbiology; ↑: increasing concentrations; ↓: decreasing concentrations; infect: infectious disease; micro: microbiology

provides further evidence that PCT will respond to the same insult differently during the course of the disease, and hence values should be interpreted with care.

To put these considerations into a clinical context, two very common scenarios will be discussed, which are summarized in two decision trees (Figs. 1 and 2). Figure 1 shows how PCT can help in decision-making when infection is suspected. If the patient is hemodynamically unstable and infection is likely, by definition he/she has septic shock or at least one cannot exclude it, hence antibiotic therapy should not be delayed but has to be commenced immediately, regardless of the PCT or any biomarker value [16]. However, if the patient is stable hemodynamically, and PCT is 'low' or decreasing (based on the problems with absolute PCT values, discussed in detail above, we deliberately avoid giving exact numbers), then we can wait, observe the patient and reassess later (Fig. 1; [3]).

The next scenario demonstrates the reevaluation of the situation when microbiological data become available, which usually takes place 2–3 days after specimens were sent to the laboratory and antibiotics have been started (Fig. 2). There are several issues to consider. A multimodal approach considering the presence or absence of clinical improvement, combined with microbiological and PCT results, can help in decisions as to whether to continue, reconsider or change antibiotics and/or reassess organ support and most importantly, to stop antibiotics if they are considered unnecessary (for more explanation see Fig. 2).

This multimodal evaluation could be called the MET-concept: Measure, Evaluate and Treat, which may help to individualize suspected infection management in the early course of sepsis on the ICU.

Evaluating Antibiotic Appropriateness

Once it has been decided that empirical antibiotic therapy should be started, it is of utmost importance to confirm the appropriateness, type and dose, or change treatment if needed as soon as possible, because antibiotic therapy is a double-edged sword: on the one hand, we have some evidence that in septic shock every hour delay in starting adequate antibiotic therapy could have a serious effect on survival [16]; on the other hand, unnecessary overuse of antibiotics can cause harm, such as increased bacterial resistance, the occurrence of multi-resistant strains, invasive fungal infections, adverse effects of the drug itself, and increased costs [29]. International guideline-based local protocols and antibiotic stewardship may help in choosing the right medication. Unfortunately, it seems that inappropriate empirical antibiotic therapy is still a common feature on the ICU and in the hospital in general, and can be as high as 25–30% [28, 30]. The gold standard for proving the appropriateness of antibiotic therapy is microbiological confirmation of the bacteria and its susceptibility. However, these results may come far too late, in reality days after the specimen had been sent, and treatment cannot be delayed. At present there is very little to help clinicians identify appropriate antibiotic treatment at the early stage of patient care. In a recent pilot study, we measured PCT before initiating antibiotics (t_0), and then 8 hourly (t_8, t_{16}, t_{24}) after commencing empirical antibiotic therapy, and found that there was a significant difference in PCT kinetics between patients who received appropriate compared to those who received inappropriate antibiotic therapy (Molnar et al., unpublished data). Receiver operating characteristic (ROC) curve analysis revealed that a PCT elevation $\geq 55\%$ within the first 16 h (i.e., from t_0-t_{16}) had an area under the curve (AUC) for predicting inappropriate antibiotic treatment of 0.78 (95% CI: 0.66–0.85), $p < 0.001$; from t_0-t_{24} a $\geq 70\%$ increase had an AUC of 0.85 (0.75–0.90), $p < 0.001$. These data suggest that early response of PCT within the first 24 h of commencing empirical antibiotics in critically ill patients may help the clinician to evaluate the appropriateness of therapy, a concept which certainly will have to be tested in the future. Hospital mortality was 35% in the appropriate and 65% in the inappropriate group ($p = 0.001$), which provides further evidence that choosing inappropriate antibiotic therapy seriously affects survival.

Stopping Antibiotic Therapy

PCT, mainly due to its favorable kinetic profile, can potentially also be a useful biomarker for stopping antibiotic treatment [31]. In the PRORATA study [4], PCT-guided antibiotic management was tested in an ICU population. Similar to the study by Christ-Crain et al. [3], antibiotics were encouraged when PCT concentrations were elevated, and discouraged when concentrations were low. The novelty of this trial was that investigators were encouraged to discontinue antibiotics when the PCT concentration was less than 80% of the peak value or when an absolute concentration of less than 0.5 ng/ml was reached. This approach shortened antibiotic exposure by 23% and by almost 3 days in the PCT-group compared to conventionally treated patients. It is very important, however, to acknowledge that patients in the PCT-group also received antibiotics for a shorter period of time as recommended by guidelines and local protocols. Despite the significantly shorter antibiotic therapy, the researchers were unable to show any difference in outcome between the groups; in other words, patients did not suffer harm from not receiving antibiotics for the length of time recommended by guidelines. In two other studies, on high-risk surgical patients with suspected infection, PCT-guided therapy during the postoperative period in the ICU resulted in significant reduction of antibiotic therapy and length of ICU stay [32, 33].

In a recent, large, multicenter study by Shehabi et al., the authors found no significant differences between PCT-guided and conventional groups, although PCT-managed patients received a median of 2 days fewer (9 vs 11 day) antibiotics, which in fact was the main outcome measure [7]. However, as was clearly stated by the authors, the study was powered for a very ambitious 25% reduction in the length of antibiotic treatment based on an estimated 9 days of antibiotic therapy, which in fact translated after the final analysis into an almost 4 day reduction in the study arm, with 11 antibiotic treatment days being the baseline in the control arm.

Conclusion

In this deadly battle of fighting the burden of serious infections on the ICU, we often keep missing the point. Although sepsis exists, just like critical illness, precisely defining it is probably impossible because of its diversity in etiology, pathomechanisms and clinical manifestation. Therefore, interpreting the results of sepsis studies is a daunting task. PCT is definitely one of the most reliable inflammatory markers in the critically ill to date, and there is also convincing evidence that its use to guide antibiotic therapy can rationalize the starting, escalating and stopping of antibiotic therapy. Furthermore, when the concept highlighted in this chapter is applied, PCT may also become cost-effective, because of the effects of not starting antibiotic therapy or stopping it early. However, starting or stopping antibiotic treatment is more complex than just treating a single value or even the kinetics of PCT concentrations. A multimodal, individualized concept, consisting of recognizing organ dysfunction, identifying the possible source, following the clinical picture, and taking PCT and PCT-kinetics into account, is necessary in order to correctly interpret PCT concentrations and optimize everyday patient management.

References

1. Dellinger RP, Levy MM, Rhodes A et al (2013) Surviving sepsis campaign: international guidelines for management of severe sepsis and septic shock, 2012. Intensive Care Med 39:165–228
2. Pierrakos C, Vincent JL (2010) Sepsis biomarkers: a review. Crit Care 14:R15
3. Christ-Crain M, Jaccard-Stolz D, Bingisser R et al (2004) Effect of procalcitonin-guided treatment on antibiotic use and outcome in lower respiratory tract infections: cluster-randomised, single-blinded intervention trial. Lancet 21:600–607
4. Bouadma L, Luyt CE, Tubach F et al (2010) Use of procalcitonin to reduce patients' exposure to antibiotics in intensive care units (PRORATA trial): a multicentre randomised controlled trial. Lancet 375:463–474
5. Layios N, Lambermont B, Canivet JL et al (2012) Procalcitonin usefulness for the initiation of antibiotic treatment in intensive care unit patients. Crit Care Med 40:2304–2309
6. Jensen JU, Lundgren B, Hein L et al (2008) The Procalcitonin and Survival Study (PASS) – a randomised multi-centre investigator initiated trial to investigate whether daily measurements biomarker procalcitonin and pro-active diagnostic and therapeutic responses to abnormal procalcitonin levels, can improve survival in intensive care unit patients. Calculated sample size (target population): 1000 patients. BMC Infect Dis 8:91–101
7. Shehabi Y, Sterba M, Garrett PM et al (2014) Procalcitonin algorithm in critically ill adults with undifferentiated infection or suspected sepsis. A randomized controlled trial. Am J Respir Crit Care Med 190:1102–1110
8. Bone RC, Fisher CJ Jr, Clemmer TP, Slotman GJ, Metz CA, Balk RA (1987) A controlled clinical trial of high-dose methylprednisolone in the treatment of severe sepsis and septic shock. N Engl J Med 317:653–658
9. Bone RC, Fisher CJ Jr, Clemmer TP, Slotman GJ, Metz CA, Balk RA (1989) Sepsis syndrome: a valid clinical entity. Methylprednisolone Severe Sepsis Study Group. Crit Care Med 17:389–393

10. American College of Chest Physicians, Society of Critical Care Medicine (1992) Consensus Conference: definitions for sepsis and organ failure and guidelines for the use of innovative therapies in sepsis. Crit Care Med 20:864–874

11. Vincent JL, Opal SM, Marshall JC, Tracey KJ (2013) Sepsis definitions: time for change. Lancet 381:774–775

12. Sartori M, Cosmi B, Legnani CJ et al (2012) The Wells rule and D-dimer for the diagnosis of isolated distal deep vein thrombosis. J Thromb Haemost 10:2264–2269

13. Cavaillon JM, Adrie C, Fitting C, Adib-Conqui M (2005) Reprogramming of circulatory cells in sepsis and SIRS. J Endotoxin Res 11:311–320

14. Cavaillon JM, Adib-Conquy M (2006) Bench-to-bedside review: endotoxin tolerance as a model of leukocyte reprogramming in sepsis. Crit Care 10:233

15. Zhang Q, Raoof M, Chen Y (2010) Circulating mitochondrial DAMPs cause inflammatory responses to injury. Nature 464:104–107

16. Kumar A, Roberts D, Wood KE et al (2006) Duration of hypotension before initiation of effective antimicrobial therapy is the critical determinant of survival in human septic shock. Crit Care Med 34:1589–1596

17. Dandona P, Nix D, Wilson MF et al (1994) Procalcitonin increase after endotoxin injection in normal subjects. J Clin Endocrinol Metab 79:1605–1608

18. Meisner M (2010) Procalcitonin – Biochemistry and Clinical Diagnosis, 1st edn. UNI-MED Science, Germany

19. Müller B, Becker KL, Schächinger H et al (2000) Calcitonin precursors are reliable markers of sepsis in a medical intensive care unit. Crit Care Med 28:977–983

20. Jensen JU, Heslet L, Jensen TH, Espersen K, Steffensen P, Tvede M (2006) Procalcitonin increase in early identification of critically ill patients at high risk of mortality. Crit Care Med 34:2596–2602

21. Pupelis G, Drozdova N, Mukans M, Malbrain ML (2014) Serum procalcitonin is a sensitive marker for septic shock and mortality in secondary peritonitis. Anaesthesiol Intensive Ther 46:262–273

22. Clec'h C, Ferriere F, Karoubi P et al (2004) Diagnostic and prognostic value of procalcitonin in patients with septic shock. Crit Care Med 32:1166–1169

23. Clec'h C, Fosse JP, Karoubi P et al (2006) Differential diagnostic value of procalcitonin in surgical and medical patients with septic shock. Crit Care Med 34:102–107

24. Tsangaris I, Plachouras D, Kavatha D et al (2009) Diagnostic and prognostic value of procalcitonin among febrile critically ill patients with prolonged ICU stay. BMC Infect Dis 9:213

25. Nemeth M, Trasy D, Osztroluczki A et al (2013) Increase in procalcitonin kinetics may be a good indicator of starting empirical antibiotic treatment in critically ill patients (a pilot study). Intensive Care Med 39(S2):80

26. Schuetz P, Christ-Crain M, Thomann R et al (2009) Effect of procalcitonin-based guidelines vs standard guidelines on antibiotic use in lower respiratory tract infections: the ProHOSP randomized controlled trial. JAMA 302:1059–1066

27. Rau BM, Frigerio I, Büchler MW et al (2007) Evaluation of procalcitonin for predicting septic multiorgan failure and overall prognosis in secondary peritonitis: a prospective, international multicenter study. Arch Surg 142:134–142

28. Charles PE, Tinel C, Barbar S et al (2009) Procalcitonin kinetics within the first days of sepsis: relationship with the appropriateness of antibiotic therapy and the outcome. Crit Care 13:R38

29. Ohl CA, Luther VP (2011) Antimicrobial stewardship for inpatient facilities. J Hosp Med 1:S4–S15

30. Mettler J, Simcock M, Sendi P et al (2007) Empirical use of antibiotics and adjustment of empirical antibiotic therapies in a university hospital: a prospective observational study. BMC Infect Dis 7:21

31. Gogos CA, Drosou E, Bassaris HP, Skoutelis A (2000) Pro- versus anti-inflammatory cytokine profile in patients with severe sepsis: a marker for prognosis and future therapeutic options. J Infect Dis 181:176–180

32. Hochreiter M, Kohler T, Schweiger AM et al (2009) Procalcitonin to guide duration of antibiotic therapy in intensive care patients: a randomized prospective controlled trial. Crit Care 13:R83
33. Schroeder S, Hochreiter M, Koehler T et al (2009) Procalcitonin (PCT)-guided algorithm reduces length of antibiotic treatment in surgical intensive care patients with severe sepsis: results of a prospective randomized study. Langenbecks Arch Surg 394:221–226

Reducing Antibiotic Use in the ICU: A Time-Based Approach to Rational Antimicrobial Use

P. O. Depuydt, L. De Bus, and J. J. De Waele

Introduction

Antibiotics are life-saving drugs and among the most important therapeutic weapons of the intensive care unit (ICU) physician. In severe bacterial infection, community-acquired, healthcare-associated and hospital-acquired, timely administration of antibiotic therapy active against the causal pathogen is one of the main determinants of a favorable patient outcome. On the other hand, it is an undeniable fact that antibiotics need to be used judiciously, as the induction and rapid spread of resistance threatens to reduce their lifespan. Trying to spare our current antibiotic armamentarium has become urgent, as development of new antibiotics has lagged completely behind the emergence of resistance [1]. As such, the ICU physician faces a daily dilemma: Using antibiotics may improve individual patient outcome (inasmuch as clinical deterioration is due to bacterial infection), but will induce selection pressure and potential harm to future patients or to the same patient in the future, whereas withholding antibiotics will avoid selection pressure but may put the individual patient at increased risk of harm caused by an untreated infection. This dilemma is made worse by the fact that, in critically ill patients, clinical presentation of hospital-acquired infection may be subtle or atypical at the time when the decision of whether or not to start antibiotics has to be made. Moreover, at that time, the causative pathogen is usually not identified but assumed to be potentially resistant to multiple antibiotics. These uncertainties lead ICU physicians to err on the side of caution for the immediate benefit of the individual patient and to accept a certain overuse of broad-spectrum antibiotics. However, as the ecological impact of antibiotic consumption is escalating, efforts have been made to reconcile maximum short-term patient safety (the least number of 'missed' infections or 'missed' pathogens) with a reduction in overall antibiotic use.

P. O. Depuydt · L. De Bus · J. J. De Waele (✉)
Department of Critical Care Medicine, Ghent University Hospital
Ghent, Belgium
email: jan.dewaele@ugent.be

© Springer International Publishing Switzerland 2016
J.-L. Vincent (ed.), *Annual Update in Intensive Care and Emergency Medicine 2016*,
DOI 10.1007/978-3-319-27349-5_2

As no biomarkers have been identified that can reliably distinguish bacterial infection from other disease at an early stage, the general approach to antibiotic decision-making in the ICU is that of an upfront broad-spectrum regimen followed by deescalation. Basically, this strategy consists of having a low threshold for starting antibiotics (often several in combination) at clinical suspicion of infection, covering a wide spectrum of potential pathogens and resistance mechanisms, and subsequently reevaluating when microbiological data become available. This reevaluation considers whether there is a need to continue antibiotic therapy and, if so, whether the initial broad-spectrum antibiotic can be replaced by a narrower-spectrum drug tailored to the identified causal pathogen but causing less selection pressure [2]. The main concept underlying this approach is to strike a balance between immediate patient safety ('more antibiotics') and preserving ecology ('less antibiotics') at each time point, using all the information that progressively becomes available [3].

Although this strategy sounds attractive and logical, there is general agreement that antibiotics are overused in critical care. Indeed, many empirical antibiotic treatments include broad-spectrum agents and deescalation is performed in only a minority of patients; overall treatment duration is also often longer than deemed necessary. Antibiotic stewardship programs have been introduced to counter these trends and have been advocated by several societies. Practical implementation of these concepts at the bedside is difficult, however. In this chapter, we propose a

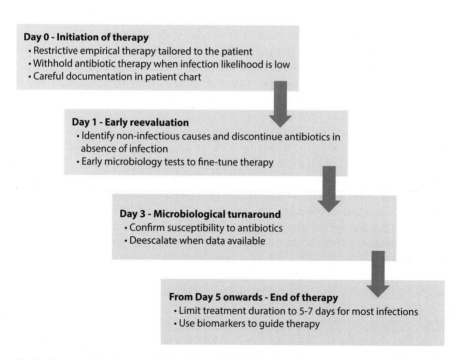

Day 0 - Initiation of therapy
• Restrictive empirical therapy tailored to the patient
• Withhold antibiotic therapy when infection likelihood is low
• Careful documentation in patient chart

Day 1 - Early reevaluation
• Identify non-infectious causes and discontinue antibiotics in absence of infection
• Early microbiology tests to fine-tune therapy

Day 3 - Microbiological turnaround
• Confirm susceptibility to antibiotics
• Deescalate when data available

From Day 5 onwards - End of therapy
• Limit treatment duration to 5-7 days for most infections
• Use biomarkers to guide therapy

Fig. 1 Opportunities for stewardship during antibiotic decision-making in the ICU

time-based approach to antibiotic use including the concept of dynamic reevaluation, and we present four key time points at which to (re)consider antibiotic therapy in the ICU (Fig. 1). In this way, antibiotic stewardship philosophy is integrated into the clinical decision-making process.

Time Point 1: Day 0 – Start of Empirical Antibiotic Therapy

Obviously the start of empirical therapy is a first crucial moment of the antibiotic course. The first hurdle to take in an ICU environment is to distinguish sepsis, severe sepsis or septic shock from a systemic inflammatory response syndrome (SIRS) (with or without one or more organ dysfunctions) caused by a non-infectious condition, e.g., in surgical, burn, pancreatitis and trauma patients. If the infectious origin is obvious, there is no doubt that initiation of antibiotics should be an integral component of early treatment. There may be situations, however, in which the infectious origin of the clinical picture is not (yet) clear, and antibiotics may be withheld. The Surviving Sepsis Campaign (SSC) recommendation is largely based on a retrospective cohort study of septic shock patients in which mortality increased per hour delay in administration of adequate antibiotic therapy [4], and should not be lightly extrapolated to patients without septic shock. A recent meta-analysis that included 11,017 patients with severe sepsis or septic shock could not confirm the mortality benefit of starting antibiotics within 1 h of shock recognition and challenges the current SSC recommendation [5]. A multicenter randomized controlled trial (RCT) suggested that the exact timing of antibiotics may be less important when early aggressive resuscitation is achieved [6]. These data support the concept that prompt resuscitation is primordial in any unstable patient, but also that a watchful waiting strategy regarding antibiotic administration beyond the proposed 1-h timeframe may be safe in selected patients when the likelihood of infection is low.

Fears of missing this window of presumed opportunity for life-saving treatment and peer as well as societal pressure to start antibiotics, together with the difficulties in the early recognition of infection, may tempt the physician to take the 'safe and easy' path and start antibiotic therapy from the moment a suspicion of infection is raised. Essentially, the SSC recommendations are for patients who present with severe sepsis or septic shock. On the other hand, patients can suffer from an obvious infection, e.g., peritonitis due to gastrointestinal perforation, without the necessary SIRS criteria, and the need for early antibiotic treatment is not really questioned. However, infection may not always be evident. A before and after observational cohort study – excluding septic shock patients – compared aggressive initiation of antibiotic treatment with a treatment strategy where initiation was withheld until more objective data, particularly microbiological evidence, were obtained [7]. The rate of initial appropriate therapy was higher in the less aggressive arm and mortality was lower, suggesting that a more reserved approach to starting antibiotics in the hemodynamically stable patient with possible infection may be justified. In the Sepsis Occurrence in Acutely ill Patients (SOAP) study, more than half of the patients who received antibiotic treatment during their ICU stay did not have severe sepsis [8], implying that a substantial number of patients may in fact be candidates for a more restricted antibiotic initiation as described above.

If the decision to start antibiotics is made, it is important to select an adequate antibiotic regimen covering all expected pathogens. Inevitably in a setting where multidrug resistance (MDR) is problematic, this will require an antibiotic scheme that includes all potential pathogens even if this exceeds the spectrum of the pathogens that are eventually identified. As an example, international guidelines, such as those published by the Infectious Diseases Society of America (IDSA), propose empirical broad-spectrum and, as a rule, combination therapy for hospital-acquired pneumonia [2]. However, it is pointless to cover microorganisms that are very unlikely given the patient profile and local ecology. Guidelines tailoring empirical therapy to local susceptibility data resulted in increased appropriateness and reduced use of broad-spectrum combination therapy [9, 10]. Furthermore, mapping the patient's colonization status by surveillance cultures may reduce the use of broad-spectrum regimens [11, 12]. Therefore, in the current situation of a worldwide, but very inhomogeneous spread of MDR, customizing these (inter)national guidelines to local institutional and patient ecology may offer an opportunity to reduce antibiotic use from the very start.

This decision-making process is complex and, as such, should be carefully recorded in the patient's file. To facilitate decision-making later in the course of therapy, it is essential to obtain all relevant microbiological cultures at this stage and preferably before the start of antibiotics to document the infection and identify the causative pathogen.

Time Point 2: Day 1 – Early Reevaluation

After 24 h of antibiotic therapy, we advocate a systematic clinical reevaluation of the patient to confirm (or not) the presence of infection. As signs and symptoms suggesting infection in critically ill patients may be non-specific, alternative diagnoses should always be considered from the very start, whether or not clinical deterioration calls for immediate start of antibiotics. A 24 h window may be a good moment to reevaluate the patient, as the evolution of the clinical picture often allows better differentiation between infectious and non-infectious causes of deterioration or SIRS. This offers an opportunity to discontinue antibiotics that were – in retrospect – initiated inappropriately and will depend on the level of certainty that infection was present when antibiotics were initiated. In patients who are not improving, a careful search for an alternative diagnosis is important and is to be preferred to blind escalation of antibiotic therapy when clinical signs and symptoms do not respond favorably early after start of antibiotics. If there is another clear cause of the current condition or deterioration of the patient, then antibiotics should not be continued. A typical example of this would be a patient with pancreatitis, who may present with acute abdominal pain and who may receive early empirical antibiotic therapy for suspected infection but who is found to have pancreatitis only, without signs of infection and without the need for antibiotic therapy.

At this point also, the results of microbiological studies may become available, which can help to guide therapy. These include simple techniques such as direct examination with Gram-stain and direct antibiogram but also more sophisticated techniques, including matrix assisted laser desorption ionization time-of-flight (MALDI-TOF)- and polymerase chain reaction (PCR)-based techniques. The cost-effectiveness of these techniques at this point is unclear. Using this approach creates a second opportunity to treat less obvious pathogens and may also allow the identification of MDR pathogens, such as *Acinetobacter* and *Stenotrophomonas* spp. or fungi, which may not be covered by the spectrum of the antibiotic administered.

Direct Examination and Gram-stain of Samples

Although the information that can be obtained from a Gram-stain may appear limited, it may assist the clinician in directing empirical antibiotic therapy as well as in assessing the need for other interventions. This technique can be applied to several types of samples, including respiratory and abdominal samples. Direct examination may suggest the presence of microorganisms that are not covered by the initial treatment strategy and this is, therefore, particularly helpful in a restricted empirical antibiotic strategy.

Direct Susceptibility Testing

Rather than the susceptibility of one pathogen, direct susceptibility testing reflects the susceptibility of the microbial community in a sample. Although there are some limitations to this technique, direct susceptibility testing using direct inoculation of the clinical sample may provide early information on susceptibility and reduce turnaround time by 24 h [13].

MALDI-TOF

This recently introduced proteomics-based technique allows rapid determination of pathogens after culture [14]. Again this may not provide any details on susceptibility but may point the clinician to the presence of unexpected pathogens.

PCR-based Techniques

Several commercial tests have been developed in recent years and most allow identification of pathogens with 8 h of sampling. A recent systematic review and meta-analysis of the available studies on one of the most studied tests found the test to be of limited value to exclude infection in the critically ill [15]; nevertheless, this test may allow identification of pathogens that have limited susceptibility to the empirical regimen. Susceptibility information is not available from these PCR-based techniques (except for the presence of the MecA gene for methicillin-resistant *Staphylococcus aureus* (MRSA)). It should be noted that most of the studies in this field have been conducted in patients with blood stream infection only and the value in other infections remains to be determined.

Time Point 3: Day 3 – Microbiological Turnaround

At 72 h the picture is usually complete, with all relevant culture results available in most situations. This is the pivotal moment for reassessing likelihood of infection as well as streamlining antibiotic therapy.

Similar to the 24 h time point, the presence of infection may be reconfirmed but again alternative diagnoses may be considered. Clinicians may decide, based on the available information, that infection may not have been present, and stopping antibiotics is definitely an option in selected patients. Although there is often reluctance to stop antibiotic therapy once started, an RCT from 2,000 already showed this to be safe [16].

This is usually also the time point when the susceptibility pattern of the pathogen is available and definite antibiotic therapy can be decided. Apart from changing the antibiotic in case of resistance to the pathogen, this offers an opportunity to stop unnecessary antibiotics – antibiotics that do not cover the pathogen involved but were part of multidrug empirical antibiotic therapy, e.g., vancomycin as part of an empirical broad-spectrum regimen for hospital-acquired pneumonia. Similarly, in patients who have been treated with combination therapy, e.g., a beta-lactam antibiotic plus an aminoglycoside, it may be the appropriate time to stop the more toxic antibiotic.

Deescalation of antibiotic therapy, or changing the antibiotic to another agent with a smaller spectrum, has been advocated as an essential element of antibiotic stewardship programs [17]. As such, it will reduce the use of broad-spectrum agents and presumably reduce selection pressure. In clinical practice, however, deescalation is only used in 13 to 43% of patients in most studies [18]. Deescalation has been associated with decreased mortality in critically ill patients [19] but a causal effect is unlikely.

Time Point 4: From Day 5 Onwards – End of the Antibiotic Course

If antibiotics are continued beyond 72 h, it is assumed that infection is present and that a complete antibiotic course is necessary. However, the optimal duration of such a course is at present not known and is probably dependent on pathogen load and susceptibility, focus and tissue extension of the infection, host defense mechanisms and whether or not some form of source control can be achieved. Extending antibiotic therapy must balance the possible benefit of achieving better microbial control against the harm of promoting resistance by prolonging selection pressure. As most of the current evidence relates patient outcome to treatment determinants that appear at the 'head' of antibiotic therapy (timing/initiation of therapy, appropriate empirical choice), the 'tail' of antibiotic therapy may offer the best opportunities to reduce overall antibiotic exposure without compromising patient outcome. As such, in the more recently published literature, there is a clear tendency to decrease duration of antibiotic courses. This trend is best documented for pneumonia. A landmark RCT in patients with ventilator-associated pneumonia (VAP) found that an 8-day antibiotic course did not result in worse patient outcome as compared to a 15-day course; the rate of infection recurrence was higher for *Pseudomonas* infections, but this was not associated with increased mortality or length of stay [20]. This result provides firm ground for the recommendation to set a stop at day 8 of antibiotic therapy for pneumonia, counting from the first day of appropriate therapy. Although data from RCTs are lacking, the SSC recommend a similar 7 to 10 day course of antibiotic therapy as a standard for all nosocomial infections, to be modified in the light of clinical response and microbiological data [17, 21]. However, these guidelines are only slowly changing daily practice, as the mean duration of a 'usual care' antibiotic course in the ICU (gleaned from observational studies and control arms of interventional studies) still exceeds these times [22, 23]. Recommendations for shorter antibiotic treatment courses may be most effective when translated into a default stop date for antibiotic therapy, with continuation of antibiotics beyond this date only for selected indications or clinical situations. Apart from some clearly defined clinical infections for which prolonged antibiotic treatment is standard of care (such as endocarditis or prosthetic joint infection), longer antibiotic courses may be required in situations with extensive and persistent tissue inflammation together with lack of microbial eradication, such as necrotizing pulmonary infections, persistent gastrointestinal leaks or inaccessible infection foci. For this latter category, however, it should be recognized that there is no evidence that prolonged antibiotic courses improve outcome beyond standard courses, and continued efforts to achieve source control (preferably as early as possible in the course of the treatment) may be more effective [24]. As mentioned before, a decision to stop or continue antibiotics should be formally noted in the patient's clinical files to allow subsequent reevaluation.

Several RCTs have compared antibiotic courses prescribed as usual care with an approach focusing on antibiotic stopping, using algorithms taking into account the evolution of biomarkers or clinical parameters. Serial measurements of procalcitonin (PCT) with an algorithm recommending that antibiotics be stopped when PCT concentrations decrease below a certain threshold or percentage from its peak value, can be used to reduce the duration of the antibiotic course to a median of 6 days [25]. When PCT is not available, serial clinical evaluations may achieve the same goal, at least for respiratory infections [26]. Most importantly, during daily clinical rounds in the ICU, all ongoing antibiotic prescriptions should receive a critical evaluation by the attending physician.

Conclusion

Decision-making about initiation, changing and stopping antibiotic therapy in the ICU is a complex activity due to its dual goal – eradicating pathogenic bacteria causing serious infection versus minimizing promotion of antimicrobial resistance caused by selection pressure – and due to the uncertainties surrounding clinical diagnosis of infection and its causal pathogen(s). There are, however, several opportunities to reduce unnecessary antibiotic exposure while preserving patient outcome. The principle of deescalation is currently the main answer to this diagnostic and therapeutic problem. However, it is important to tailor this principle to the individual clinical case and avoid unnecessary antibiotics as much as possible. This goal is best achieved by a dynamic approach with critical reassessments of the need for and choice of antibiotics at preset time points while actively pursuing diagnostics and integrating all the available information. This proposed time-based approach is a convenient way to translate different aspects of antimicrobial stewardship into clinical practice at the bedside.

References

1. Spellberg B, Guidos R, Gilbert D et al (2008) The epidemic of antibiotic-resistant infections: a call to action for the medical community from the Infectious Diseases Society of America. Clin Infect Dis 46:155–164
2. American Thoracic Society and Infectious Diseases Society of America (2005) Guidelines for the management of adults with hospital-acquired, ventilator-associated, and healthcare-associated pneumonia. Am J Respir Crit Care Med 171:388–416
3. Niederman MS (2006) Use of broad-spectrum antimicrobials for the treatment of pneumonia in seriously ill patients: maximizing clinical outcomes and minimizing selection of resistant organisms. Clin Infect Dis 42(Suppl 2):S72–S81
4. Kumar A, Roberts D, Wood KE et al (2006) Duration of hypotension before initiation of effective antimicrobial therapy is the critical determinant of survival in human septic shock. Crit Care Med 34:1589–1596
5. Sterling SA, Miller WR, Pryor J, Puskarich MA, Jones AE (2015) The impact of timing of antibiotics on outcomes in severe sepsis and septic shock: A systematic review and meta-analysis. Crit Care Med 43:1907–1915
6. Puskarich MA, Trzeciak S, Shapiro NI et al (2011) Association between timing of antibiotic administration and mortality from septic shock in patients treated with a quantitative resuscitation protocol. Crit Care Med 39:2066–2071
7. Hranjec T, Rosenberger LH, Swenson B et al (2012) Aggressive versus conservative initiation of antimicrobial treatment in critically ill surgical patients with suspected intensive-care-unit-acquired infection: a quasi-experimental, before and after observational cohort study. Lancet Infect Dis 12:774–780
8. Vincent JL, Sakr Y, Sprung CL et al (2006) Sepsis in European intensive care units: results of the SOAP study. Crit Care Med 34:344–353
9. Beardsley JR, Williamson JC, Johnson JW, Ohl CA, Karchmer TB, Bowton DL (2006) Using local microbiologic data to develop institution-specific guidelines for the treatment of hospital-acquired pneumonia. Chest 130:787–793
10. Becher RD, Hoth JJ, Rebo JJ, Kendall JL, Miller PR (2012) Locally derived versus guideline-based approach to treatment of hospital-acquired pneumonia in the trauma intensive care unit. Surg Infect (Larchmt) 13:352–359

11. De Bus L, Saerens L, Gadeyne B et al (2014) Development of antibiotic treatment algorithms based on local ecology and respiratory surveillance cultures to restrict the use of broad-spectrum antimicrobial drugs in the treatment of hospital-acquired pneumonia in the intensive care unit: a retrospective analysis. Crit Care 18:R152

12. Michel F, Franceschini B, Berger P et al (2005) Early antibiotic treatment for BAL-confirmed ventilator-associated pneumonia: a role for routine endotracheal aspirate cultures. Chest 127:589–597

13. Coorevits L, Boelens J, Claeys G (2015) Direct susceptibility testing by disk diffusion on clinical samples: a rapid and accurate tool for antibiotic stewardship. Eur J Clin Microbiol Infect Dis 34:1207–1212

14. Patel R (2013) Matrix-assisted laser desorption ionization-time of flight mass spectrometry in clinical microbiology. Clin Infect Dis 57:564–572

15. Dark P, Blackwood B, Gates S et al (2015) Accuracy of LightCycler(®) SeptiFast for the detection and identification of pathogens in the blood of patients with suspected sepsis: a systematic review and meta-analysis. Intensive Care Med 41:21–33

16. Singh N, Rogers P, Atwood CW, Wagener MM, Yu VL (2000) Short-course empiric antibiotic therapy for patients with pulmonary infiltrates in the intensive care unit. A proposed solution for indiscriminate antibiotic prescription. Am J Respir Crit Care Med 162:505–511

17. Dellinger RP, Levy MM, Rhodes A et al (2013) Surviving sepsis campaign: international guidelines for management of severe sepsis and septic shock, 2012. Intensive Care Med 39:165–228

18. De Waele JJ, Bassetti M, Martin-Loeches I (2014) Impact of de-escalation on ICU patients' prognosis. Intensive Care Med 40:1583–1585

19. Garnacho-Montero J, Gutierrez-Pizarraya A, Escoresca-Ortega A et al (2014) De-escalation of empirical therapy is associated with lower mortality in patients with severe sepsis and septic shock. Intensive Care Med 40:32–40

20. Chastre J, Wolff M, Fagon JY et al (2003) Comparison of 8 vs 15 days of antibiotic therapy for ventilator-associated pneumonia in adults: a randomized trial. JAMA 290:2588–2598

21. Dellinger RP, Carlet JM, Masur H et al (2004) Surviving Sepsis Campaign guidelines for management of severe sepsis and septic shock. Intensive Care Med 30:536–555

22. Bouadma L, Luyt C-E, Tubach F et al (2010) Use of procalcitonin to reduce patients' exposure to antibiotics in intensive care units (PRORATA trial): a multicentre randomised controlled trial. Lancet 375:463–474

23. Rello J, Ulldemolins M, Lisboa T et al (2011) Determinants of prescription and choice of empirical therapy for hospital-acquired and ventilator-associated pneumonia. Eur Respir J 37:1332–1339

24. Tabah A, Koulenti D, Laupland K et al (2012) Characteristics and determinants of outcome of hospital-acquired bloodstream infections in intensive care units: the EUROBACT International Cohort Study. Intensive Care Med 38:1930–1945

25. Agarwal R, Schwartz DN (2011) Procalcitonin to guide duration of antimicrobial therapy in intensive care units: a systematic review. Clin Infect Dis 53:379–387

26. Micek ST, Ward S, Fraser VJ, Kollef MH (2004) A randomized controlled trial of an antibiotic discontinuation policy for clinically suspected ventilator-associated pneumonia. Chest 125:1791–1799

Plasmacytoid Dendritic Cells in Severe Influenza Infection

B. M. Tang, M. Shojaei, and A. S. McLean

Introduction

Plasmacytoid dendritic cells are the main producers of interferon-alpha (IFNα), the most powerful endogenous anti-viral molecule, which suppresses influenza virus replication [1, 2]. During influenza infection, plasmacytoid dendritic cells are the earliest cells to enter the bronchoalveolar space, followed by other immune cells [3]. After capturing influenza virus, plasmacytoid dendritic cells are activated and release a massive amount of IFNα at a magnitude that is 1,000 times more than any other cell type [4]. In addition to this unparalleled anti-viral potency, plasmacytoid dendritic cells communicate with key immune cells (e.g., CD8 T cells) to coordinate the adaptive immune response [5, 6]. This adaptive immune response results in the clearance of the virus and ultimately the resolution of the primary influenza infection.

The above highlights three important tasks performed by plasmacytoid dendritic cells, namely (1) pathogen recognition, (2) production of anti-viral IFN, (3) coordination of the immune response. Given these central roles in host response, plasmacytoid dendritic cells are ideal targets for immune modulation. Immune modulation therapy can restore immune homeostasis in viral and autoimmune diseases [7, 8]. Immune modulation of plasmacytoid dendritic cells in influenza infection represents a novel class of anti-influenza therapy. Here, we review the basic science of plasmacytoid dendritic cells, their roles in influenza pathogenesis and the ther-

B. M. Tang (✉)
Department of Intensive Care Medicine, Nepean Hospital
Sydney, Australia
Center for Immunology and Allergy Research, Westmead Millennium Institute
Sydney, Australia
email: benjamin.tang@sydney.edu.au

M. Shojaei · A. S. McLean
Department of Intensive Care Medicine, Nepean Hospital
Sydney, Australia

© Springer International Publishing Switzerland 2016
J.-L. Vincent (ed.), *Annual Update in Intensive Care and Emergency Medicine 2016*,
DOI 10.1007/978-3-319-27349-5_3

apeutic implications of plasmacytoid dendritic cell modulation in severe influenza pneumonitis.

The Functional Plasticity of Plasmacytoid Dendritic Cells

The plasmacytoid dendritic cell is a unique member of the dendritic cell family because it has features of lymphocytes and of classical dendritic cells [9]. In the decade since the discovery of the plasmacytoid dendritic cell as a distinct immune cell type, extensive evidence has shown that plasmacytoid dendritic cells differ from other dendritic cells in their ability to display functional plasticity – i.e., they can differentiate into different morphological states, each associated with a distinctive immune profile that may be either harmful or beneficial to host response [10]. This functional dichotomy has implications for the treatment of influenza infection because plasmacytoid dendritic cell modulation may play either beneficial or harmful roles in the host response.

Evidence for Beneficial Roles of Plasmacytoid Dendritic Cells

The host response plays a critical role in the containment and ultimately clearance of influenza virus infection. A successful host response is a tightly controlled process in which the activation and recruitment of key immune cells (e.g., CD8 T cells) is proportional to the viral load and the degree of tissue damage. Plasmacytoid dendritic cells play a central role in regulating this process. In fact, many published studies have provided evidence (1) that plasmacytoid dendritic cells play important roles in immune regulation in viral infections (influenza virus, human immunodeficiency virus [HIV], hepatitis C virus [HCV], herpes virus, human papilloma virus and Epstein-Barr virus) [11, 12], and (2) that plasmacytoid dendritic cells interact with and regulate immune cells in both normal and diseased states [1]. In addition to immune regulation, plasmacytoid dendritic cells are the most potent producers of IFNα, which has powerful anti-viral effects. There is a large published literature demonstrating that IFNα suppresses virus replication and reduces the spread of the virus to uninfected cells in the respiratory tract [13–15].

Evidence for Harmful Roles of Plasmacytoid Dendritic Cells

At the onset of influenza infection, the influenza virus triggers a cascade of immune pathways including the release of cytokines (macrophages), killing of virus infected cells (CD8 T cells) and resolution of inflammation (T-regulatory cells) [6]. Plasmacytoid dendritic cells are involved in the modulation of all three immune cells, namely, macrophages, CD8 cells and T-regulatory cells [9]. Not surprisingly, three lines of evidence support the potential deleterious role of plasmacytoid dendritic cells:

(1) In a murine model of influenza infection, plasmacytoid dendritic cell depletion improved macrophage recruitment and enhanced inflammatory response (tumor necrosis factor (TNF)-α/interleukin (IL)-6 increased 5–35 fold), suggesting that plasmacytoid dendritic cells may have a restrictive role in the inflammatory response of macrophages [16].

(2) In infected mice, plasmacytoid dendritic cells reduced CD8 cells by inducing FasL-dependent apoptosis, which subsequently increased mortality [17].

(3) In another murine model, plasmacytoid dendritic cells induced Treg responses, which suppressed antigen-specific CD8 cells, further limiting CD8 cell number [18].

Collectively, this evidence shows that plasmacytoid dendritic cells may either restrict the inflammatory response or augment immunosuppression and that they do so by influencing key immune cells, including macrophages, CD8 T cells and T-regulatory cells.

The Therapeutic Implications

The dichotomy of plasmacytoid dendritic cells (normal vs. harmful) described above has therapeutic implications because variations in plasmacytoid dendritic cell states can affect therapeutic effect (i.e., the same drug may have an opposing effect, dependent on underlying plasmacytoid dendritic cell activity). In *in vitro* experiments studying drug response, the plasmacytoid dendritic cell transcriptome displays a divergent activation program in response to therapeutic agents, with significant differences in resultant inflammatory cytokine production [10]. This finding is confirmed *in vivo*, where plasmacytoid dendritic cells can be either pro-inflammatory or immunosuppressive [19]. Consequently, if a drug is given without due consideration to the underlying plasmacytoid dendritic cell state, it will increase the risk of dampening desirable plasmacytoid dendritic cell responses or exacerbating immunosuppression.

New Anti-influenza Therapy to Target Plasmacytoid Dendritic Cells

Currently, there is no effective therapeutic agent for influenza pneumonia; management is mainly supportive (oxygen therapy and intravenous fluid). Antiviral agents, such as oseltamivir (Tamiflu), can reduce viral load. However, sufficient evidence has demonstrated that even if viral replication has been suppressed by antivirals, the dysregulated inflammatory process triggered by the infection will continue to drive immunopathologic progression [20]. Effective therapy for influenza pneumonia therefore requires an additional agent that restores immune homeostasis. Global immune suppressors, such as systemic steroids, do not restore immune homeostasis. In fact, recent evidence showed that steroids may be harmful in severe influenza pneumonitis [21, 22]. This observation is in keeping with animal studies, in which cytokine-knockout mice or steroid-treated wild-type mice did not show a survival advantage over wild-type mice after a viral challenge [20].

Modulation of plasmacytoid dendritic cells may restore homeostasis. Unlike systemic steroids, plasmacytoid dendritic cell modulation therapy does not result in global immune suppression. Furthermore, plasmacytoid dendritic cell therapy offers much greater cellular specificity and molecular precision [23]. Newer therapeutic agents, such as Toll-like receptor (TLR)7 or TLR9 agonists, can specifically target plasmacytoid dendritic cell pathways (TLR7 and TLR9 are the dominant pathway in these cells) [13]. Such agents have entered clinical trials and hold promise as a new class of anti-influenza therapy [8].

Biomarker-guided Therapy for Plasmacytoid Dendritic Cells

The dichotomy of dendritic cell state, as discussed previously, has implications for the new plasmacytoid dendritic cell modulation therapy, since the same therapy can exert opposing effects, dependent on the underlying plasmacytoid dendritic cell state. In other words, indiscriminate modulation of plasmacytoid dendritic cells will cause diminution of true therapeutic effects or, worse, unexpected toxicity. Consequently, determination of the plasmacytoid dendritic cell state in each patient is clinically important. A central requirement of future immunomodulation therapy is therefore to better understand the plasmacytoid dendritic cell dichotomy and to develop a method to measure plasmacytoid dendritic cell state. This would allow clinicians to identify patients with a favorable plasmacytoid dendritic cell state (appropriate IFNα production and immune homeostasis) and distinguish them from patients with an undesirable plasmacytoid dendritic cell state (excessive immune suppression). This approach would thus enable clinicians to apply therapy in patients in whom plasmacytoid dendritic cell therapy is indicated, as opposed to an uninformed approach of administering therapy to all patients regardless of underlying plasmacytoid dendritic cell status. However, there is one problem with this approach – there is no laboratory test currently available that can detect the transition between a robust immune response supported by healthy plasmacytoid dendritic cells and immune suppression driven by anomalous plasmacytoid dendritic cell activity.

New Biomarker to Measure Plasmacytoid Dendritic Cells

To address this unmet clinical need, we need a biomarker that measures virus-activated plasmacytoid dendritic cell states (activation vs. suppression). Plasmacytoid dendritic cells *per se* are not suitable biomarkers because they represent less than 0.8% of peripheral blood mononuclear cells, making it difficult to reliably measure them at the bedside. However, it is possible to identify an IFN-derived biomarker to measure plasmacytoid dendritic cell activity. Plasmacytoid dendritic cells are

Fig. 1 The mechanism of interferon-alpha-inducible protein 27 (IFI27) expression in plasmacytoid dendritic cells. TLR: Toll-like receptor

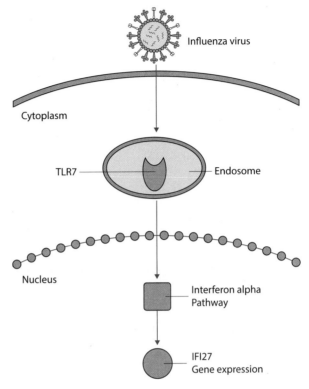

equipped with the pathogen recognition receptor, TLR7, which recognizes RNA viruses (e.g., influenza virus). Upon encounter with influenza virus, the endosomal TLR7 pathway is activated [24]. This results in the IFNα response described previously, leading to upregulation of IFN-stimulated genes, many of which are signature genes of RNA virus infection [25].

Using *in vitro* studies, we recently identified a signature IFN-stimulated gene that correlated with plasmacytoid dendritic cell activity – namely, IFNα-inducible protein 27 (IFI27) (Fig. 1). The discovery of the IFI27 gene-expression biomarker makes it possible to detect virus-activated plasmacytoid dendritic cells. To further translate this finding into clinical practice, we recently developed a peripheral blood IFI27 assay (which requires only 2.5 ml of blood) that could track plasmacytoid dendritic cell states in critically ill patients. This assay allows clinicians to determine whether the patient has increased activation of plasmacytoid dendritic cells or has a repressed plasmacytoid dendritic cell state (Fig. 2).

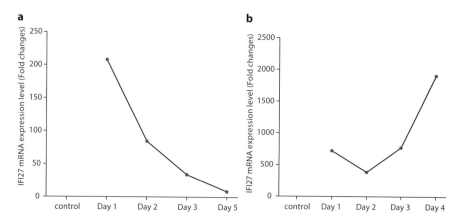

Fig. 2 Tracking of plasmacytoid dendritic cell state in critically ill patients is possible by serial interferon-alpha-inducible protein 27 (IFI27) measurements. Panel **a** represents daily IFI27 measurement in a patient who recovered from influenza viral pneumonitis. Panel **b** represent daily IFI27 measurement in a patient who subsequently died from influenza pneumonitis. IFI27 measurements were performed in peripheral blood samples using real time polymerase chain reaction (PCR) with the magnitude of IFI27 changes expressed in fold changes (relative to GAPDH housekeeping genes)

Advantage of the IFI27 Assay over Virus Detection Assays

The IFI27 biomarker has an advantage over conventional virus detection assay in that it identifies the immune response associated with the infection. Upon infection by influenza virus, plasmacytoid dendritic cells initiate the immune response in the infected lung. The virus-activated plasmacytoid dendritic cells then migrate to regional lymph nodes and subsequently traffic into circulating blood where their expressed IFI27 signals are detected (Fig. 3). Therefore, the peripheral blood IFI27 assay measures the immune response originating in the lung. Our recent study also

Fig. 3 Detection of plasmacytoid dendritic cell activation state by measuring interferon-alpha-inducible protein 27 (IFI27) gene-expression level in peripheral blood

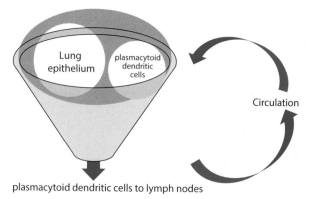

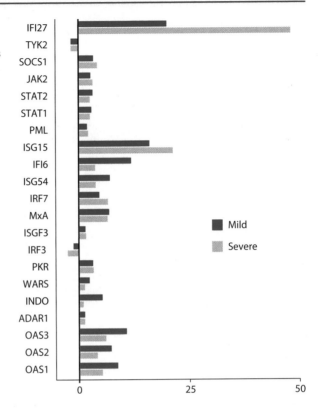

Fig. 4 Interferon-alpha-inducible protein 27 (IFI27) and other IFN-derived genes in mild and severe influenza infection

shows that, in influenza infected patients, peripheral blood IFI27 levels correlated with 20 IFN-derived genes that are implicated in the immune response against influenza virus (unpublished data; Fig. 4). These data indicate that: (1) IFI27 reflects a key component of the immune response against influenza virus; and (2) IFI27 may better reflect disease activity than virus load. In contrast, virus load has not been shown to correlate with disease severity or predict clinical outcomes [26, 27].

Conclusion

Dendritic cell therapy has emerged as a new avenue to restore immune homeostasis in viral and autoimmune diseases. However, indiscriminate dendritic cell inhibition/augmentation (e.g., plasmacytoid dendritic cell modulation) can inadvertently affect appropriate physiological functions performed by dendritic cells (e.g., antiviral IFNα production). This concern is particularly important in critically ill patients, who often have concomitant multiple organ impairment and therefore are highly susceptible to decompensation. For successful application of plasmacytoid dendritic cell modulation, clinicians need to know what level of plasmacytoid dendritic cell activity is commensurate with a beneficial host response and what level correlates with immunopathology. In other words, we need tools at the bedside to quantify variations in plasmacytoid dendritic cell activity (from normal to immunopathological). Such tools will assist the decision about whether to administer immune therapy and the timing of such therapy. The recently discovered gene-expression biomarker (IFI27) could provide this information by quantifying plasmacytoid dendritic cell suppression or augmentation states in critically ill patients. This biomarker represents an important first step in developing plasmacytoid dendritic cell therapy for influenza infection. Further research is urgently needed to define plasmacytoid dendritic cell states in all critically ill patients, in order to better inform clinical decision-making in treating influenza pneumonia with plasmacytoid dendritic cell therapy.

References

1. Reizis B, Bunin A, Ghosh HS, Lewis KL (2011) Plasmacytoid dendritic cells: recent progress and open questions. Annu Rev Immunol 29:163–183
2. Kugel D, Kochs G, Obojes K et al (2009) Intranasal administration of alpha interferon reduces seasonal influenza A Virus Morbidity in ferrets. J Virol 83:3843–3851
3. Lambrecht BN, Hammad H (2012) Lung dendritic cells in respiratory viral infection and asthma: from protection to immunopathology. Annu Rev Immunol 30:243–270
4. Colonna M, Trinchieri G, Liu YJ (2004) Plasmacytoid dendritic cells in immunity. Nat Immunol 5:1219–1226
5. Waithman J, Mintern JD (2012) Dendritic cells and influenza A virus infection. Virulence 3:603–608
6. Kreijtz JHCM, Fouchier RAM, Rimmelzwaan GF (2011) Immune responses to influenza virus infection. Virus Res 162:19–30
7. Lee SMY, Yen HL (2012) Targeting the host or the virus: Current and novel concepts for antiviral approaches against influenza virus infection. Antiviral Res 96:391–404
8. Guiducci C, Coffman RL, Barrat FJ (2009) Signalling pathways leading to IFN-α production in human plasmacytoid dendritic cell and the possible use of agonists or antagonists of TLR7 and TLR9 in clinical indications. J Intern Med 265:43–57
9. Barchet W, Cella M, Colonna M (2005) Plasmacytoid dendritic cells – virus experts of innate immunity. Semin Immunol 17:253–261
10. Iparraguirre A, Tobias JW, Hensley SE et al (2008) Two distinct activation states of plasmacytoid dendritic cells induced by influenza virus and CpG 1826 oligonucleotide. J Leukoc Biol 83:610–620
11. Swiecki M, Colonna M (2010) Accumulation of plasmacytoid DC: Roles in disease pathogenesis and targets for immunotherapy. Eur J Immunol 40:2094–2098
12. Jegalian AG, Facchetti F, Jaffe ES (2009) Plasmacytoid dendritic cells: physiologic roles and pathologic states. Adv Anat Pathol 16:392–404
13. Ito T, Wang YH, Liu YJ (2005) Plasmacytoid dendritic cell precursors/type I interferon-producing cells sense viral infection by Toll-like receptor (TLR) 7 and TLR9. Springer Semin Immunpathol 26:221–229
14. Sadler AJ, Williams BRG (2008) Interferon-inducible antiviral effectors. Nature Rev Immunol 8:559–568
15. Schoggins JW, Rice CM (2011) Interferon-stimulated genes and their antiviral effector functions. Curr Opin Virol 1:519–525
16. Soloff AC, Weirback HK, Ross TM, Barratt-Boyes SM (2012) Plasmacytoid dendritic cell depletion leads to an enhanced mononuclear phagocyte response in lungs of mice with lethal influenza virus infection. Comp Immunol Microbiol Infect Dis 35:309–317

17. Langlois RA, Legge KL (2010) Plasmacytoid dendritic cells enhance mortality during lethal influenza infections by eliminating virus-specific CD8 T cells. J Immunol 184:4440–4446
18. Moseman EA, Liang X, Dawson AJ et al (2004) Human plasmacytoid dendritic cells activated by CpG oligodeoxynucleotides induce the generation of CD4+CD25+ regulatory T cells. J Immunol 173:4433–4442
19. Björck P, Leong HX, Engleman EG (2011) Plasmacytoid dendritic cell dichotomy: identification of IFN-α producing cells as a phenotypically and functionally distinct subset. J Immunol 186:1477–1485
20. Salomon R, Hoffmann E, Webster RG (2007) Inhibition of the cytokine response does not protect against lethal H5N1 influenza infection. Proc Natl Acad Sci USA 104:12479–12481
21. Martin-Loeches I, Lisboa T, Rhodes A et al (2011) Use of early corticosteroid therapy on ICU admission in patients affected by severe pandemic (H1N1)v influenza A infection. Intensive Care Med 37:272–283
22. Zhang Y, Sun W, Svendsen ER et al (2015) Do corticosteroids reduce the mortality of influenza A (H1N1) infection? A meta-analysis. Crit Care 19:46
23. Sabado RL, Bhardwaj N (2013) Dendritic cell immunotherapy. Ann N Y Acad Sci 1284:31–45
24. Lund JM, Alexopoulou L, Sato A et al (2004) Recognition of single-stranded RNA viruses by Toll-like receptor 7. Proc Natl Acad Sci USA 101:5598–5603
25. Liu YJ (2005) IPC: Professional type 1 interferon-producing cells and plasmacytoid dendritic cell precursors. Annu Rev Immunol 23:275–306
26. Wu UI, Wang JT, Chen YC, Chang SC (2011) Severity of pandemic H1N1 2009 influenza virus infection may not be directly correlated with initial viral load in upper respiratory tract. Influenza Other Respir Viruses 6:367–373
27. Oshansky CM, Gartland AJ, Wong SS et al (2014) Mucosal immune responses predict clinical outcomes during influenza infection independently of age and viral load. Am J Respir Crit Care Med 189:449–462

Critically Ill Patients with Middle East Respiratory Syndrome Coronavirus Infection

H. M. Al-Dorzi, S. Alsolamy, and Y. M. Arabi

Introduction

The Middle East respiratory syndrome coronavirus (MERS-CoV) is an emerging virus that may lead to severe acute respiratory illness frequently associated with multiorgan failure and death. The objective of this chapter is to summarize the current state of knowledge regarding the pathogenesis, clinical manifestations, diagnosis, management and outcomes of MERS-CoV infection focusing on the critically ill.

Epidemiology

The virus was first isolated from a patient with fatal pneumonia and acute kidney injury in Jeddah, Saudi Arabia in June 2012 [1]. After its identification, the virus was linked to a healthcare-associated cluster of respiratory illnesses in Jordan dat-

H. M. Al-Dorzi
Intensive Care Department, King Saud bin Abdulaziz University for Health Sciences (KSAU-HS)
Riyadh, Saudi Arabia
King Abdullah International Medical Research Center (KAIMRC)
Riyadh, Saudi Arabia

S. Alsolamy
Emergency Medicine and Intensive Care Departments, King Saud bin Abdulaziz University for Health Sciences (KSAU-HS)
Riyadh, Saudi Arabia
King Abdullah International Medical Research Center (KAIMRC)
Riyadh, Saudi Arabia

Y. M. Arabi (✉)
Intensive Care Department, King Saud bin Abdulaziz University for Health Sciences (KSAU-HS)
Riyadh, Saudi Arabia
King Abdullah International Medical Research Center (KAIMRC)
Riyadh, Saudi Arabia
email: arabi@ngha.med.sa

© Springer International Publishing Switzerland 2016
J.-L. Vincent (ed.), *Annual Update in Intensive Care and Emergency Medicine 2016*,
DOI 10.1007/978-3-319-27349-5_4

ing back to March 2012 [2]. The disease epidemiology has been characterized by sporadic cases throughout the year with surges of cases occurring because of hospital outbreaks. As of December 27, 2015, the World Health Organization (WHO) had reported 1,621 laboratory-confirmed cases, including at least 584 (36%) related deaths [3]. Cases of MERS-CoV have occurred in 26 countries, with all cases linked to residence in or travel to the Arabian Peninsula.

The majority of cases have occurred in Saudi Arabia (80%) and South Korea (12%) [3]. In Saudi Arabia, multiple hospital outbreaks occurred in Alahsa (April–May 2013) [4], Jeddah (April and May 2014) [5], and Riyadh (August–September 2015) [3]. The outbreak in the Republic of Korea started in May 2015 and resulted from a case with travel history to the Middle East (Saudi Arabia, Qatar, United Arab Emirates and Bahrain). Subsequently, human-to-human transmission occurred to close contacts (family members, patients sharing a room or ward with infected patients and healthcare workers caring for infected patients) and led to 185 cases of MERS-CoV infection [3]. The last laboratory-confirmed case in Korea was on 4 July 2015 [3].

Pathogenesis

Coronaviruses are a family of enveloped, single-stranded RNA viruses [6]. They can infect animals and humans and have the propensity to cross species [6]. They cause a variety of illnesses that range from the common cold to severe respiratory illnesses [6]. The Severe Acute Respiratory Syndrome coronavirus (SARS-CoV) was the first coronavirus identified to cause widespread outbreaks of critical illness. It caused a worldwide outbreak during the winter of 2002–2003, eventually leading to 8096 confirmed cases, including 774 deaths [7]. The SARS epidemic was contained in 2003 [7]. SARS-CoV belongs to lineage B of the betacoronavirus [8], whereas MERS-CoV belongs to lineage C of the same genus. MERS-CoV enters cells via a common receptor, the dipeptidyl peptidase-4 (DPP4), also known as CD26, and replicates in bronchial, bronchiolar and type I and II alveolar epithelial cells [9, 10]. The virus has primarily been detected in respiratory secretions, with the highest viral loads in the lower respiratory tract [11]. In MERS-CoV cases, one study showed that approximately 70% of patients had continued respiratory shedding for > 30 days [12]. MERS-CoV infection often manifests with acute kidney injury (AKI), the pathogenesis of which remains unknown, although direct viral infection is a possibility since the DPP4 receptor is heavily expressed in human kidneys [13]. Viral shedding has also been detected in the urine and stool of infected patients [14].

There is accumulating evidence that camels are the primary source for animal-to-human transmission of MERS-CoV. The virus has been isolated from dromedary camels [15]. The high viral loads in the upper respiratory tract of infected camels suggest that transmission to humans occurs through close camel contact [15]. Transmission through ingestion of camel products (meat and milk) is possible but has never been confirmed. In a cross-sectional serosurveillance study of 10,009 individuals in Saudi Arabia, positive serology was documented in only 0.15% [16]. Seropositivity was more common in men than in women, in central than in coastal provinces and in shepherds and slaughterhouse workers than in others [16]. This may explain, at least in part, the sporadic community-acquired cases seen at low rates throughout the year.

Human-to-human transmission of MERS-CoV has been demonstrated among close household contacts and family members [17]. However, sustained community-based transmission has not been reported. Secondary transmission within healthcare settings has been described with already-hospitalized patients and healthcare workers acquiring the disease [18, 19]. This has been attributed to overcrowding, movement of infected patients who did not yet have a diagnosis and breaches of infection prevention and control practices [3]. A study evaluated the stability of MERS-CoV under different environmental conditions and found that the virus was more stable at low temperature/low humidity than at higher temperature/ higher humidity conditions [20]. MERS-CoV could be recovered after 48 h at a 20 °C/40% relative humidity condition [20]. During MERS-CoV aerosolization, no decrease in stability was observed at the 20 °C/40% relative humidity condition [20]. The prolonged environmental presence suggests that MERS-CoV may be transmitted via contact or fomites [20], although this has not been confirmed.

Clinical Manifestations

The disease spectrum ranges from asymptomatic infection to rapidly progressive severe respiratory failure with multiorgan failure. Symptomatic cases manifest after an incubation period of 2–14 days [21]. Most severe cases have been reported in adults with chronic comorbidities, including diabetes mellitus, chronic cardiac disease, chronic lung disease, end-stage kidney disease, or immunosuppression [21, 22]. However, severe infection may also occur among younger patients, including healthcare workers [18]. Compared with SARS-CoV, MERS-CoV affects older patients, men more than women, and people with comorbid illnesses. The healthcare-associated MERS-CoV infections occurred within the first week of the index case illness, while for SARS they occurred mainly in the second week, likely due to the different timings of peak viral load [23]. The current literature suggests that children are rarely affected by MERS-CoV [24].

The most common clinical features in critically ill patients with MERS-CoV are fever (71%), cough (68%), dyspnea (66%), and gastrointestinal symptoms (32%) [21]. Common laboratory abnormalities include leukopenia, lymphocytopenia, and thrombocytopenia, elevated serum creatinine and lactate dehydrogenase, and altered liver enzymes [21]. Initial chest radiographs are abnormal in most symptomatic patients and findings range from minimal abnormalities to extensive bilateral infiltrates [21]. Figure 1 shows the chest radiographs of four patients with MERS-CoV pneumonia on the first day of intubation and demonstrates different patterns of lung infiltrates. Computed tomography (CT) findings have included bi-

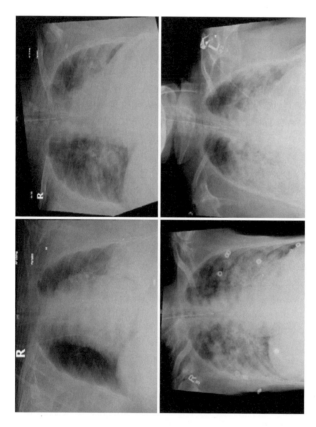

Fig. 1 Chest radiographs on the first day of endotracheal intubation of four patients with Middle East respiratory syndrome coronavirus (MERS-CoV) pneumonia

lateral airspace opacities predominantly in the subpleural and basilar lung regions with more extensive ground-glass opacities than consolidation [25].

Rapid progression to hypoxemic respiratory failure requiring intubation usually occurs within the first week after symptom onset [26]. In one observational study at a single center in Saudi Arabia (October 1, 2012 to May 31, 2014), severe infection requiring ICU admission occurred in 49 (70%) of 70 cases with 46 (66%) requiring invasive mechanical ventilation. In the univariate analysis, factors associated with severe infection requiring ICU admission were age ≥ 65 years (odds ratio [OR] 9.47, 95% confidence interval [CI] 2.45–36.56), male sex (OR 3.05, 95% CI 1.05–8.84), higher age-adjusted Charlson comorbidity index (OR 1.35, 95% CI 1.11–1.65), the presence of bilateral pulmonary infiltrates on chest radiograph (OR 4.89, 95% CI 1.16–20.47), concomitant infections (OR 12.66, 95% CI 2.65–60.46), and serum albumin < 35 g/l at MERS-CoV diagnosis (OR 8.0, 95% CI 1.97–32.46) [19]. Severe neurologic syndrome, including altered level of consciousness, ranging from confusion to coma, ataxia, and focal motor deficit, has been reported in three critically ill MERS-CoV patients, with brain magnetic resonance imaging (MRI) showing widespread, bilateral hyperintense lesions on T2-weighted images in the white matter and subcortical areas of different brain areas [27].

Diagnosis

The WHO has issued guidance for the definition of MERS-CoV cases, based on clinical criteria, exposure history and diagnostic findings as shown in Table 1 [3]. The clinical and radiological manifestations do not differentiate MERS-CoV infection from other causes of respiratory infection. Diagnosis is, therefore, based on molecular testing by real-time reverse-transcription polymerase chain reaction (rRT-PCR) for two sites in the virus genome: the upstream E protein (upE) for screening and the open reading frame (ORF) 1a or 1b for confirmation [28]. Lower respiratory tract specimens have a higher sensitivity than upper respiratory tract specimens for detecting MERS-CoV [29]. The success of rRT-PCR testing depends on the experience and expertise of laboratory personnel, avoidance of contamination and the type and specimen condition. Gene sequencing targeting *RdRp* (present in all corona viruses) and *N* (specific to MERS-CoV) gene fragments can be used for confirmation [28]. MERS-CoV can be also diagnosed by seroconversion on two samples two weeks apart. Enzyme-linked immunosorbent assay can be used for screening and immunofluorescence assay (IFA) or neutralization for confirmation [28]. Several MERS-CoV-specific serologic assays have been developed but need validation [28]. The MERS-CoV virus can be cultured in commonly available cell lines [28]; however, this requires specialized biosafety level 3 laboratories.

Table 1 Interim case definitions for Middle East respiratory syndrome coronavirus (MERS-CoV) infection (as of 14 July 2015) [3]

Probable case	An acute respiratory illness with fever and clinical, radiological, or histopathological evidence of pulmonary involvement **AND** Direct epidemiologic link with a confirmed MERS-CoV case **AND** MERS-CoV testing is unavailable, negative on a single inadequate specimen or inconclusive
	An acute respiratory illness with fever and clinical, radiological, or histopathological evidence of pulmonary involvement **AND** The person lives in or has travelled to Middle Eastern countries or countries where MERS-CoV is known to be circulating in dromedary camels or where human MERS-CoV infections have recently occurred **AND** MERS-CoV testing is inconclusive
	An acute febrile respiratory illness of any severity **AND** Direct epidemiologic link with a confirmed MERS-CoV case **AND** MERS-CoV testing is inconclusive
Confirmed case	A person with laboratory-confirmed MERS-CoV infection irrespective of clinical signs and symptoms

Management

At present, there is no proven specific therapy for MERS-CoV infection. Therefore, the mainstay of management of critically ill patients with MERS-CoV infection is supportive evidence-based care. Admission to the ICU is frequently required for close monitoring (e.g., patients with high oxygen requirements) or organ support. The WHO has issued interim guidance for the management of suspected and confirmed MERS-CoV infection [30].

Infection Prevention and Control

Because of the risk of transmission within the healthcare setting, appropriate patient isolation and strict implementation of infection prevention and control measures are crucial in the management of MERS-CoV cases. For suspected cases, the WHO recommends droplet and contact precautions [30]. When performing an aerosol generating procedure (e.g., aspiration or open suctioning of respiratory tract, intubation, bronchoscopy, cardiopulmonary resuscitation) airborne precautions should be additionally applied [30]. The Centers for Disease Control and Prevention (CDC) recommends that droplet precautions should be added to standard precautions when providing care to all patients with symptoms of acute respiratory infection and that a suspected or confirmed MERS-CoV case should be isolated in an airborne infection isolation room that is constructed and maintained according to current guidelines [31]. If such a room is not available, the patient should be transferred as soon as is feasible to a facility where one is available [31]. Until transfer, the patient should wear a facemask and should be isolated in a room with the door closed [31]. Healthcare workers should adhere to standard contact and airborne precautions. Hand hygiene should be performed appropriately and personal protective equipment, including respirators, should be applied correctly [31]. In addition, visitation should be restricted and controlled [31]. Hospitals should also develop protocols to be ready for a potential increase in the need to isolate patients with suspected or confirmed MERS-Cov infection.

Management of Respiratory Failure

Early supportive management includes supplemental oxygen for hypoxemia, respiratory distress and shock and early invasive mechanical ventilation for significant respiratory distress or persistent hypoxemia [30]. Patients with acute respiratory distress syndrome (ARDS) should receive evidence-based care that includes a lung-protective ventilation strategy [32]: targeting a tidal volume of 6 ml/kg of predicted body weight, a plateau airway pressure $\leq 30\,cmH_2O$ and SpO_2 88–93% or PaO_2 55–80 mmHg. Moderate to severe ARDS cases (PaO_2:FiO_2 < 150 mmHg) are candidates for early prone positioning [33] and early neuromuscular blockade for 48 h [34]. Proning is recommended within 36 h of ARDS onset for at least 16 h, since this approach was associated with reduced mortality compared with managing patients in the supine position [33]. A 48-h infusion of intravenous cisatracurium within 48 h of ARDS onset has also been associated with reduced mortality compared with placebo [34]. Extracorporeal membrane oxygenation (ECMO) is an option for patients with refractory hypoxemia [35, 36], and has been successfully used in young patients with severe H1N1 influenza with refractory hypoxemia [36] as well as in MERS-CoV patients [11]. Systematic corticosteroids should generally be avoided unless indicated for other established reasons [30]. The effect of corticosteroids on the outcome of MERS-CoV patients is unknown; however, corticosteroid use has been associated with increased morbidity in patients with SARS-CoV and severe influenza [37, 38].

High-flow oxygen, non-invasive ventilation and high-frequency oscillatory ventilation should probably be avoided or used with caution in MERS patients because of the potential to generate aerosols and lack of effectiveness in patients with ARDS [39]. A systematic review found that the following procedures were associated with an increased risk of acute respiratory infection transmission to healthcare workers through aerosol-generation: endotracheal intubation, non-invasive ventilation, tracheotomy, and manual ventilation [39]. Strict infection prevention practices should, therefore, be employed when these interventions are performed.

Management of Acute Kidney Injury

Conservative fluid management is advocated especially in the presence of hypoxemia and the absence of shock. When renal replacement therapy (RRT) should be started in patients with AKI is controversial. However, the presence of fluid overload at the start of RRT has been associated with a worse outcome [40]. Starting ultrafiltration at lower degrees of fluid overload and early targeting of a negative balance may be beneficial [41, 42].

Feeding

Early trophic feeding for 7 days in ARDS patients [43] and permissive underfeeding for up to 14 days in mechanically ventilated patients [44] have been shown to be equivalent to target feeding for most outcomes including survival. Underfeeding may be preferred for patients in the prone position.

Specific Therapies

To date, there is no effective specific treatment for MERS-CoV infection. Data on ribavirin, interferon, and convalescent plasma are limited [21]. A study in rhesus macaques found that a combination of interferon-α2b and ribavirin was associated with a reduction in MERS-CoV replication and improved outcome [45]. Clinical studies on combined ribavirin and interferon showed inconsistent results [46]. Convalescent sera from patients who have recovered may be useful. A post-hoc meta-analysis of 32 studies on SARS-CoV and severe influenza found reduced mortality after antibody treatment compared with placebo or no treatment (pooled OR 0.25, 95% CI 0.14–0.45), but the included studies were of low or very low quality [47]. Three studies from separate laboratories have reported the development of fully human neutralizing monoclonal antibodies against MERS-CoV but no clinical data are currently available [48]. Repurposed commonly-used drugs, such as statins, mycophenolic acid, and anti-tumor necrosis factor agents, which have potential anti-inflammatory or antiviral effects against MERS-CoV and at the same time an excellent safety record, may be treatment options. However, these drugs are not recommended for clinical use outside clinical trials [49]. There are no currently licensed MERS-CoV vaccines; however, work is ongoing to develop effective vaccines [50].

Outcomes

The overall case fatality rate of MERS-CoV infection is ~35% [3]. However, the mortality rate of patients with severe illness requiring critical care is higher (58–84%) [19, 22, 26]. Requirement for ICU admission for hospitalized patients is frequent (45–70%) [19, 22]. In an observational study, 41 out of 49 (84%) cases requiring ICU admission died, with 33 (78.6%) having a progressive disease course until death [19]. In a multivariable regression analysis, only the presence of a concomitant infection (OR 14.13, 95% CI 1.58–126.09) and a low serum albumin (OR 6.31, 95% CI 1.24–31.90) were associated with the need for ICU admission [19]. The multivariable analysis showed age ≥ 65 years to be the only independent risk factor for increased mortality (OR 4.39, 95% CI 2.13–9.05) [19]. AKI (41%), hepatic dysfunction (31%) and cardiac arrhythmias (16%), such as tachyarrhythmias and severe bradycardia requiring temporary pacemaker insertion, were common complications [19]. Another observational study of 12 critically ill cases found that barotrauma occurred in 17%, vasopressors were needed in 92% and RRT was performed in 58% [26]. The median time from onset of symptoms to intubation was 4.5 days (range 0–33 days). The median ICU and hospital lengths of stay were 30 (7–104) days and 41 (8–96) days, respectively, and 25% of patients had a tracheostomy [26]. The 28-day and 90-day mortality rates were 42 and 58%, respectively [26].

It should be noted that the mortality of MERS-CoV cases during the Korean outbreak (May–July 2015) was only 19% compared with ~42% in Saudi Arabia (as at Sept 11, 2015) [3]. However, the composition of the two cohorts was different in the relative percentages of asymptomatic and mildly symptomatic cases. The Korean healthcare authorities applied widespread screening and intensified public health measures, such as contact tracing, quarantine and isolation of suspected cases and all contacts for at least 14 days [3]. The identification of asymptomatic or mildly symptomatic patients and differences in patient characteristics, such as comorbid conditions, may have led to an overall lower mortality rate in Korea.

Conclusions and Future Directions

More than three years after its identification, MERS-CoV remains a major global threat. Infection with MERS-CoV is frequently severe and associated with significant morbidity and mortality. Although our understanding of this virus and its disease continues to evolve, large knowledge gaps remain. The Arabian Peninsula remains the most affected region, but there is concern about the spread of this virus to other countries and globally. Until zoonotic transfer of the virus from animals to humans is stopped, the risk of additional domestic and perhaps international outbreaks persists. Moreover, there is an urgent need for larger epidemiologic and outcome studies and randomized controlled trials examining different therapeutic interventions. Collaboration between international health authorities and research centers is necessary and is crucial to achieve these goals.

References

1. Zaki AM, van Boheemen S, Bestebroer TM, Osterhaus AD, Fouchier RA (2012) Isolation of a novel coronavirus from a man with pneumonia in Saudi Arabia. N Engl J Med 367:1814–1820

2. Hijawi B, Abdallat M, Sayaydeh A et al (2013) Novel coronavirus infections in Jordan, April 2012: epidemiological findings from a retrospective investigation. East Mediterr Health J 19(Suppl 1):S12–S18

3. World Health Organization (2015) Middle East respiratory syndrome coronavirus (MERS-CoV). http://www.who.int/csr/disease/coronavirus_infections/case_definition/en/. Accessed December 2015

4. Assiri A, McGeer A, Perl TM et al (2013) Hospital outbreak of Middle East respiratory syndrome coronavirus. N Engl J Med 369:407–416

5. Oboho IK, Tomczyk SM, Al-Asmari AM et al (2015) 2014 MERS-CoV outbreak in Jeddah – a link to health care facilities. N Engl J Med 372:846–854

6. Abdel-Moneim AS (2014) Middle East respiratory syndrome coronavirus (MERS-CoV): evidence and speculations. Arch Virol 159:1575–1584

7. World Health Organization (2003) Summary of probable SARS cases with onset of illness from 1 November 2002 to 31 July 2003. http://www.who.int/csr/sars/country/table2004_04_21/en/. Accessed December 2015

8. van Boheemen S, de Graaf M, Lauber C et al (2012) Genomic characterization of a newly discovered coronavirus associated with acute respiratory distress syndrome in humans. MBio 3:1–9

9. Hocke AC, Becher A, Knepper J et al (2013) Emerging human middle East respiratory syndrome coronavirus causes widespread infection and alveolar damage in human lungs. Am J Respir Crit Care Med 188:882–886

10. Chan RW, Chan MC, Agnihothram S et al (2013) Tropism of and innate immune responses to the novel human betacoronavirus lineage C virus in human ex vivo respiratory organ cultures. J Virol 87:6604–6614

11. Guery B, Poissy J, el Mansouf L et al (2013) Clinical features and viral diagnosis of two cases of infection with Middle East Respiratory Syndrome coronavirus: a report of nosocomial transmission. Lancet 381:2265–2272

12. Memish ZA, Assiri AM, Al-Tawfiq JA (2014) Middle East respiratory syndrome coronavirus (MERS-CoV) viral shedding in the respiratory tract: an observational analysis with infection control implications. Int J Infect Dis 29:307–308

13. Eckerle I, Muller MA, Kallies S, Gotthardt DN, Drosten C (2013) In-vitro renal epithelial cell infection reveals a viral kidney tropism as a potential mechanism for acute renal failure during Middle East Respiratory Syndrome (MERS) Coronavirus infection. Virol J 10:359

14. Drosten C, Seilmaier M, Corman VM et al (2013) Clinical features and virological analysis of a case of Middle East respiratory syndrome coronavirus infection. Lancet Infect Dis 13:745–751

15. Azhar EI, El-Kafrawy SA, Farraj SA et al (2014) Evidence for camel-to-human transmission of MERS coronavirus. N Engl J Med 370:2499–2505

16. Muller MA, Meyer B, Corman VM et al (2015) Presence of Middle East respiratory syndrome coronavirus antibodies in Saudi Arabia: a nationwide, cross-sectional, serological study. Lancet Infect Dis 15:559–564

17. Memish ZA, Zumla AI, Al-Hakeem RF, Al-Rabeeah AA, Stephens GM (2013) Family cluster of Middle East respiratory syndrome coronavirus infections. N Engl J Med 368:2487–2494

18. Memish ZA, Zumla AI, Assiri A (2013) Middle East respiratory syndrome coronavirus infections in health care workers. N Engl J Med 369:884–886

19. Saad M, Omrani AS, Baig K et al (2014) Clinical aspects and outcomes of 70 patients with Middle East respiratory syndrome coronavirus infection: a single-center experience in Saudi Arabia. Int J Infect Dis 29:301–306

20. van Doremalen N, Bushmaker T, Munster VJ (2013) Stability of Middle East respiratory syndrome coronavirus (MERS-CoV) under different environmental conditions. Euro Surveill 18:1–4
21. Alsolamy S (2015) Middle East respiratory syndrome: knowledge to date. Crit Care Med 43:1283–1290
22. Al-Tawfiq JA, Hinedi K, Ghandour J et al (2014) Middle East respiratory syndrome coronavirus: a case-control study of hospitalized patients. Clin Infect Dis 59:160–165
23. Hui DS, Memish ZA, Zumla A (2014) Severe acute respiratory syndrome vs. the Middle East respiratory syndrome. Curr Opin Pulm Med 20:233–241
24. Memish ZA, Al-Tawfiq JA, Assiri A et al (2014) Middle East respiratory syndrome coronavirus disease in children. Pediatr Infect Dis J 33:904–906
25. Ajlan AM, Ahyad RA, Jamjoom LG, Alharthy A, Madani TA (2014) Middle East respiratory syndrome coronavirus (MERS-CoV) infection: chest CT findings. AJR Am J Roentgenol 203:782–787
26. Arabi YM, Arifi AA, Balkhy HH et al (2014) Clinical course and outcomes of critically ill patients with Middle East respiratory syndrome coronavirus infection. Ann Intern Med 160:389–397
27. Arabi YM, Harthi A, Hussein J et al (2015) Severe neurologic syndrome associated with Middle East respiratory syndrome corona virus (MERS-CoV). Infection 43:495–501
28. Corman VM, Muller MA, Costabel U et al (2012) Assays for laboratory confirmation of novel human coronavirus (hCoV-EMC) infections. Euro Surveill 17:1–9
29. Lee JH, Lee CS, Lee HB (2015) An appropriate lower respiratory tract specimen is essential for diagnosis of Middle East Respiratory Syndrome (MERS). J Korean Med Sci 30:1207–1208
30. World Health Organization (2015) Clinical management of severe acute respiratory infection when Middle East respiratory syndrome coronavirus (MERS-CoV) infection is suspected – Interim guidance. www.who.int/csr/disease/coronavirus_infections/case-management-ipc/en/. Accessed December 2015
31. Centers for Disease Control and Prevention (2014) Interim Infection Prevention and Control Recommendations for Hospitalized Patients with Middle East Respiratory Syndrome Coronavirus (MERS-CoV). http://www.cdc.gov/coronavirus/mers/infection-prevention-control.html. Accessed December 2015
32. Petrucci N, De Feo C (2013) Lung protective ventilation strategy for the acute respiratory distress syndrome. Cochrane Database Syst Rev 2:CD003844
33. Guerin C, Reignier J, Richard JC et al (2013) Prone positioning in severe acute respiratory distress syndrome. N Engl J Med 368:2159–2168
34. Papazian L, Forel JM, Gacouin A et al (2010) Neuromuscular blockers in early acute respiratory distress syndrome. N Engl J Med 363:1107–1116
35. Peek GJ, Mugford M, Tiruvoipati R et al (2009) Efficacy and economic assessment of conventional ventilatory support versus extracorporeal membrane oxygenation for severe adult respiratory failure (CESAR): a multicentre randomised controlled trial. Lancet 374:1351–1363
36. Davies A, Jones D, Bailey M et al (2009) Extracorporeal membrane oxygenation for 2009 Influenza A (H1N1) acute respiratory distress syndrome. JAMA 302:1888–1895
37. Martin-Loeches I, Lisboa T, Rhodes A et al (2011) Use of early corticosteroid therapy on ICU admission in patients affected by severe pandemic (H1N1)v influenza A infection. Intensive Care Med 37:272–283
38. Stockman LJ, Bellamy R, Garner P (2006) SARS: systematic review of treatment effects. PLoS Med 3:1525–1531
39. Tran K, Cimon K, Severn M, Pessoa-Silva CL, Conly J (2012) Aerosol generating procedures and risk of transmission of acute respiratory infections to healthcare workers: a systematic review. PLoS One 7:e35797

40. Bellomo R, Cass A, Cole L et al (2012) An observational study fluid balance and patient outcomes in the Randomized Evaluation of Normal vs. Augmented Level of Replacement Therapy trial. Crit Care Med 40:1753–1760
41. Ronco C, Ricci Z, De Backer D et al (2015) Renal replacement therapy in acute kidney injury: controversy and consensus. Crit Care 19:146
42. Han F, Sun R, Ni Y et al (2015) Early initiation of continuous renal replacement therapy improves clinical outcomes in patients with acute respiratory distress syndrome. Am J Med Sci 349:199–205
43. Rice TW, Wheeler AP, Thompson BT et al (2012) Initial trophic vs full enteral feeding in patients with acute lung injury: the EDEN randomized trial. JAMA 307:795–803
44. Arabi YM, Aldawood AS, Haddad SH et al (2015) Permissive underfeeding or standard enteral feeding in critically ill adults. N Engl J Med 372:2398–2408
45. Falzarano D, de Wit E, Rasmussen AL et al (2013) Treatment with interferon-alpha2b and ribavirin improves outcome in MERS-CoV-infected rhesus macaques. Nat Med 19:1313–1317
46. Al-Tawfiq JA, Momattin H, Dib J, Memish ZA (2014) Ribavirin and interferon therapy in patients infected with the Middle East respiratory syndrome coronavirus: an observational study. Int J Infect Dis 20:42–46
47. Mair-Jenkins J, Saavedra-Campos M, Baillie JK et al (2015) The effectiveness of convalescent plasma and hyperimmune immunoglobulin for the treatment of severe acute respiratory infections of viral etiology: a systematic review and exploratory meta-analysis. J Infect Dis 211:80–90
48. Ying T, Li H, Lu L, Dimitrov DS, Jiang S (2015) Development of human neutralizing monoclonal antibodies for prevention and therapy of MERS-CoV infections. Microbes Infect 17:142–148
49. Zumla A, Azhar EI, Arabi Y et al (2015) Host-directed therapies for improving poor treatment outcomes associated with the middle east respiratory syndrome coronavirus infections. Int J Infect Dis 40:71–74
50. Zhang N, Jiang S, Du L (2014) Current advancements and potential strategies in the development of MERS-CoV vaccines. Expert Rev Vaccines 13:761–774

Part II
Sepsis

Immunomodulation: The Future for Sepsis?

T. Girardot, F. Venet, and T. Rimmelé

Introduction

Despite significant advances over the last decades, sepsis remains the leading cause of death in the intensive care unit (ICU), with a mortality rate of 40% [1]. In addition to infection control, which associates early and appropriate antimicrobial agents and sometimes surgery, treatment has long been limited to the supportive care of organ dysfunction. The complex host immune response to sepsis is progressively becoming understood [2]. Numerous lines of evidence describing the association between sepsis-induced immune alterations and increased risk of death or nosocomial infections have supported the rationale for several innovative therapies in this field [3]. The goal of these therapies is to restore adequate immune homeostasis in these patients, either by pharmacological agents or by extracorporeal blood purification techniques.

Early after sepsis onset, the activation of immune cells results in the intense release of pro- and anti-inflammatory cytokines. Essential and beneficial to the host when controlled and adapted, this "cytokine storm" can become harmful when unbalanced. Whereas patients whose immune status remains close to homeostasis are more likely to survive, uncontrolled over-inflammation leads to capillary leak and multiorgan failure, responsible for early deaths. On the compensatory anti-inflammatory hand, severe sepsis is responsible for the development of marked immune cell anergy [2]. This immunoparalysis, if persistent, increases the risk of nosoco-

T. Girardot · T. Rimmelé (✉)
Department of Anesthesiology and Critical Care Medicine, Edouard Herriot Hospital, Hospices Civils de Lyon, University Claude Bernard Lyon 1
Lyon, France
email: th.rimmele@gmail.com

F. Venet
Cellular Immunology Department, Edouard Herriot Hospital, Hospices Civils de Lyon, University Claude Bernard Lyon 1
Lyon, France

© Springer International Publishing Switzerland 2016
J.-L. Vincent (ed.), *Annual Update in Intensive Care and Emergency Medicine 2016*,
DOI 10.1007/978-3-319-27349-5_5

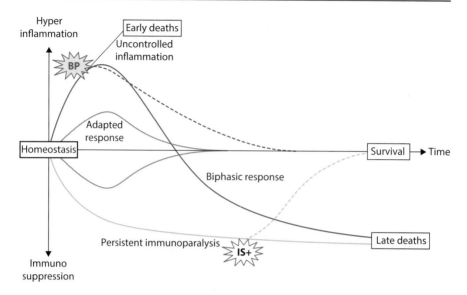

Fig. 1 Host immune response to sepsis and impact of immunomodulation therapies. *Continuous lines*: possible patient immune status; *dotted lines*: potential effects of therapies; BP: blood purification techniques; IS+: immunostimulant drugs

mial infections and viral reactivation, and impedes the patient from clearing the infection. Most sepsis-related deaths occur during this secondary phase [4].

The two therapeutic approaches discussed below aim to restore immune homeostasis, which may contribute to enhance survival. Overwhelming inflammation may be controlled by extracorporeal blood purification techniques and immunostimulating drugs could resolve immune system incompetence (Fig. 1).

Extracorporeal Blood Purification Techniques

Several extracorporeal blood purification techniques, most of them derived from renal replacement therapy (RRT) techniques, have been proposed to modulate the host response to sepsis. The removal of inflammatory mediators from the blood could limit their cytotoxic effects, and also restore the cytokine/chemokine gradient between blood and the infected locus, hence promoting leukocyte migration to the correct place. These techniques could also modify the phenotype of immune cells, heavily altered in sepsis [5].

High-volume Hemofiltration

High volume hemofiltration (HVHF) is defined as the use of ultrafiltration rates greater than those used for renal support, i.e. > 50 ml/kg/h. High or very high ultrafiltration flows have been proposed to enhance the purge of middle molecular weight molecules, such as cytokines [6, 7].

HVHF has long been the most widely used blood purification technique, supported by encouraging animal and preclinical studies. In a porcine model of bile-induced pancreatitis, HVHF restored the normal expression of several markers of immunoparalysis. A beneficial effect on mortality was even suggested [8]. Nevertheless, in the IVOIRE randomized trial, comparing ultrafiltration flow rates of 35 versus 70 ml/kg/h in septic shock patients with acute kidney injury (AKI), there was no benefit on mortality or on secondary endpoints [9]. Combined with two recent meta-analyses upholding these negative results [10, 11], the IVOIRE trial may put an end to the use of HVHF for sepsis.

Cascade Hemofiltration

HVHF has, in addition, significant limitations, such as massive losses of low molecular weight molecules (vitamins, nutrients, antibiotics ...), elevated costs, and high nursing workload. With two different hemofilters, the cascade circuit can provide an answer to all these drawbacks. Its original concept allows selective elimination of middle molecular weight molecules, and return of the small solutes to the patient. The first filter, with an elevated cut-off, heads middle and low molecular weight molecules to a second filter. This second, low cut-off membrane allows for the return of small molecular weight molecules to the patient, then 'selectively' eliminates the middle ones (such as cytokines) in the definitive effluent (Fig. 2).

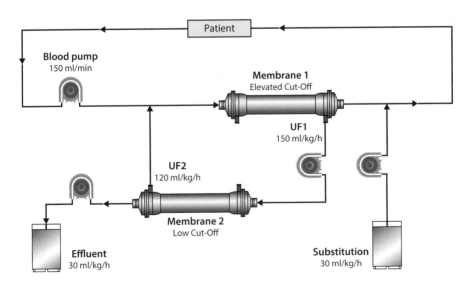

Fig. 2 Cascade hemofiltration circuit. UF: ultrafiltration

In a porcine model of septic shock, this technique decreased the required epinephrine doses and improved biological parameters compared with standard HVHF [12]. A clinical trial evaluating the hemodynamic effects of this technique in patients with septic shock has recently been completed (NCT 00922870).

Plasma Exchange

Plasma exchange consists of the removal of the native plasma and its replacement by fluids. It may, therefore, theoretically be very efficient for cytokine removal from the patient's blood. Consequently, it has been proposed for blood purification and showed interesting results when applied early in Gram-negative infections [13]. This efficient removal of cytokines may be responsible for the demonstrated lowering of inflammatory markers of sepsis and organ failure [14]. In a randomized trial, plasma exchange also increased survival when associated with conventional therapies of septic shock, but only in intra-abdominal infections. However, this result was only obtained in a *post-hoc* analysis of one subgroup. Patients from the control group were older and had more severe respiratory failure, making this result controversial [15].

Hemoperfusion

Hemoperfusion, also called hemoadsorption, uses materials with particular adsorption properties. The blood circulates in direct contact with the sorbent, which attracts solutes via hydrophobic, ionic, and van der Waals interactions. Thus, high-molecular weight molecules, sometimes exceeding the cut-off of standard high-flux hemofilters, can be removed from the blood, as they bind to the sorbent surface. Technical biocompatibility problems with these materials have been solved. One limitation lies in the fact that, unlike most blood purification techniques, hemoperfusion is not also a RRT technique at the same time [6].

In a recent meta-analysis, the beneficial effect of blood purification on mortality was mainly driven by the results of Japanese studies assessing hemoperfusion with polymyxin-B [16]. This material is the most widely used, especially for the treatment of Gram-negative infections. Beyond hemodynamic and respiratory improvements, the EUPHAS trial suggested a survival benefit for patients receiving this therapy in intra-abdominal infection-related severe sepsis [17]. However, the recent ABDO-MIX trial did not confirm these results [18]. This randomized multicenter trial was designed to assess the effect on mortality of hemoperfusion with polymyxin-B in peritonitis-induced septic-shock. There was no statistical difference between the polymyxin-B and the conventional groups and a trend towards a higher mortality rate in polymyxin-B-treated patients was noticed. Secondary outcomes and subgroup analysis did not demonstrate any benefit of this technique either [18]. The EUPHRATES trial, currently ongoing (NCT 01046669), will provide additional information about the potential usefulness of polymyxin-B hemoperfusion in sepsis.

In other countries, a cartridge filled with divinylbenzene beads has been proposed. *Ex vivo,* this material has proved its capacity to remove activated innate and adaptive immune cells from the blood, and to modify cytokine expression profiles [5]. In a rat model of septic shock, its use was associated with decreased interleukin (IL)-6 and IL-10 concentrations and prolonged survival [19].

Coupled Plasma Filtration and Adsorption

Combining the above described possibilities, coupled plasma filtration and adsorption (CPFA) is an original, promising technique that could find its place in the arsenal of extracorporeal blood purification [20]. Plasma is first extracted from the whole blood through a plasmafilter. Its inability to coagulate allows very slow circulation over the adsorbent material, hence optimizing the adsorption process. Thereafter, the purified plasma is mixed with the blood from which it has been separated earlier, and is directed towards a second hemofilter, which interestingly adds to this so-called "hybrid" technique a standard continuous RRT circuit (Fig. 3) [21].

In a pilot study on patients with severe sepsis and multiple organ dysfunction syndrome, CPFA was more efficient than HVHF at reversing immunoparaly-

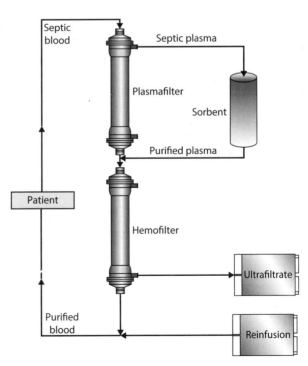

Fig. 3 Coupled plasma filtration and adsorption circuit

sis. Notably, it enhanced the expression of HLA-DR on monocytes and restored lipopolysaccharide (LPS)-induced tumor necrosis factor (TNF) production [22]. In the COMPACT-1 trial, CPFA was combined with standard care of septic shock for 5 days. Unfortunately, issues of circuit coagulation limited the volume of plasma treated, leading to numerous protocol violations. Nevertheless, a dose-response relationship may exist: the subgroup of patients who received the higher 'dose' of CPFA had a lower mortality rate compared with controls [23]. The ongoing COMPACT-2 trial (NCT 01639664) was designed to answer this question. With regional citrate circuit anticoagulation preventing coagulation drawbacks, this ongoing study aims to evaluate the effects of high doses of CPFA (> 0.2 l/kg/d of plasma) in septic shock.

Highly Adsorptive Membranes

RRT membranes can be modified to serve as a blood purification device themselves [24]. For example, adding a positively charged polymer to a classic polyacrylonitrile membrane enhances its adsorption capacities for LPS and inflammatory cytokines. In a porcine model of septic shock, a 6-h session of HVHF with this particular membrane improved hemodynamics, when compared with a standard membrane [25].

High Cut-off Membranes

Other properties of the membrane can also be modified. Increasing their cut-off should allow the removal of a larger spectrum of middle molecules. These membranes were first used with hemofiltration, and showed hemodynamic improvements in sepsis [26]. However, loss of proteins, such as albumin, represents the main drawback of this technique. In addition to the continuing optimization of all the other technical parameters of these membranes, their use with diffusive (and not convective) techniques greatly reduces albumin leakage [27]. Innovative filters such as "super-high flux" membranes are now available, allowing for the preservation of albumin and purification of cytokines [5].

Pharmacological Approaches

The second strategy for modulation of the host immune response to sepsis is pharmacologic. After the recent failure of hydrocortisone and activated protein C, some new molecules have shown very promising preliminary results [28, 29]. These molecules could influence multiple septic alterations of immune cells: their number, their phenotype, and their function, thus contributing to an appropriate, adaptive response.

IL-7

Essential for lymphocyte survival and involved in many leukocyte functions, IL-7 may be an interesting adjuvant therapy in sepsis. In a murine peritonitis model, recombinant human IL-7 (rhIL-7) was shown to block apoptosis of CD4+ and CD8+ T cells, restore interferon (IFN)γ production, and improve leukocyte trafficking to the infected nidus *via* increased expression of the adhesion molecules lymphocyte function-associated antigen (LFA)-1 and very late antigen (VLA)-4. It also enhanced survival in septic mice [30]. This capacity to restore immune functions of lymphocytes was confirmed in an *ex vivo* study, demonstrating that rhIL-7 also increased STAT-5 (signal transducer and activator of transcription 5) phosphorylation and B-cell lymphoma 2 induction after stimulation [31]. After these encouraging preclinical results, a French/American clinical trial of rhIL-7 in well-selected immunocompromised septic shock patients should begin soon.

Granulocyte Macrophage-Colony Stimulating Factor

In a small clinical trial in patients with sepsis-induced immunosuppression, defined by a decreased expression of monocyte HLA-DR, granulocyte macrophage-colony stimulating factor (GM-CSF) was shown to restore HLA-DR expression. It also restored *ex vivo* Toll-like receptor (TLR) 2/4-induced pro-inflammatory monocytic cytokine production. Clinical outcomes (duration of mechanical ventilation, organ dysfunctions, and length of ICU and hospital stay) were also improved in the GM-CSF group [32].

To confirm these interesting results, a large phase 3, double-blind randomized controlled trial named GRID (GM-CSF to decrease ICU-acquired infections) is just about to begin (NCT 02361528). The investigators will assess the effects of GM-CSF on the prevention of secondary infections and other clinical outcomes.

IFNγ

As with GM-CSF, *ex vivo* IFNγ can restore the immune functions of stimulated leukocytes from septic patients. In healthy volunteers receiving intravenous LPS, IFNγ limited the reduction of the LPS-induced TNF response, compared with placebo. It also increased monocyte HLA-DR expression [33]. In small case series, IFNγ, when added to standard care, seemed to hasten the cure of invasive fungal infections and restore immune function [34, 35]. An ongoing randomized controlled trial in septic shock patients (NCT 01649921) may provide insight into the effects of recombinant IFNγ on immune function and relevant clinical outcomes.

PD-1 and PD-L1, and CTLA-4 Antagonists

Increased expression of programmed death cell-1 (PD-1) in septic lymphocytes may play a major role in the T-cell anergy associated with sepsis. Blockade of this pathway was tested in a murine model of fungal sepsis. Antagonist antibodies for PD-1 and its ligand (PD-L1) restored the expression of IFNγ and HLA-DR, but also improved the survival of infected mice [36]. Considering the rapid development of therapies targeting this pathway in cancer, clinical trials testing these treatments in sepsis might also start soon [37].

In the same trial [36], the authors blocked the cytotoxic T-lymphocyte antigen-4 (CTLA-4), a negative costimulatory molecule that acts like PD-1 to suppress T-cell function. This blockade reproduced the immunologic effects on IFNγ and HLA-DR expression, and the clinically beneficial effect on mouse mortality [36].

Intravenous Immunoglobulins

Intravenous immunoglobulins (IVIG) are used in many immunological diseases to modify the inflammatory response. Standard or IgM-enriched polyclonal IVIG could be useful in sepsis as an adjunctive therapy for immunomodulation. A recent meta-analysis concluded that these agents were associated with a significant reduction in the mortality rate when compared with placebo or no intervention. However, when considering only trials with a low risk of bias, this beneficial effect disappeared [38]. In addition, in some of the trials included in this meta-analysis, the standard care of the control group did not fit the bundle of evidence published by the Surviving Sepsis Campaign [39].

Conclusion

Significant progress on sepsis-related mortality and morbidity has been achieved in the past decade [40, 41]. Progressive improved understanding of sepsis-induced immunosuppression leads to the development of adjunctive therapies that aim to modulate the pathologic inflammatory response and limit its deleterious consequences. Several extracorporeal techniques and pharmacological approaches have been proposed. Some of them may be of interest to help control the burden of sepsis.

These therapies acting on patients' immune responses may be selected according to the status of each patient. Monocyte HLA-DR expression is, to date, the gold standard to identify patients who could benefit from immunostimulation, but further research may identify other relevant and suitable markers for daily clinical practice [42].

Finally, genetic background plays a leading role in the high heterogeneity of host reactions to the infectious insult. The development of transcriptomics will help to explore the pathways involved in immunosuppression, and to adapt future therapies to each patient [43].

References

1. Quenot JP, Binquet C, Kara F et al (2013) The epidemiology of septic shock in French intensive care units: the prospective multicenter cohort EPISS study. Crit Care 17:R65
2. Hotchkiss RS, Monneret G, Payen D (2013) Sepsis-induced immunosuppression: from cellular dysfunctions to immunotherapy. Nat Rev Immunol 13:862–874
3. Lukaszewicz A-C, Grienay M, Resche-Rigon M et al (2009) Monocytic HLA-DR expression in intensive care patients: interest for prognosis and secondary infection prediction. Crit Care Med 37:2746–2752
4. Venet F, Lukaszewicz A-C, Payen D, Hotchkiss R, Monneret G (2013) Monitoring the immune response in sepsis: a rational approach to administration of immunoadjuvant therapies. Curr Opin Immunol 25:477–483
5. Rimmelé T, Kaynar AM, McLaughlin JN et al (2013) Leukocyte capture and modulation of cell-mediated immunity during human sepsis: an ex vivo study. Crit Care 17:R59
6. Rimmelé T, Kellum JA (2012) High-volume hemofiltration in the intensive care unit: a blood purification therapy. Anesthesiology 116:1377–1387
7. Kellum JA, Johnson JP, Kramer D, Palevsky P, Brady JJ, Pinsky MR (1998) Diffusive vs. convective therapy: effects on mediators of inflammation in patient with severe systemic inflammatory response syndrome. Crit Care Med 26:1995–2000
8. Yekebas EF, Eisenberger CF, Ohnesorge H et al (2001) Attenuation of sepsis-related immunoparalysis by continuous veno-venous hemofiltration in experimental porcine pancreatitis. Crit Care Med 29:1423–1430
9. Joannes-Boyau O, Honoré PM, Perez P et al (2013) High-volume versus standard-volume haemofiltration for septic shock patients with acute kidney injury (IVOIRE study): a multicentre randomized controlled trial. Intensive Care Med 39:1535–1546
10. Clark E, Molnar AO, Joannes-Boyau O, Honoré PM, Sikora L, Bagshaw SM (2014) High-volume hemofiltration for septic acute kidney injury: a systematic review and meta-analysis. Crit Care 18:R7
11. Borthwick EMJ, Hill CJ, Rabindranath KS, Maxwell AP, McAuley DF, Blackwood B (2013) High-volume haemofiltration for sepsis. Cochrane Database Syst Rev 1:CD008075
12. Rimmelé T, Hayi-Slayman D, Page M, Rada H, Monchi M, Allaouchiche B (2009) Cascade hemofiltration: principle, first experimental data. Ann Fr Anesth Reanim 28:249–252
13. Hjorth V, Stenlund G (2000) Plasmapheresis as part of the treatment for septic shock. Scand J Infect Dis 32:511–514
14. Reeves JH, Butt WW, Shann F et al (1999) Continuous plasmafiltration in sepsis syndrome. Plasmafiltration in Sepsis Study Group. Crit Care Med 27:2096–2104
15. Busund R, Koukline V, Utrobin U, Nedashkovsky E (2002) Plasmapheresis in severe sepsis and septic shock: a prospective, randomised, controlled trial. Intensive Care Med 28:1434–1439
16. Zhou F, Peng Z, Murugan R, Kellum JA (2013) Blood purification and mortality in sepsis: a meta-analysis of randomized trials. Crit Care Med 41:2209–2220
17. Cruz DN, Antonelli M, Fumagalli R et al (2009) Early use of polymyxin B hemoperfusion in abdominal septic shock: the EUPHAS randomized controlled trial. JAMA 301:2445–2452
18. Payen DM, Guilhot J, Launey Y et al (2015) Early use of polymyxin B hemoperfusion in patients with septic shock due to peritonitis: a multicenter randomized control trial. Intensive Care Med 41:975–984
19. Peng ZY, Carter MJ, Kellum JA (2008) Effects of hemoadsorption on cytokine removal and short-term survival in septic rats. Crit Care Med 36:1573–1577
20. Joannes-Boyau O, Honore PM, Boer W, Collin V (2009) Are the synergistic effects of high-volume haemofiltration and enhanced adsorption the missing key in sepsis modulation? Nephrol Dial Transplant 24:354–357
21. Ronco C, Brendolan A, Lonnemann G et al (2002) A pilot study of coupled plasma filtration with adsorption in septic shock. Crit Care Med 30:1250–1255

22. Mao HJ, Yu S, Yu XB et al (2009) Effects of coupled plasma filtration adsorption on immune function of patients with multiple organ dysfunction syndrome. Int J Artif Organs 32:31–38
23. Livigni S, Bertolini G, Rossi C et al (2014) Efficacy of coupled plasma filtration adsorption (CPFA) in patients with septic shock: A multicenter randomised controlled clinical trial. BMJ Open 4:e003536
24. Honore PM, Jacobs R, Joannes-Boyau O et al (2013) Newly designed CRRT membranes for sepsis and SIRS – a pragmatic approach for bedside intensivists summarizing the more recent advances: a systematic structured review. ASAIO J 59:99–106
25. Rimmelé T, Assadi A, Cattenoz M et al (2009) High-volume haemofiltration with a new haemofiltration membrane having enhanced adsorption properties in septic pigs. Nephrol Dial Transplant 24:421–427
26. Morgera S, Haase M, Kuss T et al (2006) Pilot study on the effects of high cutoff hemofiltration on the need for norepinephrine in septic patients with acute renal failure. Crit Care Med 34:2099–2104
27. Haase M, Bellomo R, Baldwin I et al (2007) Hemodialysis membrane with a high-molecular-weight cutoff and cytokine levels in sepsis complicated by acute renal failure: a phase 1 randomized trial. Am J Kidney Dis 50:296–304
28. Sprung CL, Annane D, Keh D et al (2008) Hydrocortisone therapy for patients with septic shock. N Engl J Med 358:111–124
29. Martí-Carvajal AJ, Solà I, Gluud C, Lathyris D, Cardona AF (2012) Human recombinant protein C for severe sepsis and septic shock in adult and paediatric patients. Cochrane Database Syst Rev 12:CD004388
30. Unsinger J, McGlynn M, Kasten KR et al (2010) IL-7 promotes T cell viability, trafficking, and functionality and improves survival in sepsis. J Immunol 184:3768–3779
31. Venet F, Foray A-P, Villars-Méchin A et al (2012) IL-7 restores lymphocyte functions in septic patients. J Immunol 189:5073–5081
32. Meisel C, Schefold JC, Pschowski R et al (2009) Granulocyte-macrophage colony-stimulating factor to reverse sepsis-associated immunosuppression: a double-blind, randomized, placebo-controlled multicenter trial. Am J Respir Crit Care Med 180:640–648
33. Leentjens J, Kox M, Koch RM et al (2012) Reversal of immunoparalysis in humans in vivo: a double-blind, placebo-controlled, randomized pilot study. Am J Respir Crit Care Med 186:838–845
34. Armstrong-James D, Teo IA, Shrivastava S et al (2010) Exogenous interferon-gamma immunotherapy for invasive fungal infections in kidney transplant patients. Am J Transplant 10:1796–1803
35. Delsing CE, Gresnigt MS, Leentjens J et al (2014) Interferon-gamma as adjunctive immunotherapy for invasive fungal infections: a case series. BMC Infect Dis 14:166
36. Chang KC, Burnham C-A, Compton SM et al (2013) Blockade of the negative co-stimulatory molecules PD-1 and CTLA-4 improves survival in primary and secondary fungal sepsis. Crit Care 17:R85
37. Brahmer JR, Tykodi SS, Chow LQM et al (2012) Safety and activity of anti-PD-L1 antibody in patients with advanced cancer. N Engl J Med 366:2455–2465
38. Alejandria MM, Lansang MAD, Dans LF, Mantaring JB (2013) Intravenous immunoglobulin for treating sepsis, severe sepsis and septic shock. Cochrane Database Syst Rev 9:CD001090
39. Dellinger RP, Levy MM, Rhodes A et al (2013) Surviving Sepsis Campaign: international guidelines for management of severe sepsis and septic shock, 2012. Intensive Care Med 39:165–228
40. Kaukonen K-M, Bailey M, Suzuki S, Pilcher D, Bellomo R (2014) Mortality related to severe sepsis and septic shock among critically ill patients in Australia and New Zealand, 2000–2012. JAMA 311:1308–1316
41. Stevenson EK, Rubenstein AR, Radin GT, Wiener RS, Walkey AJ (2014) Two decades of mortality trends among patients with severe sepsis: a comparative meta-analysis. Crit Care Med 42:625–631

42. Monneret G, Venet F (2015) Sepsis-induced immune alterations monitoring by flow cytometry as a promising tool for individualized therapy. Cytometry B Clin Cytom (in press)
43. Monteiro Sousa C, Boissel JP, Gueyffier F, Olivera-Botello G (2015) Comparative transcriptomic analysis between an artificially induced SIRS in healthy individuals and spontaneous sepsis. C R Biol 338:635–642

Norepinephrine in Septic Shock: Five Reasons to Initiate it Early

M. Jozwiak, X. Monnet, and J.-L. Teboul

Introduction

Septic shock is one of the main causes of admission and death in critically ill patients [1]. Septic shock is characterized by a combination of hypovolemia, peripheral vascular dysfunction resulting in hypotension and abnormalities in the local/regional distribution of blood flow, cardiac failure and cell dysfunction. Importantly, the hemodynamic profile differs from patient to patient. In some septic patients, hypovolemia is predominant. In others, a marked decrease in vascular tone or myocardial depression is in the forefront of the hemodynamic failure. A variety of combinations can thus exist. In addition to macrocirculatory disorders, microcirculatory abnormalities contribute to tissue hypoxia through altered oxygen extraction. Whatever the macro- and microcirculatory disturbances, the prognosis of septic shock is tightly linked to how soon antibiotic therapy and hemodynamic management are initiated, including administration of fluid and of vasopressors to target a mean arterial pressure (MAP) > 65 mmHg [1]. Currently, the early use of vasopressors is one of the emerging concepts in the hemodynamic management of septic shock that may change our practice. In this chapter, we will set out five reasons to support early initiation of vasopressors, and namely, of norepinephrine (Box 1).

M. Jozwiak · X. Monnet
Service de réanimation médicale, Hôpital de Bicêtre, Université Paris-Sud; Faculté de Médecine, Université Paris-Saclay
Le Kremlin-Bicêtre, France
Inserm UMR_S 999, Hôpital Marie Lannelongue
Le Plessis-Robinson, France

J.-L. Teboul (✉)
Service de réanimation médicale, Hôpitaux universitaires Paris-Sud, Hôpital de Bicêtre
Le Kremlin-Bicêtre, France
Inserm UMR_S 999, Hôpital Marie Lannelongue
Le Plessis-Robinson, France
email: jean-louis.teboul@aphp.fr

© Springer International Publishing Switzerland 2016
J.-L. Vincent (ed.), *Annual Update in Intensive Care and Emergency Medicine 2016*,
DOI 10.1007/978-3-319-27349-5_6

Box 1. Five Reasons to Initiate Vasopressors Early in Septic Shock

1. The duration and the degree of hypotension are associated with increased mortality.
2. Delayed initiation of vasopressors is associated with increased mortality.
3. Early administration of norepinephrine also increases cardiac output by increasing preload.
4. Early administration of norepinephrine in severely hypotensive patients improves the microcirculation.
5. Early administration of norepinephrine prevents harmful fluid overload.

Five Arguments to Support Early Initiation of Norepinephrine

1. The Duration and the Degree of Hypotension Are Associated with Increased Mortality

Varpula et al. retrospectively assessed the impact of hemodynamic variables in the first six hours and in the first 48 hours of management of septic shock patients on 30-day mortality [2]. The hemodynamic management included fluid resuscitation, norepinephrine as first-line vasopressor and dobutamine as first-line inotropic agent, in order to target a MAP > 65 mmHg and a mixed venous oxygen saturation $(SvO_2) > 65\%$ [2]. The area of MAP under the threshold of 65 mmHg during the first 48 h was the best predictor of 30-day mortality [2]. This result was one of the major arguments on which the recommendations of the Surviving Sepsis Campaign in terms of initial MAP target were based [1]. Thereafter, in another retrospective study, Dünser et al. confirmed the association between the time spent below a certain level of MAP in the first 24 h of management of septic shock and 28-day mortality [3]. In this study, a level of MAP of 60 mmHg, and not 65 mmHg as in the study by Varpula et al. [2], was found to be the best threshold to discriminate survivors and non-survivors at day-28.

In a prospective observational study including 65 patients in septic shock, Benchekroune et al. reported that the diastolic arterial pressure was an independent prognostic factor of in-hospital mortality [4]. They also showed that the mortality decreased when a diastolic arterial pressure (DAP) > 50 mmHg was restored with norepinephrine within the first 48 h after the onset of septic shock [4]. This finding makes sense, because the DAP is mainly related to the arterial tone so that a low DAP reflects global vasoplegia. Taken together, these results [2–4] indicate that arterial blood pressure should not be allowed to decrease too low or for too long. These findings support early use of norepinephrine in severe hypotension, especially when the DAP is low, as is recommended by the Surviving Sepsis Campaign [1].

2. Delayed Initiation of Vasopressors is Associated with Increased Mortality

The Surviving Sepsis Campaign recommends that an MAP > 65 mmHg should be achieved by using fluids and norepinephrine in the first six hours of septic shock resuscitation [1]. The timing of norepinephrine administration within these six hours is crucial. On the one hand, delayed initiation of vasopressors could lead to prolonged hypotension in the context of severely depressed vascular tone, because fluid infusion alone cannot restore vascular tone. As previously mentioned, prolonged hypotension is associated with increased mortality in patients with septic shock [2–4]. On the other hand, it has been suggested that initiating vasopressors before adequate fluid resuscitation may lead to microcirculatory disturbances and further peripheral ischemia [5]. In a retrospective study, Bai et al. assessed the relationship between the delay in norepinephrine administration and the hospital mortality [6]. In that study, the timing of norepinephrine administration was left to the discretion of the attending physician: when hypotension was considered as refractory to fluid resuscitation, norepinephrine was started. Almost 20% of patients received norepinephrine in the first hour of resuscitation. At day-28, survivors had received norepinephrine significantly earlier and for a shorter period than non-survivors [6]. Patients in whom norepinephrine was administered within two hours after the onset of resuscitation received fewer fluids and the duration of hypotension was shorter. Moreover, there was a relationship between the delay in norepinephrine administration and mortality: for each hour delay in norepinephrine initiation (within the first six hours), the mortality rate increased by 5.3%. Finally, in a multivariate logistic regression analysis, the time from the onset of resuscitation to norepinephrine initiation was an independent determinant of 28-day mortality [6]. Although this study was retrospective and observational, the results argue that initiation of norepinephrine in septic shock should not be delayed. Another interesting finding is that administering norepinephrine earlier may result in an earlier withdrawal and/or a decrease in the total dose of this drug. It can be postulated that reversing hypotension early may prevent further hypotension-related macro/microcirculatory disorders such that a reduced vasopressor load would be necessary to maintain the targeted MAP. This effect could be considered as beneficial, because vasopressor load was suggested to be a factor associated with increased morbidity/mortality in a retrospective study analyzing data from the 1990s [7].

3. Early Administration of Norepinephrine also Increases Cardiac Output by Increasing Preload

In addition to increasing arterial blood pressure, norepinephrine may have some interesting hemodynamic effects when administered early. Indeed, norepinephrine can increase systemic venous return, resulting in an increase in right atrial pressure and cardiac preload [8, 9]. In 105 patients with septic shock who had already received volume expansion, norepinephrine was administered for life-threatening hypotension and then titrated to obtain an MAP > 65 mmHg [8]. All patients were monitored with transpulmonary thermodilution. Norepinephrine significantly increased MAP, cardiac index and the global end-diastolic volume (GEDV), which is considered as a static marker of preload [8]. In patients fully adapted to their ventilator, pulse pressure variation was calculated and shown to decrease with norepinephrine, suggesting a decrease in preload dependence. This result was in line with a previous study showing a decrease in pulse pressure variation after norepinephrine administration in an experimental model of hemorrhagic shock in dogs [10]. In another clinical study in 25 patients with septic shock, the effects of early administration of norepinephrine on preload-dependence were assessed using a passive leg raising (PLR) test [9]. Patients were included if they still had preload-dependence at a first PLR test in spite of early fluid resuscitation and if they remained hypotensive (MAP < 65 mmHg) with a DAP < 40 mmHg, [9]. In this study, norepinephrine induced an increase in cardiac preload, as demonstrated by the increase in central venous pressure (CVP), left ventricular end-diastolic area and GEDV [9]. Simultaneously, cardiac output increased in all patients. Interestingly, the PLR performed with norepinephrine increased cardiac output to a lesser extent than the earlier PLR, suggesting that norepinephrine decreased the degree of preload-dependence [9]. The norepinephrine-induced effects on cardiac preload and cardiac output in preload-dependent patients are quite similar to the effects of fluid infusion. An increase in cardiac output induced by norepinephrine was also reported in recent clinical studies in which norepinephrine was initiated early [11–13]. It is important to highlight that in older studies no effect of norepinephrine on cardiac output was found [14–16]. These discrepancies could be explained by the fact that these earlier studies were conducted before the publication of the Surviving Sepsis Campaign guidelines and that at that time patients received norepinephrine only when large amounts of fluid had been infused and no preload-dependence was supposed to persist. In this regard, high values of cardiac output were reported before initiation of norepinephrine [14–16].

Recent studies have addressed the mechanisms of an increase in venous return and cardiac preload with norepinephrine [17, 18]. According to Guyton's theory, venous return depends on the mean systemic pressure, which is the upstream pressure of venous return, and on the resistance to venous return. Persichini et al. studied the effect of norepinephrine on venous return in 16 mechanically ventilated patients with septic shock, in whom the dose of norepinephrine was decreased because their hemodynamic status improved [17]. The mean systemic pressure and the resistance to the venous return were estimated by plotting the relationship between the CVP and cardiac output, measured at two different levels of positive end-expiratory pressure (PEEP), before and during end-inspiratory and end-expiratory ventilator occlusions. Such abrupt changes in intrathoracic pressure were performed with the aim of abruptly changing CVP and cardiac output. Assuming a linear relationship between the CVP and the cardiac output, the mean systemic pressure was estimated as the pressure corresponding to the x-intercept of the linear regression. The resistance to the venous return was estimated from the inverse of the slope of the regression line. The decrease in norepinephrine induced a decrease in cardiac output, a decrease in cardiac preload as assessed by a decrease in GEDV and in CVP [17]. Moreover, the decrease in norepinephrine induced a decrease in the estimated mean systemic pressure and a decrease in the resistance to the venous return to a lesser extent, resulting in a decrease in the venous return [17]. In other words, the lowest dose of norepinephrine was associated with the lowest mean systemic pressure and the lowest venous return. Finally, the increase in cardiac output induced by PLR performed after decreasing the dose of norepinephrine was larger than that observed at baseline, suggesting an increase in unstressed blood volume at the lowest dose of norepinephrine [17]. In agreement with these results, Maas et al. found in cardiac surgical patients that increasing the dose of norepinephrine increased the mean systemic pressure and the resistance to the venous return to a lesser extent, which resulted in an increase in venous return [18].

Taking these results together, one can conclude that norepinephrine increases the mean systemic pressure due to venous blood redistribution from unstressed to stressed volume. This increases cardiac preload and hence cardiac output in patients with preload-dependence. This hemodynamic effect is of importance in patients with septic shock, since unstressed volume is abnormally increased during sepsis and can be further overfilled by fluid administration.

4. Early Administration of Norepinephrine in Severely Hypotensive Patients Improves the Microcirculation

Septic shock is characterized by microcirculatory disturbances even in patients with preserved or corrected macrocirculatory variables [19, 20]. These disturbances are more severe in non-survivors [19] and are independent prognostic factors of mortality [20]. Several authors have studied the effects of norepinephrine on the microcirculation in patients with shock in whom hypotension was already corrected by fluid and norepinephrine. Increasing the dose of norepinephrine further in order to increase MAP from 65 mmHg to 75, 85 or 90 mmHg was never shown to worsen sublingual microvascular flow assessed with sidestream darkfield (SDF) imaging [12, 13, 21]. Some studies even found better microcirculatory variables at 85 or 90 mmHg than at 65 mmHg [13], especially when the microcirculation was severely impaired at baseline (MAP at 65 mmHg).

Data concerning the effects of norepinephrine administered at an earlier phase of human septic shock when hypotension is profound are scarcer, because the studies are more difficult to perform. Georger et al. assessed the microcirculatory effects of early administration of norepinephrine in patients with septic shock and severe hypotension despite initial fluid resuscitation [22]. All the patients had low DAP, suggesting a depressed vascular tone. Microcirculation was assessed at the level of the thenar eminence muscles using a near-infrared spectroscopy (NIRS) device. Restoration of a MAP > 65 mmHg with norepinephrine resulted in a significant increase in tissue oxygen saturation (StO_2). Vascular occlusion tests were performed before and after introducing norepinephrine (or increasing its dose) to test the local hyperemic response to transient ischemia of the occluded vascular bed. Norepinephrine administration resulted in a significant increase in the StO_2 recovery slope [22], which reflects the capacity of microvessels to dilate and/or to be recruited in response to the local ischemic stimulus, and represents an important prognostic factor in patients with septic shock [23]. In other words, early correction of hypotension with norepinephrine resulted in improved muscle tissue oxygenation and microcirculatory reserve capacities. It is noteworthy that the associated increase in cardiac output (cardiac preload effect) may have contributed to the observed positive effects of early norepinephrine initiation on the microcirculation. Additionally, it could be postulated that increasing MAP in severely hypotensive patients also increased the perfusion pressure and thus improved microvascular blood flow in pressure-dependent vascular beds. In this regard, sublingual microvascular perfusion indices and MAP were shown to be correlated in the first six hours of management of septic shock [24]. Thus, early administration of norepinephrine could be of interest in patients with septic shock in order to correct MAP and microcirculatory disorders.

5. Early Administration of Norepinephrine Prevents Harmful Fluid Overload

It is now well established that a positive fluid balance [25–27] is an independent risk factor for mortality in patients with septic shock: the higher the positive fluid balance, the poorer the prognosis. In this regard, an experimental study in a murine model of endotoxic shock showed that the early use of norepinephrine associated with volume expansion resulted in a decrease in the amount of fluid infused [28]. These results were confirmed in patients with septic shock, in the retrospective study by Bai et al. [6]. Patients in whom norepinephrine was administered within the first two hours of resuscitation received less fluid than patients with delayed norepinephrine administration.

Conclusion

As recommended by the Surviving Sepsis Campaign guidelines, in septic shock patients, norepinephrine should be started early in the face of life-threatening hypotension, even when hypovolemia has not been yet resolved [1]. At least five arguments, described in this article, support this recommendation, although no randomized clinical trial comparing early *versus* delayed administration has been conducted. A low DAP, as a marker of depressed vascular tone, is an easy way to identify which patients are eligible for early initiation of this vasopressor.

References

1. Dellinger RP, Levy MM, Rhodes A et al (2013) Surviving Sepsis Campaign: international guidelines for management of severe sepsis and septic shock, 2012. Intensive Care Med 39:165–228
2. Varpula M, Tallgren M, Saukkonen K, Voipio-Pulkki LM, Pettila V (2005) Hemodynamic variables related to outcome in septic shock. Intensive Care Med 31:1066–1071
3. Dunser MW, Takala J, Ulmer H et al (2009) Arterial blood pressure during early sepsis and outcome. Intensive Care Med 35:1225–1233
4. Benchekroune S, Karpati PC, Berton C et al (2008) Diastolic arterial blood pressure: a reliable early predictor of survival in human septic shock. J Trauma 64:1188–1195
5. LeDoux D, Astiz ME, Carpati CM, Rackow EC (2000) Effects of perfusion pressure on tissue perfusion in septic shock. Crit Care Med 28:2729–2732
6. Bai X, Yu W, Ji W et al (2014) Early versus delayed administration of norepinephrine in patients with septic shock. Crit Care 18:532
7. Dunser MW, Ruokonen E, Pettila V et al (2009) Association of arterial blood pressure and vasopressor load with septic shock mortality: a post hoc analysis of a multicenter trial. Crit Care 13:R181
8. Hamzaoui O, Georger JF, Monnet X et al (2010) Early administration of norepinephrine increases cardiac preload and cardiac output in septic patients with life-threatening hypotension. Crit Care 14:R142
9. Monnet X, Jabot J, Maizel J, Richard C, Teboul JL (2011) Norepinephrine increases cardiac preload and reduces preload dependency assessed by passive leg raising in septic shock patients. Crit Care Med 39:689–694
10. Nouira S, Elatrous S, Dimassi S et al (2005) Effects of norepinephrine on static and dynamic preload indicators in experimental hemorrhagic shock. Crit Care Med 33:2339–2343
11. Deruddre S, Cheisson G, Mazoit JX, Vicaut E, Benhamou D, Duranteau J (2007) Renal arterial resistance in septic shock: effects of increasing mean arterial pressure with norepinephrine on the renal resistive index assessed with Doppler ultrasonography. Intensive Care Med 33:1557–1562
12. Dubin A, Pozo MO, Casabella CA et al (2009) Increasing arterial blood pressure with norepinephrine does not improve microcirculatory blood flow: a prospective study. Crit Care 13:R92
13. Thooft A, Favory R, Salgado DR et al (2011) Effects of changes in arterial pressure on organ perfusion during septic shock. Crit Care 15:R222
14. Desjars P, Pinaud M, Potel G, Tasseau F, Touze MD (1987) A reappraisal of norepinephrine therapy in human septic shock. Crit Care Med 15:134–137
15. Martin C, Papazian L, Perrin G, Saux P, Gouin F (1993) Norepinephrine or dopamine for the treatment of hyperdynamic septic shock? Chest 103:1826–1831
16. Martin C, Viviand X, Arnaud S, Vialet R, Rougnon T (1999) Effects of norepinephrine plus dobutamine or norepinephrine alone on left ventricular performance of septic shock patients. Crit Care Med 27:1708–1713
17. Persichini R, Silva S, Teboul JL et al (2012) Effects of norepinephrine on mean systemic pressure and venous return in human septic shock. Crit Care Med 40:3146–3153
18. Maas JJ, Pinsky MR, de Wilde RB, de Jonge E, Jansen JR (2013) Cardiac output response to norepinephrine in postoperative cardiac surgery patients: interpretation with venous return and cardiac function curves. Crit Care Med 41:143–150
19. De Backer D, Creteur J, Preiser JC, Dubois MJ, Vincent JL (2002) Microvascular blood flow is altered in patients with sepsis. Am J Respir Crit Care Med 166:98–104
20. De Backer D, Donadello K, Sakr Y et al (2013) Microcirculatory alterations in patients with severe sepsis: impact of time of assessment and relationship with outcome. Crit Care Med 41:791–799

21. Jhanji S, Stirling S, Patel N, Hinds CJ, Pearse RM (2009) The effect of increasing doses of norepinephrine on tissue oxygenation and microvascular flow in patients with septic shock. Crit Care Med 37:1961–1966
22. Georger JF, Hamzaoui O, Chaari A, Maizel J, Richard C, Teboul JL (2010) Restoring arterial pressure with norepinephrine improves muscle tissue oxygenation assessed by near-infrared spectroscopy in severely hypotensive septic patients. Intensive Care Med 36:1882–1889
23. Creteur J, Carollo T, Soldati G, Buchele G, De Backer D, Vincent JL (2007) The prognostic value of muscle StO2 in septic patients. Intensive Care Med 33:1549–1556
24. Trzeciak S, Dellinger RP, Parrillo JE et al (2007) Early microcirculatory perfusion derangements in patients with severe sepsis and septic shock: relationship to hemodynamics, oxygen transport, and survival. Ann Emerg Med 49:88–98 (98 e81–82)
25. Vincent JL, Sakr Y, Sprung CL et al (2006) Sepsis in European intensive care units: results of the SOAP study. Crit Care Med 34:344–353
26. Boyd JH, Forbes J, Nakada TA, Walley KR, Russell JA (2011) Fluid resuscitation in septic shock: a positive fluid balance and elevated central venous pressure are associated with increased mortality. Crit Care Med 39:259–265
27. Acheampong A, Vincent JL (2015) A positive fluid balance is an independent prognostic factor in patients with sepsis. Crit Care 19:251
28. Sennoun N, Montemont C, Gibot S, Lacolley P, Levy B (2007) Comparative effects of early versus delayed use of norepinephrine in resuscitated endotoxic shock. Crit Care Med 35:1736–1740

Myths and Facts Regarding Lactate in Sepsis

M. Nalos, A. S. McLean, and B. Tang

Introduction

Lactate has a questionable reputation amongst professionals caring for patients with sepsis. The concern is partly justified, as lactate is indeed a sentinel marker of shock and poor prognosis in sepsis [1]. Traditionally, elevated serum lactate is synonymous of tissue hypoxia, in particular when associated with metabolic acidosis and frequently clinicians guide fluid resuscitation or inotrope/vasopressor use based on that premise [2]. The concept is based on the distinction between two types of glycolysis: aerobic and anaerobic (insufficient oxygen availability for mitochondrial ATP production), the latter being regarded as the main source of increased lactate [2, 3]. In this chapter, we argue that such a view of pathophysiology in sepsis is more a "habit of mind" then a real phenomenon and has limited clinical relevance [4]. We will argue that lactate is a crucial molecule in energy metabolism, acid base homeostasis and cellular signaling in sepsis largely independent of tissue oxygenation.

M. Nalos (✉) · A. S. McLean
Department of Intensive Care Medicine, Nepean Hospital
Penrith, Australia
Department of Intensive Care Medicine, University of Sydney, Nepean Clinical School
Penrith, Australia
email: mareknalos@gmail.com

B. Tang
Department of Intensive Care Medicine, University of Sydney, Nepean Clinical School
Penrith, Australia
Centre for Immunology and Allergy Research, Westmead Millennium Institute
Sydney, Australia

© Springer International Publishing Switzerland 2016
J.-L. Vincent (ed.), *Annual Update in Intensive Care and Emergency Medicine 2016*,
DOI 10.1007/978-3-319-27349-5_7

The Physiology of Lactate

Lactate, a natural molecule produced in relatively large quantities (~ 20 mmol/kg/day), is a conjugate base of lactic acid, first isolated from sour milk and later discovered to be produced in muscles during exertion. At physiological pH, lactic acid is almost fully dissociated and is constantly produced during glycolysis from pyruvate under aerobic conditions. The cytosolic lactate dehydrogenase (LDH)-catalyzed reaction runs in both directions depending on the isoform present and the respective concentrations of its substrates, pyruvate and lactate (Eq. 1; [5]).

$$\text{Pyruvate} + \text{NADH} + \text{H}^+ \rightarrow \text{Lactate} + \text{NAD}^+ \tag{1}$$

Pyruvate is formed from glucose as well as from alanine, α-ketoglutarate and partial oxidation of glutamine [6]. Importantly, the cytosolic lactate production by LDH regenerates nicotinamide adenine dinucleotide (NAD^+) required for the glyceraldehyde 3-phosphate dehydrogenase (GADPH) reaction of glycolysis. The only other significant NAD^+ regeneration occurs in the mitochondrial respiratory chain [7].

Depending on the tissue concerned, lactate is shuttled either out of the cells ('glycolytic' cells) mainly by the monocarboxylate transporter-4 (MCT-4) or into the intramembranous mitochondrial space via MCT-1 in 'oxidative cells' [8, 9]. In the mitochondria, lactate is converted back to pyruvate by mitochondrial LDH forming NADH in the mitochondrial inter-membranous space. This pathway, admittedly still controversial, provides direct transport of lactate into the mitochondria for oxidation and ATP production [9, 10].

Lactate and Acidosis

Lactate is also regarded as the cause of metabolic acidosis in sepsis. This view, based on the correlation of acidosis with lactate levels, however, lacks direct causative evidence [5, 7]. Robergs et al. [5] argued that lactic acid, as a cause of acidosis in exercise physiology, is a myth, highlighting that the majority of the acidifying protons come from ATP hydrolysis and the GAPDH reaction of glycolysis, the main source of glycolytic proton release (Eqs. 2 and 3).

$$\text{ATP}^{-4} + \text{H}_2\text{O} \rightarrow \text{ADP}^{-3} + \text{HPO}_4^{-2} + \text{H}^+ \tag{2}$$

$$\begin{aligned} \text{C}_6\text{H}_{12}\text{O}_6 + 2\text{NAD}^+ + 2\text{ADP}^{-3} + 2\text{HPO}_4^{-2} \\ \rightarrow 2\text{CH}_3\text{COCOO}^- + 2\text{H}^+ + 2\text{NADH} + 2\text{ATP}^{-4} + 2\text{H}_2\text{O} \end{aligned} \tag{3}$$

Lactate in fact could not be the source of acidosis because the reduction of pyruvate to lactate actually absorbs a proton (Eq. 1). Indeed, the pKa of lactic acid is higher (pKa 3.86) than that of pyruvic acid (pKa 2.50). Robergs et al. [5] also pointed out that lactate production is not associated with a stoichiometrically equivalent net production of protons. Although glycolysis releases two protons, when seen in isolation the protons are absorbed in the mitochondrial generation of ATP and released during subsequent hydrolysis of ATP. When the rate of ATP hydrolysis exceeds the mitochondrial ATP synthesis, protons accumulate causing metabolic acidosis. Furthermore, the high ADP/ATP ratio activates glycolysis thus increasing cytosolic ATP and lactate production. Under such conditions, lactate formation via LDH is essential for recovery of NAD^+ and the absorption of protons, functioning as a temporal and spatial buffer between glycolytic and oxidative metabolism [11, 12]. Without lactate, the glycolytic process would halt and intracellular pH compatible with cellular function would not be maintained [7].

Therefore, instead of causing acidosis, lactate delays its onset: first, when lactate is formed from pyruvate; second by being shuttled into mitochondria; and third when lactate is transported across the cellular membrane in a 1:1 stoichiometric relationship with proton via MCTs, the role of which has been extensively reviewed [8]. The irony for the reputation of lactate is, however, that while the transport via MCTs delays intracellular accumulation of protons it does contribute to extracellular acidosis and hyperlactatemia [13, 14]. Under normal conditions, however, the acidosis is only transient as lactate is taken up by oxidative or gluconeogenic cells in local or distant tissues [13]. An important consideration in shock is that the transport capacity of MCTs is not infinite and that impaired tissue perfusion limits the functionality of the intra- and inter-organ lactate shuttle. For example, during exhaustive exercise, the rapidly rising intracellular lactate slows down the activity of LDH by a mass effect with consequent cellular acidosis. More lactate accumulation means lower rates of lactate production via LDH, leading to lower rates of pyruvate production, and so on, such that flux through the entire glycolytic pathway is inhibited. Reduced cytosolic NAD^+ availability limits cytosolic ATP formation and leads to energetic failure [7]. From the above, it is clear that lactate formation, oxidation, export out of cells and further transport to distant organs play a pivotal role in cellular metabolism, acid-base and energy balance.

Lactate and Sepsis

Blood lactate concentration increases when the rate of lactate production exceeds the rate of lactate utilization. Increased lactate production in sepsis is due to enhanced cellular glycolysis usually in the presence of reduced mitochondrial oxidative capacity. Adrenergic stress response, inflammation and the proliferation needs of injured tissues are the main drivers of glycolysis [15–17]. On the other hand, tissue oxygen levels in sepsis are mostly sufficient for mitochondrial ATP production and are not related to lactate production [18, 19]. Reduction in the number, altered structure, function and content of mitochondria, rather than hypoxia, are responsible for diminished mitochondrial ATP production [18].

Adrenergic State: Rapid Increase in Cellular ATP Needs

Mitochondrial ATP production is an efficient process of extracting energy from metabolic substrates but the process is relatively slow and limited by the rate of NADH shuttling from the cytosol to the mitochondrial electron transport chain [20]. In comparison, the ubiquitous glycolysis is capable of very fast ATP production albeit with less efficiency, similar to a turbo in a combustion engine. During exercise, glycolysis rapidly provides ATP for calcium sequestration and sodium extrusion from the skeletal muscle. The associated increase in lactate formation regenerates cytosolic NAD^+ thus maintaining cytosolic redox and sustaining high glycolytic rates. At the same time, lactate buffers the protons produced during increased ATP breakdown, enabling intra/interorgan redox potential exchange at times when mitochondrial ATP production in active muscle lags utilization of $NADH + H^+$ potential within the cell [7, 10, 12]. During exercise, the sympatho-adrenal system is responsible for the increased glycolytic rates by activating Na^+-K^+-ATPase via the β_2-receptor [21]. This lowers the ATP/ADP ratio in the cytosol leading to further activation of glycolysis. The same physiological mechanism is functional in sepsis as evidenced by similar or higher levels of epinephrine in the plasma of critically ill patients in comparison to athletes exercising at maximum intensity [21, 22]. β_2-receptor-mediated hyperlactatemia is in fact a well-documented phenomenon in sepsis [22, 23].

Inflammation

An important cause of raised glycolytic rates and lactate production in sepsis is the activation of inflammation. It is well known that starvation and glucose deprivation impair immune function by limiting leukocyte activation, proliferation, and cytokine production [17]. Activated leukocytes upregulate glycolysis and glutaminolysis to meet their high energy, anti-oxidant and proliferation needs [17, 24]. The provision of substrates and $NADPH(H^+)$ for biosynthetic processes and for regeneration of glutathione via the pentose-phosphate pathway is vital for an effective immune response [17, 25, 26]. When the rate of glycolysis exceeds mitochondrial capacity to regenerate NAD^+, lactate is increasingly produced and exported from activated leukocytes [17, 24]. Haji-Michael et al. clearly showed increased lactate production due to leukocyte activation in sepsis and demonstrated that upon stimulation with lipopolysaccharide (LPS) almost half of blood lactate is attributed to an enhanced glycolytic rate in leukocytes [16]. The situation is even more dramatic in the liver where Kupffer cells and infiltrating leukocytes account for more than half of hepatic glucose utilization [27]. A novel mechanistic insight for those observations can be derived from gene expression studies. In a comprehensive metabolic map of LPS-activated murine macrophages, Tannahill et al. demonstrated upregulation of glycolytic and downregulation of mitochondrial genes, which correlated directly with the expression profiles of altered metabolites [28]. We measured the transcriptome profiles of canonical metabolic pathways in leukocytes obtained from

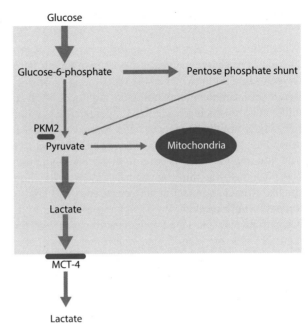

Fig. 1 Schematic illustration of metabolic reprogramming in activated leukocytes. MCT: monocarboxylate transporter; PKM2: isoform of pyruvate kinase

the arterial circulation in normoxic septic intensive care unit (ICU) patients. Similarly, we observed a significant increase in the expression of mRNA coding for key enzymes of glycolysis and the pentose-phosphate pathway, whereas the gene expression of enzymes in the mitochondrial tricarboxylic acid (TCA) cycle was significantly reduced, confirming a shift towards cytosolic glycolysis and the pentose-phosphate pathway despite a normal oxygen milieu (Fig. 1) We documented increased gene expression of MCT-4 and strikingly, pyruvate kinase isoform (PKM2) that is not present in normal tissues or quiescent leukocytes but is common in embryonic tissues and in tumors (unpublished data). In murine macrophages, Yang et al. documented that PKM2 interacts with hypoxia-inducible factor-1α (HIF-1α) to allow transcription of enzymes necessary for glycolysis. Knockdown of PKM2, HIF-1α and glycolysis-related genes decreased macrophage lactate production [29]. Interestingly, in a mouse model, Cheng et al. documented that the preference for glycolysis in monocytes is necessary for trained immunity against bacterial sepsis [30]. Michalek et al. reported that T effector lymphocytes, as opposed to T regulatory cells, in particular rely on enhanced glycolytic rates for their proliferation and function [24]. The increased lactate production by glycolytic T cells may also serve as a natural feedback mechanism for metabolic inhibition of leukocyte activation [31]. High lactate levels associated with adrenergic response to sepsis may thus contribute to the suppression of lymphocyte functions and participate in the impairment of adaptive immune responses by inhibiting cellular lactate transport and glycolysis [32, 33]. The recent discovery of the G-protein-coupled lactate receptor, GPR81, on a variety of blood cells could represent an alternative mechanism [34].

Cancer

Many cancer cells display increased rates of glycolysis and lactate production, the so-called 'Warburg' metabolic phenotype. Even in the presence of an adequate oxygen supply, tumors metabolize the majority of glucose through glycolysis into lactate [35]. Similar to inflammation, high rates of glycolysis are required to support tumor cell growth and NADPH(H$^+$) generation via the pentose-phosphate pathway [26, 35]. Specifically, cancer cells express pyruvate kinase isoform, PKM2, and upregulate pyruvate dehydrogenase (PDH) kinase 1 (PDK1), both limiting pyruvate flux into the TCA in order to divert glycolytic intermediates into the pentose-phosphate pathway. Several other factors cause the high glycolytic rates, including genetic alterations affecting key oncogenes and HIF-1α over-expression by many tumors. The increased rate of lactate production by the tumor may contribute to high lactate levels in septic patients with cancer [32, 35].

Hypoxia

Traditionally, exercise-induced hyperlactatemia is thought to be the result of tissue hypoxia when 'anaerobic' glycolysis leads to lactate release causing muscle fatigue. Nevertheless, when the effects of hypoxia were studied across a range of incremental exercise, the net blood lactate efflux was unrelated to intramuscular PO$_2$ but linearly related to epinephrine concentration, O$_2$ consumption and intracellular pH [36]. While this study also demonstrated that lactate release was higher during hypoxia, intramuscular PO$_2$ was not the main driver of glycolysis [36]. Rather, the systemic sympatho-adrenal activation of glycolysis was the causative factor and the glycolysis-driven increase in cellular redox potential supported oxidative phosphorylation and mitochondrial ATP formation. As more ATP is utilized than produced, proton concentration increases, as does the essential export of lactate via MCTs to buffer intracellular acidosis [7].

Although elevated lactate levels in sepsis may be associated with systemic or tissue ischemia, the assumption that elevated lactate is a result of 'anaerobic' glycolysis is inaccurate and treatment decisions should not be based on this paradigm [22]. While lactate levels reflect the balance between tissue glycolytic rates and mitochondrial ATP synthesis, reduction in mitochondrial metabolism due to absence of molecular oxygen is not a common mechanism of mitochondrial dysfunction in sepsis [18, 19]. It is rather the increased production of reactive oxygen species (ROS) by mitochondria sensing a low oxygen tension that triggers stabilization of HIF-1α, followed by enhanced expression of genes that either increase O$_2$ delivery – represented by erythropoietin and vascular endothelial growth factor (VEGF) – or decrease O$_2$ consumption – including glycolytic enzyme genes and glucose transporters [37–39]. Several of the products of glycolytic metabolism, including lactate, are in turn able to further stabilize HIF-1α leading to inhibition of the PDH complex, reduced flux through TCA, reduced oxygen consumption and reduced ROS formation by mitochondria, thus protecting cells from mitochondrial ROS toxicity and apoptosis. HIF-1α also suppresses mitochondrial biogenesis and activates protective autophagy of mitochondria thus reducing their numbers [40]. Activation of an HIF-1α-triggered cascade of events could be one of the drivers of cellular "hibernation"; a concept described by Carré and Singer [18]. For example, cells with a deleted HIF-1α gene exposed to hypoxia die as a consequence of ROS toxicity and there is extensive muscle damage in HIF-1α knockout mice subjected to repeated exercise [41]. Whereas the HIF-1α mediated response to low oxygen is an important adaptive cellular process, sufficient mechanisms must ensure proton and lactate transport out of cells during reduced mitochondrial flux. Indeed, MCT4 expression is also enhanced by hypoxia, consistent with its role in exporting protons and lactate produced by glycolysis. Under conditions of ischemia-reperfusion even MCT1, which under most conditions imports lactate, plays an important role in the restoration of intracellular pH by facilitating lactate efflux and MCT1 inhibition slows the return of the pH to normoxic values [8].

Whether HIF-1α stabilization plays an important role in sepsis and shock is, however, not clear. In an animal study, Regueira et al. measured tissue oxygenation during septic hyperlactatemia and found that systemic and hepatic oxygen consumption were well maintained, respiration of skeletal muscle and liver-isolated mitochondria were normal, and HIF-1α was not expressed in the skeletal and cardiac muscle, pancreas, lung, or kidney [42]. On the other hand, Ortega et al. found increased HIF-1α expression in the kidney of diabetic and normal mice after LPS injection [43]. Similarly, Bateman et al. reported upregulation of myocardial HIF-1α, VEGF, and glucose transporter, GLUT1, in rats after intraperitoneal LPS injection [44]. The variable results could be explained by a number of factors, such as the production of nitric oxide and other inhibitors of mitochondrial respiration that seem to prevent the stabilization of HIF-1α during hypoxia [45].

Lactate Disposal

In exercising individuals as well as in sepsis, lactate serves both as a signaling molecule and an important metabolic substrate transferring redox potential from tissues with high glycolytic rates to tissues capable of oxidative phosphorylation. The relative contribution of direct and indirect lactate oxidation to total energy expenditure is unknown in sepsis. During exercise, 75 to 80% of available lactate is oxidized as compared to approximately 50% during rest [46]. Similarly, in patients with traumatic brain injury, lactate is directly oxidized or serves as an important gluconeogenic precursor oxidized indirectly as recently demonstrated by Glenn et al. [47]. Interestingly, data on total body lactate utilization in sepsis are variable and perhaps patient specific. Investigators have found enhanced, unchanged or reduced, lactate metabolism compared to healthy individuals [48]. It is clear, however, that severe hepatic and renal dysfunction affect non-oxidative lactate utilization, unmasking elevated lactate production.

Lactate-based Resuscitation in Sepsis

Although small amounts of lactate are routinely infused in sepsis in the form of Ringer's lactate solution, few studies to date have explored the effects of predominantly lactate-based fluids in sepsis resuscitation. The use of lactate as a sodium accompanying anion in a fluid solution is an interesting alternative to chloride avoiding the undesired effects of a non-metabolizable anion. Using hypertonic sodium lactate in a porcine model of endotoxic shock, Duburcq et al. were able to achieve plasma volume expansion with improvement in hemodynamic status and microvascular reactivity while maintaining a negative fluid balance and preserving urine output [49]. Using half-molar sodium lactate solution, Somasetia et al. documented similar effects in children resuscitated from Dengue shock. The lactate-based resuscitation regime led to a neutral fluid balance, hemodynamic stability, reduced coagulopathy and endothelial inflammation accompanied by less interstitial fluid accumulation [50].

Conclusion

Although measuring lactate provides clinicians with a sentinel marker of physiological disturbance in sepsis, in particular when associated with metabolic acidosis it should not be used as a marker of tissue hypoxia and treatment decisions, such as fluid resuscitation or vasopressor/inotrope use, should not be based on this paradigm. The reasons for increased lactate production in sepsis are adrenergic and inflammatory responses rather than tissue hypoxia, an assertion strengthened by recent studies using gene expression profiling of metabolic pathways in various tissues.

References

1. Bakker J, Coffernils M, Leon M, Gris P, Vincent JL (1991) Blood lactate levels are superior to oxygen-derived variables in predicting outcome in human septic shock. Chest 99:956–962
2. Jones AE, Shapiro NI, Trzeciak S et al (2010) Lactate clearance vs central venous oxygen saturation as goals of early sepsis therapy: a randomized clinical trial. JAMA 303:739–746
3. Andersen LW, Mackenhauer J, Roberts JC, Berg KM, Cocchi MN, Donnino MW (2013) Etiology and therapeutic approach to elevated lactate levels. Mayo Clin Proc 88:1127–1140
4. Schurr A (2014) Cerebral glycolysis: a century of persistent misunderstanding and misconception. Front Neurosci 8:360
5. Robergs RA, Ghiasvand F, Parker D (2004) Biochemistry of exercise-induced metabolic acidosis. Am J Physiol Regul Integr Comp Physiol 287:R502–R516
6. Board M, Humm S, Newsholme EA (1990) Maximum activities of key enzymes of glycolysis, glutaminolysis, pentose phosphate pathway and tricarboxylic acid cycle in normal, neoplastic and suppressed cells. Biochem J 265:503–509
7. Robergs RA (2011) Nothing 'evil' and no 'conundrum' about muscle lactate production. Exp Physiol 96:1097–1098
8. Halestrap AP (2013) Monocarboxylic acid transport. Compr Physiol 3:1611–1643

9. Elustondo PA, White AE, Hughes ME, Brebner K, Pavlov E, Kane DA (2013) Physical and functional association of lactate dehydrogenase (LDH) with skeletal muscle mitochondria. J Biol Chem 288:25309–25317
10. Kane DA (2014) Lactate oxidation at the mitochondria: a lactate-malate-aspartate shuttle at work. Front Neurosci 8:366
11. Rogatzki MJ, Ferguson BS, Goodwin ML, Gladden LB (2015) Lactate is always the end product of glycolysis. Front Neurosci 9:22
12. Bergersen LH (2015) Lactate transport and signaling in the brain: potential therapeutic targets and roles in body-brain interaction. J Cereb Blood Flow Metab 35:176–185
13. Gladden LB (2008) A "lactatic" perspective on metabolism. Med Sci Sports Exerc 40:477–485
14. Fencl V, Jabor A, Kazda A, Figge J (2000) Diagnosis of metabolic acid base disturbances in critically ill patients. Am J Respir Crit Care Med 162:2246–2251
15. Levy B, Desebbe O, Montemont Ch, Gibot S (2008) Increased aerobic glycolysis through beta-2 stimulation is a common mechanism involved in lactate formation during shock states. Shock 4:417–421
16. Haji-Michael PG, Ladrière L, Sener A, Vincent JL, Malaisse WJ (1999) Leukocyte glycolysis and lactate output in animal sepsis and ex vivo human blood. Metabolism 48:779–785
17. Newsholme EA, Crabtree B, Ardawi MS (1985) The role of high rates of glycolysis and glutamine utilization in rapidly dividing cells. Biosci Rep 5:393–400
18. Carré JE, Singer M (2008) Cellular energetic metabolism in sepsis: the need for a systems approach. Biochim Biophys Acta 1777:763–771
19. Ronco JJ, Fenwick JC, Tweeddale MG et al (1993) Identification of the critical oxygen delivery for anaerobic metabolism in critically iii septic and nonseptic humans. JAMA 270:1724–1730
20. Bauer DE, Harris MH, Plas DR et al (2004) Cytokine stimulation of aerobic glycolysis in hematopoietic cells exceeds proliferative demand. FASEB 18:1303–1305
21. Febbraio MA, Lambert DL, Starkie RL, Proietto J, Hargreaves M (1998) Effect of epinephrine on muscle glycogenolysis during exercise in trained men. J Appl Physiol 84:465–470
22. James JH, Luchette FA, McCarter FD, Fischer JE (1999) Lactate is an unreliable indicator of tissue hypoxia in injury or sepsis. Lancet 354:505–508
23. Levy B, Desebbe O, Montemont C, Gibot S (2008) Increased aerobic glycolysis through beta-2 stimulation is a common mechanism involved in lactate formation during shock states. Shock 4:417–421
24. Michalek RD, Gerriets VA, Jacobs SR et al (2011) Cutting edge: distinct glycolytic and lipid oxidative metabolic programs are essential for effector and regulatory CD4+ T cell subsets. J Immunol 186:3299–3303
25. MacIver NJ, Jacobs SR, Wieman HL, Wofford JA, Coloff JL, Rathmell JC (2008) Glucose metabolism in lymphocytes is a regulated process with significant effects on immune cell function and survival. J Leukoc Biol 84:949–957
26. Chen X, Qian Y, Wu S (2015) The Warburg effect: Evolving interpretations of an established concept. Free Radic Biol Med 79C:253–263
27. Meszaros K, Bojta J, Bautista AR, Lang CH, Spitzer JJ (1991) Glucose utilisation by Kupffer cells, endothelial cells and granulocytes in endotoxemic rat liver. Am J Physiol 1260:G7–G12
28. Tannahill GM, Curtis AM, Adamik J et al (2013) Succinate is an inflammatory signal that induces IL-1β through HIF-1α. Nature 496:238–242
29. Yang L, Xie M, Yang M et al (2014) PKM2 regulates the Warburg effect and promotes HMGB1 release in sepsis. Nat Commun 5:4436
30. Cheng SC, Quintin J, Cramer RA et al (2014) mTOR- and HIF-1α-mediated aerobic glycolysis as metabolic basis for trained immunity. Science 345:1250684
31. Durrbach A, Francois H (2013) Intracellular lactate flux: a new regulator of the allogenic immune response. Transpl Int 26:20–21
32. Fischer K, Hoffmann P, Voelkl S et al (2007) Inhibitory effect of tumor cell-derived lactic acid on human T cells. Blood 109:3812–3819

33. Parnell GP, Tang BM, Nalos M et al (2013) Identifying key regulatory genes in the whole blood of septic patients to monitor underlying immune dysfunctions. Shock 40:166–174
34. Hoque R, Farooq A, Ghani A, Gorelick F, Mehal WZ (2014) Lactate reduces liver and pancreatic injury in Toll-like receptor- and inflammasome-mediated inflammation via GPR81-mediated suppression of innate immunity. Gastroenterology 146:1763–1774
35. Bui T, Thompson CB (2006) Cancer's sweet tooth. Cancer Cell 9:419–420
36. Richardson RS, Noyszewski EA, Leigh JS, Wagner (1998) Lactate efflux from exercising human skeletal muscle: role of intracellular PO2. J Appl Physiol 85:627–634
37. Mason S, Johnson RS (2007) The role of HIF-1 in hypoxic response in the skeletal muscle. Adv Exp Med Biol 618:229–244
38. Chandel NS, Maltepe E, Goldwasser E, Mathieu CE, Simon MC, Schumacker PT (1998) Mitochondrial reactive oxygen species trigger hypoxia-induced transcription. Proc Natl Acad Sci 95:11715–11720
39. Semenza GL (2002) HIF-1 and tumor progression: pathophysiology and therapeutics. Trends Mol Med 8:S62–S67
40. Zhang H, Bosch-Marce M, Shimoda LA et al (2008) Mitochondrial autophagy is a HIF-1-dependent adaptive metabolic response to hypoxia. J Biol Chem 283:10892–10903
41. Mason SD, Howlett RA, Kim MJ et al (2004) Loss of skeletal muscle HIF-1alpha results in altered exercise endurance. PLoS Biol 2:e288
42. Regueira T, Djafarzadeh S, Brandt S et al (2012) Oxygen transport and mitochondrial function in porcine septic shock, cardiogenic shock, and hypoxaemia. Acta Anaesthesiol Scand 56:846–859
43. Ortega A, Fernández A, Arenas MI et al (2013) Outcome of acute renal injury in diabetic mice with experimental endotoxemia: role of hypoxia-inducible factor-1 α. J Diabetes Res 2013:254529
44. Bateman RM, Tokunaga C, Kareco T, Dorscheid DR, Walley KR (2007) Myocardial hypoxia-inducible HIF-1alpha, VEGF, and GLUT1 gene expression is associated with microvascular and ICAM-1 heterogeneity during endotoxemia. Am J Physiol Heart Circ Physiol 293:H448–H456
45. Hagen T, Taylor CT, Lam F, Moncada S (2003) Redistribution of intracellular oxygen in hypoxia by nitric oxide: effect on HIF1alpha. Science 302:1975–1978
46. Emhoff CA, Messonnier LA, Horning MA, Fattor JA, Carlson TJ, Brooks GA (2013) Direct and indirect lactate oxidation in trained and untrained men. J Appl Physiol 115:829–838
47. Glenn TC, Martin NA, Horning MA et al (2015) Lactate: brain fuel in human traumatic brain injury: a comparison with normal healthy control subjects. J Neurotrauma 32:820–832
48. Garcia-Alvarez M, Marik P, Bellomo R (2014) Sepsis-associated hyperlactatemia. Crit Care 18:503
49. Duburcq T, Favory R, Mathieu D et al (2014) Hypertonic sodium lactate improves fluid balance and hemodynamics in porcine endotoxic shock. Crit Care 18:467
50. Somasetia DH, Setiati TE, Sjahrodji AM et al (2014) Early resuscitation of dengue shock syndrome in children with hyperosmolar sodium-lactate: a randomized single-blind clinical trial of efficacy and safety. Crit Care 18:466

Part III
Renal Issues

Creatinine-Based Definitions: From Baseline Creatinine to Serum Creatinine Adjustment in Intensive Care

S. De Rosa, S. Samoni, and C. Ronco

Introduction

There is still controversy in the literature regarding the diagnosis of acute kidney injury (AKI), despite the latest definition provided by the Kidney Disease – Improving Global Outcomes (KDIGO) working group created in 2012. Standardized definitions of AKI, using changes in serum creatinine (SCr) and urine output, have enabled a better evaluation of the epidemiology of intensive care unit (ICU)-acquired AKI, including long-term outcomes in patients who have experienced AKI [1]. Very few studies have considered the correlation of baseline renal function with increased creatinine concentrations during the episode of AKI [2]. Although the AKIN (Acute Kidney Injury Network), KDIGO and ERBP (European Renal Best Practice) groups have contributed to standardizing the diagnosis and staging of AKI, the lack of a joint approach to baseline serum creatinine (bSCr) concentration has influenced the creatinine-based AKI definitions. This concept is complicated by other factors, such as: (i) the absence of standardized laboratory methods for quantification of SCr; (ii) arbitrary cut-offs for SCr in the diagnosis of AKI, which compromises the validity of studies because of the different classifications used [3, 4]; (iii) the presence of pre-existing undiagnosed chronic kidney disease (CKD) in a large part of the population; (iv) unknown baseline status of renal function in patients affected by AKI. All these reasons participate to the inability to define a 'universal bSCr'. The absence of a shared approach has resulted in variability among centers, with different interpretations of the SCr value for the definition and classification of AKI. Moreover, in the ICU setting, fluid overload and muscle wasting can delay recognition of AKI by affecting the true value of the SCr. Recent studies have demonstrated the effect of fluid balance on SCr: a positive fluid balance can dilute SCr, decreasing the ability to identify the development of AKI

S. De Rosa (✉) · S. Samoni · C. Ronco
International Renal Research Institute, San Bortolo Hospital
Vicenza, Italy
email: derosa.silvia@ymail.com

© Springer International Publishing Switzerland 2016
J.-L. Vincent (ed.), *Annual Update in Intensive Care and Emergency Medicine 2016*,
DOI 10.1007/978-3-319-27349-5_8

[5–8]. In terms of muscle wasting, there are no data available regarding its effect on SCr and, moreover, ICU-acquired myopathy is rarely recognized because of insufficient diagnostic criteria or methodological limitations [9, 10]. Despite these limits, SCr is still considered the standard for assessing acute changes in renal function. The present review details the existing evidence related to the importance of bSCr in ICU patients, describing in particular the limits of the non-shared approach. We also attempt to highlight the effects of fluid balance and muscle wasting on SCr based on recent evidence.

Estimating Baseline Serum Creatinine

In 2004, recommendations drawn up by the Acute Dialysis Quality Initiative (ADQI) working group defined a value of estimated glomerular filtration rate (eGFR) [75–100 ml/min / 1.73 m^2], that was useful for defining the value of bSCr using the Modification of Diet in Renal Disease (MDRD) equation (back-estimation) in patients with unknown baseline renal function and in the absence of prior renal disease [11]. The back-estimation formula is:

$$\text{Serum creatinine} = (75/[186 \times (\text{age}^{-0.203}) \times (0.742 \text{ if female}) \times (1.21 \text{ if black})])^{-0.887}.$$

Unfortunately, in patients with suspected CKD, the back-estimation formula overestimates the incidence of AKI and should not be used [3]. This method, although used in several epidemiological studies, lacks scientific validation [12, 13]. Two other methods are used to determine the bSCr: the first SCr measured at admission; and the nadir (the lowest measured value) of SCr during the first three days of the ICU stay. RIFLE and KDIGO suggest using the back-estimation formula, whereas AKIN recommends using the first measurement of SCr [3, 14, 15]. ERBP and NICE (The National Institute for Health and Care Excellence) guidelines suggest using the admission SCr value because of the correlation of this value with patient outcomes, such as mortality and need for renal replacement therapy (RRT). In a large study, Broce et al. estimated the baseline renal function in patients with AKI using the nadir SCr measured in the first three days of hospitalization. Hospital-acquired AKI was defined according to the difference between the nadir and the subsequent peak SCr. Different thresholds of nadir-to-peak SCr were independently associated with increased in-hospital mortality. In addition, the time lag between the nadir SCr and the peak SCr was seven days [16]. Several authors have demonstrated an over-estimation of 50% using MDRD back-estimation in different patient populations [3]. In a cohort study, Siew et al. estimated bSCr in a population of almost 5000 hospitalized patients using the three different methods [15]. The MDRD equation and nadir SCr overestimated the incidence of AKI by at least 50% and the admission SCr underestimated it by 46% [4, 15]. The use of admission SCr had the lowest sensitivity for diagnosis of hospital-acquired AKI [3] and missed the diagnosis of community-acquired AKI. For this reason, admission SCr should be used with caution, especially in AKI stage 1 [16]. Moreover, in addition to these three estimation methods, some authors have also considered the pre-admission SCr when it is available, but few have defined the timing of this measurement. For example, Matheny et al. proposed a time-period of a maximum of 365 days and minimum of 7 days from the moment of hospital admission [14, 17]. Unfortunately, pre-admission SCr is often not available [1]. Recent data support a bidirectional relationship between AKI and CKD. Some patients with AKI can develop CKD because their renal function does not return to normal. For this reason, it is important to identify patients at risk of developing CKD or at risk of progressing to end-stage renal disease (ESRD). In order to improve the use of SCr for diagnosing AKI and CKD, biomarkers of renal function could be helpful.

Baseline Serum Creatinine in Cardiac Surgery and Pediatrics

Cardiac Surgery

The development of AKI in the cardiac surgery setting is complex: exposure to nephrotoxins (e.g., radio-contrast from cardiac catheterization, antibiotics), pre-existing conditions (e.g., diabetes mellitus, CKD), and exposure to intraoperative events (e.g., duration of cardiopulmonary bypass [CPB], hypotension) can all influence the risk of AKI and patient outcomes [18]. Elevated preoperative SCr is an independent risk factor for morbidity and mortality after cardiac surgery [19]. Small postoperative increases in SCr of 20–25% from preoperative baseline are associated with adverse outcomes [20–22]. However, SCr values are poor predictors of AKI in the early period after cardiac surgery [23]. In this setting, creatinine-based AKI definitions are not easy to use and very often the bSCr value used is the preadmission or admission SCr. Meersch et al. [24] defined the bSCr as the median of all values available from six months to one day prior to cardiac surgery; if this was not possible, the SCr value determined one day before cardiac surgery was used. Renal recovery from AKI was defined as an SCr value at hospital discharge equal to or less than the bSCr [23]. Other recent studies have shown that use of the bSCr from the MDRD equation (back-estimation) overestimated the incidence of AKI in patients undergoing cardiac surgery [15, 25]. One possible explanation could be that in these special populations, the average patient age is high and there is a large prevalence of vascular disease and consequently more CKD than in the general population. When these classes of patients are excluded, the overestimation decreases. Indeed, as explained earlier, the MDRD equation (back-estimation) can be used in patients with normal or nearly normal premorbid GFR, but it overestimates AKI in populations with an increased prevalence of mild CKD.

Pediatrics

In children, the bSCr is often unknown and little information is available concerning outcomes after AKI. Variations in estimating bSCr have led to clinically significant differences in ascertainment of AKI incidence. Zappitelli et al. [26] showed that, depending on which bSCr measurement was used, AKI patterns, incidence and outcome associations differed substantially. The authors suggested that change in estimated creatinine clearance (eCrCl) be used to define AKI and, when bSCr is unknown, the Schwartz eCrCl of 120 ml/min per $1.73 \, m^2$ should be used to estimate baseline renal function. In another study [27], the authors showed that bSCr was unknown in over 50% of the study population. They used center-specific age- and sex-based normative values in all patients versus only in those with an unknown bSCr. Results showed that normative estimated bSCr might be a reasonable alternative when 'true' bSCr data are unavailable, which is particularly likely to occur in population-based studies. In addition, they showed that in many children who develop AKI, SCr had not returned to bSCr values at the last pediatric ICU SCr assessment and that values were less likely to return to bSCr values in those with worse AKI. These children could be at risk of long-term renal disease [25, 26]. In a pediatric cardiac surgery setting, peaks in SCr levels following CPB are not evident until 24–48 h after surgery. In a prospective observational study, Mamikonian et al. defined AKI as a doubling in SCr from preoperative baseline and using the pediatric-modified RIFLE criteria. Their results showed a significant increase in SCr as early as 2 h following completion of CPB, with peak SCr levels occurring at 6 h after bypass [28].

Factors Influencing Serum Creatinine Values

Fluid Overload

In ICU patients, early and appropriate goal-directed fluid therapy is fundamental but is almost always associated with a certain degree of fluid overload responsible for tissue edema and progressive organ dysfunction. In this scenario, a positive fluid balance and lower urine volume are important factors associated with mortality of AKI patients [5, 29]. However, fluid management influences SCr and, using creatinine-based definitions, 'unrecognized' AKI could be identified after adjusting SCr concentration for positive fluid balance. A reanalysis of data from the Fluid and Catheter Treatment Trial demonstrated that correction of SCr for fluid balance unmasked the presence of AKI in some patients and led to a strong association between AKI and increased morbidity [6]. The adjustment of SCr concentration was performed using the following formula:

$$\text{Corrected SCr} = \text{measured SCr} \times \left[1 + \left(\frac{\text{accumulated net FB}}{\text{TBW}} \right) \right]$$

where FB is fluid balance and TBW is total body water. The TBW is defined as: TBW = 0.6 × weight (kg).

Basu et al. analyzed the impact of this correction on pediatric AKI in a cardiac surgery setting using the same formula: the presence of AKI was associated with increased duration of mechanical ventilation, prolonged postoperative ICU length of stay, and hospital length of stay. In addition, patients with AKI had increased net fluid balance and required increased inotropic support [7]. In another study, Moore et al. [8] analyzed the effect of positive fluid balance on the incidence and the outcome of AKI in adult cardiac surgery patients. The authors adjusted the SCr concentration using the same formula, and then categorized patients into three groups based on the presence or absence of AKI using AKIN criteria and pre- and post-the adjustment: Group A, with no AKI pre or post-adjustment for fluid balance; Group B, with no AKI pre- but AKI post-adjustment for fluid balance; Group C, with AKI pre- and post-adjustment for fluid balance. The results showed that the adjustment of SCr for fluid balance was associated with outcomes that were midway between those of patients with and without AKI by standard criteria. This means that these patients may have less severe but still significant AKI but unfortunately have been incorrectly defined as AKI-free because of dilution of SCr [8].

Muscle Wasting

SCr is a metabolite of creatine phosphate, an energy store found in skeletal muscle, and in normal subjects it is produced at a constant rate. A decrease in muscle mass could decrease SCr levels, and conversely SCr may be falsely increased with higher muscle mass [30]. SCr concentrations are extremely variable among el-

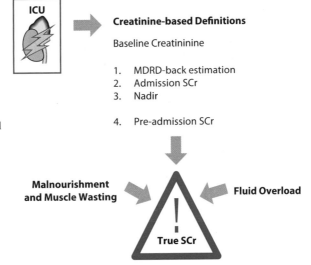

Fig. 1 Factors influencing creatinine-based definitions of acute kidney injury. Creatinine-based definitions can be influenced by baseline creatinine estimation, fluid overload, malnourishment and muscle wasting. SCr: serum creatinine; MDRD: Modification of Diet in Renal Disease

derly individuals and in children, as well as in critically ill patients. In this latter group of patients, muscle wasting starts already within the first week and is strongly related to poor outcome. Nevertheless, the early detection of muscle wasting is difficult. In a critical care setting, many conditions may lead to muscle wasting (e.g., malnourishment, immobilization, mechanical ventilation) [31], thus affecting SCr concentration, which may, therefore, appear to be within the reference range despite marked renal impairment. Consequently, the sensitivity of SCr for the early detection of AKI in these patients is poor. Fluid overload and malnutrition can seriously affect early creatinine-based AKI diagnosis and prognosis (Fig. 1). It is mandatory that the treating physician takes these factors into account when managing the critically ill patient at risk of AKI. Future studies should address the effect of fluid overload and muscle wasting on the true SCr concentration.

Susceptibility to Kidney Damage

The diagnosis of subclinical AKI through the early identification of damage markers may lead to earlier initiation of AKI treatment or to adjustment of care, thus mitigating the adverse effects of AKI until renal function recovery. This approach could be relevant for risk stratification regarding future injury or subsequent CKD development. Emerging biomarkers have been identified that detect renal tubular damage, even in the absence of an increase in SCr, and extend the spectrum of acute renal failure to early diagnostic evaluation and treatment of renal disorders [32]. In this scenario, the renal functional reserve (RFR) may be a relevant tool to predict the evolution of renal function. The RFR represents the capacity of intact nephron mass to increase GFR in response to stress and hence the difference between the peak stress CrCl induced by protein load and the baseline CrCl [33]. In physiological (e.g., pregnancy, solitary kidney) or pathological (e.g., diabetes mellitus, nephrotic syndrome) hyperfiltration states, the RFR allows the GFR to increase through mechanisms that are still unclear and under investigation. A recent theory suggests the presence of a population of "dormant cortical nephrons" uninvolved in filtration during resting conditions and potentially recruitable in response to stress; nevertheless these nephrons have never been demonstrated. Glomerular hyperfiltration, which may be considered another potential mechanism, is still controversial. Indeed, in most studies, the filtration fraction appears to be unaltered [34, 35], although some authors found an increase in the transcapillary hydraulic pressure gradient [36, 37]. However, whether we consider the hypothetical recruitment of dormant cortical nephrons or the increase in net glomerular ultrafiltration pressure, these factors are both related to afferent vasodilation [34–36, 38], a mechanism which all authors agree on. Because pre-surgical kidney function is one of the most important determinants of both mortality and AKI outcomes [20, 39], it is reasonable to assume that the RFR plays a role in a patient's susceptibility to develop AKI.

Conclusion

The absence of a shared approach to AKI definitions has resulted in variability among centers, with different interpretations of SCr concentrations. The three possible methods used to define bSCr under- or over-estimate renal function in both cardiac surgery and ICU settings. In pediatrics, some authors have suggested the use of changes in eCrCl to define AKI, and when the bSCr is unknown, use of the Schwartz eCrCl of 120 ml/min per 1.73 m^2 could be useful to estimate baseline renal function. More studies and improved methods to estimate bSCr are clearly needed. Fluid overload and muscle wasting, often present in critically ill patients, can influence SCr and mask a diagnosis of AKI. Future investigations should address the estimation of true SCr values and the use of RFR as an important supportive tool for screening and prediction of kidney function recovery or progression to CKD.

References

1. Koyner JL (2012) Assessment and diagnosis of renal dysfunction in the ICU. Chest 141:1584–1594
2. Roy AK, Mc Gorrian C, Treacy C et al (2013) A comparison of traditional and novel definitions (RIFLE, AKIN, and KDIGO) of acute kidney injury for the prediction of outcomes in acute decompensated heart failure. Cardiorenal Med 3:26–37
3. Bagshaw SM, Uchino S, Cruz D et al (2009) A comparison of observed versus estimated baseline creatinine for determination of RIFLE class in patients with acute kidney injury. Nephrol Dial Transplant 24:2739–2744
4. Lafrance JP, Miller DR (2010) Defining acute kidney injury in database studies: the effects of varying the baseline kidney function assessment period and considering CKD status. Am J Kidney Dis 56:651–660
5. Teixeira C, Garzotto F, Piccinni P et al (2013) Fluid balance and urine volume are independent predictors of mortality in acute kidney injury. Crit Care 17:R14
6. Liu KD, Thompson BT, Ancukiewicz M et al (2011) Acute kidney injury in patients with acute lung injury: impact of fluid accumulation on classification of acute kidney injury and associated outcomes. Crit Care Med 39:2665–2671
7. Basu RK, Andrews A, Krawczeski C et al (2013) Acute kidney injury based on corrected serum creatinine is associated with increased morbidity in children following the arterial switch operation. Pediatr Crit Care Med 14:e218–e224
8. Moore E, Tobin A, Reid D et al (2015) The impact of fluid balance on the detection, classification and outcome of acute kidney injury after cardiac surgery. J Cardiothorac Vasc Anesth 29:1229–1235
9. Puthucheary ZA, Rawal J, McPhail M et al (2013) Acute skeletal muscle wasting in critical illness. JAMA 310:1591–1600
10. Larsson L (2008) Acute quadriplegic myopathy: an acquired "myosinopathy". Adv Exp Med Biol 642:92–98
11. Bellomo R, Ronco C, Kellum JA, Mehta RL, Palevsky P (2004) Acute renal failure – definition, outcome measures, animal models, fluid therapy and information technology needs: the Second International Consensus Conference of the Acute Dialysis Quality Initiative (ADQI) Group. Crit Care 8:R204–212
12. Bagshaw SM, George C, Bellomo R (2008) A comparison of the RIFLE and AKIN criteria for acute kidney injury in critically ill patients. Nephrol Dial Transplant 23:1569–1574

13. Joannidis M, Metnitz B, Bauer P et al (2009) Acute kidney injury in critically ill patients classified by AKIN versus RIFLE using the SAPS 3 database. Intensive Care Med 35:1692–1702

14. Siew ED, Ikizler TA, Matheny ME et al (2012) Estimating baseline kidney function in hospitalized patients with impaired kidney function. Clin J Am Soc Nephrol 7:712–719

15. Siew ED, Matheny ME, Ikizler TA et al (2010) Commonly used surrogates for baseline renal function affect the classification and prognosis of acute kidney injury. Kidney Int 77:536–542

16. Broce JC, Price LL, Liangos O, Uhlig K, Jaber BL (2011) Hospital-acquired acute kidney injury: an analysis of nadir-to-peak serum creatinine increments stratified by baseline estimated GFR. Clin J Am Soc Nephrol 6:1556–1565

17. Matheny ME, Peterson JF, Eden SK et al (2014) Laboratory test surveillance following acute kidney injury. PloS One 9:e103746

18. Rosner MH, Okusa MD (2006) Acute kidney injury associated with cardiac surgery. Clin J Am Soc Nephrol 1:19–32

19. Nashef SA, Roques F, Sharples LD et al (2012) EuroSCORE II. Eur J Cardiothorac Surg 41:734–744

20. Wijeysundera DN, Karkouti K, Dupuis JY et al (2007) Derivation and validation of a simplified predictive index for renal replacement therapy after cardiac surgery. JAMA 297:1801–1809

21. Chertow GM, Levy EM, Hammermeister KE, Grover F, Daley J (1998) Independent association between acute renal failure and mortality following cardiac surgery. Am J Med 104:343–348

22. Mangano CM, Diamondstone LS, Ramsay JG, Aggarwal A, Herskowitz A, Mangano DT (1998) Renal dysfunction after myocardial revascularization: risk factors, adverse outcomes, and hospital resource utilization. The Multicenter Study of Perioperative Ischemia Research Group. Ann Intern Med 128:194–203

23. Wagener G, Jan M, Kim M et al (2006) Association between increases in urinary neutrophil gelatinase-associated lipocalin and acute renal dysfunction after adult cardiac surgery. Anesthesiology 105:485–491

24. Meersch M, Schmidt C, Van Aken H et al (2014) Urinary TIMP-2 and IGFBP7 as early biomarkers of acute kidney injury and renal recovery following cardiac surgery. PloS One 9:e93460

25. Candela-Toha AM, Recio-Vazquez M, Delgado-Montero A et al (2012) The calculation of baseline serum creatinine overestimates the diagnosis of acute kidney injury in patients undergoing cardiac surgery. Nefrologia 32:53–58

26. Zappitelli M, Parikh CR, Akcan-Arikan A, Washburn KK, Moffett BS, Goldstein SL (2008) Ascertainment and epidemiology of acute kidney injury varies with definition interpretation. Clin J Am Soc Nephrol 3:948–954

27. Alkandari O, Eddington KA, Hyder A et al (2011) Acute kidney injury is an independent risk factor for pediatric intensive care unit mortality, longer length of stay and prolonged mechanical ventilation in critically ill children: a two-center retrospective cohort study. Crit Care 15:R146

28. Mamikonian LS, Mamo LB, Smith PB, Koo J, Lodge AJ, Turi JL (2014) Cardiopulmonary bypass is associated with hemolysis and acute kidney injury in neonates, infants, and children. Pediatr Crit Care Med 15:e111–e119

29. Bouchard J, Soroko SB, Chertow GM et al (2009) Fluid accumulation, survival and recovery of kidney function in critically ill patients with acute kidney injury. Kidney Int 76:422–427

30. Baxmann AC, Ahmed MS, Marques NC et al (2008) Influence of muscle mass and physical activity on serum and urinary creatinine and serum cystatin C. Clin J Am Soc Nephrol 3:348–354

31. Lodeserto F, Yende S (2014) Understanding skeletal muscle wasting in critically ill patients. Crit Care 18:617

32. Haase M, Kellum JA, Ronco C (2012) Subclinical AKI – an emerging syndrome with important consequences. Nat Rev Nephrol 8:735–739

33. Sharma A, Mucino MJ, Ronco C (2014) Renal functional reserve and renal recovery after acute kidney injury. Nephron Clin Pract 127:94–100
34. Hostetter TH (1986) Human renal response to meat meal. Am J Physiol 250:F613–F618
35. Solling K, Christensen CK, Solling J, Christiansen JS, Mogensen CE (1986) Effect on renal haemodynamics, glomerular filtration rate and albumin excretion of high oral protein load. Scand J Clin Lab Invest 46:351–357
36. Chan AY, Cheng ML, Keil LC, Myers BD (1988) Functional response of healthy and diseased glomeruli to a large, protein-rich meal. J Clin Invest 81:245–254
37. Rodriguez-Iturbe B, Herrera J, Garcia R (1988) Relationship between glomerular filtration rate and renal blood flow at different levels of protein-induced hyperfiltration in man. Clin Sci (Lond) 74:11–15
38. ter Wee PM, Geerlings W, Rosman JB et al (1985) Testing renal reserve filtration capacity with an amino acid solution. Nephron 41:193–199
39. Thakar CV, Arrigain S, Worley S, Yared JP, Paganini EP (2005) A clinical score to predict acute renal failure after cardiac surgery. J Am Soc Nephrol 16:162–168

Detrimental Cross-Talk Between Sepsis and Acute Kidney Injury: New Pathogenic Mechanisms, Early Biomarkers and Targeted Therapies

S. Dellepiane, M. Marengo, and V. Cantaluppi

Introduction

Acute kidney injury (AKI) complicates about 3–50% of hospital admissions [1] depending on patient comorbidities and on medical procedures performed during the stay. The greatest incidence of AKI is observed in the intensive care unit (ICU): indeed, critically ill patients with hospital-acquired AKI have a greater in-hospital mortality (30–70%) and a more than double risk of severe adverse outcomes even 5 years after discharge, including an increased incidence of end-stage chronic kidney disease (CKD), than patients without AKI [2]. The most common cause of in-hospital AKI is sepsis, the systemic inflammatory response to infection that is often complicated by multiple organ failure and death [3]. In recent years, experimental and clinical studies have provided new insights into the pathogenic mechanisms of sepsis-associated AKI, also explaining how the loss of renal function may impair the immune system and lead to the subsequent development of sepsis. In this chapter, we review the recent findings on the detrimental cross-talk between sepsis and AKI and the identification of new, early biomarkers and targeted therapies aimed at improving the outcome of these critically ill patients.

S. Dellepiane
Dept of Medical Science, AOU Città Della Salute e Della Scienza, Turin University
Turin, Italy

M. Marengo
S.C. Nefrologia e Dialisi, Dipartimento Area Medica, ASLCN1
Cuneo, Italy

V. Cantaluppi (✉)
Dept of Translational Medicine, "Maggiore della Carità" University Hospital, University of Eastern Piedmont
Novara, Italy
email: vincenzo.cantaluppi@med.uniupo.it

© Springer International Publishing Switzerland 2016
J.-L. Vincent (ed.), *Annual Update in Intensive Care and Emergency Medicine 2016*,
DOI 10.1007/978-3-319-27349-5_9

New Pathogenic Mechanisms of Sepsis-Associated AKI: The 'Liaison Dangereuse' Revisited

Major advances have been made in our understanding of the detrimental connection between the systemic inflammatory response to infection and the acute loss of kidney function with consequent improvements in clinical practice. In particular, recent findings have challenged the dogma that in the course of severe sepsis and septic shock, AKI is merely a consequence of ischemic damage due to tissue hypoperfusion (Fig. 1).

Renal Overflow Rather Than Hypoperfusion

According to old theories, tissue hypoperfusion associated with sepsis causes renal ischemia and consequently acute tubular necrosis. By contrast, AKI is also found in the early phases of severe sepsis even in absence of an impaired cardiac output and in milder infectious diseases without manifest systemic signs. In a large prospective study including more than 1800 patients, Murugan et al. reported that AKI was frequent in patients with non-severe pneumonia, including those not transferred to the ICU and without hemodynamic instability [3]. In addition, the few studies reporting data on biopsies or autopsies from patients who developed sepsis-associated AKI have demonstrated that tubular necrosis is not common. Moreover, the number of apoptotic cells is significantly lower than that observed in any other types of AKI and not related to the severity of renal dysfunction [4]. On this basis, it is now accepted that septic AKI is only in part sustained by renal hypoperfusion. Di Giantomasso and coworkers elegantly proved this new theory in a sepsis model of sheep subjected to invasive monitoring of renal blood flow (RBF) [5]. Interestingly, these authors found that RBF was normal or even increased in sepsis and proposed the new model of hyperdynamic septic AKI [5]. Furthermore, increased RBF in septic AKI has also been observed in humans using thermodilution and magnetic resonance imaging (MRI) [6]. As a proof of concept, other studies have confirmed *in vitro* that plasma obtained from patients with sepsis-associated AKI induced tubular epithelial cell dysfunction without the contribution of any ischemia-reperfusion injury [7].

Based on these data, septic AKI is currently considered to be the consequence of several concomitant factors: a dysfunction of the renal microvascular system; direct interaction of pathogen fragments with renal resident cells; the cytotoxic effect of the sepsis-induced cytokine storm; and, finally, the deleterious cross-talk between injured organs. All these changes are sustained by fascinating intracellular mechanisms that may be targeted by new therapeutic approaches.

Microvascular and Glomerular Changes in Septic AKI

The parenchymal distribution of blood flow during sepsis is still far from being completely understood: the only incontestable point is the concomitant reduction in the

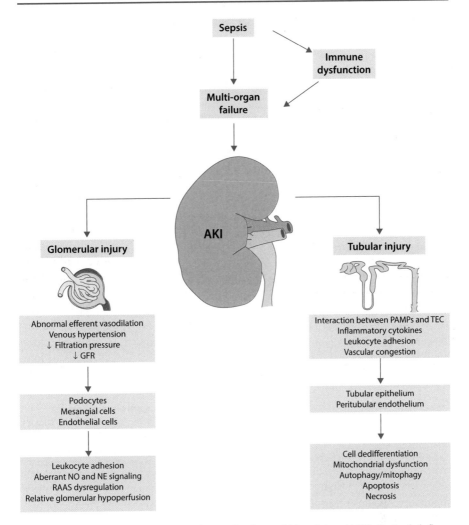

Fig. 1 Pathogenetic mechanisms of sepsis-associated acute kidney injury (AKI). Systemic inflammation coupled with multi-organ failure induces renal injury through several mechanisms: renal hemodynamic changes, activation of immune cells, massive release of inflammatory molecules and endocrine dysregulation. All contribute to glomerular and tubular cell injury. NO: nitric oxide; NE: norepinephrine; RAAS: renin-angiotensin-aldosterone system; GFR: glomerular filtration rate; PAMP: pathogen-associated molecular pattern; TEC: tubular epithelial cells; ↓: decreased

glomerular filtration rate (GFR). For this reason, several studies have focused on the mechanisms that decouple RBF from GFR. It has been shown that sepsis triggers a redistribution of RBF that leads to relative cortical hypoperfusion and to medullary overflow: this effect is enhanced by administration of norepinephrine [8]. Nevertheless, peritubular flow has been found to be sluggish and congested, probably as the result of a high capacity and low resistance circulation [9]. Other theories about the GFR decline during sepsis have focused on the reduction of filtration pressure not necessarily associated with glomerular hypoperfusion; renal and central (CVP) venous pressures are frequently increased in sepsis as a possible consequence of the so-called fluid challenge of septic patients in the first hours after ICU admission. This relative venous hypertension may induce microvascular congestion and tissue edema, thus affecting GFR. In support of this hypothesis, a retrospective analysis of 105 ICU patients found a linear correlation between the CVP and AKI incidence or duration [10]. Moreover, it has been shown that fluid overload in septic patients is independently associated with death and worse renal outcomes [11]. Another theory is based on the presence of efferent arteriole over-dilation as a consequence of altered angiotensin signaling or regional differences in nitric oxide (NO) and norepinephrine production and/or sensitivity [8]. The role of norepinephrine seems particularly relevant within the renal parenchyma: preliminary clinical and experimental studies have reported that the use of sympatholytic agents, such as clonidine or the α-2 receptor antagonist, dexmedetomidine, improves outcomes in septic AKI [12]. It has also been proposed that inflammation-activated shunt systems may directly connect afferent and efferent arterioles, thus decreasing GFR. However, although this effect is present in experimental studies in large animals subjected to sepsis, it has not been yet recognized in humans [8]. Finally, tubular cell dysfunction (see next paragraph) may induce the back-leakage of filtered substances and a resultant GFR decrease completely independent from glomerular physiology.

Systemic Inflammation Directly Affects Tubular Cell Function

Sepsis comprises the concomitant presence of an invasive infection and a host systemic inflammatory response syndrome (SIRS). SIRS is characterized by an over-inflammatory state due to a massive and deregulated activation of innate and adaptive immunity usually followed by an equally massive and deleterious counter-regulatory response leading to the so-called 'immune paralysis'. Accordingly, a bi-modal trend in patient mortality has been described with a first early phase due to SIRS and a second late phase caused by immunosuppression and lymphocyte exhaustion [13].

As stated above, renal inflammatory injury may be consequent to the direct interaction of resident cells with pathogens as well as with molecules released following the deregulated host immune response. Different pathogen-associated molecular patterns (PAMPs), such as lipopolysaccharide (LPS), lipoteichoic acid and porins, may directly interact with resident kidney cells. In particular, tubular epithelial cells express Toll-like receptor 4 (TLR4), the molecule with the highest affinity for LPS. It has been shown that LPS reduces the expression of the endocytic receptors megalin and cubilin in the apical compartment of proximal tubular epithelial cells, leading to an interference with the normal processes of protein re-absorption, thus contributing to the typical low molecular weight proteinuria of septic patients [7].

Renal resident endothelial and tubular cells directly communicate with the immune system: indeed, these cells not only express cytokine receptors, but they are also able to release several inflammatory proteins and to increase the expression of specific adhesion molecules able to recruit circulating cells that perpetuate tissue damage. It has also been demonstrated that tubular epithelial cells can recruit T cells by expressing vascular cell adhesion molecules (VCAMs) and intercellular cell adhesion molecules (ICAMs) and that they are consequently able to activate lymphocytes via the co-stimulatory molecule CD40 [14].

Circulating inflammatory cytokines directly affect the renal parenchyma and are associated with an increased risk of mortality in AKI patients [15]. The prominent role of cytokines in septic patients was further highlighted by a recent randomized controlled trial based on the administration of afelimomab (an anti-tumor necrosis factor [TNF]-α monoclonal antibody). Patients with higher basal levels of interleukin (IL)-6 had a small but significant mortality reduction when treated with this monoclonal antibody and, although the authors did not focus on AKI incidence, a significant improvement in the overall sequential organ failure assessment (SOFA) score was observed 48 h after the infusion [16]. Of interest, some of these inflammatory mediators, such as TNF-α, IL-6, CD40-ligand and Fas-ligand, can directly interact with specific counter-receptors located on tubular epithelial cells causing loss of function and apoptotic cell death.

A further mechanism of renal injury in the course of sepsis is probably linked to detrimental organ crosstalk. Apart from the validated models of hepatorenal and cardiorenal syndromes, recent studies have highlighted the effect of lung, brain and bone marrow as sources of potential nephrotoxic molecules. Indeed, studies performed *in vivo* and *in vitro* using plasma derived from patients treated with mechanical invasive ventilation showed that pneumocytes produce IL-1β, IL-6, IL-8 and TNF-α after ventilator-induced biotrauma and that the release of these cytokines promoted tubular cell apoptosis and consequently AKI. Moreover, the massive cytokine release observed after traumatic brain injury is a putative further cause of tubular cell dysfunction and has been associated with renal injury and consequent delayed graft function after donation for kidney transplantation [14]. The mechanisms of interaction between systemic inflammation and tubular epithelial cells and the potential clinical consequences of sepsis-associated AKI are shown in detail in Fig. 2.

Mechanisms of Cellular Dysfunction

All the hemodynamic and cytotoxic alterations described in the previous paragraphs directly affect kidney cell survival and function. Several types of cellular injury occur in the course of AKI, including necrosis, apoptosis or their combined form, necroptosis. This latter type of cellular injury is a highly immunogenic form of programmed cell death that normally represents a defense against viruses expressing caspase-8 inhibitors, but may also be triggered by cytokine imbalance [14]. The role of this pathway in AKI has not been completely investigated.

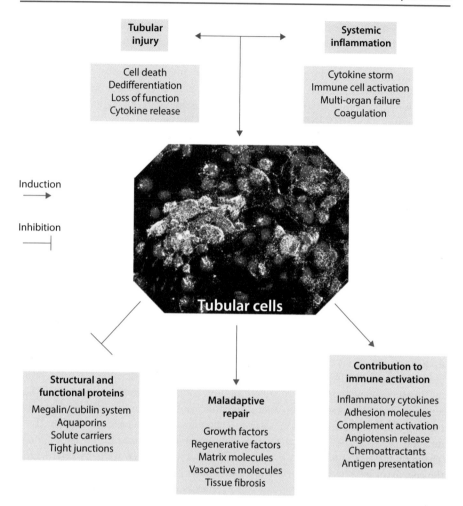

Fig. 2 Interplay between tubular epithelial cells and systemic inflammation. Tubular epithelial cells are directly targeted by inflammation through specific membrane receptors able to modulate cytokines, activated immune cells and bacterial products. In response to these deleterious stimuli, tubular cells dedifferentiate and release a plethora of paracrine factors as an ultimate effort to induce tissue regeneration. On the other hand, tubular cells directly contribute to systemic inflammation by carrying out immune functions, such as cytokine release and leukocyte recruitment and activation

As noted earlier, at biopsy or autopsy, septic patients have a significantly lower rate of tubular apoptosis than other ICU patients with AKI. Furthermore, the amount of necrosis also seems to be marginal. In addition, both apoptosis and necrosis are found in a few limited parenchymal areas and do not correlate with renal dysfunction and AKI duration. The direct consequence of these observations is that septic AKI is probably associated with a series of cell dysfunctions rather than cell death.

Available histological data have demonstrated mostly tubular cell vacuolization and mitochondrial rarefaction, possible consequences of autophagy and mitophagy, respectively. Based on these findings, it has been proposed that tubular epithelial cells react to injury by regressing to a dedifferentiated and energy-saving state. Accordingly, it has been found that during sepsis, renal oxygen consumption is significantly reduced [17]. The auto-digestion of energy-consuming organelles (autophagy), including the mitochondria (mitophagy), is one of the key passages of this biological phenomenon. Moreover, it has been shown that tubular cells exposed to septic plasma lose cell polarity and the expression of the endocytic receptor, megalin [7]. These alterations confirmed the transition of tubular cells toward a dedifferentiated state with the consequent loss of preservation of two distinct fluid-filled compartments characterized by precise electrolyte concentrations. As a consequence of tubular dysfunction, both electrolyte reabsorption and protein trafficking are almost completely abolished during septic AKI [7].

Another energy-sparing strategy is the arrest of the cell cycle. This phenomenon has been demonstrated in tubular cells subjected to a septic microenvironment. Accordingly, two of the most promising urine early biomarkers of AKI (tissue inhibitor of metalloproteinases [TIMP]-2 and insulin-like growth factor-binding protein [IGFBP]-7) are proteins involved in the G1-S phase transition arrest [18]. A further mechanism of tubular dysfunction may depend on the horizontal cross signaling between proximal and distal segments. Kalakeche et al. reported that cellular uptake of LPS in the S1 segment caused oxidative stress at both S2 and S3 levels [19].

Finally, recent data suggest that AKI may contribute to the development and aggravation of a systemic inflammatory state. Indeed, tubular cells are immunologically active, because they are able to act as antigen-presenting cells and are devoted to the clearance of various soluble mediators involved in inflammation. These findings may at least in part explain the pathogenic mechanisms underlying the accelerating development of sepsis and multiple organ failure when patients lose tubular cell function. In this setting, Naito et al. elegantly proved the direct influence of LPS on tubular cell gene expression. These authors demonstrated *in vivo* increased RNA-polymerase II density at TNF-α, monocyte chemotactic protein-1 (MCP-1) and heme oxygenase-1 (HO-1) loci after LPS injection in mice. This effect was related to selective histone methylation and was enhanced by different nephrotoxic stimuli [20]. These AKI-associated epigenetic alterations of tubular cells may be responsible for the above-mentioned increase in circulating inflammatory mediators.

Biomarkers of Sepsis-Associated AKI

AKI is currently defined using the Risk, Injury, Failure, Loss of kidney function, and End-stage kidney disease (RIFLE), Acute Kidney Injury Network (AKIN) and Kidney Disease – Improving Global Outcomes (KDIGO) criteria [21]: all these systems are based on the levels of serum creatinine (SCr), estimated GFR (eGFR) and on urine output. However, these parameters are insensitive, non-specific and have a substantial latency, in particular in patients with sepsis-associated AKI. Indeed, sepsis *per se* is known to decrease creatinine production; moreover, the fluid overload that frequently characterizes septic patients may be responsible for a further delay in SCr increase. Urine output is also influenced by several confounding factors: its rapid decrease not associated with changes in GFR is currently classified as 'transient' or 'subclinical' AKI, with uncertain clinical significance and not consistent with the presence of parenchymal injury [22].

Several molecules have recently been proposed for the early diagnosis of sepsis-associated AKI. However, numerous problems confound the validation of these molecules in the clinical setting. First, these biomarkers are always compared to the above-mentioned defective classifications. Moreover, the current scarcity of effective therapies limits the effect of early diagnosis on the achievement of hard clinical endpoints. These two aspects concur to underestimate the diagnostic accuracy of these new identified molecules. Finally, some of the AKI biomarkers are (or are functionally associated with) acute phase proteins and are influenced by the inflammatory state. On this basis, the cytokine storm observed during sepsis may lead to a false-positive interpretation. However, despite these limits, several studies have demonstrated substantial diagnostic improvements using different molecules.

Neutrophil gelatinase-associated lipocalin (NGAL) is a 25 kDa protein belonging to the lipocalins, a class of soluble factors involved in small molecule traffic. NGAL binds to prokaryotic and eukaryotic siderophora, iron-chelating molecules involved in bacterial growth and tissue differentiation, respectively. During the course of AKI, NGAL is increased in both serum and urine. Serum NGAL is mainly produced by hepatocytes and immune cells, whereas urinary NGAL derives in part from serum NGAL filtered by glomeruli and in part from NGAL released by kidney tubular epithelial cells following injury. NGAL is the most extensively studied biomarker in septic AKI and is also frequently used as the control molecule when other proteins are investigated. NGAL has a bimodal trend with a first peak before and a second peak 24–48 h after AKI onset [23]. A limitation of clinical NGAL use is that its increase in both serum and urine may be related to the presence of a systemic inflammatory state including sepsis and not only to the development of AKI. Indeed, it has been shown that patients developing only sepsis or only AKI have similar serum and urinary NGAL levels: by contrast, non-AKI non-septic patients and those affected by both clinical conditions are clearly classified [21]. To summarize these studies, urinary and serum NGAL levels are more associated with sepsis severity (and the presence of multiple organ failure) than with AKI incidence. To reduce this limitation, some authors propose to strengthen NGAL performance by combining it with sepsis-specific biomarkers. Lentini et al. measured circulating levels of NGAL together with advanced oxidation protein products (AOPP) in 98 consecutive ICU patients. The authors found that NGAL values were slightly higher in patients with only AKI than in those with only sepsis without any significant difference: however, AOPP levels were able to distinguish between septic and non-septic subjects and allowed a correct classification for most patients. Similar results were obtained coupling serum NGAL levels with endotoxin activity assay (EAA) results, which can identify LPS-induced neutrophilic responses in Gram-negative bacteria, septic shock [21]. Despite these encouraging data, a key point for NGAL measurement still remains unresolved: three different forms of NGAL have been isolated – a 25 kDa monomer, a 45 kDa dimer and a 135 kDa heterodimer, conjugated with gelatinase. Currently, no commercially available assays can discriminate between the monomer, mainly released from tubular epithelial cells, and the dimer, originating from neutrophils [22]. Future development in this context may further increase the diagnostic accuracy of this molecule.

Triggering receptor expressed on myeloid cells (TREM)-1 is a membrane receptor belonging to the immunoglobulin superfamily and expressed on neutrophils and monocytes. Its soluble form, sTREM, is massively released in body fluids during sepsis, pneumonia, septic arthritis, meningitis, peritonitis, and uterine cavity infections. In septic patients, urinary sTREM is increased 24–48 h before clinical evidence of AKI, whereas a continuous increase in sTREM independently correlates with sepsis progression and with a worse outcome [24]. However, similar to NGAL, sTREM correlates with AKI as well as with systemic inflammation and more studies are needed to detect possible confounding factors.

The host SIRS is the cornerstone of sepsis development: SIRS is caused by an immune system over-reaction to pathogens and induces a 'cytokine storm'. Additionally, recent findings have demonstrated that several cytokines are involved in AKI development and some are directly produced by renal cells. In a cohort of ICU patients, Cho et al. found that IL-8 and IL-10 were increased in AKI patients independent of the presence of sepsis. Interestingly, the authors found a significant increase in soluble CD25 (IL-2 receptor) in septic AKI [15]. Soluble CD25 is a marker of T regulatory cell activity and it may correlate with the development of a counter-regulatory response leading to immune paralysis.

The combined use of urinary IGFBP-7 and TIMP-2 has recently been approved by the FDA as an early indicator of AKI [18]. Other new biomarkers of AKI include liver fatty acid binding protein (L-FABP), IL-18, netrin-1, kidney injury molecule-1 (KIM-1) and α1-microglobulin. Other circulating mediators, including CD40-ligand, Fas-ligand, angiopoietin-2 and presepsin (soluble CD14) have been validated in septic patients as indicators of mortality [21, 25]. In the next few years, the evolving field of 'omics' technologies (genomics, transcriptomics, proteomics, and metabolomics) may lead to a system biology-based approach that could improve diagnostic strategies for sepsis-associated AKI.

Targeted Therapeutic Approaches for Sepsis-Associated AKI

Several clinical trials in patients with severe sepsis and septic shock have failed to show an improvement in outcomes. Despite the initial benefits of so-called early goal-directed therapies, a prolonged series of therapeutic failures of promising strategies including corticosteroids, activated protein C and the use of standard renal replacement therapies (RRT) has been observed. Septic patients still have an unacceptable high mortality and, excluding antimicrobial agents, clinical management is almost exclusively based on supportive therapies that are not able to interfere with the underlying pathogenic mechanisms of concomitant tissue damage and immunoparalysis. In this section, we summarize the more recent advances in the therapeutic treatment of experimental and clinical sepsis-associated AKI.

Pharmacological Agents

The severity of injury and the poor outcomes associated with septic AKI worsen with delayed recognition of renal dysfunction. Early identification of AKI in septic patients is crucial because employed supportive and therapeutic strategies are frequently nephrotoxic (e.g., antibiotics, such as vancomycin and aminoglycosides, use of vasopressor therapy without adequate fluid resuscitation, etc.) and may additionally worsen the extent of the renal injury. A recent clinical trial by Sood et al. [26] showed that septic patients who had reversible or improved AKI within 24 h of diagnosis had better survival rates than patients who did not recover from AKI and even than those who did not develop AKI at all. Most of the available interventions for AKI are based on prevention of further renal insult or organ support (early administration of appropriate antimicrobial therapy, restoration of tissue perfusion and optimization of the hemodynamic status), but these standard treatment approaches have not been effective in significantly reducing the incidence of septic AKI. Furthermore, the emergence of antibiotic-resistant microbes as well as the increased clinical complexity of patients emphasizes the need to understand and to develop novel pharmacologic approaches to successfully treat sepsis-associated AKI.

The paradigm of sepsis-associated organ dysfunction and AKI has focused largely on specific cytokines and their modulation or removal for improving outcome. However, therapeutic approaches based on targeting specific pathways known to contribute to the pathogenesis of septic AKI have failed. Indeed, clinical trials focused on antagonizing a single detrimental mediator including anti-endotoxin (LPS), TNF-α, IL-1β, and TLR-4 did not show any significant results [27]. These failures may be, at least in part, explained by the early-deregulated host immune response mediated by the activation of innate immunity followed by a state of immunosuppression. For this reason, therapeutic approaches should consider the temporal profile of the immune status in sepsis: the early blockade of pro-inflammatory pathways should be followed by distinct therapies aimed at triggering the late activation of immunity. On this basis, Swaminathan et al. recently reviewed emerging therapeutic approaches in septic AKI, focusing on targeting early pro-inflammatory and late anti-inflammatory processes [28]. The suppression of early inflammation during sepsis-associated AKI could be obtained by using alkaline phosphatase. This enzyme is able to reduce inflammation through dephosphorylation and thereby 'detoxification' of LPS, which is a key mediator of sepsis-induced organ failure, including AKI. Furthermore, alkaline phosphatase catalyzes the conversion of adenosine triphosphate into adenosine, a potent anti-inflammatory factor. The administration of recombinant alkaline phosphatase reduced inflammation and the incidence of septic AKI, but no changes in mortality rate were observed [29].

In order to attenuate the early inflammatory response, some authors have also proposed the use of cannabinoid 2 (CB2) receptor agonists [30]. CB2 receptors are expressed on leukocytes and regulate the immune system: their activation attenuates leukocyte-endothelial cell interaction and the recruitment of leukocytes, thus reducing the amount of circulating pro-inflammatory mediators. Fibrates, which are peroxisome proliferator-activated receptor-α (PPARα) agonists, have been shown to ameliorate sepsis induced by Gram-negative bacteria by promoting neutrophil recruitment [28]. Experimental studies recently described the role of the cholinergic anti-inflammatory pathway: stimulation of the vagus nerve may attenuate cytokine release in sepsis, ischemia-reperfusion injury and other states of inflammation [31]. Moreover, nicotine (an α7 nicotinic acetylcholine receptor agonist) has been shown to reduce mortality in sepsis [28]. Other studies have demonstrated that soluble thrombomodulin was effective in preventing and treating established AKI, an effect associated with reduced leukostasis and endothelial cell permeability [32].

Later in the course of sepsis, the marked immunosuppressive state requires interventions that can stimulate the immune response. IL-7, which is critical for T-cell development and function, enhances immunity by increasing the expression of cell adhesion molecules, facilitating leukocyte trafficking to sites of infection [33]. Granulocyte macrophage-colony stimulating factor (GM-CSF) restores monocyte function and shortens the duration of mechanical ventilation and length of ICU stay [34].

Extracorporeal Blood Purification Techniques

In the last few decades, many studies have evaluated the clinical and biological effects of different extracorporeal blood purification techniques in sepsis-associated AKI. The use of RRT in septic patients has been evaluated both for renal support and immunomodulation. Traditional RRT indications are uremia, metabolic disturbances, fluid overload and electrolyte derangements. However, several authors have proposed the use of different RRT techniques to remove inflammatory mediators potentially involved in AKI and distant organ damage. Large clinical trials have suggested that, in septic AKI, early initiation of RRT and the use of continuous and not intermittent strategies are associated with a better hemodynamic profile and outcome. However, the timing of RRT initiation remains heterogeneous in clinical practice and is not yet definitely supported by consistent scientific evidence. Excessive delays in RRT initiation have been associated with higher mortality rates and with worsening of renal function. However, the only published randomized controlled trial available showed no significant differences in renal outcomes or patient survival between early and late initiation of dialysis [11]. The ongoing IDEAL-ICU study (Initiation of Dialysis EArly versus Late in the Intensive Care Unit) will help define the optimal timing of RRT in septic AKI patients [35]. The use of continuous renal replacement therapies (CRRT) in septic AKI is still preferred because of their relationship with better hemodynamic tolerability and with enhanced renal recovery compared to intermittent modalities. In a retrospective study examining patients undergoing continuous therapies versus daily hemofiltration, Sun et al. suggested that patients undergoing continuous veno-venous hemofiltration (CVVH) had a significant improvement in renal function, although the all-cause mortality rates were similar at 60 days [36].

Another relevant issue in RRT for sepsis-associated AKI is the dose of renal support, which has been evaluated in different randomized clinical trials since the initial data from the Vicenza study in which a dose of 35 ml/kg/h was associated with a better survival of AKI patients, in particular in the presence of sepsis [37]. Unfortunately, subsequent studies, including the RENAL and the Acute Renal Failure Trial Network (ATN) trials, did not confirm these encouraging results [38, 39]. The RENAL study [38] compared a dose of 25 vs. 40 ml/kg/h in continuous veno-venous hemodiafiltration (CVVHDF), whereas the ATN study [39] compared 20 vs. 35 ml/kg/h in 3 times/week intermittent or continuous dialysis. Both studies showed that an increased intensity of the RRT dose had no beneficial effect on outcome (mortality was the primary endpoint of both studies). However, in the RENAL study, a *post-hoc* analysis of septic patients showed a tendency toward a reduction in mortality rate in the group of patients treated with the higher-intensity approach (40 ml/kg/h) [38]. Recently, the multicenter randomized controlled trial, IVOIRE (hIgh VOlume in Intensive caRE) evaluated the impact of high-volume hemofiltration (HVHF) on 28-day mortality in critically ill patients with septic shock and AKI. In this study, the authors did not observe a reduction in 28-day mortality or an early improvement in hemodynamic profile or organ function using HVHF at 70 ml/kg/h compared to standard-volume hemofiltration at 35 ml/kg/h [40]. Even though the above-mentioned studies led to negative results in sepsis-associated AKI, they have helped define an optimal dose of dialysis, taking into consideration the difference between prescribed and delivered doses.

As stated before, the application of RRT in patients with septic AKI also has the purpose of increasing the clearance of inflammatory mediators involved in tissue injury. Over the years, different extracorporeal techniques have been developed leading to a wide range of possible therapeutic approaches.

1. Standard RRT techniques (CVVH, CVVHD and CVVHDF) using high molecular flow membranes (HFM) or membranes with enhanced adsorption capacity. HFM have an average cut-off value of approximately 30–40 kDa and are capable of eliminating significant amounts of inflammatory mediators including chemokines and cytokines in the middle-molecular weight category. Adsorptive membranes, such as polymethyl methacrylate (PMMA) and AN69ST, have also been used to enhance endotoxin and cytokine clearance and some clinical trials are underway in septic patients with AKI [41]. However, we must emphasize that these inflammatory mediators have a very high generation rate: for this reason, studies using CVVH failed to show any significant modulation of plasma levels of different cytokines [41].

2. Convection-based high-volume techniques (HVHF) are defined by a flow rate of more than 35 ml/kg/h. Use of HVHF was the subject of a recent Cochrane

review [11]: selected trials comparing HVHF with a standard dialysis dose did not show any improvement in patient outcomes. Despite a reported increase in hemodynamic stability and the absence of relevant adverse effects, these studies did not support a strong recommendation for the use of HVHF in critically ill patients with severe sepsis and septic shock. Furthermore, the application of HVHF may potentially cause increased clearance of antibiotics and other drugs, electrolyte disturbances and depletion of micronutrients, which may all lead to a less favorable outcome.

3. High cut-off (HCO) membranes: these membranes are porous enough to achieve the removal of larger molecules (30–60 kDa) mainly by diffusion. Several studies showed benefits of using HCO therapy, such as improved immune cell function, removal of inflammatory cytokines, and a reduction in catecholamine dosage. An undesired effect is albumin loss, which can be attenuated by albumin replacement or by using HCO membranes in a diffusive and not convective manner [42].

4. Hemoperfusion, hemoadsorption and plasma-adsorption: these techniques involve placement of a sorbent, often a resin, in direct contact with blood or plasma through an extracorporeal circuit. Most of these devices are designed to combine the adsorption strategy with standard RRT. The biocompatibility of these devices is the main limitation for their use and thrombocytopenia and bleeding risk are the most relevant adverse effects [43].

Polymyxin B (PMX-B) is a cationic polypeptide antibiotic with activity against Gram-negative bacteria and high affinity for endotoxin, but its intravenous use has been limited due to the well-known nephrotoxicity and neurotoxicity. PMX-B has been fixed and immobilized onto polystyrene fiber in a hemoperfusion column cartridge that allows endotoxin removal without toxic effects [44]. The main mechanism of action is through removal of circulating endotoxin, although its effects are likely pleiotropic including the entrapment of inflammatory cells, such as monocytes and neutrophils, and the clearance of cytokines TNF-α and IL-6 with a consequent reduction in the intracellular mechanisms of apoptosis. Cruz et al. [44] published a meta-analysis showing that PMX-B hemoperfusion used in patients with severe sepsis led to an improvement in hemodynamics as measured by mean arterial pressure as well as in oxygenation. These results were observed in the Early Use of Polymyxin Hemoperfusion in Abdominal Septic shock (EUPHAS) trial in Europe that confirmed preliminary data coming from the Japanese experience [45]. However, the sample size of these studies was small and confirmation of these clinical benefits in larger studies is still awaited. The first randomized, controlled, diagnostic-directed and theragnostic trial, named EUPHRATES (Evaluating the Use of Polymyxin B Hemoperfusion in a Randomized controlled trial of Adults Treated for Endotoxemia and Septic shock) is still ongoing in the US and Canada [46].

The LPS adsorber is a medical device designed for extracorporeal use, which contains a series of porous polyethylene plates coated with a peptide specific to endotoxin. Yaroustovsky et al. compared the LPS adsorber and PMX-B hemoperfusion in patients with Gram-negative sepsis and reported no significant differences in outcome (small number of enrolled patients) [47].

CytoSorb is a highly adsorptive and biocompatible polymer able to remove multiple inflammatory mediators from the bloodstream. Animal studies have elegantly shown that therapeutic apheresis using CytoSorb can restore chemokine gradients toward infected tissue and away from healthy organs through a sort of leukocyte trafficking control [48].

Coupled plasma filtration adsorption (CPFA) is an extracorporeal treatment based on non-specific adsorption of cytokines and other pro-inflammatory mediators onto a specially designed resin cartridge that is in direct contact with filtered plasma. This system is coupled in series with a standard RRT circuit. Some studies have shown interesting results concerning an improvement in hemodynamics, microvascular derangement and respiratory parameters during the course of CPFA [49].

5. The existing extracorporeal techniques are mainly based on plasma filtration and consequently on substitution of the glomerular function of the kidney. However, standard RRT techniques did not allow some specific functions of transport, metabolic and endocrine activities of tubular epithelial cells to be replaced. To overcome this limitation, Tumlin and coworkers developed a renal assist device (RAD) using a polysulfone filter containing living kidney tubular epithelial cells coupled with a conventional RRT circuit. These authors validated this bio-engineered device in several *in vivo* models demonstrating that septic animals affected by AKI and treated with the RAD maintained reabsorption of K^+, $HCO3^-$, and glucose, as well as the excretion of ammonia and normal levels of 1,25-OH-vitamin D3 [50]. Moreover, the RAD modulates systemic inflammation by regulating circulating levels of several cytokines. Based on these preclinical studies, a randomized controlled trial was performed and showed that the RAD induced about a 50% reduction in 180-day mortality when compared to standard CVVH [50]. Moreover, the RAD was able to modulate plasma levels of several cytokines, including G-CSF, IL-6, and IL-10, thus improving both the early SIRS and late immunoparalysis typical of septic AKI. Of interest, the clinical trial with the RAD was prematurely interrupted because the investigators also observed a significant decrease in mortality using a sham cartridge not containing viable tubular cells. Following this observation, the same authors developed the so-called selective cytophoretic device (SCD) able to sequestrate activated leukocytes within the membrane, inhibiting the release of harmful mediators. Preliminary studies indicated that, when coupled to a standard hemofilter, SCD reduced mortality and dialysis dependence in septic patients. However, the beneficial effects of SCD were observed only when citrate but not heparin was used as the anticoagulant strategy [51]. This finding emphasizes the potential anti-inflammatory properties of citrate, which may at least in part explain the data on a reduction in mortality in clinical trials in ICU patients subjected to RRT with citrate [51].

Stem Cell Therapies

Stem cell-based therapies have been proposed in almost all fields of medicine with controversial success. One of the major limitations of this approach comes from the host immune reaction as well as from the possibility of cell dysplasia and tumorigenesis or other maladaptive responses including maldifferentiation, tissue fibrosis, calcification and innate immunity dysregulation. For these reasons, despite a large number of experimental studies, effective clinical results are still lacking, even in the field of sepsis [52].

Bone marrow-derived stem cells of both mesenchymal and hematopoietic origin have been extensively studied in different experimental models of AKI. Mesenchymal stem cells are a heterogeneous population that can be isolated from a variety of adult tissues of mesodermal origin, including bone marrow, adipose tissue, placenta, umbilical cord, dental pulp and synovia. For their regenerating and immune-modulatory effects, mesenchymal stem cells have been tested in several experimental models of acute tissue injury models including AKI and kidney transplantation [52]. Mesenchymal stem cells are able to sense inflammation through the expression of cytokine receptors and adhesion molecules. Mesenchymal stem cells can induce M2 macrophages as well as T-regulatory cells [52]. Mesenchymal stem cell-related anti-inflammatory M2 macrophages have also been induced in sepsis models. Moreover, mesenchymal stem cells improved monocyte and neutrophil phagocytosis and reduced bacterial load in different organs (peritoneal cavity, blood, spleen and liver) [53].

Endothelial progenitor cells are circulating committed cells involved in vascular regeneration processes. The therapeutic use of endothelial progenitor cells may be of particular interest in sepsis because of their major role in protection from endothelial dysfunction. Moreover, sepsis is associated with a severe depletion in the endothelial progenitor cell circulating pool and this impairment independently correlates with a worse outcome [54].

Recent studies have suggested that most of the beneficial effects of mesenchymal stem cell and endothelial progenitor cell infusions are observed in the absence of cell engraftment within injured tissues [55]. In addition, the infusion of stem cell supernatants induced a protective effect similar to that observed after whole cell transplantation [55]. Taken together, these results suggest that endocrine/paracrine factors promote the regenerative effects of stem cells. In this setting, recent studies have demonstrated the potential role of microvesicles released from stem cells in tissue regeneration following AKI. Microvesicles are cell fragments involved in cell-to-cell communication that are able to shuttle different RNA subsets (mRNA and microRNA), proteins and lipids. In different experimental AKI models, microvesicle administration was associated with improved renal function, histological lesions and survival, preventing the progression toward end-stage CKD [56]. These regenerative effects were partially due to the epigenetic reprogramming of target injured renal cells through the horizontal transfer of mRNA and microRNA [57].

Conclusion

Experimental and clinical studies have proven the presence of a detrimental cross-talk between sepsis, the systemic inflammatory response to infection, and the development of AKI. Sepsis represents the main cause of renal dysfunction in critically ill patients admitted to the ICU. From a pathogenic point of view, it has been shown that the damage of renal endothelial and tubular epithelial cells during sepsis occurs in the absence of evident signs of tissue hypoperfusion. Indeed, septic AKI develops in the presence of a normal or even increased RBF. These results suggest that the pathogenic mechanisms of septic AKI are associated with the detrimental activity of circulating pro-inflammatory and pro-apoptotic mediators that directly bind to renal resident cells. In particular, the onset of apoptosis, necrosis, necroptosis, autophagy, mitophagy and cell cycle arrest has been identified as the main mechanism of tubular injury during sepsis. Early identification of sepsis-associated AKI using new biomarkers ('omics' technologies) may improve patient outcomes. Moreover, new therapeutic strategies based on pharmacological agents, extracorporeal blood purification techniques and stem cell infusion have been developed and exciting clinical results are expected in the next few years.

References

1. Gomez H, Ince C, De Backer D et al (2014) A unified theory of sepsis-induced acute kidney injury: inflammation, microcirculatory dysfunction, bioenergetics, and the tubular cell adaptation to injury. Shock 41:3–11
2. Glodowski SD, Wagener G et al (2015) New insights into the mechanisms of acute kidney injury in the intensive care unit. J Clin Anesth 27:175–180
3. Murugan R, Karajala-Subramanyam V, Lee M et al (2010) Genetic and Inflammatory Markers of Sepsis (GenIMS) Investigators: Acute kidney injury in non-severe pneumonia is associated with an increased immune response and lower survival. Kidney Int 77:527–535
4. Lerolle N, Nochy D, Guérot E et al (2010) Histopathology of septic shock induced acute kidney injury: apoptosis and leukocytic infiltration. Intensive Care Med 36:471–478
5. Di Giantomasso D, May CN, Bellomo R (2003) Vital organ blood flow during hyperdynamic sepsis. Chest 124:1053–1059
6. Brenner M, Schaer GL, Mallory DL, Suffredini AF, Parrillo JE (1990) Detection of renal blood flow abnormalities in septic and critically ill patients using a newly designed indwelling thermodilution renal vein catheter. Chest 98:170–179
7. Mariano F, Cantaluppi V, Stella M et al (2008) Circulating plasma factors induce tubular and glomerular alterations in septic burns patients. Crit Care 12:R42
8. Di Giantomasso D, Morimatsu H, May CN, Bellomo R (2003) Intrarenal blood flow distribution in hyperdynamic septic shock: Effect of norepinephrine. Crit Care Med 31:2509–2513
9. Holthoff JH, Wang Z, Seely KA, Gokden N, Mayeux PR (2012) Resveratrol improves renal microcirculation, protects the tubular epithelium, and prolongs survival in a mouse model of sepsis-induced acute kidney injury. Kidney Int 81:370–378
10. Legrand M, Dupuis C, Simon C et al (2013) Association between systemic hemodynamics and septic acute kidney injury in critically ill patients: a retrospective observational study. Crit Care 17:R278
11. Borthwick EMJ, Hill CJ, Rabindranath KS, Maxwell AP, McAuley DF, Blackwood B (2013) High-volume haemofiltration for sepsis. Cochrane Database Syst Rev CD008075

12. Taniguchi T, Kurita A, Kobayashi K, Yamamoto K, Inaba H (2008) Dose- and time-related effects of dexmedetomidine on mortality and inflammatory responses to endotoxin-induced shock in rats. J Anesth 22:221–228

13. Boomer JS, To K, Chang KC et al (2011) Immunosuppression in patients who die of sepsis and multiple organ failure. JAMA 306:2594–2605

14. Cantaluppi V, Quercia AD, Dellepiane S, Ferrario S, Camussi G, Biancone L (2014) Interaction between systemic inflammation and renal tubular epithelial cells. Nephrol Dial Transplant 29:2004–2011

15. Cho E, Lee JH, Lim HJ et al (2014) Soluble CD25 is increased in patients with sepsis-induced acute kidney injury. Nephrol Carlton Vic 19:318–324

16. Panacek EA, Marshall JC, Albertson TE et al (2014) Efficacy and safety of the monoclonal anti-tumor necrosis factor antibody F(ab')2 fragment afelimomab in patients with severe sepsis and elevated interleukin-6 levels. Crit Care Med 32:2173–2182

17. Yang R, Wang X, Liu D, Liu S (2014) Energy and oxygen metabolism disorder during septic acute kidney injury. Kidney Blood Press Res 39:240–251

18. Gocze I, Koch M, Renner P et al (2015) Urinary biomarkers TIMP-2 and IGFBP7 early predict acute kidney injury after major surgery. PloS One 10:e0120863

19. Kalakeche R, Hato T, Rhodes G et al (2011) Endotoxin uptake by S1 proximal tubular segment causes oxidative stress in the downstream S2 segment. J Am Soc Nephrol 22:1505–1516

20. Naito M, Bomsztyk K, Zager RA (2008) Endotoxin mediates recruitment of RNA polymerase II to target genes in acute renal failure. J Am Soc Nephrol 19:1321–1330

21. Lentini P, de Cal M, Clementi A, D'Angelo A, Ronco C (2012) Sepsis and AKI in ICU patients: the role of plasma biomarkers. Crit Care Res Pract 2012:856401

22. Vanmassenhove J, Glorieux G, Lameire N et al (2015) Influence of severity of illness on neutrophil gelatinase-associated lipocalin performance as a marker of acute kidney injury: a prospective cohort study of patients with sepsis. BMC Nephrol 16:18

23. Si Nga H, Medeiros P, Menezes P, Bridi R, Balbi A, Ponce D (2015) Sepsis and AKI in Clinical Emergency Room Patients: The Role of Urinary NGAL. BioMed Res Int 2015:413751

24. Su L, Feng L, Zhang J et al (2011) Diagnostic value of urine sTREM-1 for sepsis and relevant acute kidney injuries: a prospective study. Crit Care 15:R250

25. Bagshaw SM, Langenberg C, Haase M, Wan L, May CN, Bellomo R (2007) Urinary biomarkers in septic acute kidney injury. Intensive Care Med 33:1285–1296

26. Sood MM, Shafer LA, Ho J et al (2014) Cooperative Antimicrobial Therapy in Septic Shock (CATSS) Database Research Group: Early reversible acute kidney injury is associated with improved survival in septic shock. J Crit Care 29:711–717

27. Opal SM, Laterre P-F, Francois B et al (2013) ACCESS Study Group: Effect of eritoran, an antagonist of MD2-TLR4, on mortality in patients with severe sepsis: the ACCESS randomized trial. JAMA 309:1154–1162

28. Swaminathan S, Rosner MH, Okusa MD (2015) Emerging therapeutic targets of sepsis-associated acute kidney injury. Semin Nephrol 35:38–54

29. Pickkers P, Heemskerk S, Schouten J et al (2012) Alkaline phosphatase for treatment of sepsis-induced acute kidney injury: a prospective randomized double-blind placebo-controlled trial. Crit Care 16:R14

30. Sardinha J, Kelly MEM, Zhou J, Lehmann C (2014) Experimental cannabinoid 2 receptor-mediated immune modulation in sepsis. Mediators Inflamm 2014:978678

31. Rosas-Ballina M, Olofsson PS, Ochani M et al (2011) Acetylcholine-synthesizing T cells relay neural signals in a vagus nerve circuit. Science 334:98–101

32. Sharfuddin AA, Sandoval RM, Berg DT et al (2009) Soluble thrombomodulin protects ischemic kidneys. J Am Soc Nephrol 20:524–534

33. Unsinger J, McGlynn M, Kasten KR et al (2010) IL-7 promotes T cell viability, trafficking, and functionality and improves survival in sepsis. J Immunol 184:3768–3779

34. Meisel C, Schefold JC, Pschowski R et al (2009) Granulocyte-macrophage colony-stimulating factor to reverse sepsis-associated immunosuppression: a double-blind, randomized, placebo-controlled multicenter trial. Am J Respir Crit Care Med 180:640–648
35. Barbar SD, Binquet C, Monchi M, Bruyère R, Quenot JP (2014) Impact on mortality of the timing of renal replacement therapy in patients with severe acute kidney injury in septic shock: the IDEAL-ICU study (initiation of dialysis early versus delayed in the intensive care unit): study protocol for a randomized controlled trial. Trials 15:270
36. Sun Z, Ye H, Shen X, Chao H, Wu X, Yang J (2014) Continuous venovenous hemofiltration versus extended daily hemofiltration in patients with septic acute kidney injury: a retrospective cohort study. Crit Care 18:R70
37. Ronco C, Bellomo R, Homel P et al (2000) Effects of different doses in continuous veno-venous haemofiltration on outcomes of acute renal failure: a prospective randomised trial. Lancet 356:26–30
38. Bellomo R, Cass A, Cole L et al (2009) Intensity of continuous renal-replacement therapy in critically ill patients. N Engl J Med 361:1627–1638
39. Palevsky PM, Zhang JH, O'Connor TZ et al (2008) Intensity of renal support in critically ill patients with acute kidney injury. N Engl J Med 359:7–20
40. Joannes-Boyau O, Honore PM, Perez P et al. (2013) High-volume versus standard volume haemofiltration for septic shock patients with acute kidney injury (IVOIRE study): a multicenter randomized controlled trial. Intensive Care Med 39:1535–1546
41. Honore PM, Jacobs R, Joannes-Boyau O et al (2013) Newly designed CRRT membranes for sepsis and SIRS – a pragmatic approach for bedside intensivists summarizing the more recent advances: a systematic structured review. ASAIO J 59:99–106
42. Haase M, Bellomo R, Baldwin I et al (2007) Hemodialysis membrane with a high-molecular-weight cutoff and cytokine levels in sepsis complicated by acute renal failure: a phase 1 randomized trial. Am J Kidney Dis 50:296–304
43. Winchester JF, Kellum JA, Ronco C et al (2003) Sorbents in acute renal failure and the systemic inflammatory response syndrome. Blood Purif 21:79–84
44. Cruz DN, Perazella MA, Bellomo R et al (2007) Effectiveness of polymyxin B-immobilized fiber column in sepsis: a systematic review. Crit Care 11:R47
45. Cruz DN, Antonelli M, Fumagalli R et al (2009) Early use of polymyxin B hemoperfusion in abdominal septic shock: the EUPHAS randomized controlled trial. JAMA 301:2445–2452
46. Klein DJ, Foster D, Schorr CA, Kazempour K, Walker PM, Dellinger RP (2014) The EUPHRATES trial (Evaluating the Use of Polymyxin B Hemoperfusion in a Randomized controlled trial of Adults Treated for Endotoxemia and Septic shock): study protocol for a randomized controlled trial. Trials 15:218
47. Yaroustovsky M, Abramyan M, Popok Z et al (2009) Preliminary report regarding the use of selective sorbents in complex cardiac surgery patients with extensive sepsis and prolonged intensive care stay. Blood Purif 28:227–233
48. Peng Z-Y, Bishop JV, Wen X-Y et al (2014) Modulation of chemokine gradients by apheresis redirects leukocyte trafficking to different compartments during sepsis, studies in a rat model. Crit Care 18:R141
49. Livigni S, Bertolini G, Rossi C et al (2014) Efficacy of coupled plasma filtration adsorption (CPFA) in patients with septic shock: A multicenter randomised controlled clinical trial. BMJ Open 4:e003536
50. Tumlin J, Wali R, Williams W et al (2008) Efficacy and safety of renal tubule cell therapy for acute renal failure. J Am Soc Nephrol 19:1034–1040
51. Tumlin JA, Chawla L, Tolwani AJ et al (2013) The effect of the selective cytopheretic device on acute kidney injury outcomes in the intensive care unit: a multicenter pilot study. Semin Dial 26:616–623
52. Camussi G, Cantaluppi V, Deregibus MC, Gatti E, Tetta C (2011) Role of microvesicles in acute kidney injury. Contrib Nephrol 174:191–199

53. Németh K, Leelahavanichkul A, Yuen PST et al (2009) Bone marrow stromal cells attenuate sepsis via prostaglandin E(2)-dependent reprogramming of host macrophages to increase their interleukin-10 production. Nat Med 15:42–49

54. Cribbs SK, Sutcliffe DJ, Taylor WR et al (2012) Circulating endothelial progenitor cells inversely associate with organ dysfunction in sepsis. Intensive Care Med 38:429–436

55. Camussi G, Deregibus MC, Bruno S et al (2011) Exosome/microvesicle-mediated epigenetic reprogramming of cells. Am J Cancer Res 1:98–110

56. Bruno S, Grange C, Collino F et al (2012) Microvesicles derived from mesenchymal stem cells enhance survival in a lethal model of acute kidney injury. PloS One 7:e33115

57. Cantaluppi V, Medica D, Mannari C et al (2015) Endothelial progenitor cell-derived extracellular vesicles protect from complement-mediated mesangial injury in experimental anti-Thy1.1 glomerulonephritis. Nephrol Dial Transplant 30:410–422

Timing of Acute Renal Replacement Therapy

A. Jörres

Introduction

The optimal timing of acute renal replacement therapy (RRT) in patients with acute kidney injury (AKI) remains a subject of intense discussion. Whilst there is agreement that RRT should be initiated if urgent clinical indications are present, such as life-threatening changes in fluid, electrolyte, and acid-base balance that cannot be managed by conservative therapy, the question of when therapy should ideally be initiated in order to prevent the occurrence of these emergency situations largely remains unanswered. The current AKI guidelines [1, 2] advise that the broader clinical context, the presence of conditions that can be modified with RRT, and trends in laboratory test results, rather than single blood urea nitrogen (BUN) and creatinine thresholds alone, should be considered when making the decision to start RRT, thus leaving plenty of room for individualized clinical decision-making.

The present chapter discusses the current state-of-the-art derived from clinical studies that may assist in this decision, and also offers some practical guidance of how to approach this question in patients with AKI.

Clinical Studies Comparing 'Early' and 'Late' Start of Acute RRT

Most of the previous clinical studies in this area are observational, thereby applying arbitrary cut-off variables such as serum creatinine (SCr), serum urea or urine output in order to distinguish 'early' from 'late' start of RRT. Other authors have used time from ICU admission or AKI stage to make this distinction; however, the large heterogeneity of definitions used and the variable quality of these studies have made the interpretation of their results difficult. This is nicely reflected by

A. Jörres (✉)
Med. Klinik m.S. Nephrologie und internistische Intensivmedizin, Virchow-Klinikum,
Charité-Universitätsmedizin Berlin Campus
Berlin, Germany
email: achim.joerres@charite.de

© Springer International Publishing Switzerland 2016
J.-L. Vincent (ed.), *Annual Update in Intensive Care and Emergency Medicine 2016*,
DOI 10.1007/978-3-319-27349-5_10

a systematic review which concluded that 'earlier' initiation of acute RRT in critically ill patients may have a beneficial impact on survival, however, the paucity of randomized controlled trials, use of variable definitions of early RRT, and publication bias precluded definitive conclusions [3], a notion that was supported by another more recent review and meta-analysis [4]. Moreover, the application of different definitions may lead to controversial results in the same study cohort. The BEST Kidney (Beginning and Ending Supportive Therapy) investigators performed a large prospective observational study in 54 centers from 23 countries comparing early vs. late start of RRT in 1,238 patients with AKI [5]. 'Early' RRT was defined as start within the first 2 days of ICU admission, with a serum urea ≤ 24.2 mmol/l or with an SCr ≤ 309 μmol/l; 'late' RRT was defined as start at least 5 days after ICU admission, with a serum urea > 24.2 mmol/l or with an SCr > 309 μmol/l. Interestingly, the authors found no difference in patient survival with early vs. late start defined by serum urea; however, there was a better survival with late start as defined by SCr. By contrast, for timing relative to ICU admission, late RRT was associated with greater crude and covariate-adjusted mortality (odds ratio [OR] 1.95, 95% CI 1.30–2.92, p = 0.001). The conclusion of this study was that timing of acute RRT, a potentially modifiable factor, might have an important influence on patient survival, however, this largely depended on its definition [5].

Other studies have suggested that BUN may indeed serve as a discriminating parameter. Liu and colleagues [6] performed an analysis of survival as a function of the BUN before initiation of acute RRT in 243 patients from the PICARD study (multicenter observational Program to Improve Care in Acute Renal Disease) and found a median pre-RRT BUN of 76 mg/dl. In patients with BUN < 76 mg/dl at the time of initiation of RRT, survival at 14 and 28 days was 80 and 65%, respectively, as compared with 75 and 59% for patients whose BUN was > 76 mg/dl at the time of RRT initiation (p = 0.09). Similarly, in a retrospective analysis of 130 patients with sepsis and AKI, Carl and colleagues [7] found that an 'early' start at BUN of 66 ± 20.4 mg/dl was associated with better survival than 'late' start at BUN of 137 ± 28.4 mg/dl. In contrast, a recent prospective randomized clinical study from a tertiary-care center in western India in 208 adults with community-acquired AKI and progressively worsening azotemia found no differences in survival or dialysis dependency at 3 months between an 'early-start' group according to BUN and/or SCr or a 'usual-start' group who received dialysis when clinically indicated [8]. However, these findings may not be generalizable to central European circumstances as, in both groups, the entry values were rather high suggesting rather late initiation in the two groups (early start: BUN 71.76 ± 21.7 mg/dl and SCr 7.46 ± 5.3 mg/dl; usual start BUN 100.96 ± 32.6 mg/dl and SCr 10.41 ± 63.3 mg/dl).

Ostermann and Chang [9] performed a large retrospective analysis of demographic and physiologic data in 1,847 patients who received acute RRT for AKI in 22 ICUs in the UK and Germany between 1989 and 1999. They found that 54.1% of patients who received acute RRT died in the ICU. Survivors were younger, had a lower APACHE II score and fewer failed organ systems on admission to the ICU. Oligo-anuria, acidosis and concomitant dysfunction of other organs at the time of

RRT were associated with poor survival. In contrast, SCr and serum urea levels only had a weak correlation with outcome after RRT. Their conclusion was that the decision when to start RRT for AKI should be guided more by associated dysfunction of other organ systems, urine output and serum pH rather than absolute SCr and/or urea levels.

Is There a Role for 'Pre-Emptive' RRT?

Several studies have tested the hypothesis that 'pre-emptive' initiation of RRT, that is, well before clinical indications are present, may lead to better outcomes. Bouman and colleagues [10] performed a prospective, randomized clinical study in 106 severely ill mechanically ventilated patients who remained oliguric despite fluid resuscitation, inotropic support, and high-dose intravenous diuretics. Patients were randomized to receive either early high-volume continuous veno-venous hemofiltration (CVVH, 72–96 l/24 h), early low-volume CVVH (24–36 l/24 h), or late low-volume CVVH (24–36 l/24 h). 'Early' CVVH was started within 12 h after the patient fulfilled eligibility criteria (urine output of < 30 ml/h for >6 h despite aggressive fluid resuscitation); the 'late' group received CVVH when conventional (clinical) criteria for RRT were present. On average, CVVH was started 7 h after inclusion in the early groups and 42 h after inclusion in the late group. The authors found that survival at 28 days as well as recovery of renal function were not improved by using high ultrafiltrate volumes or by early initiation of CVVH.

Two studies investigated the effect of CVVH initiation in patients with septic shock, when considering the potential value of CVVH as adjunctive treatment of sepsis. Cole and colleagues [11] randomized 24 patients with septic shock to receive 48 h of isovolemic CVVH (2 l/h fluid exchange) in addition to usual care or to usual care only and found no benefit of early CVVH in terms of organ dysfunction, nor was there a reduction in circulating cytokines or anaphylotoxins. Payen and colleagues [12] reported on a prospective multicenter randomized study in patients with severe sepsis/septic shock who were included in the study within 24 h after their first organ failure. Patients either received CVVH (25 ml/kg/h) for a 96-h period, or conventional care without CVVH. The study was stopped following an interim analysis with 76 patients randomized. The number and severity of organ failures were significantly higher in the CVVH group ($p < 0.05$), and again no effect on plasma cytokine levels could be detected. These findings suggested that early application of standard-dose CVVH may even be deleterious in severe sepsis and septic shock when applied in patients without a 'renal' indication.

More recently, Vaara and colleagues [13] presented results from a substudy of the FINNAKI (Finnish Acute Kidney Injury) study that was conducted in 2011–2012 with 2,901 patients from 17 Finnish ICUs. The patients were classified as "pre-emptive" (no conventional indications) or "classic" (one or more indications) RRT recipients. Patients with "classic" RRT initiation were further divided into the subgroups of "classic-urgent" (RRT initiated ≤ 12 h from manifesting indications) and "classic-delayed" (RRT > 12 h from first indication) start. Additionally, 2,450 patients treated without RRT were matched to patients with "pre-emptive" RRT. Of the 239 patients treated with RRT, 134 fulfilled at least one conventional indication before commencing RRT treatment. These patients had higher crude and adjusted 90-day mortality compared with patients without conventional indications. The highest mortality was observed in the group with delayed RRT (> 24 h) and classic indications, suggesting a benefit for the pre-emptive initiation of RRT in critically ill patients.

By contrast, a recent propensity-matched cohort study comparing dialysis and nondialysis in patients with AKI suggested that pre-emptive dialysis may be putting some patients in harm's way who would otherwise recover without RRT. Wilson and colleagues [14] studied 6,119 adults who were admitted to one of three acute care hospitals within the University of Pennsylvania Health System 2004–2010 and who subsequently developed severe AKI. Of these, 602 received acute dialysis. Demographic, clinical, and laboratory variables were used to generate a time-varying propensity score representing the daily probability of initiation of dialysis for AKI, and not-yet-dialyzed patients were matched to each dialyzed patient according to day of AKI and propensity score. The results indicated that RRT was associated with increased survival when initiated in patients with AKI who had a more elevated creatinine level but was associated with increased mortality when initiated in patients who had lower creatinine values.

Overall the present data suggest that the benefits of RRT, such as the control of metabolic, electrolyte, and volume homeostasis, must be weighed on an individual patient basis against the potential complications of extracorporeal treatments, such as catheter-related complications, bleeding due to anticoagulation, and problems related to under-dosing of medication because of extracorporeal drug elimination.

Conclusion: Practical Approach to Individualized Initiation of RRT

Until conclusive results from ongoing prospective randomized studies comparing early versus delayed RRT, e.g., STARRT-AKI (STandard versus Accelerated initiation of RRT in AKI) [15] or IDEAL-ICU (Initiation of Dialysis EArly versus Late in the Intensive Care Unit) [16], are available, 'pre-emptive' RRT initiation cannot be recommended as a general approach. Instead, the decision to start RRT should remain a clinical decision based on the fluid, electrolyte and metabolic status of each individual patient, with the aim of initiating acute therapy once AKI is established but before overt complications have developed. The British Renal Association AKI guidelines [17] also suggest that the threshold for initiating RRT should be lowered when AKI occurs as part of multiorgan failure, which seems sensible as these patients are at increased risk of suffering from fluid/electrolyte/acid base derangements and at the same time usually have a lower chance of recovering kidney function without dialysis as compared to a patient with isolated AKI.

Box 1. Clinical/Laboratory Indications for the Initiation of Acute Renal Replacement Therapy (RRT).

Urgent
- Uremic organ symptoms (e.g., pericarditis, encephalopathy, neuropathy, myopathy, uremic bleeding)
- Refractory hyperkalemia ($K^+ > 6.5$ mmol/l; typical electrocardiogram [EKG] abnormalities)
- Refractory oligo-anuria and volume overload
- Refractory metabolic acidosis (pH < 7.1)

Relative
- Metabolic control (urea; uremic toxins; electrolytes; acid-base balance)
- Volume management, e.g., creating intravascular space for infusions, blood products or nutrition
- Refractory electrolyte abnormalities: hyponatremia, hypernatremia or hypercalcemia
- Tumor lysis syndrome with hyperuricemia and hyperphosphatemia
- Refractory lactic acidosis
- Severe poisoning or drug overdose
- Severe hypothermia or hyperthermia

Thus, the suggested approach in a patient with isolated AKI would include:

- Check for clinical RRT indications (see Box 1).
- Restore fluid status and correct electrolyte/acid base abnormalities.
- Treat underlying problems, avoid/discontinue nephrotoxins.
- Observe trends in laboratory values.
- Re-evaluate RRT indications regularly (at least daily).
- Consider RRT if oliguria persists and/or creatinine/urea continue to rise over several days.

In a patient with AKI as part of multiorgan failure, the suggested approach would be to:

- Check for clinical RRT indications (see Box 1).
- Restore fluid status and circulation, correct electrolyte/acid base abnormalities.
- Treat underlying problems, avoid/discontinue nephrotoxins.
- If oliguria persists despite adequate fluid resuscitation and hemodynamic management, consider starting RRT without further delay (i.e., within 12–24 h).

On the other hand, the initiation of RRT may be deferred if the underlying clinical condition is improving and there are early signs of renal recovery (e.g., an increase in urine output is observed).

References

1. KDIGO (2012) Clinical practice guideline for acute kidney injury. Kidney Int Suppl 2(2012):89–115
2. Jörres A, John S, Lewington A et al (2013) A European Renal Best Practice (ERBP) position statement on the Kidney Disease Improving Global Outcomes (KDIGO) Clinical Practice Guidelines on Acute Kidney Injury: part 2: renal replacement therapy. Nephrol Dial Transplant 28:2940–2945
3. Seabra VF, Balk EM, Liangos O, Sosa MA, Cendoroglo M, Jaber BL (2008) Timing of renal replacement therapy initiation in acute renal failure: a meta-analysis. Am J Kidney Dis 52:272–284
4. Karvellas CJ, Farhat MR, Sajjad I et al (2011) A comparison of early versus late initiation of renal replacement therapy in critically ill patients with acute kidney injury: a systematic review and meta-analysis. Crit Care 15:R72
5. Bagshaw SM, Uchino S, Bellomo R et al (2009) Timing of renal replacement therapy and clinical outcomes in critically ill patients with severe acute kidney injury. J Crit Care 24:129–140
6. Liu KD, Himmelfarb J, Paganini E et al (2006) Timing of initiation of dialysis in critically ill patients with acute kidney injury. Clin J Am Soc Nephrol 1:915–919
7. Carl DE, Grossman C, Behnke M, Sessler CN, Gehr TW (2010) Effect of timing of dialysis on mortality in critically ill, septic patients with acute renal failure. Hemodial Int 14:11–17
8. Jamale TE, Hase NK, Kulkarni M et al (2013) Earlier-start versus usual-start dialysis in patients with community-acquired acute kidney injury: a randomized controlled trial. Am J Kidney Dis 62:1116–1121
9. Ostermann M, Chang RW (2009) Correlation between parameters at initiation of renal replacement therapy and outcome in patients with acute kidney injury. Crit Care 13:R175
10. Bouman CS, Oudemans-Van Straaten HM, Tijssen JG, Zandstra DF, Kesecioglu J (2002) Effects of early high-volume continuous venovenous hemofiltration on survival and recovery of renal function in intensive care patients with acute renal failure: a prospective, randomized trial. Crit Care Med 30:2205–2211
11. Cole L, Bellomo R, Hart G et al (2002) A phase II randomized, controlled trial of continuous hemofiltration in sepsis. Crit Care Med 30:100–106
12. Payen D, Mateo J, Cavaillon JM, Fraisse F, Floriot C, Vicaut E (2009) Impact of continuous venovenous hemofiltration on organ failure during the early phase of severe sepsis: a randomized controlled trial. Crit Care Med 37:803–810
13. Vaara ST, Reinikainen M, Wald R, Bagshaw SM, Pettila V (2014) Timing of RRT based on the presence of conventional indications. Clin J Am Soc Nephrol 9:1577–1585
14. Wilson FP, Yang W, Machado CA et al (2014) Dialysis versus nondialysis in patients with AKI: a propensity-matched cohort study. Clin J Am Soc Nephrol 9:673–681
15. Smith OM, Wald R, Adhikari NK, Pope K, Weir MA, Bagshaw SM (2013) Standard versus accelerated initiation of renal replacement therapy in acute kidney injury (STARRT-AKI): study protocol for a randomized controlled trial. Trials 14:320
16. Barbar SD, Binquet C, Monchi M, Bruyere R, Quenot JP (2014) Impact on mortality of the timing of renal replacement therapy in patients with severe acute kidney injury in septic shock: the IDEAL-ICU study (initiation of dialysis early versus delayed in the intensive care unit): study protocol for a randomized controlled trial. Trials 15:270
17. Lewington A, Kanagasundaram S (2011) Renal Association Clinical Practice Guidelines on acute kidney injury. Nephron Clin Pract 118(Suppl 1):349–390

(Multiple) Organ Support Therapy Beyond AKI

Z. Ricci, S. Romagnoli, and C. Ronco

Introduction

More than 30 years ago, extracorporeal treatment was used in the intensive care unit (ICU) for the first time in order to deliver hemodialysis. Due to improvements in medical and surgical standards of care and an increase in the average age of patients, clinicians are today facing a significant increase in patients' severity of illness at ICU admission and the frequent occurrence of multiple organ failure (MOF) with the simultaneous dysfunction of two or more organs. Extracorporeal treatments to support different organs (kidneys, liver, lungs, heart, septic blood) are now common in the ICU. However, paralleling the evolution of continuous dialytic treatments over the last two decades, in recent years, multiple organ support therapy (MOST) has been delivered as a "Christmas-tree like" addition of one system on another (e.g., continuous renal replacement therapy [CRRT] on extracorporeal membrane oxygenation [ECMO] or molecular adsorbent recycling system [MARS] on CRRT). Current developments and the future of MOST foresee the application of dedicated

Z. Ricci (✉)
Department of Cardiology and Cardiac Surgery, Bambino Gesù Children's Hospital
Rome, Italy
email: z.ricci@libero.it

S. Romagnoli
Department of Health Science, Section of Anesthesiology and Intensive Care, University of Florence
Florence, Italy
Department of Anesthesia and Intensive Care, Azienda Ospedaliero-Universitaria Careggi
Florence, Italy

C. Ronco
Department of Nephrology, Dialysis and Transplantation, San Bortolo Hospital
Vicenza, Italy
International Renal Research Institute, San Bortolo Hospital
Vicenza, Italy

© Springer International Publishing Switzerland 2016   117
J.-L. Vincent (ed.), *Annual Update in Intensive Care and Emergency Medicine 2016*,
DOI 10.1007/978-3-319-27349-5_11

and integrated multipurpose advanced platforms for the support of patients with MOF. This review will detail extracorporeal blood purification treatments that can be delivered for dysfunction of organs other than the kidneys.

Sepsis

Although mortality related to sepsis has significantly decreased throughout the last decade, it still represents a major challenge for healthcare systems from clinical and economical points of view [1, 2]. The broad heterogeneity of clinical presentations and the complex interplay of host pro-inflammatory and anti-inflammatory processes are among the principal obstacles for further reduction in sepsis-related morbidity and mortality. Since the imbalance between hyper-inflammation and immunosuppression is supposed to be a key factor in determining outcomes, during recent years most research on sepsis has been focused on re-establishing an equilibrium in the cytokine-mediated inflammation by clearing them from the blood using CRRT-based techniques [3].

High-Volume Hemofiltration

It has been speculated that CRRT 'pushed' to doses higher than usual (>45 ml/kg/h; high volume hemofiltration, HVHF) may play a role in blood purification in septic patients by clearing the bloodstream of cytokines. Animal models of severe sepsis demonstrated a beneficial effect of HVHF on hemodynamics, proportional to the intensity of ultrafiltration [4] and, based on this hypothesis, different protocols have been developed and tested [5]. A Cochrane analysis published in 2013, including randomized controlled trials (RCTs) and quasi-randomized trials, that compared HVHF to standard dialysis in adult ICU patients, concluded that the evidence was still insufficient to recommend its use in septic critically ill patients [6]. A systematic review and meta-analysis of studies performed between 1966 and 2013 was recently published [7]. The analysis included four RCTs (470 participants) that compared HVHF (effluent rate >50 ml/kg/h) and standard hemofiltration (HF) in patients with sepsis and septic shock. Pooled analysis for 28-day mortality did not show any difference between HVHF and HF in kidney recovery, improvement in hemodynamics or reduction in ICU or hospital lengths of stay. In addition, significant side effects, including hypophosphatemia and hypokalemia, were more common in the HVHF group. Based on the current literature, HVHF cannot be recommended for routine use in sepsis and septic acute kidney injury (AKI). Moreover, adverse effects should be carefully monitored when more intense doses of CRRT are used in septic and non-septic patients.

Polymyxin B Hemoperfusion

High levels of endotoxin activity, a basic component of the outer membrane of Gram-negative bacteria, have been associated with worse clinical outcomes [8]. Polymyxin B hemoperfusion (PMX-HP) is a technique based on the high affinity for polymyxin B of endotoxin, which, during extracorporeal hemoperfusion, remains bound to the filter. In 2009, a multicenter randomized controlled study [9] showed, in 64 patients with severe sepsis or septic shock, that PMX-HP, added to conventional therapy, significantly improved hemodynamics and organ dysfunction and reduced 28-day mortality. More recently, a larger multicenter randomized controlled study including 232 patients with septic shock (119 vs 113 controls) did not confirm the previous findings [10]: there was no difference in 28-day mortality between the study group and the control patients. By contrast, a recent retrospective analysis, part of an ongoing study (EUPHAS2; PMX-HP in abdominal vs non-abdominal sepsis), showed that the sequential organ failure assessment (SOFA) score decreased significantly 72 h after PMX-HP in patients with abdominal sepsis ($p < 0.001$), 28-day mortality was 35% in abdominal sepsis vs 49% in patients with non-abdominal sepsis, and in-hospital mortality was 44% in abdominal sepsis vs 55% in non-abdominal sepsis [11]. Based on the current evidence, the efficacy of PMX-HP is currently being questioned and new data are absolutely necessary to clarify its role in abdominal and non-abdominal septic patients.

High Cut-Off Hemofiltration

Because of the role of the humoral mediators of the immune system in the pathogenesis of sepsis, many attempts have been made to remove the cytokines from the bloodstream [12]. High cut-off (HCO) membranes have pore diameters ($> 0.01\,\mu m$) that allow molecules up to 60 kDa to pass [13]. A review that included 23 publications on HCO hemofiltration (HCO-HF), showed that a reduction in inflammatory and anti-inflammatory cytokines (interleukin [IL]-4, IL-6, IL-1 receptor antagonist [IL-1ra], IL-8, IL-10, IL-12, tumor necrosis factor [TNF]-α) was common in all the studies [13]. Moreover, cytokine removal was associated with significant improvement in hemodynamics, oxygenation, and organ dysfunction [13]. A 16-ICU multicenter observational study, designed to evaluate changes in inflammatory biomarkers and tissue oxygenation/perfusion indexes in septic ICU patients with AKI during HCO-CVVHD, has recently been concluded and preliminary results released [14]. A significant improvement in organ function was demonstrated but there was no reduction in mortality. Before drawing definitive conclusions on the effects of HCO-HF in sepsis, some factors need to be considered: first, the current literature is biased by the lack of a standardized definition and classification of HCO dialysis membranes making comparison among studies difficult [13, 15]; second, heterogeneity of the clinical picture of septic patients requires strict patient selection; third, which mediators should be removed and which should not during different phases of sepsis has not been established [16]; and, finally, technology that can select specific molecules has not been developed so far.

Coupled Plasma Filtration Adsorption

Coupled plasma filtration adsorption (CPFA) is a complex extracorporeal blood purification technique: plasma, separated from blood by a plasma-filter, is run through a synthetic resin cartridge (with adsorption capacity for inflammatory mediators) and then returned to the blood circuit where a hemofilter removes excess fluid and allows renal replacement [17, 18]. In other words, CPFA is a sorbent technology based on RRT for removal of endotoxin, bacterial products and both pro- and anti-inflammatory endogenous substances in septic patients with AKI [19]. In 2014, Livigni and colleagues, published the results from a multicenter, randomized trial comparing CPFA with standard care in the treatment of critically ill patients with septic shock [20]. There were no statistically significant differences in hospital mortality secondary endpoints (occurrence of new organ failure), or free-ICU days during the first 30 days. The authors suggested that the technical difficulties occurring during the treatments (early clotting) may have biased the results. A new trial, including only patients achieving the prescribed CPFA treatment is currently ongoing: in order to limit clotting-related treatment failure, only citrate is now allowed as anticoagulant [20]. Technical difficulties, frequently met during CPFA application, should be carefully weighed with potential, theoretical advantages. New generation machines, implementing default citrate anticoagulation, have recently been released into the market. In a recent study, including 15 critically ill patients with septic shock, citrate pharmacokinetics during CPFA were evaluated [21]. The study showed that high doses of citrate (needed for this complex treatment) can be safely managed with predilution hemodiafiltration and pre/postdilution hemofiltration.

Although promising, the results from studies in septic patients undergoing blood purification therapies are totally inconclusive. It is possible that key factors to improve extracorporeal treatment for sepsis will be the identification of a selected population of patients, targeting the clearance of a specific molecular pattern, and improved understanding of the optimal timing for such treatments.

Lung

The majority of ICU patients with AKI are affected by MOF and many patients need respiratory and renal support [22–25]. Patients who develop severe AKI are burdened by extrarenal complications and respiratory function is frequently impaired because of pulmonary congestion and increased vascular permeability [26]. At the same time, mechanical ventilation itself causes negative effects on kidney function through hemodynamic impairment, biohumoral mediators, blood gas disorders, and biotrauma (one of the components of ventilator-induced lung injury [VILI]) highlighting a clear negative organ crosstalk [27, 28]. Barotrauma (high volumes leading to high transpulmonary pressures), volutrauma (alveolar overdistention), atelectrauma (repetitive opening and closing of alveoli) represent the other components of VILI often associated with mechanical ventilation [28]. All these physical and biochemical stresses, mutually and simultaneously interacting, lead to local and systemic inflammatory reactions that negatively impact distal organs and promote the development of MOF [29, 30]. A landmark study published in 2000 [31] in patients with acute respiratory distress syndrome (ARDS), strongly contributed to highlight that mechanical ventilation may further worsen already injured lungs and stimulated the practice of protective ventilation [32]. The concept of protective ventilation relies on the observation that 'less aggressive' ventilation – low tidal volumes and airway pressures – limits pulmonary damage and respiratory complications [28, 33, 34]. On the other hand, when protective ventilation cannot maintain normal values of partial pressure of carbon dioxide in the arterial blood ($PaCO_2$), so-called 'permissive hypercapnia' is usually tolerated as a "lesser evil" [35]. Although permissive hypercapnia has proved advantages and benefits [36], it may also exert multiple negative effects [37–39]. In order to limit excessive CO_2 accumulation, devices for extracorporeal CO_2 removal ($ECCO_2R$), have been developed. The general concept of an $ECCO_2R$ system is very close to the hemofiltration circuit: the blood is drained from the patients, CO_2 is cleared by a membrane and blood is then re-injected into the systemic circulation. Apart from the first attempts to remove CO_2 through hemodialysis [40, 41], currently $ECCO_2R$ is mainly applied in two clinical conditions: chronic obstructive pulmonary disease (COPD) patients with hypercapnic respiratory failure who fail non-invasive ventilation (NIV) [42, 43] and ARDS patients with excessive hypercapnia [44]. From a technical point of view, two principal $ECCO_2R$ systems can be considered (Table 1): the arteriovenous (AV) and the veno-venous (VV) configurations. The AV modality does not need an artificial pump because it uses the AV pressure gradient to generate flow through a low resistance membrane [45]. Two main drawbacks limit this pumpless system: the need for an AV pressure gradient, which is unsuitable for hemodynamically unstable patients, and the cannulation of a major artery, which can result in distal ischemia [46]. The VV configuration, adopted in newer $ECCO_2R$ devices, uses 14–18 French (Fr) venous double cannulas in a pumped system (which generates a blood flow rate of 300–500 ml/min) equipped with a membrane (gas exchanger) that allows the elimination of CO_2 [47]. In order to clear CO_2, $ECCO_2R$ requires higher pump flow rates than RRT. By contrast, during ECMO, blood oxygenation is delivered with blood flows exceeding 3 l/min [48, 49]. $ECCO_2R$ (lowflow) may be integrated into a CRRT system, possibly using the same extracorporeal circuit (Table 1). Although pioneering attempts date to about 25 years ago [50], modern applications with (easy-to-use) standard pump-driven RRT-circuits are very recent: Godet and coworkers [51] instrumented five adult female healthy pigs with a low flow CO_2 removal device (PrismaLung®, Hospal®) integrated on a CRRT platform (a device based on a Prismaflex® system). The gas exchanger membrane was connected into the CRRT circuit, in place of the hemofilter. Satisfactory CO_2 clearance was obtained (*in vivo* mean decrease of 14%) demonstrating the applicability of the system. Forster and colleagues, in a pilot study, applied a CRRT

Table 1 Currently available CO_2 removal systems

Device	Company	ECCO$_2$R/ CRRT/ECMO	Characteristics	Information
iLA-membrane ventilator®	Novalung, Germany	ECCO$_2$R	Membrane ventilator for pumpless (AV configuration) extrapulmonary lung support. Surface area of gas exchange membrane 1.3 m^2	www.novalung.com
Novalung iLA activve®	Novalung, Germany	From ECCO$_2$R to ECMO	Small portable diagonal pump and operational console. It may run at low or high flow rates (0.5 to >4.5 l/min) covering wide range of respiratory support from CO$_2$ clearance to complete oxygenation and ventilation support (depending on the gas exchanger installed)	www.novalung.com
PALP™	Maquet, Germany	ECCO$_2$R	Low-flow system based on Maquet's Cardiohelp console (portable heart-lung support system – ECMO)	www.maquet.com
Hemolung®	A-lung Technologies, USA	ECCO$_2$R	Small (0.67 m^2) surface area. Specifically designed for CO$_2$ removal generally recommended for COPD patients	www.alung.com
Decap®	Hemodec, Italy	ECCO$_2$R	Uses a membrane lung (0.3 to 1.35 m^2) connected in series with a hemodialysis filter. Flow rates < 500 ml/min. Useful for patients requiring both pulmonary and renal support	www.hemodec.com
Abylcap®	Bellco, Italy	ECCO$_2$R (insertable in Lynda®-CPFA®)	Membrane surface area 0.67 m^2, blood flow 280 to 350 ml/min, phosphorylcholine coated	www.bellco.net
Prisma-Lung®	Medos Medizintechnik AG	ECCO$_2$R-CRRT	The gas exchanger (0.32 m^2, heparin coated, maximal blood flow rate 450 ml/min) can be used in presence or in absence of the hemodialyzer	www.gambro.com
Aferetica®	Aferetica. Purification therapy, Italy	ECCO$_2$R-CRRT	Blood flows 30–450 ml/min. Infusion fluid in post-dilution: after the HF and before the ECCO$_2$R. The kit allows the CO$_2$ removal treatment to be performed for 5 days	www.aferetica.com

iLA: interventional lung assist; *PALP*: pump-assisted lung protection; *ECCO$_2$R*: extracorporeal CO$_2$ removal; *CO$_2$*: carbon dioxide; *ECMO*: extracorporeal membrane oxygenation; *COPD*: chronic obstructive pulmonary disease; *AV*: arterio-venous; *CPFA*: coupled plasma filtration adsorption; *HF*: hemofilter.

system, with a ECCO$_2$R device, in 10 critically ill patients with combined respiratory-renal failure [52]. A standard CRRT system was integrated, in series, with a hollow-fiber gas. This "lung-assisting renal replacement system" gave encouraging results since the treatment allowed a mean 28.1% decrease in PaCO$_2$ with a blood flow of 378 ml/min. Finally, Quintard and colleagues, in 16 mechanically ventilated patients with respiratory acidosis and AKI requiring ongoing CRRT, applied a gas exchanger originally designed for pediatric use [53]. The system significantly reduced the PaCO$_2$ (−31% at 6 h and −39% at 12 h) and increased arterial pH (+0.16 at 6 h and +0.23 at 12 h) without complications.

Liver

Acute liver dysfunction in the ICU is not a rare occurrence although its incidence may vary significantly, depending on whether or not liver disease referral centers are considered. The main cause of acute liver failure (ALF) is acetaminophen toxicity [54]. Interestingly, in critically ill patients, liver disease is frequently at the pyramid of the development of MOF, being the trigger of several pathological pathways, eventually involving lungs, kidneys and brain [54]. Essentially two kinds of hepatic syndrome can be treated in the ICU: ALF and acute-on-chronic liver failure (ACLF). ALF is defined as the development of hepatic encephalopathy within 26 weeks of jaundice and coagulopathy with an international normalized ratio (INR) > 1.5 in a patient with no previous liver disease. ACLF is an acute worsening of hepatic function in cirrhotic patients, either secondary to deterioration of initial liver injury (alcoholic hepatitis, superimposed viral hepatitis, portal vein thrombosis, drug-induced liver injury) or caused by secondary liver involvement in the context of trauma, surgery, sepsis or, more generically, MOF.

The kidneys are involved in about 50% of overall liver failure cases and AKI is an independent risk factor for mortality. In cirrhotic patients with renal involvement, a very well studied and peculiar disease has been described: hepato-renal syndrome (HRS) [55]. The definition of HRS has been recently updated to "a potentially reversible syndrome that occurs in patients with cirrhosis, ascites and liver failure that is characterized by impaired kidney function, marked alterations in cardiovascular function, and over-activity of the sympathetic nervous system and renin-angiotensin system. Severe renal vasoconstriction leads to a decrease of glomerular filtration rate. HRS may appear spontaneously or can follow a precipitating event" [55].

When extracorporeal treatments for liver or combined liver-kidney support are indicated, several options have been described: no conclusive evidence can be currently recommended since no specific extracorporeal treatment has shown a consistent increase in survival with respect to liver transplantation. Interestingly, Naka and coworkers [56], in a retrospective study, compared the effects of CVVH in liver failure patients admitted to the ICU and in patients who had received liver transplantation. The authors showed that CVVH achieved very good outcomes in transplanted patients, but was not effective in improving blood chemistry (creatinine, lactate, acidosis) or mortality in patients with persistent liver dysfunction.

Important considerations on the dialytic support of ALF patients are that: coagulation derangements have to be taken into account and that generally a low heparin approach should be considered [56]; citrate may not be well tolerated even though several authors have described satisfactory use even in ALF patients [57]; and intermittent techniques should not be recommended due to the risk of increasing intracranial pressure [58]. Very recently, with a similar rationale but using an (11 year long) RCT design, Larsen and coworkers showed that treatment with high volume plasma exchange (1–2 l/h up to 8–10 l per day for three consecutive days) improved hospital survival in ALF patients compared to standard medical treatment (59 vs 48%) [59]. By contrast with Naka's observations, this improvement was not particularly evident in patients who underwent liver transplantation but in those who were not listed to receive a transplantation: this study has the merit of being one of the first to show the benefit of extracorporeal therapy other than after liver transplantation. The authors elegantly showed that high volume plasma exchange was able to significantly blunt the inflammatory syndrome of treated patients and to correct INR, bilirubin, alanine transaminase (ALT) and ammonia levels. Interestingly plasma exchange also prevented the occurrence of AKI and need for RRT [59].

Unlike hemodialysis for the kidneys, specific liver support systems able to effectively support liver function until either recovery or transplant remain elusive [60]. Specific extracorporeal liver substitution can currently be achieved by albumin dialysis (MARS), fractionated plasma separation and adsorption (Prometheus) – classified as artificial systems- and bioartificial systems that combine plasma separation with perfusion of bio-reactors filled with human or animal hepatocytes (such as the extracorporeal liver assist device [ELAD], Vital Therapies, San Diego, California, USA). MARS and Prometheus are available commercially and have been repeatedly tested in large case series and randomized trials: neither has been shown to decrease mortality in patients with ACLF [60]. A recent important trial that compared MARS with medical therapy in patients with ALF and listed for liver transplant failed to demonstrate benefit because the median time to transplantation was too short to allow MARS enough time to exert any significant beneficial effect [61]. Improved survival of ALF and ACLF patients treated with bioartificial liver support systems has also never been clearly demonstrated [60]. At present, intense research into artificial liver support is ongoing even though there is currently little evidence to support routine clinical use in ALF.

Heart

Systemic congestion in the context of acute heart failure includes pulmonary insufficiency but also impairment of renal function. Pharmacological decongestion with loop diuretics is fundamental but has been commonly associated with AKI and type 1 cardiorenal syndrome [62]. On this background (injured kidneys due to the primary cardiac illness and to pharmacologic management) slow continuous ultrafiltration (SCUF) was described many years ago in order to artificially remove plasma water and relieve cardiopulmonary symptoms, thus bypassing the need for intense diuresis [63]. In case of a reno-cardiac syndrome (acute heart failure secondary to acute or chronic renal failure), application of artificial fluid balance control and volume unloading for pulmonary edema management to a dialytic session is a common clinical picture encountered by nephrologists [64]. SCUF is currently considered as a last chance therapy by the European Society of Cardiology guidelines for management of patients with acute heart failure that is refractory to diuretic therapy [65]. Several randomized trials have been conducted in order to verify whether extracorporeal water removal might be beneficial compared to diuretic therapy. The UNLOAD (Ultrafiltration Versus Intravenous Diuretics for Patients Hospitalized for Acute Decompensated Heart Failure) Study showed that ultrafiltration allowed a greater amount of plasma water to be removed than did furosemide [66]. Interestingly, however, more patients in the ultrafiltration group than in the diuretic arm experienced an increase in creatinine levels of 0.3 mg/dl. Of note, the timing, dose, duration and clinical target of ultrafiltration remains to be investigated. By contrast, the CARRESS-HF (Cardiorenal Rescue Study in Acute Decompensated Heart Failure) showed that ultrafiltration was not associated with a significant difference in weight loss at 96 h and, again, was associated with a significantly greater increase in creatinine levels [67]. Another small recent randomized trial (Continuous Ultrafiltration for cOngestive heaRt failure, CUORE), showed that extracorporeal ultrafiltration was associated with prolonged clinical stabilization and a greater freedom from re-hospitalization for acute heart failure [68].

Given the apparently controversial results of these trials, which are probably due to different therapeutic algorithms, clinical targets and severity of included patients, it seems reasonable to reserve ultrafiltration for use in the most severely ill patients with initial signs of diuretic resistance. Furthermore, pharmacologic and extracorporeal removal of water should not be seen as alternative approaches but may be considered as synergistic. Finally, institutional expertise with extracorporeal devices should always be taken into account, because it may have a significant impact on final outcomes. The results of the large Aquapheresis versus Intravenous Diuretics and Hospitalizations for Heart Failure (AVOID-HF) trial will likely clarify the safety and effectiveness of ultrafiltration therapy [69]. As far as worsening of renal function during decongestion therapies is concerned, it must be noted that loop diuretics and ultrafiltration have both been associated with increased creatinine levels. Extracorporeal water removal, however, has not been associated with neuro-hormonal activation and it should not activate tubulo-glomerular feedback as diuretics do [70]. Excessive intravascular depletion due to aggressive ultrafiltration prescription or a severely decreased glomerular filtration rate before ultrafiltration start may be possible reasons for the described increase in creatinine levels [70]. Furthermore, regardless of whether decongestion is achieved with drugs or ultrafiltration, a recent *post hoc* analysis of patients enrolled in the Diuretic Optimization Strategy Evaluation in Acute Decompensated Heart Failure (DOSE-AHF) and CARRESS-HF trials showed that only patients free of signs of orthodema at discharge had lower 60-day rates of death, rehospitalization, or unscheduled visits compared to those having residual orthodema [71]. The authors hypothesize that despite congestion relief, therapies might be ineffective in definitively treating orthodema during hospitalization. It can be speculated that tools, such as biomarkers, bioimpedance, echocardiography, and minimally invasive hemodynamic monitors, should also be implemented in order to improve patient care.

Conclusions

New extracorporeal therapies are conceived to provide supportive treatment beyond the classic renal indications: today, consistent artificial support can be provided to multiple organs simultaneously. Ideally, new machines will include multiple platforms in which different circuits and filters can be used in combination to support renal, heart, liver, and lung function according to increasing patient needs and severity of MOF. Similarly to what happened about 30 years ago for hemofiltration use in critically ill patients, which was initially seen as cumbersome and reserved for a few patients and has now become a routine tool, MOST may today appear somewhat naïve and burdened by an excessive rate of treatment failures: technological improvements, increased clinical experience and marked improvements in clinical results are certainly expected in the next few years.

References

1. Vincent J, Opal S, Marshall J, Tracey K (2013) Sepsis definitions: time for change. Lancet 381:774–775
2. Kaukonen K-M, Bailey M, Suzuki S et al (2014) Mortality related to severe sepsis and septic shock among critically ill patients in Australia and New Zealand, 2000–2012. JAMA 311:1308–1316
3. Remick DG (2011) The pathogenesis of sepsis. Annu Rev Pathol 6:19–48
4. Lonneman G (1999) Tumor necrosis factor-alpha during continuous high-flux hemodialysis in sepsis with acute renal failure. Kidney Int 56:S84–S87
5. Lehner GF, Wiedermann CJ, Joannidis M (2014) a systematic review and meta-analysis. Minerva Anestesiol 80:595–609
6. Borthwick E, Hill C, Rabindranath K et al (2013) High-volume haemofiltration for sepsis. Cochrane Database Syst Rev 1:CD008075
7. Clark E, Molnar AO, Joannes-Boyau O et al (2014) High-volume hemofiltration for septic acute kidney injury: a systematic review and meta-analysis. Crit Care 18:R7
8. Marshall JC, Foster D, Vincent JL et al (2004) Diagnostic and prognostic implications of endotoxemia in critical illness: results of the MEDIC study. J Infect Dis 190:527–534
9. Cruz DN, Antonelli M, Fumagalli R, Foltran F (2009) Early use of polymyxin b hemoperfusion in abdominal septic shock. JAMA 301:2445–2452
10. Payen DM, Guilhot J, Launey Y et al (2015) Early use of polymyxin B hemoperfusion in patients with septic shock due to peritonitis: a multicenter randomized control trial. Intensive Care Med 41:975–984
11. Early Use of Polymyxin B Hemoperfusion in the Abdominal Sepsis 2 Collaborative Group (2014) Polymyxin B hemoperfusion in clinical practice: The picture from an unbound collaborative registry. Blood Purif 37:22–25

12. Connolly A, Vernon D (2000) Manipulations of the metabolic response for management of patients with severe surgical illness: review. World J Surg 24:696–704
13. Villa G, Zaragoza JJ, Sharma A et al (2014) Cytokine removal with high cut-off membrane: review of literature. Blood Purif 38:167–173
14. Villa G, Chelazzi C, Valente S et al (2014) Hemodialysis with high cutoff membranes improves tissue perfusion in severe sepsis: preliminary data of the Sepsis in Florence sTudy (SIFT). Crit Care 18:401
15. Ronco C (2014) Standard nomenclature for renal replacement therapy in acute kidney injury: very much needed! Blood Purif 38:37–38
16. Hotchkiss RS, Monneret G, Payen D (2013) Sepsis-induced immunosuppression: from cellular dysfunctions to immunotherapy. Nat Rev Immunol 13:862–874
17. Ronco C, Brendolan A, Lonnemann G et al (2002) A pilot study of coupled plasma filtration with adsorption in septic shock. Crit Care Med 30:1250–1255
18. Formica M, Olivieri C, Livigni S et al (2003) Hemodynamic response to coupled plasmafiltration-adsorption in human septic shock. Intensive Care Med 29:703–708
19. Bellomo R, Tetta C, Ronco C (2003) Coupled plasma filtration adsorption. Intensive Care Med 29:1222–1228
20. Livigni S, Bertolini G, Rossi C et al (2014) Efficacy of coupled plasma filtration adsorption (CPFA) in patients with septic shock: A multicenter randomised controlled clinical trial. BMJ open 4:e003536
21. Mariano F, Morselli M, Holló Z et al (2015) Citrate pharmacokinetics at high levels of circuit citratemia during coupled plasma filtration adsorption. Nephrol Dial Transplant 30:1911–1919
22. Bone R, Balk R, Cerra F et al (2009) Definitions for sepsis and organ failure and guidelines for the use of innovative therapies in sepsis. The ACCP/SCCM Consensus Conference Committee. American College of Chest Physicians/Society of Critical Care Medicine. 1992. Chest 136(5 Suppl):e28
23. Liu KD, Matthay M (2008) Advances in critical care for the nephrologist: Acute lung injury/ARDS. Clin J Am Soc Nephrol 3:578–586
24. Esteban A, Alía I, Gordo F et al (2000) Prospective randomized trial ventilation and volume-controlled ventilation in ARDS. Chest 117:1690–1696
25. Dasta JF, Mclaughlin TP, Mody SH, Piech CT (2005) Daily cost of an intensive care unit day: The contribution of mechanical ventilation. Crit Care Med 33:1266–1271
26. Vieira JM, Castro I, Curvello-Neto A et al (2007) Effect of acute kidney injury on weaning from mechanical ventilation in critically ill patients. Crit Care Med 35:184–191
27. Kuiper JW, Groeneveld BJ, Slutsky AS, Plötz FB (2005) Mechanical ventilation and acute renal failure. Crit Care Med 33:1408–1415
28. Slutsky A, Ranieri V (2013) Ventilator-induced lung injury. N Engl J Med 369:2126–2136
29. Tremblay L, Slutsky A (1998) Ventilator-induced injury: from barotrauma to biotrauma. Proc Assoc Am Physicians 110:482–488
30. Kuiper JW, Vaschetto R, Della Corte F et al (2011) Bench-to-bedside review: Ventilation-induced renal injury through systemic mediator release – just theory or a causal relationship? Crit Care 15:228
31. ARDSNetwork (2000) Ventilation with lower tidal volumes as compared with traditional tidal volumes for acute lung injury and the acute respiratory distress syndrome. N Engl J Med 342:1301–1308
32. Fitzgerald M, Millar J, Blackwood B et al (2014) Extracorporeal carbon dioxide removal for patients with acute respiratory failure secondary to the acute respiratory distress syndrome: a systematic review. Crit Care 18:222
33. Serpa Neto A, Simonis FD, Barbas CSV et al (2015) Lung-protective ventilation with low tidal volumes and the occurrence of pulmonary complications in patients without acute respiratory distress syndrome. Crit Care Med 28:1
34. Futier E, Jaber S (2014) Lung-protective ventilation in abdominal surgery. Curr Opin Crit Care 20:426–430

35. Feihl F, Perret C (1998) Permissive hypercapnia. European Respiratory Monograph 3:162–173
36. Contreras M, Masterson C, Laffey J (2015) Permissive hypercapnia: what to remember. Curr Opin Crit Care 18:26–37
37. Brian JJ (1998) Carbon dioxide and the cerebral circulation. Anesthesiology 88:1365–86
38. Doerr CH, Gajic O, Berrios JC et al (2005) Hypercapnic acidosis impairs plasma membrane wound reseating in ventilator-injured lungs. Am J Respir Crit Care Med 171:1371–1377
39. Curley G, Contreras M, Nichol A et al (2010) Hypercapnia and acidosis in sepsis: a double-edged sword? Anesthesiology 112:462–472
40. Isobe J, Mizuno H, Matsunobe S et al (1989) A new type of low blood flow ECCO$_2$R using a hemodialysis system in apneic states. ASAIO Trans 35:638–639
41. Nolte SH, Jonitz WJ, Grau J et al (1989) Hemodialysis for extracorporeal bicarbonate/CO2 removal (ECBicCO2R) and apneic oxygenation for respiratory failure in the newborn. Theory and preliminary results in animal experiments. ASAIO Trans 35:30–34
42. Quinnell TG, Pilsworth S, Shneerson JM, Smith IE (2006) Prolonged invasive ventilation following acute ventilatory failure in COPD: weaning Results, survival, and the role of noninvasive ventilation. Chest 129:133–139
43. Menzies R, Gibbons W, Goldberg P (1989) Determinants of weaning and survival among patients with COPD who require mechanical ventilation for acute respiratory failure. Chest 95:398–405
44. Bein T, Weber-Carstens S, Goldmann A et al (2013) Lower tidal volume strategy ($\approx$3 ml/kg) combined with extracorporeal CO2 removal versus "conventional" protective ventilation (6 ml/kg) in severe ARDS: The prospective randomized Xtravent-study. Intensive Care Med 39:847–856
45. Cove ME, MacLaren G, Federspiel WJ, Kellum J (2012) Bench to bedside review: Extracorporeal carbon dioxide removal, past present and future. Crit Care 16:232
46. Bein T, Weber F, Philipp A et al (2006) A new pumpless extracorporeal interventional lung assist in critical hypoxemia/hypercapnia. Crit Care Med 34:1372–1377
47. Del Sorbo L, Pisani L, Filippini C et al (2013) Extracorporeal CO2 removal in Hypercapnic patients at risk of noninvasive ventilation failure: a matched cohort study with historical control. Crit Care Med 43:120–127
48. Ricci Z, Romagnoli S, Ronco C (2014) Extracorporeal support therapies. In: Miller R (ed) Miller's Anesthesia, 2-Volume Set, 8th edn. Elsevier, Philadelphia, pp 3158–3181
49. MacLaren G, Combes A, Bartlett R (2011) Respiratory dialysis is not extracorporeal membrane oxygenation. Crit Care Med 39:2787–2788
50. Young J, Dorrington K, Blake G, Ryder W (1992) Femoral arteriovenous extracorporeal carbon dioxide elimination using low blood flow. Crit Care Med 20:805–809
51. Godet T, Combes A, Zogheib E et al (2015) Novel CO2 removal device driven by a renal-replacement system without hemofilter. A first step experimental validation. Anaesth Crit Care Pain Med 34:135–140
52. Forster C, Schriewer J, John S et al (2013) Low-flow CO2 removal integrated into a renal-replacement circuit can reduce acidosis and decrease vasopressor requirements. Crit Care 17:R154
53. Quintard JM, Barbot O, Thevenot F, de Matteis O, Benayoun L, Leibinger F (2014) Partial extracorporeal carbon dioxide removal using a standard continuous renal replacement therapy device. ASAIO J 60:564–569
54. Siddiqui MS, Stravitz RT (2014) Intensive care unit management of patients with liver failure. Clin Liver Dis 18:957–978
55. Fagundes C, Ginès P (2012) Hepatorenal syndrome: A severe, but treatable, cause of kidney failure in cirrhosis. Am J Kidney Dis 59:874–885
56. Naka T, Wan L, Bellomo R et al (2004) Kidney failure associated with liver transplantation or liver failure: the impact of continuous veno-venous hemofiltration. Int J Artif Organs 27:949–955

57. Patel S, Wendon J (2012) Regional citrate anticoagulation in patients with liver failure – time for a rethink? Crit Care 16:153
58. Leventhal TM, Liu KD (2015) What a nephrologist needs to know about acute liver failure. Adv Chronic Kidney Dis 22:376–381
59. Larsen FS, Schmidt LE, Bernsmeier C et al (2016) High-volume plasma exchange in patients with acute liver failure: An open randomised controlled trial. J Hepatol 64:69–78
60. Willars C (2014) Update in intensive care medicine: acute liver failure. Initial management, supportive treatment and who to transplant. Curr Opin Crit Care 20:202–209
61. Saliba F, Camus C, Durand F et al (2013) Albumin dialysis with a noncell artificial liver support device in patients with acute liver failure. Ann Intern Med 159:522–531
62. Palazzuoli A, Ruocco G, Ronco C, McCullough P (2015) Loop diuretics in acute heart failure: beyond the decongestive relief for the kidney. Crit Care 19:296
63. Nalesso F, Garzotto F, Ronco C (2010) Technical aspects of extracorporeal ultrafiltration: Mechanisms, monitoring and dedicated technology. Contrib Nephrol 164:199–208
64. Ronco C, Haapio M, House A (2008) Cardiorenal syndrome. J Am Coll Cardiol 52:1527–1539
65. McMurray JJV, Adamopoulos S, Anker SD et al (2012) ESC Guidelines for the diagnosis and treatment of acute and chronic heart failure 2012: The Task Force for the Diagnosis and Treatment of Acute and Chronic Heart Failure 2012 of the European Society of Cardiology. Eur Heart J 33:1787–1847
66. Costanzo MR, Guglin ME, Saltzberg MT et al (2007) Ultrafiltration versus intravenous diuretics for patients hospitalized for acute decompensated heart failure. J Am Coll Cardiol 49:675–683
67. Bart BA, Goldsmith SR, Lee KL et al (2012) Ultrafiltration in decompensated heart failure with cardiorenal syndrome. N Engl J Med 367:2296–2304
68. Marenzi G, Muratori M, Cosentino ER et al (2014) Continuous ultrafiltration for congestive heart failure: The CUORE trial. J Card Fail 20:9–17
69. Krishnamoorthy A, Felker GM (2014) Fluid removal in acute heart failure: diuretics versus devices. Curr Opin Crit Care 20:478–483
70. Goldsmith SR, Bart BA, Burnett J (2014) Decongestive therapy and renal function in acute heart failure: Time for a new approach? Circ Heart Fail 7:531–535
71. Lala A, McNulty SE, Mentz RJ et al (2015) Relief and recurrence of congestion during and after hospitalization for acute heart failure. Circ Heart Fail 8:741–748

Part IV
Fluid Therapy

Crystalloid Fluid Therapy

S. Reddy, L. Weinberg, and P. Young

Introduction

"she filled his ancient veins with rich elixir. As he received it ... his wasted form renewed, appeared in all the vigor of bright youth, no longer lean and sallow, for new blood coursed in his well-filled veins" (Publius Ovidius Naso, Metamorphoses Book VII – The Story of Medea and Jason, 8 AD).

Our desire to find solutions that rejuvenate and resuscitate is captured in the story of Medea revitalizing Jason's elderly father by filling his veins with a specially prepared elixir. Although no such elixir exists, intravenous fluids are an integral component of the multimodal resuscitation strategy used in medicine. Intravenous fluids were first administered over 180 years ago and despite their widespread use there remains uncertainty about their relative safety and efficacy.

Worldwide, there is variation in the prescribing of resuscitative intravenous fluids and the preferred choice of fluid appears to be based on local customs, marketing, fluid costs and availability [1]. The majority of intravenous fluids were introduced into clinical practice during an era where they did not undergo the same scrutiny

S. Reddy (✉)
Medical Research Institute of New Zealand
Wellington, New Zealand
email: sumeet.reddy@mrinz.ac.nz

L. Weinberg
Department of Anesthesia, Austin Hospital
Melbourne, Australia
Departments of Surgery and Anesthesia, Perioperative Pain Medicine Unit, University of Melbourne
Melbourne, Australia

P. Young
Medical Research Institute of New Zealand
Wellington, New Zealand
Intensive Care Unit, Wellington Regional Hospital
Wellington, New Zealand

© Springer International Publishing Switzerland 2016
J.-L. Vincent (ed.), Annual Update in Intensive Care and Emergency Medicine 2016,
DOI 10.1007/978-3-319-27349-5_12

as other drugs. Hence, there is a paucity of research in this area and only recently has there been an increase in academic interest in the comparative effectiveness of different intravenous fluids.

Here, we review the composition of different crystalloid fluids, potential pathophysiological responses following crystalloid fluid infusion, evidence from animal studies, observational studies, and interventional studies comparing crystalloid fluids, and suggest future directions for research on the comparative effectiveness of various crystalloid fluids.

Unbuffered/Unbalanced Crystalloids

The composition of 0.9% saline was first mentioned by Jakob Hamburger in the 1890s. It is unknown how 0.9% saline became known as 'normal saline'; however, use of term 'normal' may have contributed to the widespread acceptance of 0.9% saline into clinical practice. Despite being referred to as 'normal', 0.9% saline is not physiologically 'normal'. First, 0.9% saline has a higher chloride concentration than plasma. Second, 0.9% saline has a different strong ion difference (SID) to plasma. According to the Stewart physiochemical approach to describing acid-base balance, fluid pH is in part determined by the SID, which is the sum of the strong cation concentrations in the solution (e.g., sodium, potassium, magnesium), minus the sum of the strong anion concentrations in the solution (e.g., chloride and lactate). The SID of the extracellular fluid is approximately 40 mEq/l, whereas the SID of 0.9% saline is zero. Following an infusion of 0.9% saline there is a net decrease in the plasma SID resulting in a metabolic acidosis.

0.9% saline is often thought of as a relatively hypertonic solution because the sum of its osmotically active components gives a theoretical *in vitro* osmolality of 308 mosmol/kg H_2O (154 mmol/l sodium plus 154 mmol/l chloride). However, 0.9% saline is more accurately referred to as an isotonic solution as its constituents – sodium and chloride – are only partially active, with an osmotic coefficient of 0.926. The calculated *in vivo* osmolality (tonicity) of saline is 285 mosmol/kg H_2O, which is the same as plasma osmolality (tonicity).

Buffered/Balanced Crystalloids

Sydney Ringer's *in vitro* experiments in the 1880s on the influence of crystalloid fluid composition on cardiac contractility led to the recognition of a potential benefit of the addition of other inorganic constituents to sodium chloride solutions. Alexis Hartmann further modified Ringer's solution through the addition of sodium lactate to act as a buffering agent in an effort to combat acidosis in dehydrated pediatric patients.

Unlike 0.9% saline, the available buffered crystalloid solutions contain physiological or near physiological amounts of chloride. One of the key differences between 0.9% saline and buffered/balanced crystalloids is the presence of additional anions, such as lactate, acetate, malate and gluconate, which act as physiological buffers to generate bicarbonate. Further, buffered fluids, such as Hartmann's solution and Ringer's lactate, have near physiologically effective *in vivo* SIDs of 27 and 29 mEq/l, respectively. In contrast, Plasma-Lyte 148® has an effective SID *in vivo* of 50 mEq/l. Despite the fact that buffered crystalloid fluids are designed to better mimic the composition of human plasma, no perfectly balanced or physiologically 'normal' crystalloid fluid is currently available (see Table 1).

Historically, sodium acetate was used during hemodialysis as an alternative to bicarbonate because of the incompatibility of bicarbonate with solutions containing calcium and magnesium salts. Early evidence suggested that sodium acetate solution was effective in restoring blood pH and plasma bicarbonate in patients suffering from metabolic acidosis [2]; however, a more recent study suggested that acetate was associated with hemodynamic instability, vasodilatation and negative inotropic affects in patients undergoing high volume renal replacement therapy (RRT) [3]. Concern about the potential for myocardial depression with acetate is supported by studies suggesting that acetate decreases myocardial contractility and blood pressure in dogs [4] and impaired contractile function in an isolated perfused rat heart model [5]. Even the small quantity of acetate present in various dialysis fluids (usually 35 mmol/l) can result in plasma acetate concentrations of 10 to 40 times the physiological level (50 to 100 μmol/l) [6]. Use of acetated solutions as a circuit prime for cardiac patients undergoing cardiopulmonary bypass (CPB) also results in short-lived supra-physiological concentrations of acetate; however, it is not clear if these have any adverse clinical effects [7].

Despite these potential concerns, there are several theoretical advantages of using acetated solutions compared to lactate-containing crystalloids. Acetate is metabolized widely throughout the body, is not reliant entirely on hepatic metabolism and is metabolized more rapidly than lactate [8]. A canine study showed that acetate metabolism was well-preserved in profound shock while lactate metabolism was significantly impaired [9]. Acetate metabolism does not result in changes in glucose or insulin concentrations, whereas exogenously administered lactate can be converted to glucose via gluconeogenesis resulting in hyperglycemia [10]. Acetate turnover shows no age-related differences [11], and acetate may protect against malnutrition by replacing fat as an oxidative fuel without affecting glucose oxidation, or causing hyperglycemia [10].

Little is known about the clinical effects of gluconate. Gluconate is largely excreted unchanged in the urine (80%). In a recent Phase II evaluation of an acetate/gluconate-based buffered solution (Plasma-Lyte 148®) versus a bicarbonate buffered crystalloid fluid for CPB circuit priming, Plasma-Lyte 148® was associated with an immediate increase in unmeasured anions of > 10 mEq/l (presumably acetate and/or gluconate), with residual elevations still present just prior to CPB cessation [12]. The clinical significance of elevated gluconate and/or acetate levels remains unclear in this setting.

Hartmann's solution or Ringer's lactate are hypotonic solutions with a calculated *in vivo* osmolality (tonicity) of approximately 254 mOsmol/kgH₂O. Perioperative administration of hypotonic fluids can represent a significant free water load that

Table 1 Characteristics of common crystalloid solutions compared to human plasma

	Plasma	0.9% saline	Compound sodium lactate (lactate buffered solution)	Ringer's lactate (lactate buffered solution)	Ionosteril® (acetate buffered solution)	Sterofundin ISO® (acetate & malate buffered solution)	Plasma-Lyte 148® (acetate & gluconate buffered solution)
Sodium (mmol/l)	136–145	154	129	130	137	145	140
Potassium (mmol/l)	3.5–5.0		5	4	4	4	5
Magnesium (mmol/l)	0.8–1.0				1.25	1	1.5
Calcium (mmol/l)	2.2–2.6		2.5	3	1.65	2.5	
Chloride (mmol/l)	98–106	154	109	109	110	127	98
Acetate (mmol/l)					36.8	24	27
Gluconate (mmol/l)							23
Lactate (mmol/l)			29	28			
Malate (mmol/l)						5	
eSID (mEq/l)	42		27	28	36.8	25.5	50
Theoretical osmolarity (mosmol/l)	291	308	278	273	291	309	295
Actual or measured *osmolality (mosmol/kg H_2O)	287	286	256	256	270	Not stated	271
pH	7.35–7.45	4.5–7	5–7	5.0–7	6.9–7.9	5.1–5.9	4–8

* Freezing point depression

Plasma-Lyte 148 manufactured by Baxter Healthcare, Toongabie, NSW, Australia

Ringer's Lactate manufactured by Baxter Healthcare, Deerfield, IL, USA

Hartmann's solution manufactured by Baxter Healthcare, Toongabie, NSW, Australia

Ionosteril manufactured by Fresenius Medical Care, Schweinfurt, Germany

Sterofundin ISO manufactured by B. Braun Melsungen AG, Melsungen, Germany

may not be easily excreted in the presence of the high anti-diuretic hormone concentrations commonly associated with physiological stress. Failure to excrete water in a timely fashion may result in postoperative positive fluid balance, edema, and weight gain. Hypotonic fluids are also contraindicated in patients with or at risk of cerebral edema.

In addition to differences in buffering agents, buffered solutions also vary in the presence and concentration of ancillary cations (sodium, potassium, calcium, magnesium), which means they are not biologically equivalent. Hartmann's solution contains 2 mmol/l of calcium and is contraindicated with blood or blood-related products due to concerns about precipitation and the possibility of coagulation and clot formation. A recent warning has been issued about mixing calcium-containing solutions, including Hartmann's solution or Ringer's lactate, with ceftriaxone causing the formation of the insoluble ceftriaxone calcium salt [13].

Although some authors have argued that hyperchloremia secondary to 0.9% saline is a benign and self-limiting phenomenon, there is some evidence that hyperchloremia is independently associated with adverse clinical outcomes [14]. The biological plausibility that 0.9% saline may affect renal function is supported by a cross-over study of 12 volunteers that reported significantly higher serum chloride levels, reduced renal artery blood velocity and reduced renal cortical tissue perfusion in subjects who received 2 l of 0.9% saline over 1 h compared to those that had received Plasma-Lyte 148® [15]. This study also found that although 0.9% saline and Plasma-Lyte 148® expanded the intravascular volume to the same degree, 0.9% saline expanded the extracellular fluid volume significantly more than did Plasma-Lyte 148® meaning that 0.9% saline may be more likely to result in fluid overload and interstitial edema.

Experimental research has identified possible hematological and gastrointestinal pathways that may be impaired with the use of 0.9% saline. *Ex vivo* testing of diluted whole blood reported that dilution with Ringer's lactate resulted in less impairment in thrombin generation and platelet activation when compared to 0.9% saline [16]. A swine study reported that metabolic acidosis significantly impaired gastropyloric motility by reducing pyloric contraction amplitude, which results in delayed gastric emptying or gastroparesis [17].

Animal Studies Comparing 0.9% Saline to Buffered Crystalloid Fluids

Recently, Zhou et al. reported decreased rates of acute kidney injury (AKI) and improved survival in rats receiving Plasma-Lyte® compared to 0.9% saline in an animal model of sepsis [18]. In this experiment, 60 rats were randomized to receive 0.9% saline or Plasma-Lyte® for 4 h (10 ml/kg for the first hour and 5 ml/kg over the next 3 h) after 18 h of cecal ligation and puncture. Rats that received 0.9% saline had higher rates of AKI (100% vs. 76%, p < 0.05) and significantly worse AKI severity based on the Risk, Injury, Failure, Loss of kidney function, End-stage kidney disease (RIFLE) criteria creatinine definitions (RIFLE-I or F: 83% vs. 28%, p < 0.001). Histopathological and biomarkers (urine cystatin C and urine neutrophil gelatinase-associated lipocalin) of AKI were also significantly worse in rats that received 0.9% saline compared to rats that received Plasma-Lyte®.

The largest animal study comparing 0.9% saline versus buffered fluid was a swine model of hemorrhagic shock that randomized 116 pigs to crystalloid fluid replacement at different percentages of replacement (0.9% saline at 14% replacement of blood loss; 0.9% saline at 100% replacement of blood loss; 0.9% saline at 300% replacement of blood loss; Ringer's lactate at 300% replacement of blood loss; Plasma-Lyte A® at 300% replacement of blood loss; Plasma-Lyte R® at 300% replacement of blood loss) [19]. In a comparison of the different 300% treatment groups, a significant difference was found in survival at 24 h in pigs that received Ringer's lactate (67%) compared to Plasma-Lyte A® (30%). No difference was found in survival rates in 0.9% saline (50%) or Plasma-Lyte R® (40%) groups.

Observational Studies Comparing 0.9% Saline to Buffered Crystalloid Fluids

The majority of evidence demonstrating potential adverse clinical effects with the use of 0.9% saline compared to buffered crystalloids originated from recent observational studies in critically unwell and surgical patients [20–22]. In a single center, open-label, sequential 6-month study of 1533 critically ill patients, the change from standard chloride-liberal fluids (0.9% saline, 4% succinylate gelatin or 4% albumin) to chloride-restrictive fluids (Hartmann's solution, Plasma-Lyte 148® and 20% albumin) was associated with a significant decrease in the risk of developing RIFLE-defined AKI (odds ratio [OR] 0.52, 95% CI 0.37–0.75, p < 0.01) and requirements for RRT while in the intensive care unit (ICU) (OR 0.52, 95% CI, 0.33–0.81, p = 0.004) [20]. No difference between groups was found in hospital mortality and hospital or ICU length of stay. A recently published extended analysis over the 12 months before and after the strategy change, which included 2994 patients, reported persistently lower rates of AKI according to the Kidney Disease: Improving Global Outcomes (KDIGO) creatinine definitions and decreased requirements of RRT [23]. Because multiple changes in fluids occurred simultaneously in this observational study it is not possible to determine what component of the fluid change strategy (if any) was responsible for the observed changes.

The two largest studies that have assessed the effects of buffered versus unbuffered crystalloid fluid were retrospective observational studies with patient data collected from centralized health-economic databases [21, 22]. The most recent study was conducted in non-surgical, adult patients with the International Classification of Disease, Ninth Edition Clinical Modification (ICD-9-CM) codes for sepsis who were receiving vasopressors in the ICU by day two, and had received three consecutive days of antibiotics and had had a blood culture [21]. In total 53,448 patients were identified from 360 hospitals over five years. Of this cohort, only 3365 patients (6.4%) had received some "balanced fluids" during their first two hospital days. This sample was compared with a propensity-matched group of 3365 patients who had "not received balanced fluids" (received either 0.9% saline or 5% dextrose). Patients who had received balanced fluids had a significantly lower in-hospital mortality (19.6% vs. 22.8%; relative risk [RR] 0.86, 95% CI 0.78–0.94, p = 0.001) compared to the group that had not received balanced fluids. No difference was found between groups in acute renal failure (defined by ICD-9-CM codes), need for dialysis and hospital or ICU length of stay. The vast majority of patients in the balanced group had received a mixture of intravenous fluids and it was reported that less than 1% of patients in the balanced fluid group had exclusively received balanced fluids. On further analysis, patients were stratified by the proportion of balanced to unbalanced fluid they had received. The relative risk of in-hospital mortality was progressively lower among patients who received a greater proportion of balanced fluid.

A similar retrospective study was conducted in adult patients who had undergone non-traumatic, open, general surgical abdominal operations who had exclusively received either 0.9% saline or a balanced fluid (defined as a calcium-free buffered fluid: Plasma-Lyte 148® or Plasma-Lyte A®) on the day of surgery [22]. In total 271,189 patients from approximately 600 hospitals had received fluids on the day of surgery. Of these patients, 30,994 received 0.9% saline and 926 received balanced fluid. Propensity matching was used to mitigate for baseline group imbalances, which included a significantly higher proportion of minorities, less commercial insurance, greater proportion of patients from non-teaching hospitals, greater proportion of admissions via the emergency department and significantly higher rates of co-morbidities (based on ICD-9-CM codes), such as renal failure, diabetes and congestive heart failure in patients that had exclusively received 0.9% saline. On matched analysis, patients who exclusively received balanced fluid had a decreased risk of major complications (OR 0.79, 95% CI 0.66–0.97, p < 0.05) including need for blood transfusion (1.8% vs. 11.5%, p < 0.001) and need for dialysis (1.0% vs. 4.8%, p < 0.001). However, those in the balanced fluid group had higher rates of minor gastrointestinal complications (OR 1.45; 95% CI 1.17–1.79, p < 0.05) and longer hospital lengths of stay (6.4 vs. 5.9 days, p < 0.001).

Overall, existing data from observational studies suggest that the use of high chloride, unbuffered crystalloid fluid may be associated with major complications following surgery and increased mortality in critically ill patients with sepsis. However, due to the retrospective nature of these studies and potential for unmeasured confounding, it is not possible to establish whether using buffered crystalloid fluid instead of 0.9% saline is beneficial or harmful on the basis of observational studies.

Interventional Studies Comparing 0.9% Saline to Buffered Crystalloid Fluids

Until 2015, all interventional studies comparing 0.9% saline to buffered crystalloid had a small sample size (n < 100) and focused primarily on short term physiological or biochemical outcomes (see Table 2). A systematic review and meta-analysis published in 2014 identified 28 prospective, randomized controlled trials with at

Table 2 Summary of the key interventional clinical studies that have compared 0.9% saline to buffered crystalloid fluid in adult patients

	Design, setting and participants	Key Findings
Acutely unwell population		
The SPLIT trial, 2015 [27]	Multicenter, double-blind, cluster randomized, double crossover trial comparing 0.9% saline with Plasma-Lyte 148®; n = 2262	– There was no significant difference between groups in rates of AKI or AKI requiring RRT – There was no significant difference between groups in survival to day 90
Smith et al. 2015 [28]	Single center, double-blind RCT comparing 0.9% saline with Plasma-Lyte A® in critically ill trauma patients; n = 18	– Patients receiving 0.9% saline had significantly lower serum chloride and bicarbonate concentration – Patients receiving Plasma-Lyte A® had a quicker fibrin build up and cross linking (α angle) at 6 h after infusion – No difference between groups in coagulation tests or blood products received at 6 h
Young et al. 2014 [29]	Single center, double-blind RCT comparing 0.9% saline with Plasma-Lyte A® in patients presenting to ED with severe acute trauma; n = 46	– Patients receiving 0.9% saline had an increase in serum chloride concentration and decrease in serum pH – No significant differences in mortality, hospital length of stay, blood transfusion requirements or utilization of resources
Cieza et al. 2013 [30]	Single center, open label RCT comparing 0.9% saline with Ringer's lactate in patients with severe dehydration secondary to choleriform diarrhea; n = 40	– Patients receiving 0.9% saline had lower serum pH at 2 and 4 h – No differences in serum creatinine, lactate or potassium concentration
Hasman et al. 2012 [31]	Single center, double-blind RCT comparing 0.9% saline, Ringer's lactate or Plasma-Lyte® in patients presenting to ED with dehydration; n = 90	– Patients receiving 0.9% saline had a significantly lower serum pH and lower serum bicarbonate concentration – No differences between groups in chloride, potassium, or sodium concentrations
Van Zyl et al. 2012 [32]	Multicenter, double-blind RCT of Ringer's lactate versus 0.9% saline in patients presenting to ED with diabetic ketoacidosis; n = 54	– There was no significant difference between groups in time interval for correction of acidosis – Patients receiving 0.9% saline had a significantly shorter time to lower blood glucose – No difference between groups in hospital length of stay
Mahler et al. 2011 [33]	Single center, double-blind RCT comparing 0.9% saline with Plasma-Lyte A® in patients presenting to ED with diabetic ketoacidosis; n = 45	– Patients receiving 0.9% saline had significantly higher serum chloride and lower bicarbonate concentration

Table 2 (Continued)

	Design, setting and participants	Key Findings
Wu et al. 2011 [34]	Multicenter, open label RCT comparing 0.9% saline with Ringer's lactate in patients diagnosed with acute pancreatitis; n = 40	– Patients receiving Ringer's lactate had lower rates of SIRS and lower CRP concentration at 24 h – No difference between groups in development of complications or hospital length of stay
Cho et al. 2007 [35]	Multicenter, single-blind RCT of Ringer's lactate versus 0.9% saline in patients presenting to ED with rhabdomyolysis; n = 28	– Patients receiving 0.9% saline had a significantly higher serum chloride and sodium concentration and lower serum pH – There was no significant difference between groups in time interval for normalization of creatine kinase
Surgical population		
The SPLIT-Major Surgery trial, 2015	Prospective phase 4, single center blinded study investigating the safety and efficacy of using 0.9% saline or Plasma-Lyte® 148 as fluid therapy in adult patients undergoing major surgery; n = 1100	– There was no significant difference between groups in rates of AKI – There were no significant differences between groups in the development of postoperative complications or length of hospital stay – Patients who received 0.9% saline developed a transient hyperchloremic metabolic acidosis on postoperative day 1
Potura et al. 2015 [36]	Single center, open label RCT comparing 0.9% saline with Elomel Isoton® (low chloride, acetate buffered crystalloid) in patients undergoing renal transplantation; n = 150	– Significantly more patients receiving 0.9% saline required intraoperative inotrope support – Patients receiving 0.9% saline had a significantly lower base excess and higher serum chloride concentration – No difference between groups in postoperative urine output, creatinine, blood urea nitrogen or need for RRT
Song et al. 2015 [37]	Single center, open label RCT comparing 0.9% saline with Plasma-Lyte® in patients undergoing spinal surgery; n = 50	– Patient receiving 0.9% saline had lower pH, base excess, and bicarbonate concentration and higher serum chloride concentration – Patients receiving Plasma-Lyte® had significantly higher urine output – No difference between groups in rotation thromboelastometry analysis, estimated blood loss or transfusion requirements
Hafizah et al. 2015 [38]	Single center, open label RCT comparing 0.9% saline with Sterofundin® ISO in patients undergoing neurosurgery (low chloride, acetate buffered crystalloid); n = 30	– Patients receiving 0.9% saline had a significantly lower serum pH and higher serum chloride and sodium concentration

Table 2 (Continued)

	Design, setting and participants	Key Findings
Kim et al. 2013 [39]	Single center, blinded RCT comparing either 0.9% saline with Plasma-Lyte® in patients undergoing renal transplantation; n = 60	– Patients receiving 0.9% saline had lower pH and base excess values – No difference between groups in postoperative urine output, creatinine or need for RRT
Modi et al. 2012 [40]	Single center, double-blind RCT comparing 0.9% saline with Ringer's lactate in patients undergoing renal transplantation; n = 74	– Patients receiving 0.9% saline had lower serum pH and base excess values – No difference between groups in postoperative urine output or creatinine
Heidari et al. 2011 [41]	Single center, double-blind RCT comparing 0.9% saline with Ringer's lactate and 5% saline in patients undergoing lower abdominal surgery; n = 90	– A higher proportion of patients who had received 0.9% saline experienced vomiting 6 h post-operatively
Hadimioglu et al. 2008 [42]	Single center, double-blind RCT comparing either 0.9% saline, Ringer's lactate or Plasma-Lyte® in patients undergoing renal transplantation; n = 90	– Patients receiving 0.9% saline had an increase in serum chloride concentration and decrease in serum pH – Patients receiving Ringer's lactate had a significantly increased serum lactate concentration – There was no significant difference between groups in postoperative creatinine or need for RRT
Khajavi et al. 2008 [43]	Single center, double-blind RCT comparing 0.9% saline with Ringer's lactate in patients undergoing renal transplantation; n = 52	– Patient receiving 0.9% saline had a significantly lower serum pH and higher serum potassium concentration at the end of the operation
Chin et al. 2006 [44]	Single center, open label RCT comparing 0.9% saline with Ringer's lactate, 0.9% saline with dextrose 5% in non-diabetic patients undergoing elective surgery; n = 50	– No difference between groups in serum urea, sodium or potassium concentration – Dextrose 5% resulted in significant, albeit transient hyperglycemia, even in non-diabetic patients
Karaca et al. 2006 [45]	Single center, single-blinded RCT comparing 0.9% saline with Ringer's lactate and 4% gelatin polysuccinate in patients undergoing transurethral prostatectomy under spinal anesthesia; n = 60	– No difference between groups in nausea, vomiting, dizziness or post-spinal hearing loss
Chanimov et al. 2006 [46]	Single center, double-blinded RCT comparing 0.9% saline with Ringer's lactate in patients undergoing Cesarean section; n = 40	– No difference between groups in inotrope requirements – No significant differences in the Apgar scores at 1 and 5 min or infant well-being

Table 2 (Continued)

	Design, setting and participants	Key Findings
O'Malley et al. 2005 [47]	Single center, double blind RCT comparing 0.9% saline with Ringer's lactate in patients undergoing renal transplantation; n = 51	– Significantly more patients receiving 0.9% saline required intra-operative treatment for metabolic acidosis and hyperkalemia – No difference between groups in postoperative urine output, creatinine or need for RRT
Takil et al. 2002 [48]	Single center, open label RCT comparing 0.9% saline with Ringer's lactate in patients undergoing spinal surgery; n = 30	– Patients receiving 0.9% saline had an increase in serum chloride, sodium concentration and decrease in serum pH – No difference between groups in intraoperative hemodynamic variables or hospital and ICU lengths of stay
Waters et al. 2001 [49]	Single center, double-blind RCT comparing 0.9% saline with Ringer's lactate in patients undergoing abdominal aortic aneurysm surgery; n = 66	– Patients receiving 0.9% saline had an increase in serum chloride, sodium concentration and decrease in serum pH – Patients receiving 0.9% saline received a greater volume of platelets – No difference between groups in estimated blood loss, postoperative complications, hospital and ICU lengths of stay
Schein-graber et al. 1999 [50]	Single center, open label RCT comparing 0.9% saline with Ringer's lactate in patients undergoing gynecological surgery; n = 24	– Patients receiving 0.9% saline had an increase in serum chloride concentration and decrease in serum pH
Ramanathan et al. 1984 [51]	Single center, open label RCT comparing 0.9% saline with Ringer's lactate, Ringer's lactate with dextrose 5% and Plasma-Lyte A® in patients undergoing Cesarean section; n = 60	– Patients receiving 0.9% saline had a decrease in serum pH – No difference between groups in blood pressure or inotrope requirements

AKI: acute kidney injury; *CRP*: C-reactive protein; *ED*: emergency department; *RCT*: randomized control trial; *RRT*: renal replacement therapy; *SIRS*: systemic inflammatory response syndrome

least 20 adult participants that had compared the effects of different crystalloid fluids [24]. Twenty-three studies that explored acid-base balance reported that 0.9% saline was associated with decreased serum pH, elevated serum chloride levels and decreased bicarbonate levels. In 11 studies that explored renal function, based on urine volume or serum creatinine, no significant difference was found between fluids. In three surgical studies (n = 156) that reported volumes of red blood cells transfused, patients who had received Ringer's lactate required significantly less volume of red blood cells than those who had received 0.9% saline (RR 0.42, 95% CI 0.11–0.73). No differences were found between Ringer's lactate and 0.9% saline in requirements for transfusion or operative blood loss, except in an exploratory subgroup analysis of "high-risk" patients that showed increased blood loss with the use of 0.9% saline in patients that were at increased risk of bleeding.

Based on the published evidence prior to 2014, the National Institute for Health and Care Excellence (NICE) guidelines on intravenous fluid therapy in adults in hospital currently recommend the use of crystalloids that contain sodium in the range 130–154 mmol/l for fluid resuscitation [25]. However, the guidelines state that the available evidence at the time of writing was limited and of "poor" quality. Research to date has been in heterogeneous populations and has been underpowered to allow for differences to be detected in clinically significant outcome measures. The NICE committee specifically identified that research comparing balanced solutions to 0.9% saline for fluid resuscitation was a high priority.

The SPLIT Program

The 0.9% saline vs. Plasma-Lyte 148® for intravenous fluid therapy research program is an investigator-initiated, bi-national collaborative research program investigating the comparative effectiveness of 0.9% saline versus a buffered crystalloid as intravenous fluid therapy. Specific details on the study design, methods of analyzing and reporting of the research program have been published previously [26]. At the time of writing, four of the six planned studies in critically unwell and elective surgical patients have been completed.

The largest study was the 0.9% Saline versus Plasma-Lyte 148® for Intensive care fluid Therapy (SPLIT) trial. The SPLIT trial was a multicenter, blinded, cluster randomized, double crossover study that compared Plasma-Lyte 148® with 0.9% saline as the routine ICU intravenous fluid [27]. All ICU patients needing crystalloid fluid therapy were eligible to be included. Patients who were on dialysis, expected to require RRT within six hours and patients admitted to the ICU solely for organ donation or for palliative care were excluded. In total, 2262 patients in four New Zealand tertiary ICUs over a 28-week period were enrolled and analyzed, with 1152 patients assigned to receive Plasma-Lyte 148® and 1110 assigned to receive 0.9% saline. The two groups of patients had similar admission diagnoses and baseline characteristics. There were no differences between patients who received Plasma-Lyte 148® compared to 0.9% saline in rates of AKI (9.6% vs. 9.2% [difference 0.4%, 95% CI −2.1%–2.9%; RR 1.04, 95% CI 0.80–1.36, p = 0.77]) or requirements for RRT (3.3% vs. 3.4% [difference 0.1%, 95% CI −1.5%–1.4%; RR 0.96, 95% CI 0.62–1.50, p = 0.91]). There were also no significant differences in need for mechanical ventilation, readmission to the ICU, ICU length of stay or in hospital mortality.

Two single-centered, pilot, nested cohort studies were also conducted in patients enrolled in the SPLIT trial. The first of these studies evaluated 251 adults who had undergone cardiac surgery: 131 were allocated to Plasma-Lyte 148® and 120 were allocated to 0.9% saline. No difference was found between groups in postoperative chest drain output or in the proportion of patients developing a major postoperative complication (death, myocardial infarction, new focal neurological deficit or renal failure requiring dialysis). However, fewer patients in the 0.9% saline group required blood products (packed red blood cells, fresh frozen plasma, platelets or cryoprecipitate) compared to patients in the Plasma-Lyte 148® group (18.3% vs. 30.5%, p = 0.03). The second nested cohort study compared gastrointestinal feeding intolerance in 69 patients (35 assigned to receive Plasma-Lyte 148® and 34 to receive 0.9% saline) expected to require mechanical ventilation for greater than 48 h and receiving enteral nutrition exclusively by a nasogastric tube. Despite no difference between groups in the proportion of patients with gastrointestinal feeding intolerance (defined as high gastric residual volume, diarrhea or vomiting while receiving nasogastric feeding in the ICU), a significantly lower proportion of patients in the Plasma-Lyte 148® group developed high gastric residual volumes (11.4% vs. 32.4%, p = 0.04).

Finally, a prospective single center blinded study investigated the safety and efficacy of using 0.9% saline or Plasma-Lyte® 148 as fluid therapy in adult patients undergoing major surgery. Trial fluid was used intraoperatively and postoperatively for three consecutive days. Inclusion criterion included patients undergoing surgery of at least two hours duration and requiring at least one overnight stay. Patients with end-stage renal disease and those undergoing liver or renal transplantation were excluded. The primary outcome measure was the proportion of patients with either acute kidney injury or failure based on creatinine levels in accordance with RIFLE-criteria during the index hospital admission. Intraoperatively, there was 100% compliance with the trial protocol. A total of 746 patients received Plasma-Lyte 148® and 634 patients received 0.9% saline. Patients in both groups had similar baseline characteristics with respect to age, sex, body mass index, American Society of Anesthesiologists (ASA) status, types and number of comorbidities, duration and types of surgery. The median amount of trial fluid received was greater in the Plasma-Lyte 148® group: 2000 ml (interquartile range [IQR] 1000, 2000) vs. 1925 ml (1000, 2000) in the 0.9% saline group (p = 0.007). Patients receiving 0.9% saline developed a transient hyperchloremic metabolic acidosis on postoperative Day 1 compared to patients receiving Plasma-Lyte 148®. Postoperatively, there were no differences in the incidence of AKI between the groups: 52 (10.9%) patients in the Plasma-Lyte 148® group developed postoperative AKI compared to 59 (9.3%) patients in the 0.9% saline group (p = 0.41, 95% CI 0.6–1.2). Patients who developed AKI were older, had larger volumes of fluid both intraoperatively and on postoperative Day 1, and had greater fluid balances intraoperatively and on postoperative Day 1. There were no differences in the development of postoperative complications between the groups. Median lengths of stay were similar between treatment groups: Plasma-Lyte 148® 5.0 days (2.77–8.98) vs. 0.9% saline 5.0 days (2.81–9.04).

Conclusion

Intravenous fluid therapy is a ubiquitous intervention in critically ill patients. While pre-clinical and observational data raise the possibility that the choice of crystalloid fluid therapy may affect patient-centered outcomes, there are currently no convincing data from interventional studies demonstrating that this is the case. Recent data suggest that 0.9% saline and Plasma-Lyte® 148 result in similar rates of renal complications when used for fluid therapy in patients undergoing major surgery and in ICU patients. Further large randomized controlled trials are needed to assess the comparative effectiveness of 0.9% saline and balanced/buffered crystalloids in high-risk populations and to measure clinical outcomes such as mortality. Moreover, given the widespread use of a range of balanced/buffered crystalloids in current clinical practice, high quality studies comparing the various buffered crystalloids available are also needed.

References

1. Finfer S, Liu B, Taylor C, Bellomo R et al (2010) Resuscitation fluid use in critically ill adults: an international cross-sectional study in 391 intensive care units. Crit Care 14:R185
2. Eliahou HE, Feng PH, Weinberg U, Iaina A, Reisin E (1970) Acetate and bicarbonate in the correction of uraemic acidosis. BMJ 4:399–401
3. Schrander-vd Meer AM, Ter Wee PM, Kan G et al (1999) Improved cardiovascular variables during acetate free biofiltration. Clin Nephrol 51:304–309
4. Kirkendol RL, Pearson JE, Bower JD, Holbert RD (1978) Myocardial depressant effects of sodium acetate. Cardiovasc Res 12:127–136
5. Jacob AD, Elkins N, Reiss OK, Chan L, Shapiro JI (1997) Effects of acetate on energy metabolism and function in the isolated perfused rat heart. Kidney Int 52:755–760
6. Coll E, Perez-Garcia R, Rodriguez-Benitez P et al (2007) Clinical and analytical changes in hemodialysis without acetate. Nefrologia 27:742–748
7. Davies PG, Venkatesh B, Morgan TJ et al (2011) Plasma acetate, gluconate and interleukin-6 profiles during and after cardiopulmonary bypass: a comparison of Plasma-Lyte 148 with a bicarbonate-balanced solution. Crit Care 15:R21
8. Mudge GH, Manning JA, Gilman A (1949) Sodium acetate as a source of fixed base. Proc Soc Exp Biol Med 71:136–138
9. Kveim M, Nesbakken R (1979) Utilization of exogenous acetate during canine haemorrhagic shock. Scand J Clin Lab Invest 39:653–658
10. Akanji AO, Bruce MA, Frayn KN (1989) Effect of acetate infusion on energy expenditure and substrate oxidation rates in non-diabetic and diabetic subjects. Eur J Clin Nutr 43:107–115
11. Skutches CL, Holroyde CP, Myers RN, Paul P, Reichard GA (1979) Plasma acetate turnover and oxidation. J Clin Invest 64:708–713
12. Morgan TJ, Power G, Venkatesh B, Jones MA (2008) Acid-base effects of a bicarbonate-balanced priming fluid during cardiopulmonary bypass: comparison with Plasma-Lyte 148. A randomised single-blinded study. Anaesth Intensive Care 36:822–829
13. Murney P (2008) To mix or not to mix – compatibilities of parenteral drug solutions. Aust Prescr 31:98–101
14. Neyra JA, Canepa-Escaro F, Li X et al (2015) Association of Hyperchloremia With Hospital Mortality in Critically Ill Septic Patients. Crit Care Med 43:1938–1944
15. Chowdhury AH, Cox EF, Francis ST, Lobo DN (2012) A randomized, controlled, double-blind crossover study on the effects of 2-L infusions of 0.9 % saline and plasma-lyte(R) 148 on renal blood flow velocity and renal cortical tissue perfusion in healthy volunteers. Ann Surg 256:18–24
16. Brummel-Ziedins K, Whelihan MF, Ziedins EG, Mann KG (2006) The resuscitative fluid you choose may potentiate bleeding. J Trauma 61:1350–1358
17. Tournadre JP, Allaouchiche B, Malbert CH, Chassard D (2000) Metabolic acidosis and respiratory acidosis impair gastro-pyloric motility in anesthetized pigs. Anesth Analg 90:74–79

18. Zhou F, Peng ZY, Bishop JV, Cove ME, Singbartl K, Kellum JA (2014) Effects of fluid resuscitation with 0.9 % saline versus a balanced electrolyte solution on acute kidney injury in a rat model of sepsis. Crit Care Med 42:270–278
19. Traverso LW, Lee WP, Langford MJ (1986) Fluid resuscitation after an otherwise fatal hemorrhage: I. Crystalloid solutions. J Trauma 26:168–175
20. Yunos NM, Bellomo R, Hegarty C, Story D, Ho L, Bailey M (2012) Association between a chloride-liberal vs chloride-restrictive intravenous fluid administration strategy and kidney injury in critically ill adults. JAMA 308:1566–1572
21. Raghunathan K, Shaw A, Nathanson B et al (2014) Association between the choice of IV crystalloid and in-hospital mortality among critically ill adults with sepsis. Crit Care Med 42:1585–1591
22. Shaw AD, Bagshaw SM, Goldstein SL et al (2012) Major complications, mortality, and resource utilization after open abdominal surgery: 0.9 % saline compared to Plasma-Lyte. Ann Surg 255:821–829
23. Yunos NM, Bellomo R, Glassford N, Sutcliffe H, Lam Q, Bailey M (2015) Chloride-liberal vs. chloride-restrictive intravenous fluid administration and acute kidney injury: an extended analysis. Intensive Care Med 41:257–264
24. Orbegozo Cortes D, Rayo Bonor A, Vincent JL (2014) Isotonic crystalloid solutions: a structured review of the literature. Br J Anaesth 112:968–981
25. Padhi S, Bullock I, Li L, Stroud M (2013) Intravenous fluid therapy for adults in hospital: summary of NICE guidance. BMJ 347:f7073
26. Reddy SK, Young PJ, Beasley RW et al (2015) Overview of the study protocols and statistical analysis plan for the Saline versus Plasma-Lyte 148 for Intravenous Fluid Therapy (SPLIT) research program. Crit Care Resusc 17:29–36
27. Young P, Bailey M, Beasley R et al (2015) Effect of a buffered crystalloid solution vs saline on acute kidney injury among patients in the intensive care unit. The SPLIT randomized clinical trial. JAMA 314:1701–1710
28. Smith CA, Gosselin RC, Utter GH et al (2015) Does saline resuscitation affect mechanisms of coagulopathy in critically ill trauma patients? An exploratory analysis. Blood Coagul Fibrinolysis 26:250–254
29. Young JB, Utter GH, Schermer CR et al (2014) Saline versus Plasma-Lyte A in initial resuscitation of trauma patients: a randomized trial. Ann Surg 259:255–262
30. Cieza JA, Hinostroza J, Huapaya JA, Leon CP (2013) Sodium chloride 0.9 % versus Lactated Ringer in the management of severely dehydrated patients with choleriform diarrhoea. J Infect Dev Ctries 7:528–532
31. Hasman H, Cinar O, Uzun A, Cevik E, Jay L, Comert B (2012) A randomized clinical trial comparing the effect of rapidly infused crystalloids on acid-base status in dehydrated patients in the emergency department. Int J Med Sci 9:59–64
32. Van Zyl DG, Rheeder P, Delport E (2012) Fluid management in diabetic-acidosis – Ringer's lactate versus normal saline: a randomized controlled trial. QJM 105:337–343
33. Mahler SA, Conrad SA, Wang H, Arnold TC (2011) Resuscitation with balanced electrolyte solution prevents hyperchloremic metabolic acidosis in patients with diabetic ketoacidosis. Am J Emerg Med 29:670–674
34. Wu BU, Hwang JQ, Gardner TH et al (2011) Lactated Ringer's solution reduces systemic inflammation compared with saline in patients with acute pancreatitis. Clin Gastroenterol Hepatol 9:710–717
35. Cho YS, Lim H, Kim SH (2007) Comparison of lactated Ringer's solution and 0.9 % saline in the treatment of rhabdomyolysis induced by doxylamine intoxication. Emerg Med J 24:276–280
36. Potura E, Lindner G, Biesenbach P et al (2015) An acetate-buffered balanced crystalloid versus 0.9 % saline in patients with end-stage renal disease undergoing cadaveric renal transplantation: a prospective randomized controlled trial. Anesth Analg 120:123–129

37. Song JW, Shim JK, Kim NY, Jang J, Kwak YL (2015) The effect of 0.9 % saline versus plasmalyte on coagulation in patients undergoing lumbar spinal surgery; a randomized controlled trial. Int J Surg 20:128–134

38. Hafizah M, Liu CY, Ooi JS (2016) Normal saline versus balanced-salt solution as intravenous fluid therapy during neurosurgery: Effects on acid-base balance and electrolytes. J Neurosurg Sci (in press)

39. Kim SY, Huh KH, Lee JR, Kim SH, Jeong SH, Choi YS (2013) Comparison of the effects of normal saline versus Plasmalyte on acid-base balance during living donor kidney transplantation using the Stewart and base excess methods. Transplant Proc 45:2191–2196

40. Modi MP, Vora KS, Parikh GP, Shah VR (2012) A comparative study of impact of infusion of Ringer's Lactate solution versus normal saline on acid-base balance and serum electrolytes during live related renal transplantation. Saudi J Kidney Dis Transpl 23:135–137

41. Heidari SM, Saryazdi H, Shafa A, Arefpour R (2011) Comparison of the effect of preoperative administration of Ringer's solution, normal saline and hypertonic saline 5 % on postoperative nausea and vomiting: a randomized, double blinded clinical study. Pak J Med 27:771–774

42. Hadimioglu N, Saadawy I, Saglam T, Ertug Z, Dinckan A (2008) The effect of different crystalloid solutions on acid-base balance and early kidney function after kidney transplantation. Anesth Analg 107:264–269

43. Khajavi MR, Etezadi F, Moharari RS et al (2008) Effects of normal saline vs. lactated ringer's during renal transplantation. Ren Fail 30:535–539

44. Chin KJ, Macachor J, Ong KC, Ong BC (2006) A comparison of 5 % dextrose in 0.9 % normal saline versus non-dextrose-containing crystalloids as the initial intravenous replacement fluid in elective surgery. Anaesth Intensive Care 34:613–617

45. Karaca BSM, Yildiz TS, Ozkarakas H, Toker K (2006) Effects of various loading solutions on postspinal hearing loss. J Turk Anesthesiol Reanim Soc 36:156–161

46. Chanimov M, Gershfeld S, Cohen ML, Sherman D, Bahar M (2006) Fluid preload before spinal anaesthesia in Caesarean section: the effect on neonatal acid-base status. Eur J Anaesthesiol 23:676–679

47. O'Malley CM, Frumento RJ, Hardy MA et al (2005) A randomized, double-blind comparison of lactated Ringer's solution and 0.9 % NaCl during renal transplantation. Anesth Analg 100:1518–1524

48. Takil A, Eti Z, Irmak P, Yilmaz Gogus F (2002) Early postoperative respiratory acidosis after large intravascular volume infusion of lactated ringer's solution during major spine surgery. Anesth Analg 95:294–298

49. Waters JH, Gottlieb A, Schoenwald P, Popovich MJ, Sprung J, Nelson DR (2001) Normal saline versus lactated Ringer's solution for intraoperative fluid management in patients undergoing abdominal aortic aneurysm repair: an outcome study. Anesth Analg 93:817–822

50. Scheingraber S, Rehm M, Sehmisch C, Finsterer U (1999) Rapid saline infusion produces hyperchloremic acidosis in patients undergoing gynecologic surgery. Anesthesiology 90:1265–1270

51. Ramanathan S, Masih AK, Ashok U, Arismendy J, Turndorf H (1984) Concentrations of lactate and pyruvate in maternal and neonatal blood with different intravenous fluids used for prehydration before epidural anesthesia. Anesth Analg 63:69–74

Part V
Bleeding

Emergency Reversal Strategies for Anticoagulants and Antiplatelet Agents

M. Levi

Introduction

Anticoagulant agents are frequently used for prevention and treatment of a wide range of cardiovascular diseases. The most often used anticoagulants are heparin or its derivatives, vitamin K antagonists (such as warfarin or coumadin) and, increasingly, new oral anticoagulants directly inhibiting factor Xa (e.g., rivaroxaban or apixaban) or factor IIa (e.g., dabigatran). Even more patients use antiplatelet agents, including aspirin and thienopyridine derivatives, such as clopidogrel or prasugrel. A myriad of clinical studies has demonstrated that these agents (alone or in combination) can prevent or treat acute or chronic thromboembolic complications [1]. The most important complication of treatment with anticoagulants is hemorrhage, which may be serious, may cause long-term debilitating disease, or may even be life-threatening [2]. In a large series of 34,146 patients with acute ischemic coronary syndromes, anticoagulant-associated bleeding was associated with a 5-fold increased risk of death during the first 30 days and a 1.5-fold higher mortality between 30 days and 6 months [3]. Major bleeding was an independent predictor of mortality across all subgroups that were analyzed. In some clinical situations, the incidence of serious bleeding complications associated with antithrombotic agents may be so high that despite high efficacy in prevention of thrombotic complications the overall effect on outcome is still negative, as was demonstrated in the secondary prevention of patients with ischemic stroke using vitamin K antagonists [4]. Nevertheless, in many situations, clinical studies show a favorable balance between efficacy and safety in favor of anticoagulant treatment. However, if severe bleeding occurs or if a patient needs to undergo an urgent invasive procedure, such as emergency surgery, it may be necessary to reverse the anticoagulant effect of the various agents. Depending on the clinical situation, i.e., the severity of the bleed-

M. Levi (✉)
Dept. of Medicine, Academic Medical Center, University of Amsterdam
Amsterdam, Netherlands
email: m.m.levi@amc.uva.nl

© Springer International Publishing Switzerland 2016
J.-L. Vincent (ed.), *Annual Update in Intensive Care and Emergency Medicine 2016*,
DOI 10.1007/978-3-319-27349-5_13

ing or the urgency and estimated risk of the invasive procedure, this reversal may take place over a few hours, but in some cases immediate reversal is necessary [5]. Generally, each (immediate) reversal of anticoagulant treatment needs also to take into consideration the indication for the antithrombotic agents. For example, the

Table 1 Reversing agents for currently available anticoagulants and antiplatelet agents

	Time until restoration of hemostasis after cessation of therapeutic dose	Reversing agent	Remark
Vitamin K antagonists	Warfarin: 60–80 h Acenocoumarol: 18–24 h Phenprocoumon: 8–10 days	Vitamin K i.v: reversal in 12–16 h Vitamin K orally: reversal in 24 h PCCs: immediate reversal	Dose of vitamin K or PCCs depends on INR and bodyweight
Heparin	3–4 h	Protamine sulfate 25–30 mg; immediate reversal	1 mg of protamine per 100 anti-Xa units given in the last 2–3 h
LMW heparin	12–24 h	(Partially) protamine sulfate 25–50 mg; immediate (partial) reversal	1 mg of protamine per 100 anti-Xa units given in the last 8 h
Pentasaccharides	Fondaparinux: 24–30 h Idraparinux: 5–15 days Idrabiotaparinux: 5–15 days	Recombinant factor VIIa 90 ug/kg; immediate thrombin generation* Avidin for idrabiotaparinux*	Based on laboratory end-points, no systematic experience in bleeding patients
Oral factor Xa inhibitors	Dependent on compound, usually within 12 h	Prothrombin complex concentrate (3000 U)*	Based on laboratory end-points, no systematic experience in bleeding patients
Oral thrombin inhibitors	Dependent on compound, usually within 12 h	Idracizumab*	
Aspirin	5–10 days (time to produce unaffected platelets)	DDAVP (0.3–0.4 ug/kg) and/or platelet concentrate; reversal in 15–30 min	Cessation not always required, also dependent on clinical situation and indication
Clopidogrel Prasugrel	1–2 days	Platelet concentrate, possibly in combination with DDAVP (0.3–0.4 ug/kg); reversal in 15–30 min	Cessation not always desirable, also dependent on clinical situation and indication

* = Experimental treatment;
LMW heparin; low molecular weight heparin; *PCC*: prothrombin complex concentrate; *DDAVP*: de-amino d-arginine vasopressin or desmopressin; *INR*: international normalized ratio

interruption of combined aspirin and clopidogrel treatment in a patient in whom an intracoronary stent has recently been inserted will markedly increase the risk of acute stent thrombosis with consequent downstream cardiac ischemia or infarction. Likewise, in a patient with a prosthetic mitral valve and atrial fibrillation, interruption of vitamin K antagonists may increase the risk of valve thrombosis and cerebral or systemic embolism. Each of these specific clinical situations requires a careful and balanced assessment of the benefits and risks of reversing anticoagulants (and potential strategies to keep the period of reversal as short as possible). In this chapter, we will briefly describe the epidemiology of bleeding complications due to anticoagulants and various strategies to reverse the anticoagulant effect of antithrombotic agents (Table 1), eventually focusing on the new generation of anticoagulants.

Incidence and Risk Factors for Bleeding in Patients on Anticoagulants

Currently, vitamin K antagonists (VKAs) (such as warfarin, coumadin, acenocoumarol or phenprocoumon) are frequently used anticoagulant agents for long-term prevention and treatment of a wide range of cardiovascular diseases. In well-controlled patients in clinical trials, treatment with VKAs increases the risk of major bleeding by 0.5%/year and the risk of intracranial hemorrhage by about 0.2%/year [6]. However, in three real-life surveys this incidence varied from 1.35%/year to 3.4%/year [7]. The incidence of intracranial hemorrhage was 0.2%/year in the clinical trials compared to 0.4–0.6%/year in the unselected samples. One needs to realize that trial populations may poorly reflect the real-life setting in which anticoagulants are prescribed. For example, in 6 pivotal trials that demonstrated the superiority of warfarin over placebo in the prevention of thromboembolic complications in patients with atrial fibrillation, 28,787 patients were screened but only 12.6% of these patients were included in the studies [8]. The incidence of hemorrhagic complications with the use of the new generation of oral anticoagulants with direct inhibitory properties towards thrombin or factor Xa is not very different. For dabigatran, a clear relationship between dose and incidence of bleeding complications was demonstrated in a clinical study in patients with atrial fibrillation [9] and all other new anticoagulants have demonstrated a similar dose-adverse event relationship as well [10].

The most important risk factor for hemorrhage in users of anticoagulants is the intensity of the anticoagulant effect [6]. Studies indicate that with a target international normalized ratio (INR) of > 3.0, the incidence of major bleeding is twice as large as in studies with a target INR of 2.0–3.0 [11]. In a meta-analysis of studies in patients with prosthetic heart valves, a lower INR target range resulted in a lower frequency of major bleeding and intracranial hemorrhage with a similar antithrombotic efficacy [12]. A retrospective analysis of outpatients using warfarin who presented with intracranial hemorrhage demonstrated that the risk of this complication doubled for each 1 unit increment in the INR [13]. For low molecular weight (LMW) heparin, the bleeding risk is also related to its dose. Low-dose prophylactic heparin doubles the risk of major hemorrhage, although the absolute incidence is very low [14]. Higher doses of (LMW) heparin are usually given for short time periods but are also associated with major bleeding: in a retrospective analysis from a study of patients with acute coronary syndromes it was shown that with every 10 s prolongation of the activated partial thromboplastin time (aPTT) the incidence of major hemorrhage increased by 7% [15].

Patient characteristics constitute another important determinant of the bleeding risk. Elderly patients have a 2-fold increased risk of bleeding [16] and the relative risk of intracranial hemorrhage (in particular at higher intensities of anticoagulation) was 2.5 (95% CI 2.3–9.4) in patients >85 years compared to patients 70–74 years old [17]. Comorbidity, such as renal or hepatic insufficiency, may also significantly increase the risk of bleeding. A case-control study in 1986 patients receiving VKAs showed that this comorbidity increased the risk of bleeding by about 2.5 [8]. Another very important determinant of the risk of bleeding is the combined use of medication that affects both the coagulation system and platelet function. Two meta-analyses, comprising respectively 6 trials with a total of 3874 patients [18] and 10 trials with a total of 5938 patients [19], found a relative risk of major bleeding when antithrombotic agents were combined with aspirin of 2.4 (95% CI 1.2–4.8) and 2.5 (95% CI 1.7–3.7), respectively. A population-based case-control study confirmed the high risk of upper gastrointestinal bleeding in patients using anticoagulants in combination with aspirin and/or clopidogrel [20]. Non-steroidal anti-inflammatory agents (NSAIDs) are also associated with an enhanced risk of gastrointestinal bleeding. The combined use of anticoagulants and NSAIDs may result in an 11-fold higher risk of hospitalization for gastrointestinal bleeding as compared to the general population [21]. This risk is not significantly lower when using selective inhibitors of cyclooxygenase (COX)-2.

Reversal of Vitamin K Antagonists

When interrupting the administration of VKAs, important differences in the half-lives of the various agents (9 h for acenocoumarol, 36–42 h for warfarin, and 90 h for phenprocoumon, respectively) need to be taken into account [22]. The most straightforward intervention to counteract the effect of VKAs is the administration of vitamin K [23]. A recent randomized controlled trial found no difference in bleeding or other complications in non-bleeding patients with INR values of 4.5 to 10 who were treated with vitamin K or placebo [24]. In patients with clinically significant bleeding, however, administration of vitamin K is crucial to reverse the anticoagulant effect of VKAs. Vitamin K can be given orally or intravenously, but the parenteral route has the advantage of a more rapid onset of treatment [25]. After the administration of intravenous vitamin K, the INR will start to decrease within 2 h and will be completely normalized within 12–16 h [26], whereas after oral administration it will take up to 24 h to normalize the INR [23]. An often voiced concern with the use of parenteral vitamin K is the occurrence of anaphylactic reactions; however, with the more modern micelle preparations, the incidence of this complication is very low [27]. In case of very serious or even life-threatening bleeding, immediate correction of the INR is mandatory and can be achieved by the administration of vitamin K-dependent coagulation factors. Prothrombin complex concentrates (PCCs), containing all vitamin K-dependent coagulation factors, are more useful. In prospective studies in patients using VKAs and presenting with bleeding, administration of PCCs resulted in satisfactory and sustained hemostasis in 98% [28, 29]. In recent years, the safety of PCCs, in particular regarding the transmission of blood-borne infectious diseases, has markedly improved owing to several techniques, such as pasteurization, nanofiltration, and addition of solvent detergent.

Reversal of Heparin and Heparin Derivatives

Heparin has a relatively short half-life of about 60–90 min and therefore the anti-coagulant effect of therapeutic doses of heparin will be mostly eliminated at 3–4 h after termination of continuous intravenous administration. The anticoagulant effect of high-dose subcutaneous heparin, however, will take a longer time to abolish. If a more immediate neutralization of heparin is required, intravenous protamine sulfate is the antidote of choice. Protamine, derived from fish sperm, binds to heparin to form a stable biologically inactive complex. Each mg of protamine will neutralize approximately 100 units of heparin. Hence, the protamine dose in a patient on a stable therapeutic heparin dose of 1000–1250 U/h should be about 25–30 mg (sufficient to block the amount of heparin given in the last 2–3 h). The reversal of LMW heparin is more complex, as protamine sulfate will only neutralize the anti-factor IIa activity and has no or only partial effect on the smaller heparin fragments causing the anti-factor Xa activity of the compound. A practical approach is to give 1 mg of protamine per 100 anti-factor Xa units of LMW heparin given in the last 8 h (whereas 1 mg of enoxaparin equals 100 anti-factor Xa units). If bleeding continues, a second dose of 0.5 mg per 100 anti-factor Xa units can be given. There are some other strategies to reverse (mostly unfractionated) heparin, such as platelet factor-4, heparanase, or extracorporeal heparin-removal devices, but none of these approaches has been properly evaluated and they are not currently approved for clinical use [5].

Pentasaccharides are recently developed synthetic compounds that effectively bind and potentiate antithrombin to block factor Xa. Since they lack the additional glycosaminoglycan saccharide residues to bind to thrombin, they have an effect exclusively on factor Xa. The prototype pentasaccharide is fondaparinux and the longer acting idraparinux has also been introduced. The main difference between these two agents is the elimination half-life, which is 15–20 h for fondaparinux and 5½ days for idraparinux. This means that idraparinux can be administered once weekly, which renders the subcutaneous route of administration for long-term treatment less cumbersome. Pentasaccharides were shown to be effective in the prophylaxis and treatment of venous thromboembolism and are currently licensed for prophylaxis of thrombosis [30]. The bleeding risk with pentasaccharides is dependent on the dose and is generally comparable with (LMW) heparin. The (very) long half-life of pentasaccharides necessitates the availability of a suitable antidote if major bleeding complicates the treatment. The only agent that has been systematically evaluated to reverse the anticoagulant effect of pentasaccharides is recombinant factor VIIa (rVIIa). Two randomized placebo-controlled studies in healthy volunteers tested the hypothesis that rVIIa may be useful as a suitable reversing agent for pentasaccharide anticoagulation [31]. Recently, a newly biotinylated form of idraparinux (idrabiotaparinux) has been developed. This modification enables rapid elimination of the molecule when avidin, which binds tightly to biotin, is given. In a first clinical study, the efficacy and safety of idrabiotaparinux was comparable to that of idraparinux [32].

Reversal of New Direct Factor Xa Inhibitors

In recent years, a large number of new antithrombotic agents has been developed and tested in clinical trials and many of these new agents have become widely available for clinical practice. One of the main advantages of these new agents is the relatively stable pharmacokinetic and pharmacodynamic properties, which obviate the need for repeated control of the intensity of anticoagulation and dose-adjustments.

Some of these new classes of anticoagulants are directed at factor Xa. Prototypes of these agents are rivaroxaban, edoxaban and apixaban, which have shown good efficacy and safety profiles in clinical studies [33, 34]. Rivaroxaban was also studied in patients with acute coronary syndromes and showed a dose-dependent efficacy but also increased rates of major bleeding at higher doses [35]. Apixaban showed a similar pattern and exhibited 2.5 fold increased bleeding rates, in particular in patients using simultaneous antiplatelet agents [36]. Taken together, compared to LMW heparin, direct factor Xa inhibitors have, at doses achieving equivalent efficacy, a lower bleeding risk and at doses achieving higher efficacy a similar bleeding risk. This means that for some clinical situations these drugs may represent an important improvement, however, the risk of (major) bleeding is still present. It should be noted that the combined use of the new anticoagulant agents and antiplatelet agents was discouraged in the clinical trials, whereas this is increasingly common in clinical practice and may also have a serious impact on the risk of hemorrhage.

Dependent on the severity of the clinical situation and in view of the half-life of the direct Xa inhibitors, cessation of medication may be sufficient to reverse the anticoagulant effect in case of bleeding. However, if immediate reversal of anticoagulation is required, no solid evidence is available for the efficacy of any reversing agent on the anticoagulant effect of any of these orally available factor Xa inhibitors. The administration of PCC resulted in a correction of the prolonged prothrombin time and restored depressed thrombin generation after rivaroxaban treatment in healthy human subjects [37, 38]. In view of the relatively wide availability of

PCCs, this approach would be an interesting option if the results can be confirmed in patients on oral factor Xa inhibitors who present with bleeding complications. More specific reversal can be achieved with a new agent that competitively binds to the anti-Xa agents and that is currently in development [39, 40]. Monitoring of the reversal of the anticoagulant effect of factor Xa inhibitors is most simply done by measuring the prothrombin time, although there is some variability between pro-thrombin time reagents and for some agents the anti-factor Xa assay is more reliable [41].

Reversal of New Direct Thrombin Inhibitors

Another important group of new anticoagulants is the class of direct thrombin (IIa) inhibitors. Thrombin is the central enzyme in the coagulation process, not only mediating the conversion of fibrinogen to fibrin, but also being the most important physiological activator of platelets and various other coagulation factors. Dabiga-tran is a direct thrombin inhibitor with good and relatively stable bioavailability after oral ingestion. In patients with atrial fibrillation, dabigatran (150 mg twice daily) showed a significantly lower rate of thromboembolic complications com-pared to warfarin (relative risk 0.66, 95% confidence interval 0.53–0.82) and a similar bleeding rate. Interestingly, a lower dose of dabigatran (110 mg twice daily) was equally protective of thromboembolic complications as VKAs but was associ-ated with a lower risk of major hemorrhage (2.7% per year in the dabigatran group versus 3.4% per year in the warfarin group) [9]. Dabigatran has also been proven safe and effective for prevention and treatment of venous thromboembolism. How-ever, the risk of major bleeding is still present and requires adequate management strategies. As mentioned for the anti-factor Xa agents, clinical trials in patients us-ing anti-thrombin agents excluded many patients with common comorbidities and discouraged the simultaneous use of agents affecting platelet function. Therefore, the risk of hemorrhage in these trials may have underestimated the real-life bleeding risk.

For each of the direct thrombin inhibitors, no established reversing agent is available in case of serious bleeding complicating the anticoagulant treatment. For-tunately, the half-life of most of the agents is relatively short, hence in cases of less serious bleeding interruption of treatment will be sufficient to reverse the anti-coagulant effect. However, if immediate reversal is required, it is not clear which would be the best strategy. The administration of PCC was associated with vari-able results in various volunteer trials and efficacy at relatively high doses in animal studies [37, 42, 43]. Monitoring of the anticoagulant effect of thrombin inhibitors in routine clinical practice is difficult. The aPTT is not very useful. An ecarin clot-ting time may be more accurate but is not readily available in most routine clinical settings. Most convenient and practically applicable for monitoring of the antico-agulant effect may be the diluted thrombin time, which needs to be standardized for the specific agent that was used [44].

Reversal of Antiplatelet Agents

Aspirin is effective in the secondary prevention of atherothrombotic disease, in particular coronary artery disease, cerebrovascular thromboembolism and peripheral arterial disease. As a consequence, aspirin is the most widely used antithrombotic agent worldwide. Aspirin increases the risk of bleeding, in particular gastrointestinal bleeding, and has been associated with a small but consistent increase in intracerebral hemorrhage. In addition, it has been shown that the use of aspirin is associated with increased perioperative blood loss in major procedures, although this does not necessarily translate into clinically relevant endpoints, such as the requirement for transfusion or re-operation [45]. Over recent years, the approach to the patient who uses aspirin and who presents with bleeding or needs to undergo an invasive procedure has changed considerably. In fact, in current clinical practice, bleeding can almost always be managed with local hemostatic procedures or conservative strategies without interrupting aspirin and most invasive procedures do not require the cessation of aspirin when adequate attention is given to local hemostasis. In contrast, interruption of aspirin has been associated with an increased risk of thromboembolic complications, potentially due to rebound hypercoagulability. Nevertheless, in special clinical circumstances, such as intracranial bleeding or the need to undergo a neurosurgical or ophthalmic procedure, the anti-hemostatic effect of aspirin needs to be reversed immediately. The most rigorous measure to achieve this is the administration of platelet concentrate after cessation of aspirin. Another approach is the administration of de-amino d-arginine vasopressin (DDAVP, desmopressin) [46]. The combined effect of platelet concentrate and subsequent administration of DDAVP has also been advocated to correct the aspirin effect on platelets. The standard dose of DDAVP is 0.3–0.4 µg/kg in 100 ml saline over 30 min and its effect is immediate.

Clopidogrel, prasugrel, and ticagrelor belong to the class of thienopyridine derivatives, which act by blocking the adenosine diphosphate (ADP) receptor on the platelet. Clinical studies have shown that clopidogrel is as good as aspirin in the secondary prevention of atherothrombotic events. Importantly, the combination of aspirin and clopidogrel is vastly superior over aspirin alone in patients who have received intracoronary stents or in other patients with high risk coronary artery disease. There is ample evidence that dual platelet inhibition of aspirin plus clopidogrel has a significantly higher efficacy than aspirin alone in patients with acute coronary syndromes who have undergone coronary interventions for at least a year (and possibly longer) after the event. However, the increased efficacy of the combined use of aspirin and clopidogrel is also associated with a significantly higher bleeding risk [47]. Prasugrel and ticagrelor are other oral thienopyridine derivatives that, after rapid and almost complete absorption, irreversibly bind to the ADP receptor. Prasugrel and ticagrelor have a stronger antiplatelet effect than clopidogrel because of more effective metabolism and less dependence on cytochrome P450 enzymes, which may be subject to genetic polymorphisms [48]. Taking the clinical evidence together, dual platelet inhibition, in particular with clopidogrel or even more with prasugrel or ticagrelor, is highly effective in high-risk patients with coronary artery disease but the bleeding risk with dual platelet inhibition must be taken into account and strategies to reverse the antiplatelet effect may be warranted in case of serious bleeding.

The decision whether or not to interrupt or even reverse antithrombotic treatment with dual platelet inhibition in case of serious bleeding or the need to perform an invasive procedure will depend on the specific clinical situation but also on the indication for the antithrombotic treatment (see above). Especially in patients with recent implantation of an intracoronary stent (in the last 6–12 weeks), cardiologists will often not or only reluctantly agree with cessation of treatment [49]. In this period, re-endothelialization of the stent has not yet occurred and the patient is very vulnerable to acute thrombotic occlusion of the stent. In patients with drug-eluting stents this period may be even longer. If, however, the decision is made to stop and even reverse the treatment with aspirin and clopidogrel, prasugrel, or ticagrelor, administration of platelet concentrate is probably the best way to correct the hemostatic defect [50]. In addition, DDAVP was shown to correct the defect in platelet aggregation caused by clopidogrel, so this may be another option [51].

Conclusion

Conventional anticoagulant treatment, such as with VKAs or heparin (derivatives), can be reversed by specific interventions when the clinical situation requires immediate correction of hemostasis. For the new generation of anticoagulants, several reversal strategies are under evaluation and specific antidotes or reversing agents are being developed, although most interventions need further evaluation in clinical trials. Antiplatelet therapy with aspirin, alone or in combination with thienopyridine derivatives, such as clopidogrel and prasugrel, can be reversed but this is often not required and sometimes not desirable in view of the indications for this treatment.

References

1. Hirsh J, Guyatt G, Albers GW, Harrington R, Schunemann HJ (2008) Antithrombotic and thrombolytic therapy: American College of Chest Physicians Evidence-Based Clinical Practice Guidelines (8th Edition). Chest 133:110S–112S
2. Mannucci PM, Levi M (2007) Prevention and treatment of major blood loss. N Engl J Med 356:2301–2311
3. Eikelboom JW, Mehta SR, Anand SS, Xie C, Fox KA, Yusuf S (2006) Adverse impact of bleeding on prognosis in patients with acute coronary syndromes. Circulation 114:774–782
4. Algra A (2007) Medium intensity oral anticoagulants versus aspirin after cerebral ischaemia of arterial origin (ESPRIT): a randomised controlled trial. Lancet Neurol 6:115–124
5. Levi MM, Eerenberg E, Lowenberg E, Kamphuisen PW (2010) Bleeding in patients using new anticoagulants or antiplatelet agents: risk factors and management. Neth J Med 68:68–76
6. Schulman S, Beyth RJ, Kearon C, Levine MN (2008) Hemorrhagic complications of anticoagulant and thrombolytic treatment: American College of Chest Physicians Evidence-Based Clinical Practice Guidelines (8th Edition). Chest 133:257S–298S

7. Jackson SL, Peterson GM, Vial JH, Daud R, Ang SY (2001) Outcomes in the management of atrial fibrillation: clinical trial results can apply in practice. Intern Med J 31:329–336

8. Levi M, Hovingh GK, Cannegieter SC, Vermeulen M, Buller HR, Rosendaal FR (2008) Bleeding in patients receiving vitamin K antagonists who would have been excluded from trials on which the indication for anticoagulation was based. Blood 111:4471–4476

9. Connolly SJ, Ezekowitz MD, Yusuf S et al (2009) Dabigatran versus warfarin in patients with atrial fibrillation. N Engl J Med 361:1139–1151

10. van Es N, Coppens M, Schulman S, Middeldorp S, Buller HR (2014) Direct oral anticoagulants compared with vitamin K antagonists for acute symptomatic venous thromboembolism: evidence from phase 3 trials. Blood 124:1968–1975

11. Saour JN, Sieck JO, Mamo LA, Gallus AS (1990) Trial of different intensities of anticoagulation in patients with prosthetic heart valves. N Engl J Med 322:428–432

12. Vink R, Kraaijenhagen RA, Hutten BA et al (2003) The optimal intensity of vitamin K antagonists in patients with mechanical heart valves: a meta-analysis. J Am Coll Cardiol 42:2042–2048

13. Hylek EM, Singer DE (1994) Risk factors for intracranial hemorrhage in outpatients taking warfarin. Ann Intern Med 120:897–902

14. Geerts WH, Bergqvist D, Pineo GF et al (2008) Prevention of venous thromboembolism: American College of Chest Physicians Evidence-Based Clinical Practice Guidelines (8th Edition). Chest 133:381S–453S

15. Anand SS, Bates S, Ginsberg JS et al (1999) Recurrent venous thrombosis and heparin therapy: an evaluation of the importance of early activated partial thromboplastin times. Arch Intern Med 159.2029–2032

16. Hutten BA, Lensing AW, Kraaijenhagen RA, Prins MH (1999) Safety of treatment with oral anticoagulants in the elderly. A systematic review. Drugs Aging 14:303–312

17. Fang MC, Chang Y, Hylek EM et al (2004) Advanced age, anticoagulation intensity, and risk for intracranial hemorrhage among patients taking warfarin for atrial fibrillation. Ann Intern Med 141:745–752

18. Hart RG, Benavente O, Pearce LA (1999) Increased risk of intracranial hemorrhage when aspirin is combined with warfarin: A meta-analysis and hypothesis. Cerebrovasc Dis 9:215–217

19. Rothberg MB, Celestin C, Fiore LD, Lawler E, Cook JR (2005) Warfarin plus aspirin after myocardial infarction or the acute coronary syndrome: meta-analysis with estimates of risk and benefit. Ann Intern Med 143:241–250

20. Hallas J, Dall M, Andries A et al (2006) Use of single and combined antithrombotic therapy and risk of serious upper gastrointestinal bleeding: population based case-control study. BMJ 333:726

21. Mellemkjaer L, Blot WJ, Sorensen HT et al (2002) Upper gastrointestinal bleeding among users of NSAIDs: a population-based cohort study in Denmark. Br J Clin Pharmacol 53:173–181

22. Ansell J, Hirsh J, Hylek E, Jacobson A, Crowther M, Palareti G (2008) Pharmacology and management of the vitamin K antagonists: American College of Chest Physicians Evidence-Based Clinical Practice Guidelines (8th Edition). Chest 133:160S–198

23. Dentali F, Ageno W, Crowther M (2006) Treatment of coumarin-associated coagulopathy: a systematic review and proposed treatment algorithms. J Thromb Haemost 4:1853–1863

24. Crowther MA, Ageno W, Garcia D et al (2009) Oral vitamin K versus placebo to correct excessive anticoagulation in patients receiving warfarin. Ann Intern Med 150:293–300

25. Crowther MA, Douketis JD, Schnurr T et al (2002) Oral vitamin K lowers the international normalized ratio more rapidly than subcutaneous vitamin K in the treatment of warfarin-associated coagulopathy. A randomized, controlled trial. Ann Intern Med 20(137):251–254

26. Lubetsky A, Yonath H, Olchovsky D, Loebstein R, Halkin H, Ezra D (2003) Comparison of oral vs intravenous phytonadione (vitamin K1) in patients with excessive anticoagulation: a prospective randomized controlled study. Arch Intern Med 163:2469–2473

27. Dentali F, Ageno W (2004) Management of coumarin-associated coagulopathy in the non-bleeding patient: a systematic review. Haematologica 89:857–862

28. Yates SG, Sarode R (2015) New strategies for effective treatment of vitamin K antagonist-associated bleeding. J Thromb Haemost 13(Suppl 1):S180–S186

29. Quinlan DJ, Eikelboom JW, Weitz JI (2013) Four-factor prothrombin complex concentrate for urgent reversal of vitamin K antagonists in patients with major bleeding. Circulation 128:1179–1181

30. Buller HR (2002) Treatment of symptomatic venous thromboembolism: improving outcomes. Semin Thromb Hemost 28(Suppl 2):41–48

31. Bijsterveld NR, Vink R, van Aken BE et al (2004) Recombinant factor VIIa reverses the anticoagulant effect of the long-acting pentasaccharide idraparinux in healthy volunteers. Br J Haematol 124:653–658

32. Equinox Investigators (2011) Efficacy and safety of once weekly subcutaneous idrabiotaparinux in the treatment of patients with symptomatic deep venous thrombosis. J Thromb Haemost 9:92–99

33. Agnelli G, Gallus A, Goldhaber SZ et al (2007) Treatment of proximal deep-vein thrombosis with the oral direct factor Xa inhibitor rivaroxaban (BAY 59-7939): the ODIXa-DVT (Oral Direct Factor Xa Inhibitor BAY 59-7939 in Patients With Acute Symptomatic Deep-Vein Thrombosis) study. Circulation 116:180–187

34. ROCKET AF Study Investigators (2010) Rivaroxaban-once daily, oral, direct factor Xa inhibition compared with vitamin K antagonism for prevention of stroke and Embolism Trial in Atrial Fibrillation: rationale and design of the ROCKET AF study. Am Heart J 159:340–347

35. Mega JL, Braunwald E, Mohanavelu S et al (2009) Rivaroxaban versus placebo in patients with acute coronary syndromes (ATLAS ACS-TIMI 46): a randomised, double-blind, phase II trial. Lancet 374:29–38

36. Alexander JH, Becker RC, Bhatt DL et al (2009) Apixaban, an oral, direct, selective factor Xa inhibitor, in combination with antiplatelet therapy after acute coronary syndrome: results of the Apixaban for Prevention of Acute Ischemic and Safety Events (APPRAISE) trial. Circulation 119:2877–2885

37. Eerenberg ES, Kamphuisen PW, Sijpkens MK, Meijers JC, Buller HR, Levi M (2011) Reversal of rivaroxaban and dabigatran by prothrombin complex concentrate: a randomized, placebo-controlled, crossover study in healthy subjects. Circulation 124:1573–1579

38. Levi M, Moore KT, Castillejos CF et al (2014) Comparison of three-factor and four-factor prothrombin complex concentrates regarding reversal of the anticoagulant effects of rivaroxaban in healthy volunteers. J Thromb Haemost 12:1428–1436

39. Ansell JE, Bakhru SH, Laulicht BE et al (2014) Use of PER977 to reverse the anticoagulant effect of edoxaban. N Engl J Med 371:2141–2142

40. Ansell J (2013) Blocking bleeding: reversing anticoagulant therapy. Nat Med 19:402–404

41. Hillarp A, Baghaei F, Fagerberg B et al (2011) Effects of the oral, direct factor Xa inhibitor rivaroxaban on commonly used coagulation assays. J Thromb Haemost 9:133–139

42. Lindahl TL, Wallstedt M, Gustafsson KM, Persson E, Hillarp A (2015) More efficient reversal of dabigatran inhibition of coagulation by activated prothrombin complex concentrate or recombinant factor VIIa than by four-factor prothrombin complex concentrate. Thromb Res 135:544–547

43. Honickel M, Maron B, van Ryn J et al (2015) Therapy with activated prothrombin complex concentrate is effective in reducing dabigatran-associated blood loss in a porcine polytrauma model. Thromb Haemost 115 (in press)

44. Lindahl TL, Baghaei F, Blixter IF et al (2011) Effects of the oral, direct thrombin inhibitor dabigatran on five common coagulation assays. Thromb Haemost 105:371–378

45. Merritt JC, Bhatt DL (2004) The efficacy and safety of perioperative antiplatelet therapy. J Thromb Thrombolysis 17:21–27

46. Mannucci PM (1997) Desmopressin (DDAVP) in the treatment of bleeding disorders: the first 20 years. Blood 90:2515–2521

47. Yusuf S, Zhao F, Mehta SR, Chrolavicius S, Tognoni G, Fox KK (2001) Effects of clopidogrel in addition to aspirin in patients with acute coronary syndromes without ST-segment elevation. N Engl J Med 345:494–502
48. Bhatt DL (2009) Prasugrel in clinical practice. N Engl J Med 361:940–942
49. Grines CL, Bonow RO, Casey DE Jr et al (2007) Prevention of premature discontinuation of dual antiplatelet therapy in patients with coronary artery stents: a science advisory from the American Heart Association, American College of Cardiology, Society for Cardiovascular Angiography and Interventions, American College of Surgeons, and American Dental Association, with representation from the American College of Physicians. Catheter Cardiovasc Interv 69:334–340
50. Vilahur G, Choi BG, Zafar MU et al (2007) Normalization of platelet reactivity in clopidogrel-treated subjects. J Thromb Haemost 5:82–90
51. Leithauser B, Zielske D, Seyfert UT, Jung F (2008) Effects of desmopressin on platelet membrane glycoproteins and platelet aggregation in volunteers on clopidogrel. Clin Hemorheol Microcirc 39:293–302

Part VI
Cardiovascular System

Bedside Myocardial Perfusion Assessment with Contrast Echocardiography

S. Orde and A. McLean

Introduction

Myocardial perfusion can be safely assessed at the bedside using contrast echocardiography. The contrast agents consist of tiny microbubbles (approximately 1–8 μm in diameter), which remain in the systemic circulation for ~ 3–5 min after venous injection. Low intensity ultrasound imaging is required to prevent the microbubbles from being destroyed. Myocardial perfusion is assessed by destroying the microbubbles with a 'flash' of higher intensity ultrasound and then analyzing the replenishment rate as the microbubbles seep back into the myocardial circulation.

There is reasonable evidence that myocardial contrast perfusion echocardiography (MCPE) can help in the detection of coronary artery disease as well as having prognostic value over regional wall motion analysis. However, there are challenges in bringing it into everyday clinical use: the imaging is challenging and relatively complicated compared to standard echocardiography; the sensitivity and specificity are not 100%; it remains an 'off-label' use of contrast echocardiography; and there are safety issues to consider. It has been investigated for more than 25 years and yet still has not made it into main-steam cardiac evaluation.

One area of considerable interest and future potential is in critically ill patients who have raised cardiac enzymes, especially troponins, with or without electrocardiogram (EKG) abnormalities or regional wall motion abnormalities, in whom the diagnosis of ischemia needs to be addressed. Examples include Takotsubo's or septic cardiomyopathy. Investigation with angiography or further imaging may be

S. Orde (✉)
Intensive Care Unit, Nepean Hospital
Sydney, Australia
email: samorde@hotmail.com

A. McLean
Intensive Care Unit, Nepean Hospital
Sydney, Australia
Sydney Medical School, University of Sydney
Sydney, Australia

© Springer International Publishing Switzerland 2016
J.-L. Vincent (ed.), *Annual Update in Intensive Care and Emergency Medicine 2016*,
DOI 10.1007/978-3-319-27349-5_14

detrimental in patients with acute renal failure or bleeding risk and there are dangers associated with unnecessary transfer. It is not suggested that MCPE would take the place of angiography or other investigations assessing myocardial perfusion, but potentially MCPE could identify patients (or at least triage them) who have normal myocardial perfusion yet abnormal troponins, EKGs and have regional wall motion abnormalities. In addition, there are exciting implications for the future use of microbubble contrast in terms of drug and gene delivery.

Contrast Echocardiography Agents

Echocardiography imaging in the critically ill can be frustratingly difficult at times. Contrast echocardiography agents were originally designed to help improve endocardial border definition, known as left ventricle opacification, as well as to enhance Doppler signals. Their use can prevent non-diagnostic studies from being inconclusive, particularly in the critically ill [1]. These contrast agents were originally described in the 1960s [2] and further development in the 1980s and '90s saw specific contrast agents designed to remain in the systemic circulation after venous injection, as well as ultrasound imaging enhancement techniques developed (such as harmonic imaging) to enhance left ventricular opacification [3–5].

The contrast agents consist of microbubbles containing a hemodynamically inert gaseous core (e.g., octafluoropropane, sulfur hexafluoride) and a stabilizing outer shell (e.g., lipid, albumin or biopolymer), which oscillate under the influence of ultrasound waves [6]. Similar to agitated saline, now in use for over 35 years to determine cardiac and intrapulmonary shunts, these contrast echocardiography microbubbles form multiple small liquid-air interfaces whose boundaries have a high acoustic impedance mismatch resulting in enhanced ultrasound reflection. A major difference of contrast microbubbles compared to saline bubbles is the size, with the bubbles small enough (1–8 µm) to traverse the pulmonary capillaries in order to enter the systemic circulation. Saline bubbles are typically 50–90 µm diameter and are destroyed as they pass into the pulmonary capillaries.

Microbubbles require specific 'activation' to be effective (different methods are required for different agents). Injected intravenously, they cross the pulmonary circulation into the system circulation. With similar behavior and rheology to red blood cells (RBCs) [7], they remain entirely within the vascular compartment and last in the circulation for approximately 3–5 min before they burst and lose their ability to produce ultrasound backscatter. Once the microbubbles are destroyed, the shell is metabolized by fatty acid metabolism if made of lipid (such as with Definity [BMS, Billerica, MA]), or by the reticulo-endothelial system. The inert gas is not metabolized and simply escapes from the lungs [8].

There are various contrast agents available, each having slightly different compositions and gas cores (Table 1). Different countries have different agents available. The first generation contrast agents, developed at the end of the 20th century, have a lipid shell with an air core, are soluble and are able to pass through the pulmonary circulation but lose their echogenicity and dissolve rapidly. The second generation

Table 1 Contrast echocardiography agents

Classification	Gas core	Shell	Trade name	Bubble size (μm)	Comments
First generation	Air	Albumin	Albunex	2–8	No longer made
	Air	Palmitic acid/galactose	Levovist (Schering, Kelinworth, NJ)	2–8	Non-cardiac use mainly
	Air	D-galactose	Echovist (Berlex, Lachine, Quebec City, Canada)	2–8	First commercially available agent
Second generation	Octafluoropropane (C_3F_8)	Albumin	Optison (GE healthcare, Chalfont St Giles, UK)	1–10	Available in USA, Europe, South America
	Octafluoropropane (C_3F_8)	Lipid	Definity (BMS, Billerica, MA)	1–10	Available in USA, Europe, South America, Canada, Australasia
	Sulfur hexafluoride (SF_6)	Lipid	Sonovue (Bracca, Milan, Italy)	1–10	Available in Europe and USA (known as Lumason)

NB: The list does not include every available contrast agent worldwide and the accuracy of the 'comments' section may change but is up to date at time of writing to the best of the authors' knowledge

contrast agents were then developed and have high-molecular weight gaseous cores, are less soluble than air, with stabilizing lipid or biopolymer shells and remain more stable under the ultrasound field and, therefore, have an increased lifespan in the circulation [9]. These preparations include the standard contrast agents used today: Definity, Optison (GE healthcare, Chalfont St Giles, UK) and Sonovue (Bracca, Milan, Italy). Third generation agents include those specifically used for research-based activities, specialized imaging or therapeutic purposes [8].

Effect of Ultrasound on Contrast Agents

Specific imaging techniques and software are required to perform MCPE to take advantage of the different ultrasound reflection properties of the contrast microspheres versus soft tissue. When ultrasound interacts with the microbubbles they oscillate and this effect is dependent on the ultrasound acoustic pressure as well as the shell and core gas properties of the agent. Ultrasound acoustic pressure is described as the 'mechanical index' and corresponds to the power output of the scanner [10]. With standard 2D echocardiography imaging the mechanical index is ~ 1.4; however, at this level the microspheres would oscillate to such a degree that they would burst and be destroyed. Therefore low mechanical index (<0.2) imaging is used with contrast imaging.

The oscillation effect of contrast echocardiography under low mechanical index ultrasound means the ultrasound reflections are different for microbubbles compared to soft tissue. This difference can be harnessed to enhance contrast versus tissue differentiation when imaging: microbubbles reflect ultrasound in a non-linear format compared to tissue, which reflects ultrasound in a linear manner. Non-linear reflection means the sound waves are reflected not only at the frequency of the original ultrasound wave but also at higher, harmonic frequencies. Soft tissue, however, produces fewer harmonics, hence reflection of the ultrasound waves in a more linear fashion. There are different methods used by various vendors to take advantage of the specific reflection properties for tissue vs contrast microbubbles, including: pulse inversion, power modulation and coherent contrast imaging to reduce the soft tissue linear reflections of the fundamental frequency [11].

Myocardial Perfusion Imaging

In the 1990s, initial studies in animals, subsequently validated in humans, investigated the hypothesis that myocardial blood flow could be assessed with contrast echocardiography by destroying the contrast microbubbles with a 'flash' of high diagnostic intensity ultrasound and then assessing the rate of replenishment of the microbubbles into the myocardium [12–14]. The replenishment is assessed by the change in intensity or brightness in a 'region of interest' (ROI). The microbubbles behave like RBCs, hence the theory that any change in signal intensity represents a change in myocardial blood flow.

With normal myocardial blood flow, 90% of the coronary circulation resides within the myocardial capillaries and RBCs travel at approximately 1 mm/sec at rest. After destruction of the contrast the signal intensity is anticipated to return to normal after approximately 5–7 cardiac cycles [13] (Fig. 1). During stress or exercise where vasodilation and increased capillary blood flow are present, the rate of return of signal intensity is faster: approximately 2–3 cardiac cycles. The rate of microbubble replenishment can be assessed qualitatively (as seen in Fig. 1), but also quantitatively by reviewing the change in signal intensity over time in a specific ROI (Fig. 2). Myocardial blood flow is considered the product of plateau signal intensity and rate of replenishment (Fig. 3). The concept being that the slower the rate of replenishment and lower the plateau signal intensity, the poorer the myocardial blood flow.

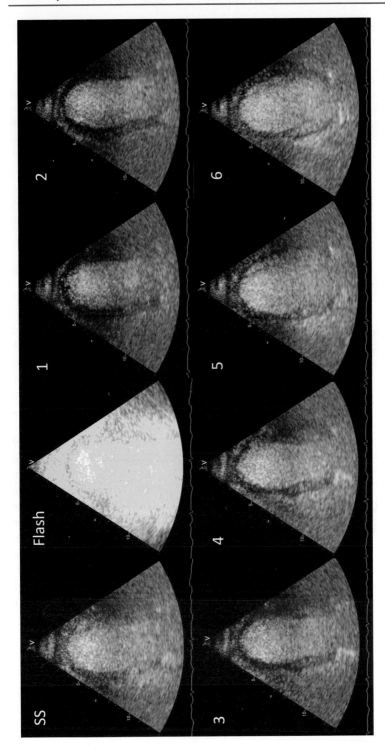

Fig. 1 Normal myocardial contrast perfusion echocardiograph: qualitative assessment. Ultrasound contrast infused until steady state achieved (SS – steady state). A 'flash' of high mechanical index ultrasound destroys the contrast microbubbles within the imaging beam. Assessment of myocardial perfusion is then made as the microbubbles return to the myocardium over subsequent cardiac cycles (1–6). Normal replenishment occurs over 5–6 cardiac cycles at rest, 2–3 cardiac cycles with stress

Fig. 2 Qualitative assessment of myocardial perfusion involves specification of a region of interest (ROI) classically corresponding to individual left ventricular myocardial segments

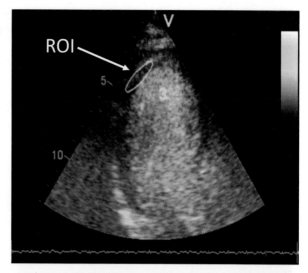

Fig. 3 Myocardial contrast perfusion echocardiography (MCPE) quantitative assessment. Regions of interest (ROI) are defined and rate of change in signal intensity assessed at end-diastolic frames. The plateau signal intensity (A) is considered to represent the myocardial capillary blood volume. The rate of replenishment (β) of the microbubbles is considered as the velocity of blood. The product of $A \times \beta$ is considered to represent the myocardial blood flow

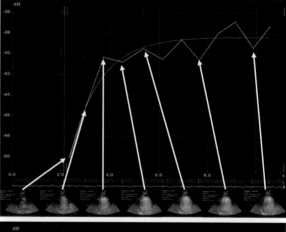

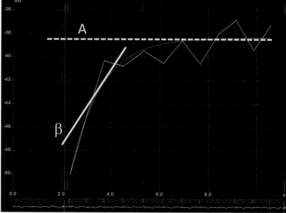

Safety Profile

The use of contrast echocardiography, extensively investigated in several large multicenter trials [15–17], has been found to be well-tolerated and safe in both non-critically ill and critically ill patients [18]. 'Black-box' warnings were issued by the US Food and Drug Administration (FDA) in 2007 but these were downgraded within 12 months. The current FDA recommendations state that if a patient has an unstable cardiopulmonary condition or pulmonary hypertension (the severity is not stated), the patient should have cardiorespiratory monitoring for 30 min after contrast agent administration [19]. In the United States, echocardiography laboratories are not accredited unless they have the ability to perform contrast echocardiography [20].

Side effects are rare and include headache, flushing or back pain. These symptoms are usually relieved on cessation of contrast agent administration. There is a 1:10000 chance of an anaphylaxis type reaction (considered secondary to the microbubble shell and possibly non-IgE related) [9]. Contraindications include previous hypersensitivity to contrast agents or to blood products (e.g., albumin), severe pulmonary hypertension and cardiac right-to-left or bidirectional shunts. These last two contraindications are under debate and evidence exists of the safety in these conditions, whereas there are only case reports of harm with recent use of ultrasound contrast [16, 21].

We consider an individualized approach of risk versus benefit is required for MCPE. Important requirements include expertise to perform and interpret the procedure, and the study should be performed in an environment with appropriate monitoring and resuscitation facilities.

Applications in the Critically Ill

Recognition of Acute Coronary Artery Disease

The diagnosis of acute coronary syndromes (ACS) in the intensive care unit (ICU) can be challenging. Critically ill patients with ischemic heart disease are at greater risk during times of stress and the classic history of central crushing chest pain can be absent as a result of acute illness, sedation and/or mechanical ventilation. Troponin elevation, EKG and regional wall motion abnormalities (RWMA) are frequently seen in conditions other than myocardial infarction [22], for example Takotsubo's and septic cardiomyopathy amongst many other causes [23]. In addition, investigating for possible ACS with angiography or single photon emission computed tomography (SPECT) can be dangerous due to the inherent risks of patient transport, contrast-induced nephropathy, radiation, access issues, anticoagulation, and delays in diagnosis. Cost and access to suitable angiographic facilities may be issues in some ICUs. Potentially, MCPE could help identify patients with ACS at the bedside in the ICU, not to replace further imaging, but rather as a triage tool or simply to add confidence to the physician's clinical acumen [24].

MCPE has been compared to SPECT, the most widely used perfusion technique for assessment of coronary artery disease. In several studies for detection of coronary artery disease, MCPE has shown excellent concordance (81% [76.4–85.6]) [25]. A meta-analysis indicated a higher sensitivity for MCPE than for SPECT and no difference was found for specificity [26]. Various clinical studies have used MCPE to quantify myocardial blood flow, trying to differentiate coronary artery ischemia from not significantly occluded coronary arteries. Senior et al. reported that MCPE could differentiate ischemic from non-ischemic cardiomyopathy (defined as <50% coronary artery stenosis) with a specificity of 89% and sensitivity of 91% [27].

Microvascular Versus Macrovascular Function Assessment

Microvascular dysfunction has been proposed in a number of cardiac conditions such as Takotsubo's [28] and septic cardiomyopathy [29] amongst others. Whether the microvascular dysfunction is a primary cause of secondary phenomena is not known. Abdelmoneim et al performed MCPE in 9 patients with angiographically confirmed Takotsubo's syndrome and were able to show reduced perfusion in the myocardium with a 71% concordance with areas of RWMA [28]. It is suggested that the microvasculature in the endocardial regional has the lowest flow reserve and is more susceptible to ischemia than the epicardium possibly due to the larger epicardially placed coronary arteries [30]. Therefore, with microvascular disorders there may be a reduction in the endocardial myocardium to a greater extent than in the epicardial myocardium (Fig. 4).

Possible Future Roles for Contrast Echocardiography

Advances in contrast microbubble formulations, imaging and post-processing analysis, indicate that the future for contrast echocardiography may include imaging of macro and microvasculature elsewhere in the body as well as targeted drug and/or gene delivery.

Contrast-Enhanced Ultrasound

Using contrast agents in a similar manner to MCPE, non-invasive and bedside perfusion assessment of organs may be possible. Schneider et al. suggested that assessing renal cortical perfusion with contrast is feasible and well-tolerated in the ICU population and that possibly a decrease in renal perfusion may occur within 24 h of surgery in patients at risk of acute kidney injury (AKI) [31]. These techniques are relatively unexplored at this time and although they hold promise, do demonstrate significant heterogeneity and the results remain unpredictable [32]. Further investigation is certainly warranted.

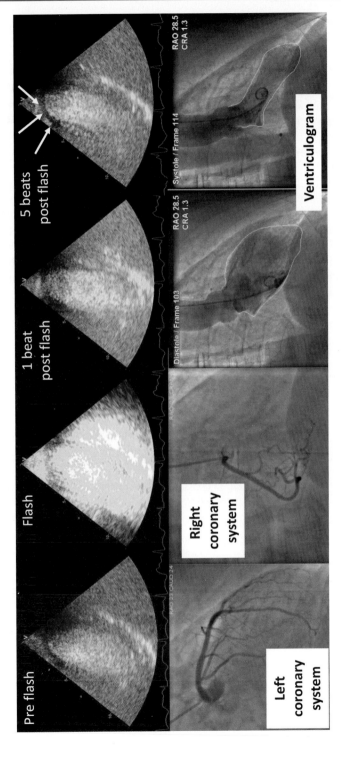

Fig. 4 Takotsubo's cardiomyopathy with microvascular dysfunction (*arrows*). Endocardial perfusion defect shown at 5 beats post flash in the apical region where transient apical hypokinesis was visualized. Coronary angiography confirmed normal vasculature and left ventriculography demonstrated apical ballooning

Targeted Drug Delivery

The property of contrast microbubbles bursting under the effect of ultrasound can be used to target drug delivery. Drugs can be attached to microbubbles by a variety of methods [10] and as long as the site is accessible to ultrasound, a burst of high mechanical index ultrasound may be able to locally deliver the drug, such as thrombolysis. Transfer of genetic material has also been suggested and has been shown to be safe and more specific than viral vectors for cDNA delivery [33].

Conclusion

The use of contrast echocardiography in the critically ill is safe compared to other contrast agents, feasible at the bedside and has the potential to rescue undiagnostic echocardiograms. Although the agents are only indicated for left ventricular opacification, the off-label use of MCPE holds promise as being a potential method to assess myocardial perfusion at the bedside. The technology has been available for over two decades and is yet to find a place in regular clinical practice, but as a result of ever evolving sophistication of microbubble agents, software and hardware still holds considerable promise. The utility of MCPE in the ICU has not been extensively considered to date but potentially may have a role in the challenging arena of accurate and timely diagnosis of ACS in the critically ill.

References

1. Kurt M, Shaikh KA, Peterson L et al (2009) Impact of contrast echocardiography on evaluation of ventricular function and clinical management in a large prospective cohort. J Am Coll Cardiol 53:802–810
2. Gramiak R, Shah PM, Kramer DH (1969) Ultrasound cardiography: contrast studies in anatomy and function. Radiology 92:939–948
3. Keller MW, Feinstein SB, Watson DD (1987) Successful left ventricular opacification following peripheral venous injection of sonicated contrast agent: an experimental evaluation. Am Heart J 114:570–575
4. Feinstein SB, Cheirif J, Cate Ten FJ et al (1990) Safety and efficacy of a new transpulmonary ultrasound contrast agent: initial multicenter clinical results. J Am Coll Cardiol 16:316–324
5. Lindner JR, Dent JM, Moos SP et al (1997) Enhancement of left ventricular cavity opacification by harmonic imaging after venous injection of Albunex. Am J Cardiol 79:1657–1662
6. Postema M, van Wamel A, Cate Ten FJ, de Jong N (2005) High-speed photography during ultrasound illustrates potential therapeutic applications of microbubbles. Med Phys 32:3707–3711
7. Keller MW, Segal SS, Kaul S, Duling B (1989) The behavior of sonicated albumin microbubbles within the microcirculation: a basis for their use during myocardial contrast echocardiography. Circ Res 65:458–467
8. Platts DG, Fraser JF (2011) Contrast echocardiography in critical care: echoes of the future? A review of the role of microsphere contrast echocardiography. Crit Care Resusc 13:44–55

9. Seol S-H, Lindner JR (2014) A primer on the methods and applications for contrast echocardiography in clinical imaging. J Cardiovasc Ultrasound 22:101–110

10. Pathan F, Marwick TH (2015) Myocardial perfusion imaging using contrast echocardiography. Prog Cardiovasc Dis 57:632–643

11. Seol S-H, Davidson BP, Belcik JT et al (2015) Real-time contrast ultrasound muscle perfusion imaging with intermediate-power imaging coupled with acoustically durable microbubbles. J Am Soc Echocardiogr 28:718–726.e2

12. Jayaweera AR, Edwards N, Glasheen WP et al (1994) In vivo myocardial kinetics of air-filled albumin microbubbles during myocardial contrast echocardiography. Comparison with radiolabeled red blood cells. Circ Res 74:1157–1165

13. Wei K, Jayaweera AR, Firoozan S et al (1998) Quantification of myocardial blood flow with ultrasound-induced destruction of microbubbles administered as a constant venous infusion. Circulation 97:473–483

14. Vogel R, Indermühle A, Reinhardt J et al (2005) The quantification of absolute myocardial perfusion in humans by contrast echocardiography: algorithm and validation. J Am Coll Cardiol 45:754–762

15. Main ML, Hibberd MG, Ryan A et al (2014) Acute mortality in critically ill patients undergoing echocardiography with or without an ultrasound contrast agent. JACC Cardiovasc Imaging 7:40–48

16. Abdelmoneim SS, Bernier M, Scott CG et al (2010) Safety of contrast agent use during stress echocardiography in patients with elevated right ventricular systolic pressure: a cohort study. Circ Cardiovasc Imaging 3:240–248

17. Wei K, Mulvagh SL, Carson L et al (2008) The safety of deFinity and Optison for ultrasound image enhancement: a retrospective analysis of 78,383 administered contrast doses. J Am Soc Echocardiogr 21:1202–1206

18. Putrino A, Platts DG (2015) Contrast echocardiography in acutely unwell patients. J Am Soc Echocardiogr 28:844

19. U.S. Food and Drug Administration (2008) Postmarket Drug Safety Information for Patients and Providers. Information for Healthcare Professionals: Micro-bubble Contrast Agents (marketed as Definity (Perflutren Lipid Microsphere) Injectable Suspension and Optison (Perflutren Protein-Type A Microspheres for Injection). Update FDA alert. http://www.fda.gov/Drugs/DrugSafety/PostmarketDrugSafetyInformationforPatientsandProviders/ucm125574.htm. Accessed Oct 2015

20. Mulvagh SL, Rakowski H, Vannan MA et al (2008) American Society of Echocardiography Consensus Statement on the Clinical Applications of Ultrasonic Contrast Agents in Echocardiography. J Am Soc Echocardiogr 21:1179–1201

21. Parker JM, Weller MW, Feinstein LM et al (2013) Safety of ultrasound contrast agents in patients with known or suspected cardiac shunts. Am J Cardiol 112:1039–1045

22. Lim W, Whitlock R, Khera V et al (2010) Etiology of troponin elevation in critically ill patients. J Crit Care 25:322–328

23. Orde SR, Pulido JN, Masaki M et al (2014) Outcome prediction in sepsis: speckle tracking echocardiography based assessment of myocardial function. Crit Care 18:R149

24. Orde SR, Huang SJ, McLean AS (2015) 2015 ASE 26th Annual Scientific Sessions. Raised Troponin in the ICU: can real-time myocardial contrast echocardiography improve recognition of acute ischaemia in the critically ill? JASE 28:B2–B134 (abst)

25. Senior R, Becher H, Monaghan M et al (2009) Contrast echocardiography: evidence-based recommendations by European Association of Echocardiography. Eur J Echocardiogr 10:194–212

26. Dijkmans PA, Senior R, Becher H et al (2006) Myocardial contrast echocardiography evolving as a clinically feasible technique for accurate, rapid, and safe assessment of myocardial perfusion: the evidence so far. J Am Coll Cardiol 48:2168–2177

27. Senior R, Janardhanan R, Jeetley P, Burden L (2005) Myocardial contrast echocardiography for distinguishing ischemic from nonischemic first-onset acute heart failure: insights into the mechanism of acute heart failure. Circulation 112:1587–1593

28. Abdelmoneim SS, Mankad SV, Bernier M et al (2009) Microvascular function in Takotsubo cardiomyopathy with contrast echocardiography: prospective evaluation and review of literature. J Am Soc Echocardiogr 22:1249–1255

29. Ait-Oufella H, Bourcier S, Lehoux S, Guidet B (2015) Microcirculatory disorders during septic shock. Curr Opin Crit Care 21:271–275

30. Linka AZ, Sklenar J, Wei K et al (1998) Assessment of transmural distribution of myocardial perfusion with contrast echocardiography. Circulation 98:1912–1920

31. Schneider AG, Goodwin MD, Schelleman A et al (2013) Contrast-enhanced ultrasound to evaluate changes in renal cortical perfusion around cardiac surgery: a pilot study. Crit Care 17:R138

32. Schneider AG, Goodwin MD, Schelleman A et al (2014) Contrast-enhanced ultrasonography to evaluate changes in renal cortical microcirculation induced by noradrenaline: a pilot study. Crit Care 18:653

33. Bhattacharyya S, Senior R (2014) The current state of myocardial contrast echocardiography: what can we read between the lines? Reply. Eur Heart J Cardiovasc Imaging 15:351–352

Pathophysiological Determinants of Cardiovascular Dysfunction in Septic Shock

F. Guarracino, R. Baldassarri, and M. R. Pinsky

Introduction

The International Sepsis Definitions consensus conference defined septic shock as the most severe clinical manifestation of sepsis [1]. Septic shock is characterized by sepsis-induced cardiovascular alterations that result in severe hypotension, tissue hypoperfusion and metabolic disorders [2]. Sepsis-induced arterial vasodilatation and the consequent loss of vascular tone are thought to be the main determinants of the altered hemodynamic state in septic shock. The introduction of echocardiography into clinical practice and the direct evaluation of heart morphology and function in septic patients emphasized the role of myocardial depression as a pathophysiological mechanism underlying hemodynamic impairment [3, 4].

The Surviving Sepsis Campaign recommends that resuscitation of patients in septic shock should be performed early and tailored to restore adequate peripheral perfusion to prevent organ injury. International guidelines strongly recommend early therapy based on fluid administration to restore cardiac output, vasopressor drugs to sustain mean arterial pressure and inotropes when cardiac dysfunction limits blood flow under pressure [2]. The mortality rate of this severe clinical manifestation of sepsis remains high (up to 50% in critically ill patients) despite the recommended therapeutic strategies and the results of several studies to determine the pathophysiological mechanisms of the altered hemodynamics in septic shock [5–8].

F. Guarracino (✉) · R. Baldassarri
Department of Cardiothoracic Anesthesia and Intensive Care Medicine, Azienda Ospedaliero Universitaria Pisana
Pisa, Italy
email: fabiodoc64@hotmail.com

M. R. Pinsky
Dept of Critical Care Medicine, University of Pittsburgh
Pittsburgh, USA
Dept of Anesthesiology, University of California, San Diego
La Jolla, USA

© Springer International Publishing Switzerland 2016
J.-L. Vincent (ed.), *Annual Update in Intensive Care and Emergency Medicine 2016*,
DOI 10.1007/978-3-319-27349-5_15

Pathophysiological determinants of cardiovascular dysfunction are receiving increased interest, with the goal of tailoring treatment options based on novel understanding of the specific pathophysiology present. This review discusses the emergent pathophysiological issues related to cardiovascular alterations in septic shock and their possible influence on clinical management.

Pathophysiology in Septic Shock

The most common hemodynamic profile in septic shock is characterized by a hyperdynamic circulation and low systemic vascular resistance (SVR), which is well characterized using pulmonary artery catheterization. A pulmonary artery catheter (PAC) allows direct and derived measures of the hemodynamic variables in septic patients by evaluating intracardiac filling pressures (e.g., central venous pressure [CVP], pulmonary artery pressure, pulmonary artery occlusion pressure [PAOP]), cardiac output and both peripheral and pulmonary vascular resistances, as well as continuous measures of mixed venous oxygen saturation (SvO_2) [9]. The lack of proven benefit associated with the known associated risks of PAC insertion have greatly limited its use in clinical practice despite the effective role of the PAC in direct hemodynamic studies in septic patients. However, the PAC remains the reference method for the continuous monitoring of cardiac output. The continuous evaluation of the hemodynamic parameters provided by the PAC allows tight monitoring of the host response to therapy and of the progression of the hemodynamic impairment.

Over the last decade, the introduction of echocardiography into the routine management of critically ill patients has provided an opportunity to enlarge understanding of the cardiovascular pathophysiological elements in altered hemodynamic states by assessing cardiac mechanics. In particular, in septic shock patients, the use of bedside echocardiography has allowed us to better understand the role of myocardial function, and very recently the non-invasive measurement of ventricular contractility by ultrasound has more deeply investigated the determinants of cardiovascular dysfunction in sepsis (Table 1).

Table 1 Derived parameter analysis based on monitoring device

PAC and arterial pressure	Echocardiography	Combined monitoring
Vasodilatation	LV function systolic and diastolic	Ventricular and arterial elastances
Hyperdynamic state	RV Function systolic and diastolic	V-A coupling

PAC: pulmonary artery catheter; *LV*: left ventricular; *RV*: right ventricular; *V-A*: ventriculo-arterial

Novel Considerations in Septic Shock

Arterial vasodilatation is the main pathophysiological mechanism for the altered hemodynamic state in septic shock, but the role of the other components of the cardiovascular system, such as cardiac contractility, in creating the observed hemodynamic impairment has only recently been recognized.

Ventricular Elastance

End-systolic ventricular elastance (Ees) is a load-independent index of left ventricular (LV) contractility. Suga [10] and Sunagawa et al. [11] defined Ees as the slope of the LV end-systolic pressure-volume relationship (ESPVR). Ees is an integrated measurement of LV systolic performance, which depends on the interactions of functional, structural and inotropic characteristics of the left ventricle because LV performance depends on intrinsic myocardial contractility (i.e., the main determinant of LV systolic function) and other LV functional and geometric properties (contractile synchrony and geometric remodeling of the cardiac chambers) [12, 13].

We reported that Ees was significantly decreased in human septic shock despite a preserved LV ejection fraction (LVEF) and a normal or even increased cardiac index (CI) [12]. These data confirm that LVEF is not a reliable index of LV systolic function. LVEF is a load-dependent index of LV function that is also influenced by the arterial system and, since arterial tone is generally decreased in septic patients, may allow LVEF to remain high despite impaired contractility. Echocardiography allows the bedside measurement of Ees, which contributes to the direct study of LV systolic performance and the assessment of ventriculo-arterial (V-A) coupling in critically ill patients by providing important information on the hemodynamic state in septic shock [12].

Myocardial Depression

Primary myocardial depression and consequent heart dysfunction occur in approximately 40–50% of patients with septic shock [14]. The most common manifestation of cardiac impairment in septic shock is combined LV systolic and diastolic failure with a significant reduction in LV stroke volume (SV). Right ventricular (RV) function may be primarily affected by sepsis-induced myocardial injury, or it may be secondarily impaired by the reduction in arterial tone and consequent decrease in RV preload (low RVEF). The eventual volume overload that is imposed on the right ventricle by fluid resuscitation can also alter RV function in the early phase of septic shock and lead to worsening LV diastolic dysfunction through ventricular interdependence [12, 15–17].

Recent literature suggests that it can be difficult to understand whether the cardiac dysfunction is due to direct myocardial injury induced by sepsis or the interaction between the heart and vascular system. But, cardiac dysfunction is a consequence of the attempt of the heart to adapt to the continuous hemodynamic changes in the vascular tree during sepsis [14]. Sepsis-induced variation in arterial tone alters preload and afterload because the increased levels of circulating cate-cholamines affect effective circulating blood volume, arterial tone and myocardial contractility [18]. Patients with preexisting cardiac failure often cannot tolerate the hemodynamic changes, and these patients are prone to worsening heart dysfunction.

Arterial Elastance

Arterial elastance (Ea) represents the total afterload that is imposed on the left ventricle during ejection. Ea depends on the association of several properties of the arteries, such as compliance, stiffness and vascular resistances. Ea can be calculated as the ratio between the LV end-systolic pressure and the LV SV. Ea is one of the two components of V-A coupling, and alterations in V-A coupling contribute significantly to impairments in cardiovascular efficiency, which lead to V-A decoupling in human septic shock [3, 12, 16]. Ea is commonly reduced in septic shock patients because of the arterial vasodilatation. The use of vasoactive drugs (e.g., norepinephrine), as recommended by the Surviving Sepsis Campaign Guidelines, to restore the mean arterial pressure (MAP) in severe hypotensive states in septic shock frequently increases Ea. Norepinephrine is the most commonly used vasopressor to quickly restore MAP in human septic shock. The normalization of systemic arterial pressure is one of the first targets of early-goal therapy in septic shock, but exaggerated peripheral vasoconstriction can result in an increase of Ea and V-A decoupling in human septic shock.

Ventricular-Arterial Coupling

Several studies recently demonstrated that V-A coupling plays a key role in determining the altered hemodynamic state in septic shock. V-A coupling has been validated as a powerful tool to evaluate cardiovascular system efficiency. Suga first defined V-A coupling as the ratio of Ea to Ees [10]. Cardiovascular performance studies demonstrated that the cardiovascular system is more efficient when it is coupled, which means that the ratio between Ea and Ees is approximately 1. Too little Ea or Ees, as occurs in beriberi, or too much Ea relative to Ees, as occurs in malignant hypertension, are both associated with acute heart failure.

Most septic shock patients present V-A decoupling because of alterations of Ea, Ees or both. Evolution in echocardiography technology has allowed bedside evaluations of Ea with the method proposed by Chen et al., enabling non-invasive calculation of V-A coupling in critically ill patients [19, 20].

Ea and Ees are generally decreased in the hemodynamic profile of septic shock patients because of severe vasoplegia and the reduction in LV contractility, respectively. A therapeutic strategy that targets the restoration of normal Ea and Ees values in this context may normalize V-A coupling in septic patients. The early therapy recommended during the immediate resuscitation of septic shock patients is based on the use of vasopressors to restore arterial tone and increase MAP to improve tissue perfusion. Vasopressor drugs increase the Ea with a consequent potential to unbalance Ea/Ees causing V-A decoupling [21].

Ees is affected by the intrinsic reduction in LV myocardial contractility, which is primarily affected by sepsis-induced myocardial injury or is impaired by the sepsis-induced hemodynamic changes in vascular tone (e.g., preload and afterload). The attempt of the heart to face the continuous changes in vascular tone and the consequent hemodynamic implications may result in LV impairment despite the eventual myocardial injury [15]. We recently reported [12] that patients with septic shock may present normal coupling when LV function is preserved (LVEF > 50%) or in cases of LV dysfunction (LVEF < 50%). Septic patients with LV dysfunction (LVEF > 50%) are generally uncoupled [12].

Novelties in Pathophysiological Understanding and Management

Recent literature has demonstrated novel and emerging issues related to the pathophysiological mechanisms of the altered hemodynamics in septic shock. V-A decoupling secondary to alterations in Ees and Ea addresses a complex and multifactorial pathophysiological hemodynamic pattern in septic shock [3, 11, 16]. These recent studies suggest that the management of the septic shock patients should be re-evaluated.

Cardiac dysfunction is a pathophysiological determinant of cardiovascular impairment in septic shock patients, and guidelines strongly recommend early fluid administration, vasopressor drugs and inotropes when cardiac dysfunction occurs, to improve cardiac performance [2].

V-A coupling plays a pivotal role in determining cardiovascular alterations in septic shock, and most septic shock patients present V-A decoupling. The efficiency of the cardiovascular system depends on the tight interaction between the heart and the arterial system to provide adequate cardiac output and tissue perfusion. Cardiovascular performance is optimal, and cardiac energies are efficient when the system is coupled. The V-A decoupling in septic patients is typically the result of combined LV dysfunction and decreased Ea. Ideally, the therapeutic strategies in human septic shock management should be based on the individual hemodynamic profile, with particular attention to the patient's Ea/Ees. The Surviving Sepsis Campaign Guidelines for the management of human septic shock recommend the use of vasoactive drugs to restore the Ea/Ees rather than improve LVEF. Paonessa et al. recently reported that septic patients with hyperdynamic LVEF exhibited increased short-term (28-day) mortality compared to patients with normal LVEF [22]. The American College of Cardiology defines hyperdynamic LVEF as an LVEF > 70% [23]. Paonessa et al. investigated patients with and without septic shock and found that hyperdynamic LVEF was more frequently reported in septic shock patients, but this finding was not specific for sepsis, as previously thought [22]. Recent reports on the use of vasoactive drugs, such as enoximone and levosimendan, in human septic shock patients have demonstrated the efficacy of these inodilators in improving V-A coupling via restoration of the Ea/Ees [12, 24, 25].

In 2013, Morelli et al. reported the use of beta-blockers (e.g., esmolol) in septic shock patients with tachycardia and high inotropic and vasopressor support [26]. The authors emphasized that the increased levels of circulating catecholamines, hyperactive sympathetic tone and dysfunction of autonomic regulation in septic shock induce myocardial dysfunction or alterations in vascular tone in septic shock patients [8, 27]. Control of the heart rate improved LV diastolic filling with a consequent increase in LV SV or coronary artery perfusion, which presumably reduced myocardial oxygen consumption and improved cardiac performance and tissue perfusion. The authors demonstrated that titrated doses of esmolol effectively decreased heart rate and significantly improved cardiac performance. This suggested that a heart rate between 80 and 94 beats/min provided adequate LV performance and tissue perfusion. Morelli and colleagues also demonstrated an improvement in short-term (28-day) mortality in the enrolled patients, but this observation was not the primary end-point of the study [26].

In our opinion, a lower heart rate in septic patients may contribute to blunting the catecholamine-induced cardiovascular stress and positively affect V-A coupling via a reduction in Ea. If resuscitation therapies aimed at increasing MAP increase Ea without also increasing Ees, then the potential exists to worsen LV contractile function. Potentially, this may be why norepinephrine, rather than phenylephrine, is the vasopressor of choice in septic shock. It will be interesting to see how well vasopressin, a pure vasoconstrictor, fares compared to norepinephrine during sepsis resuscitation in the soon to be completed clinical trial.

Conclusion

Sepsis-induced peripheral vasodilation is the primary cause of the severe hemodynamic alterations in septic shock, but a complete understanding of the pathophysiological mechanisms of the cardiovascular impairment is a challenge for clinicians. The Surviving Sepsis Campaign guidelines recommend early-goal directed therapy with fluid administration, vasopressors and inotropes to resuscitate septic patients with severe hypotension and metabolic disturbances due to organ hypoperfusion. However, the mortality rate of patients with septic shock remains high. Recent studies have reported novel determinants of the altered hemodynamic state in septic shock, and this increased understanding offers a possible re-evaluation of current therapeutic strategies. V-A decoupling is one of the most important features of the hemodynamic impairment in human septic shock. LV dysfunction and alterations in the arterial system contribute to the inefficiency of the cardiovascular system in septic shock. The management of septic shock patients should likely be tailored toward restoring adequate cardiovascular efficiency through the normalization of Ea/Ees, as reported in recent studies.

In conclusion, we advocate a more tailored diagnostic and therapeutic approach to address the underlying pathophysiological 'picture' in human septic shock.

References

1. Levy MM, Fink MP, Marshall JC et al (2003) 2001 SCCM/ESICM/ACCP/ATS/SIS International Sepsis Definitions Conference. Intensive Care Med 29:530–538
2. Dellinger RP, Levy MM, Rhodes A et al (2013) Surviving sepsis campaign: international guidelines for management of severe sepsis and septic shock: 2012. Crit Care Med 41:580–637
3. Guarracino F, Baldassarri R, Pinsky MR (2013) Ventriculo-arterial decoupling in acutely altered hemodynamic states. Crit Care 17:213
4. Vieillard-Baron A, Prin S, Chergui K, Dubourg O, Jardin F (2003) Hemodynamic instability in sepsis: bedside assessment by Doppler echocardiography. Am J Respir Crit Care Med 168:1270–1276
5. Angus DC, Linde-Zwirble WT, Lidicker J, Clermont G, Carcillo J, Pinsky MR (2001) Epidemiology of severe sepsis in the United States: analysis of incidence, outcome, and associated costs of care. Crit Care Med 29:1303–1310
6. Gu WJ, Wang F, Bakker J, Tang L, Liu JC (2014) The effect of goal-directed therapy on mortality in patients with sepsis – earlier is better: a meta-analysis of randomized controlled trials. Crit Care 18:570
7. Annane D, Bellissant E, Cavaillon JM (2005) Septic shock. Lancet 365:63–78
8. Dombrovskiy VY, Martin AA, Sunderram J, Paz HL (2007) Rapid increase in hospitalization and mortality rates for severe sepsis in the United States: a trend analysis from 1993 to 2003. Crit Care Med 35:1244–1250
9. Chatterjee K (2009) The Swan-Ganz catheters: past, present, and future. A viewpoint. Circulation 119:147–152
10. Suga H (1969) Time course of left ventricular pressure-volume relationship under various end-diastolic volume. Jap Heart J 10:509–515
11. Sunagawa K, Maughan WL, Burkhoff D, Sagawa K (1983) Left ventricular interaction with arterial load studied in isolated canine ventricle. Am J Physiol 245:H773–H780
12. Guarracino F, Ferro B, Morelli A, Bertini P, Baldassarri R, Pinsky MR (2014) Ventriculoarterial decoupling in human septic shock. Crit Care 18:R80
13. Borlaug BA, Kass DA (2008) Ventricular-vascular interaction in heart failure. Heart Fail Clin 4:23–36
14. Rudiger A, Singer M (2007) Mechanisms of sepsis-induced cardiac dysfunction. Crit Care Med 35:1599–1608
15. Parker MM, McCarthy KE, Ognibene FP, Parrillo JE (1990) Right ventricular dysfunction and dilatation, similar to left ventricular changes, characterize the cardiac depression of septic shock in humans. Chest 97:126–131
16. Antonucci E, Fiaccadori E, Donadello K, Taccone FS, Franchi F, Scolletta S (2014) Myocardial depression in sepsis: from pathogenesis to clinical manifestations and treatment. J Crit Care 29:500–511
17. Chan CM, Klinger JR (2008) The right ventricle in sepsis. Clin Chest Med 29:661–676
18. Hochstadt A, Meroz Y, Landesberg G (2011) Myocardial dysfunction in severe sepsis and septic shock: more questions than answers? J Cardiothorac Vasc Anesth 25:526–535
19. Chen CH, Fetics B, Nevo E et al (2001) Noninvasive single-beat determination of left ventricular end-systolic elastance in humans. J Am Coll Cardiol 38:2028–2034
20. Bertini P, Baldassarri R, Simone V, Amitrano D, Cariello C, Guarracino F (2014) Perioperative non-invasive estimation of left ventricular elastance (Ees) is no longer a challenge; it is a reality. Br J Anaesth 112:578
21. Schmittinger CA, Torgersen C, Luckner G, Schroder DC, Lorenz I, Dunser MW (2012) Adverse cardiac events during catecholamine vasopressor therapy: a prospective observational study. Intensive Care Med 38:950–958
22. Paonessa JR, Brennan T, Pimentel M, Steinhaus D, Feng M, Celi LA (2015) Hyperdynamic left ventricular ejection fraction in the intensive care unit. Crit Care 19:288

23. American College of Cardiology (2015) Left ventricular ejection fraction assessment. https://www.acc.org/tools-and-practice-support/clinical-toolkits/heart-failure-practice-solutions/left-ventricular-ejection-fraction-lvef-assessment-outpatient-setting. Accessed Nov 2015

24. Takaoka H, Takeuchi M, Odake M et al (1993) Comparison of the effects on arterial-ventricular coupling between phosphodiesterase inhibitor and dobutamine in the diseased human heart. J Am Coll Cardiol 22:598–606

25. Guarracino F, Cariello C, Danella A et al (2007) Effect of levosimendan on ventriculo-arterial coupling in patients with ischemic cardiomyopathy. Acta Anaesthesiol Scand 51:1217–1224

26. Morelli A, Ertmer C, Westphal M et al (2013) Effect of heart rate control with esmolol on hemodynamic and clinical outcomes in patients with septic shock: a randomized clinical trial. JAMA 310:1683–1691

27. Parker MM, Shelhamer JH, Natanson C, Alling DW, Parrillo JE (1987) Serial cardiovascular variables in survivors and nonsurvivors of human septic shock: heart rate as an early predictor of prognosis. Crit Care Med 15:923–929

Cardiovascular Response to ECMO

S. Akin, C. Ince, and D. dos Reis Miranda

Introduction

The principles of extracorporeal life support started with the first experimental efforts of Jean Baptiste Denis who circa 1693 performed a cross-transfusion of the blood of a human with the "gentle humors of a lamb" to determine whether living blood could be transmitted between two creatures [1]. However, clinical efforts to provide extracorporeal support began around 1930 with the work of John and Mary Gibbon. They developed a freestanding roller pump device for extracorporeal support after the death of a patient from a pulmonary embolus. Sixteen years later, the first human use of the device was performed in the operating room to assist during repair of an atrial septal defect in 1953. After some years, the use of the silicone membrane oxygenator, which was developed to allow recovery outside the operating room, led to the use of the term extracorporeal membrane oxygenation (ECMO). In the 1960s, with the development of gas-exchange devices, a silicone rubber membrane was interposed between the blood and the oxygen. This modification (and others) allowed the use of a heart-lung machine for days or weeks [3] reducing the threshold for their use. In 1972, Dr Bartlett successfully provided ECMO support to a two-year old boy following a Mustard procedure for correction of transposition of the great vessels with subsequent cardiac failure. The patient underwent ECMO support for 36 h until recovery. In 1975, the first neonate (Esperanza) with respiratory failure underwent ECMO support for 72 h and was successfully decannulated.

S. Akin (✉)
Department of Intensive Care, Erasmus MC, University Medical Center
Rotterdam, Netherlands
Department of Cardiology, Erasmus MC, University Medical Center
Rotterdam, Netherlands
email: sakirakin@gmail.com

C. Ince · D. dos Reis Miranda
Department of Intensive Care, Erasmus MC, University Medical Center
Rotterdam, Netherlands

© Springer International Publishing Switzerland 2016
J.-L. Vincent (ed.), *Annual Update in Intensive Care and Emergency Medicine 2016*,
DOI 10.1007/978-3-319-27349-5_16

Advances in management and monitoring of extracorporeal support therapy on the ICU are continuing. ECMO has increasingly become a part of the arsenal in the treatment of acute cardiopulmonary failure and resuscitation. Mechanical circulatory support (MCS) devices to temporarily (days to months) support heart and/or lung function (partially or totally) during cardiopulmonary failure, are functioning as a bridge to recovery or transplantation. Different varieties have been developed for specific cardiac or respiratory failure and veno-venous ECMO (VV-ECMO) for respiratory failure and veno-arterial ECMO (VA-ECMO) in cardiogenic shock, as well as during cardiopulmonary resuscitation (CPR), are growing in use.

Concerns about cardiovascular responses to different types of ECMO are inherent to the target treatment option for the failing organ. In VV-ECMO, the main issue is oxygenation of the severe hypoxic patient. VV-ECMO is used in pediatric applications, in severe respiratory distress syndrome and, since the H1N1 pandemic, use has been expanded to include severe pulmonary hypertension, hyperinflated lungs and in all conventional difficult-to-ventilate lungs.

The H1N1 flu pandemic led to a wider use of VV-ECMO, proving its power in hypoxemic emergencies and acute respiratory failure. The indications for VV-ECMO are supplemented by respiratory support as a bridge to lung transplantation, correction of lung hyperinflation during chronic obstructive pulmonary disease (COPD) exacerbation and respiratory support in patients with the acute respiratory distress syndrome (ARDS), possibly also without mechanical ventilation. In these patients, there is usually no cardiac dysfunction in need of support.

Acute severe heart failure/cardiogenic shock with a high mortality risk despite optimal conventional therapy needs VA-ECMO support. The purpose of this treatment consists primarily of recovery of the heart, bridge to a permanent support (e.g., left ventricular assist device [LVAD]) or a bridge to heart transplant. When there is acute cardiogenic shock or cardiac arrest there is an urgent need for cardiovascular blood flow indicating the need for VA-ECMO.

In VA-ECMO, oxygen rich blood is given via the artery. In VV-ECMO, venous drained blood is oxygenated and given back venously. The conventional access site is the groin although there is interest in upper body cannulation for the early mobilization of the patient. By drainage of the oxygen-poor blood from the right side of the heart to the external membrane oxygenator and back, the oxygenated blood through the arterial tube bypasses the complete cardiopulmonary system. This is comparable with cardiac surgery on cardiopulmonary bypass (CPB) except that it is for long-term support. In a cardiogenic shock patient there is severe circulatory compromise together with low cardiac output, low mean arterial pressure (MAP), tachycardia and signs of other organ failure. To achieve sufficient flow to these organs, a more or less acceptable blood pressure, tissue perfusion and coronary flow need to be achieved.

As familiarity and experience with ECMO have grown, new indications have evolved, including emergent resuscitation. This utilization has been termed extracorporeal CPR (ECPR). The literature supporting emergent cardiopulmonary support is mounting [2]. Reasonable survival rates have been achieved after initiation of support during active compressions of the chest following in-hospital cardiac arrest although there are still limitations in practice. For example, due to limitations in conventional circuits for ECMO, some centers have developed novel systems for rapid cardiopulmonary support [2]. In contrast to deteriorating heart failure or cardiogenic shock, in CPR there is no heart activity and the blood pressure (e.g. MAP, RR) is totally dependent on ECMO. This device can be implanted during resuscitation in a matter of a couple of minutes when there is insufficient flow and severe hypoxia.

After initiation of ECMO and end-organ reperfusion, reperfusion damage can occur, which has deleterious effects on the heart and blood vessels. Even though there is return of circulation, artificial usually for a couple of days, there is a high risk of thrombosis – intracardiac and intravascular – and poor cardiac contractility, reperfusion damage, inflammation and stasis in and around the great vessels/valves can persist. Conventional hemodynamic monitoring may be inadequate to identify such conditions and more sensitive monitoring modalities focusing on parenchymal perfusion and oxygenation are needed.

This chapter reviews the cardiovascular response to ECMO, with focus on (micro)circulatory alterations during ECMO support, potential consequences thereof for daily patient care and weaning of ECMO. The different influences of the daily intensive care unit (ICU) practices with different types of fluid infusion, blood transfusion and effects of ECMO on cardiopulmonary recovery and end-organ perfusion are also discussed.

Microcirculatory Alterations During ECMO

VA-ECMO, ECPR and VV-ECMO are used commonly in acute or acute-on-chronic heart or lung failure. Until now, macrocirculatory parameters have been used for clinical assessment of these patients. Tools for monitoring end-organ recovery at the end of the extracorporeal course are lacking. Measured parameters, such as lactate and mixed venous oxygen saturation (SvO_2) are still surrogates of end-organ perfusion.

Long-term ECMO support with continuous flow in the setting of the ICU is somewhat comparable to short-term CPB during cardiac surgery. Here too the systemic circulation enters the extracorporeal circulation of the heart-lung machine and the blood is exposed to non-biocompatible polymers, activating blood cells and serum proteins to cause inflammatory reactions. Other changes, including hypotension, hemodilution, hypothermia, cardiac arrest and a change from pulsatile to non-pulsatile flow, cause a detrimental effect on the parenchymal perfusion and microcirculation and can lead to tissue hypoxia and organ failure during standard coronary artery bypass graft (CABG) surgery with CPB [4–7]. Off-pump CABG can reduce the perioperative complications related to CPB. This less-invasive off-pump CABG alternative to on-pump CABG, offers pulsatile flow without the need for an extracorporeal circulation. Off-pump CABG has been associated with improved renal and pulmonary outcomes, shorter length of hospitalization and a reduction in myocardial injury compared to on-pump CABG [8–11]. Some studies have investigated the microcirculatory response to off-pump CABG. De Backer et al. for example showed that off-pump CABG was also associated with a decrease in microcirculatory perfusion [12]. Recently Bienz et al. reported that off-pump CABG did not preserve postoperative microcirculatory parameters better than on-pump CABG [13]. They showed that temperature might act as a confounding factor, because active warming of patients under CPB could have a positive effect on the microcirculation [13].

Several studies have investigated the effects of pulsatility and have generally found no advantage between pulsatile and non-pulsatile flow for end-organ perfusion [6, 14–16]. Forti et al. showed no differences in microvascular response on reduction of the CPB flow during non-pulsatile flow [17]. Consequently, there is limited evidence that pulsatility attenuates the deterioration in microvascular perfusion and there are no studies showing adverse effects of pulsatility, only studies showing an equal or better effect. Nevertheless when using pulsatile flow patterns, which mimic closely the physiological waveforms, there seems to be no advantage in terms of organ perfusion or inflammatory response. Moreover, the extent of hemolysis and capillary leak is higher compared to non-pulsatile perfusion. Efforts to optimize pulsatility therefore seem not to be justified [18].

Fluid Management in VA-ECMO

VA-ECMO patients are commonly fluid overloaded due to frequent blood transfusions and fluid infusions. The slightest form of hypovolemia results in collapse of the drainage cannula, which impairs ECMO blood flow. Usually, patients receive volume to overcome this problem. However, current evidence has shown that a positive fluid balance in the early course is highly predictive of 90-day mortality [19]. Hypotension can occur due to the reduction in blood volume, systemic inflammatory reactions, and increased vascular capacitance with warming specifically after ECPR when the patient has rewarmed after therapeutic hypothermia. Hypovolemia and/or systemic hypotension affect microcirculatory perfusion [20]. In healthy volunteers, controlled hypovolemia decreased the perfused vessel density (PVD) and microcirculatory flow index (MFI), and reduced tissue oxygenation [21]. Volume therapy using crystalloids or colloids improves cardiac output and tissue perfusion in most cases, which is why fluid therapy is considered the most important hemodynamic intervention in the postoperative period.

Whatever the fluid therapy of choice for VA-ECMO patients, fluid overload is present and is associated with increased mortality. In the setting of acute kidney injury (AKI) there will be more and earlier need for continuous renal replacement therapy (CRRT). Fluid restriction seems to be the trend in the treatment of VA-ECMO patients although transfusion restriction would be inacceptable for patients with bleeding complications. In addition, it must be kept in mind that a positive fluid balance causes hemodilution and a reduction in tissue oxygenation.

Hemodilution causes a loss of red blood cell (RBC)-filled capillaries and results in increased diffusion distances between the oxygen carrying RBCs and tissue cells.

Atasever et al. compared RBC transfusion to gelatin solutions and no infusion after cardiac surgery and studied the effects on microvascular perfusion, vascular density, hemoglobin, and oxygen saturation. They found no differences in changes in systemic oxygen delivery, oxygen uptake or oxygen extraction between the groups. RBC transfusion however, compared to gelatin or no-infusion, increased perfused microcirculatory vessel density, hemoglobin content, and saturation in the microcirculation, while microcirculatory blood flow remained unchanged [22]. Yuruk et al. showed that RBC transfusion during cardiac surgery recruited the microcirculation and led to improve PVD and tissue oxygenation [23]. A recent study by Mukaida et al. showed the presence of a compensatory mechanism in patients on CPB in which increased blood flow of the microcirculation compensated for the lack of oxyhemoglobin delivery caused by hemodilution [24]. Experiences regarding RBC function and behavior in the microcirculation in the hemodiluted cardiovascular system make it important to carefully monitor end-organ function in VA-ECMO patients and avoid the risks associated with fluid overload.

Reperfusion Damage

Experimental studies and investigations in patients with congenital heart disease have shown the usefulness of ECMO for reduction of ischemia and ischemia-induced reperfusion damage [25, 26]. The effects of cardiac arrest care on post-cardiac arrest reperfusion injury are not well known [27]. However, recent data have shown that for refractory cardiac arrest, which includes mechanical CPR, peri-arrest therapeutic hypothermia and ECMO are feasible and associated with a relatively high survival rate [28]. Several studies have shown that hyperoxemia may have deleterious effects, including a decrease in microvascular functional capillary density [29–30]. Cardiopulmonary arrest is considered as a short period of myocardial ischemia, which may cause microcirculatory deterioration. There are no studies on the microcirculatory alterations during intraoperative cardioplegia-induced arrest. Nevertheless, Elbers et al. showed that circulatory arrest in humans induced an immediate shutdown of complete sublingual small microvessels while flow in larger microvessels persisted [14]. There is also a need for studies on the microcirculation that compare ischemia and reperfusion damage in patients undergoing ECPR.

Weaning from VA-ECMO

The use of MCS devices should be anticipated, and every attempt made to initiate support before the presence of dysfunction of end organs or circulatory collapse. In an emergency, these patients can be resuscitated with ECMO and subsequently transitioned to a long-term ventricular assist device after a period of stability. But the continuing question should be how and when we can remove this MCS device. Removal of MCS devices is challenging. Despite improvements in hemodynamic monitoring some patients still die after removal of MCS devices.

Weaning from VA-ECMO is an important decision-making point in the management of these patients and should be guided by both clinical and echocardiography parameters. Echo provides the best assessment of native ventricular and valvular function in this setting. Either transthoracic echocardiography (TTE) or transesophageal echocardiography (TEE) can be used. A baseline echo is performed and any contraindications to weaning should be noted. Anticoagulation is optimized to ensure therapeutic anticoagulation unless contraindicated. A formalized weaning process should be used so that weaning evaluations can be compared.

To evaluate the success of weaning, VA-ECMO flows are reduced in a stepwise fashion. Some centers describe weaning by a set percentage of flow. Expected findings on echo to support a successful wean include evidence of recruitment of left ventricular and/or right ventricular function (qualitatively or quantitatively) and a recruitment of stroke volume demonstrated on echo by an increase in left ventricular outflow velocity time interval (VTI) [31]. In an observational study looking at the echocardiography parameters associated with successful ECMO weaning, aortic VTI ≥ 10 cm, left ventricular ejection fraction (LVEF) > 20–25% and lateral mitral annulus peak systolic velocity (TDSa) ≥ 6 cm/sec when the ECMO flow was reduced to < 1.5 l/min were predictive of successful weaning from VA-ECMO [32]. However, the main limitations in these studies are that only hemodynamically stable patients were considered eligible for such a weaning trial.

Various methods are being introduced to more effectively guide the weaning process. Recently, ECMO weaning guided by miniaturized TEE probes has been described. Tokita et al. described the usefulness of N-terminal pro-brain natriuretic peptide (NT-pro-BNP) for weaning from intra-aortic balloon pumps (IABPs) [33]. However, the usefulness of biomarkers in weaning from ECMO is very controversial. Luyt et al. reported, in contrast to previous reports, no additive value of cardiac biomarkers for weaning [34].

Microcirculatory Guided Weaning from ECMO

Current knowledge about what happens to the microcirculation during support with MCS devices is limited. Reis Miranda et al. showed that the mean pulmonary artery pressure decreased very fast after initiation of VV-ECMO in patients with respiratory distress syndrome [35]. This prompts the question as to what kind of alterations would be seen in such circumstances in the microcirculation?

In pediatric studies of VA-ECMO, there is evidence of a depressed microcirculation persisting over 24 h [36, 37]. In adults there is little literature concerning microcirculatory alterations in VV-ECMO and controversial data in VA-ECMO. ECPR is a totally new paradigm and there are no studies looking at microcirculatory alterations in ECPR patients. In our center, we are testing the hypothesis that the microcirculatory alterations measured using new-generation, handheld microscopes, called Cytocam Incident Dark Field (IDF) imaging, in response to flow reduction during ECMO can predict the likely success of weaning [38–40] (Fig. 1).

Fig. 1 The conceptual differences between sidestream dark field (SDF) and incident dark field (IDF) imaging. Previous generation SDF imaging uses light-emitting diodes (LED) optically isolated from the center-reflecting light guide and images are captured by a conventional video camera. The new generation Cytocam IDF imaging device has a wider field of illumination, a specially designed magnification lens and a computer-controlled high-resolution image sensor resulting in 30% more capillaries being observed than previous generation hand held microscopy devices. Adapted from [40]

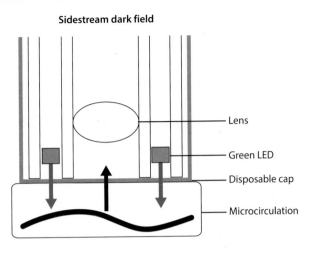

Sidestream dark field

Lens

Green LED

Disposable cap

Microcirculation

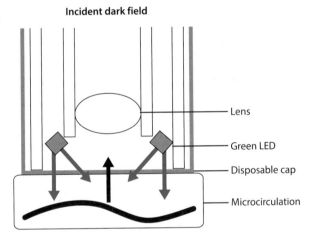

Incident dark field

Lens

Green LED

Disposable cap

Microcirculation

Cardiogenic shock is one of the most common causes of death with several underlying etiologies, including acute myocarditis, myocardial infarction, and deterioration of chronic cardiomyopathy. In these patients, ECMO provides circulatory support while awaiting cardiac recovery and allows time to consider other therapies such as heart transplantation or a long-term LVAD. The timing of weaning a 'normalized' cardiovascular system from ECMO is as important as management during ECMO, because early or late weaning can cause treatment failure and associated complications. Hemodynamic and echocardiography parameters are used to wean from ECMO. However, to date, weaning strategies following ECMO initiation for cardiogenic shock have not been reported, and only a few studies have evaluated outcome predictors following ECMO institution (e.g., [41]) (Fig. 2).

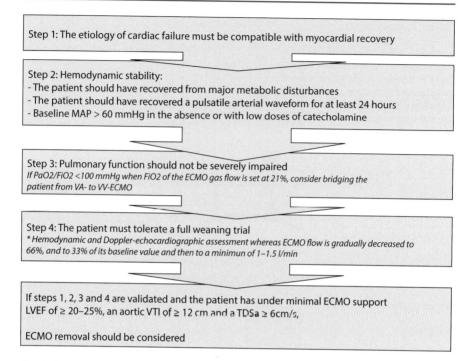

Fig. 2 Recommendations for successful weaning from ECMO. Adapted from [41] with permission. *MAP*: mean arterial pressure; *LVEF*: Left ventricular ejection fraction; *VTI*: Velocity time interval; *TDSa*: tissue Doppler lateral mitral annulus peak systolic velocity

Conclusion

In this chapter, we have briefly reviewed the cardiovascular response to ECMO, paying particular attention to the microcirculatory alterations. With the advent of ECMO, circulatory collapse can be treated effectively; however, end-organ recovery is not always successful. The appropriate timing of initiating and weaning from ECMO warrant clinical studies. The microcirculatory alterations/responsiveness to ECMO may help in these very complex clinical issues in this growing mechanical circulatory support population.

References

1. Annich GM, Lynch WR, MacLaren G, Wilson JM, Bartlett RH (2012) ECMO Extracorporeal Cardiopulmonary Support in Critical Care, 4th edn. Extracorporeal Life Support Organization, Ann Arbor
2. Cooper DS, Jacobs JP, Moore L et al (2007) Cardiac extracorporeal life support: state of the art in 2007. Cardiol Young 17(Suppl 2):104–115

3. Bartlett RH (2005) Extracorporeal life support: history and new directions. ASAIO 51:487–489
4. Kolackova M, Krejsek J, Svitek V et al (2012) The effect of conventional and mini-invasive cardiopulmonary bypass on neutrophil activation in patients undergoing coronary artery bypass grafting. Mediators Inflamm 2012:152895
5. Koning NJ, Vonk AB, van Barneveld LJ et al (2012) Pulsatile flow during cardiopulmonary bypass preserves postoperative microcirculatory perfusion irrespective of systemic hemodynamics. J Appl Physiol 1985(112):1727–1734
6. O'Neil MP, Fleming JC, Badhwar A, Guo LR (2012) Pulsatile versus nonpulsatile flow during cardiopulmonary bypass: microcirculatory and systemic effects. Ann Thorac Surg 94:2046–2053
7. Vellinga NA, Ince C, Boerma EC (2010) Microvascular dysfunction in the surgical patient. Curr Opin Crit Care 16:377–383
8. Lamy A, Devereaux PJ, Prabhakaran D et al (2012) Off-pump or on-pump coronary-artery bypass grafting at 30 days. N Engl J Med 366:1489–1497
9. Lamy A, Devereaux PJ, Prabhakaran D et al (2013) Effects of off-pump and on-pump coronary-artery bypass grafting at 1 year. N Engl J Med 368:1179–1188
10. Seguel SE, Gonzalez R, Stockins A, Alarcon CE, Concha CR (2013) Off-pump coronary surgery. Experience in 220 patients. Rev Med Chil 141:281–290
11. Thourani VH, Guyton RA (2012) Graft patency after off-pump coronary artery bypass surgery. Circulation 125:2806–2808
12. De Backer D, Dubois MJ, Schmartz D et al (2009) Microcirculatory alterations in cardiac surgery: effects of cardiopulmonary bypass and anesthesia. Ann Thorac Surg 88:1396–1403
13. Bienz M, Drullinsky D, Stevens LM, Bracco D, Noiseux N (2016) Microcirculatory response during on-pump versus off-pump coronary artery bypass graft surgery. Perfusion (in press)
14. Elbers PW, Wijbenga J, Solinger F et al (2011) Direct observation of the human microcirculation during cardiopulmonary bypass: effects of pulsatile perfusion. J Cardiothorac Vasc Anesth 25:250–255
15. Koning NJ, Vonk AB, Meesters MI et al (2014) Microcirculatory perfusion is preserved during off-pump but not on-pump cardiac surgery. J Cardiothorac Vasc Anesth 28:336–341
16. Grubhofer G, Mares P, Rajek A et al (2000) Pulsatility does not change cerebral oxygenation during cardiopulmonary bypass. Acta Anaesthesiol Scand 44:586–591
17. Forti A, Comin A, Lazzarotto N et al (2012) Pump flow changes do not impair sublingual microcirculation during cardiopulmonary bypass. J Cardiothorac Vasc Anesth 26:785–790
18. Voss B, Krane M, Jung C et al (2010) Cardiopulmonary bypass with physiological flow and pressure curves: pulse is unnecessary! Eur J Cardiothorac Surg 37:223–232
19. Schmidt M, Bailey M, Kelly J et al (2014) Impact of fluid balance on outcome of adult patients treated with extracorporeal membrane oxygenation. Intensive Care Med 40:1256–1266
20. Ince C (2014) The rationale for microcirculatory guided fluid therapy. Curr Opin Crit Care 20:301–308
21. Bartels SA, Bezemer R, Milstein DM et al (2011) The microcirculatory response to compensated hypovolemia in a lower body negative pressure model. Microvasc Res 82:374–380
22. Atasever B, van der Kuil M, Boer C et al (2012) Red blood cell transfusion compared with gelatin solution and no infusion after cardiac surgery: effect on microvascular perfusion, vascular density, hemoglobin, and oxygen saturation. Transfusion 52:2452–2458
23. Yuruk K, Bartels SA, Milstein DM et al (2012) Red blood cell transfusions and tissue oxygenation in anemic hematology outpatients. Transfusion 52:641–646
24. Mukaida H, Matsushita S, Inotani T et al (2015) Peripheral circulation evaluation with near-infrared spectroscopy in skeletal muscle during cardiopulmonary bypass. Perfusion 30:653–659
25. Amberman K, Shen I (2010) Minimizing reperfusion injuries: successful resuscitation using eCPR after cardiac arrest on a post-operative Norwood patient. J Extra Corpor Technol 42:238–241

26. Zhao L, Luo L, Chen J et al (2014) Utilization of extracorporeal membrane oxygenation alleviates intestinal ischemia-reperfusion injury in prolonged hemorrhagic shock animal model. Cell Biochem Biophys 70:1733–1740

27. Baker E, Lee G (2016) The science of reperfusion injury post cardiac arrest – Implications for emergency nurses. Int Emerg Nurs (in press)

28. Stub D, Bernard S, Pellegrino V et al (2015) Refractory cardiac arrest treated with mechanical CPR, hypothermia, ECMO and early reperfusion (the CHEER trial). Resuscitation 86:88–94

29. Joachimsson PO, Sjoberg F, Forsman M et al (1996) Adverse effects of hyperoxemia during cardiopulmonary bypass. J Thorac Cardiovasc Surg 112:812–819

30. Kamler M, Wendt D, Pizanis N et al (2004) Deleterious effects of oxygen during extracorporeal circulation for the microcirculation in vivo. Eur J Cardiothorac Surg 26:564–570

31. Aissaoui N, Luyt CE, Leprince P et al (2011) Predictors of successful extracorporeal membrane oxygenation (ECMO) weaning after assistance for refractory cardiogenic shock. Intensive Care Med 37:1738–1745

32. Cavarocchi NC, Pitcher HT, Yang Q et al (2013) Weaning of extracorporeal membrane oxygenation using continuous hemodynamic transesophageal echocardiography. J Thorac Cardiovasc Surg 146:1474–1479

33. Tokita Y, Yamamoto T, Sato N et al (2014) Usefulness of N-terminal pro-brain natriuretic peptide levels to predict success of weaning from intra-aortic balloon pumping. Am J Cardiol 114:942–945

34. Luyt CE, Landivier A, Leprince P et al (2012) Usefulness of cardiac biomarkers to predict cardiac recovery in patients on extracorporeal membrane oxygenation support for refractory cardiogenic shock. J Crit Care 27:524

35. Reis Miranda D, van Thiel R, Brodie D, Bakker J (2015) Right ventricular unloading after initiation of venovenous extracorporeal membrane oxygenation. Am J Respir Crit Care Med 191:346–348 (Correspondence)

36. Top AP, Buijs EA, Schouwenberg PH et al (2012) The microcirculation is unchanged in neonates with severe respiratory failure after the initiation of ECMO treatment. Crit Care Res Pract 2012:372956

37. Top AP, Ince C, van Dijk M, Tibboel D (2009) Changes in buccal microcirculation following extracorporeal membrane oxygenation in term neonates with severe respiratory failure. Crit Care Med 37:1121–1124

38. Aykut G, Veenstra G, Scorcella C, Ince C, Boerma C (2015) Cytocam-IDF (incident dark field illumination) imaging for bedside monitoring of the microcirculation. Intensive Care Med Exp 3:40

39. Akin S, Struijs A, van Thiel RJ, Kara A, Caliskan K, Gommers D, Ince C (2015) Can the microcirculatory alterations in response to blood flow reduction in extracorporeal membrane oxygenation predict the ability of success in weaning? Atlanta

40. van Elteren HA, Ince C, Tibboel D, Reiss IK, de Jonge RC (2015) Cutaneous microcirculation in preterm neonates: comparison between sidestream dark field (SDF) and incident dark field (IDF) imaging. J Clin Monit Comput 29:543–548

41. Aissaoui N, El-Banayosy A, Combes A (2015) How to wean a patient from veno-arterial extracorporeal membrane oxygenation. Intensive Care Med 41:902–905

Mechanical Circulatory Support in the New Era: An Overview

K. Shekar, S. D. Gregory, and J. F. Fraser

Introduction

Maximal medical therapy can no longer be seen as a justifiable end-point for refractory circulatory shock, at least in well-resourced health settings. Despite improvements in almost all other areas of cardiac and intensive care medicine, refractory cardiogenic shock, defined as cardiac and circulatory failure resulting in organ hypoperfusion [1], continues to have unacceptably high mortality and morbidity from the resultant multiple organ failure. Whilst primary cardiac pathology remains the leading cause of cardiogenic shock, acute cardiomyopathies secondary to conditions such as sepsis and toxic ingestion are not uncommon [2]. The conventional approach to supporting patients with circulatory shock includes reversal of underlying causes when feasible, mechanical ventilation, pharmacological hemodynamic support with or without intra-aortic balloon counter pulsation, renal replacement and other supportive therapy. Whilst mechanical circulatory support (MCS) has always been an attractive option when conventional approaches fail, technological limitations, suboptimal clinical application of available technology and resource limitations have all conspired against its more widespread use.

Recently, there is increasing application of extracorporeal membrane oxygenation (ECMO) technology to provide MCS in an incremental fashion either as peripheral or central venoarterial (VA)-ECMO or as univentricular or biventricular assist devices [3, 4]. The use of ECMO in cardiopulmonary resuscitation (CPR) is also expanding with experienced centers reporting favorable outcomes [5]. Other minimally invasive percutaneous ventricular assist devices (pVADs) have also been used in acute settings. Similarly, the implantable, durable, rotary blood pump-driven

K. Shekar (✉) · S. D. Gregory · J. F. Fraser
School of Medicine, The University of Queensland
Brisbane, Australia
Innovative Cardiovascular Engineering and Technology Laboratory, Critical Care Research
Group, The Prince Charles Hospital
Chermside, Australia
email: kiran.shekar@health.qld.gov.au

© Springer International Publishing Switzerland 2016
J.-L. Vincent (ed.), *Annual Update in Intensive Care and Emergency Medicine 2016*,
DOI 10.1007/978-3-319-27349-5_17

VADs have revolutionized the care of patients with chronic heart failure or those with acute heart failure who initially need to be stabilized on temporary MCS, and in whom cardiac recovery does not occur [6]. Although total artificial hearts have been used only sparsely, it is expected that their use will increase with the increasing heart failure population and rapid improvements in technology that are currently occurring [7].

In an appropriately aged critically ill patient with no absolute contraindications who is failing medical therapy for circulatory shock, especially of cardiac origin, temporary MCS strategies can now be effectively utilized as a bridge to decision, to recovery, to long-term support devices (such as VADs or total artificial hearts) and/or heart transplantation in an appropriately resourced setting. Such undertakings are resource-intensive and the risk/benefit profile of these therapies and costs are already becoming more favorable. Improved and refined technological advancements, more appropriate selection of patients and better clinical use of these devices will likewise continue.

Bridging a patient from emergent temporary MCS to long term devices and/or heart transplant is a complex multidisciplinary exercise. The choice of the initial rescue MCS strategy has significant bearing not only on limiting further iatrogenic harm in the acute setting, but also on planning long-term strategies in the absence of myocardial recovery. Most of these applications have a steep learning curve and careful planning of perfusion strategies and vascular access in a time-critical situation may be challenging. Developing predetermined institutional pathways is critical to success of such MCS programs. It should be recognized that technology has evolved sufficiently and many MCS strategies are now ready for full clinical utilization, though large multicenter trials are still lacking in many areas. Such resource intensive extraordinary therapies raise several questions in relation to resource utilization, ethics, governance, quality assurance and benchmarking, all of which need to be addressed proactively. Although evidence in this area is difficult to generate, collaboration between global centers, establishment of global registries and clinical and science research networks can facilitate the volume and quality of data needed to further augment the clinician's knowledge of when and where these technologies could and should be used. A case vignette will be used to expand on the possibilities, the problems and the pathologies that can be treated with MCS.

Case Vignette

A 28-year old, previously fit male was admitted to a peripheral intensive care unit (ICU) with cardiogenic shock of uncertain origin. Electrocardiogram (EKG) demonstrated no acute ischemic changes, but there was an increase in plasma cardiac troponin I concentration (21 ng/ml). He deteriorated rapidly following a run of ventricular arrhythmias that required brief CPR and electric cardioversion. He was subsequently commenced on inotropes and pressors and was intubated and mechanically ventilated. A transthoracic echo demonstrated an akinetic thick ventricular wall, globally diminished cardiac function with a left ventricular ejection fraction (LVEF) of 5% with no significant valvular abnormalities. An intra-aortic balloon pump (IABP) was inserted. Over the next 6 h he developed more sustained runs of ventricular arrhythmias with escalating inotrope requirement and early evidence of hepatic and renal dysfunction. The local ECMO center retrieved the patient safely, after establishing peripheral VA-ECMO support, leaving the IABP *in situ*. Upon arrival at the ECMO center, loss of pulsatility on arterial waveform suggested loss of aortic valve opening, which was confirmed by echocardiography. High intensity anticoagulation, increased inotropes, afterload reduction with nitrates and higher positive end-expiratory pressure (PEEP) were augmented with amiodarone infusion. A follow-up echocardiography hours later demonstrated a distended left ventricle with evidence of some early thrombus in the ventricle and possibly the aortic root. It was predicted that peripheral VA-ECMO was likely to fail and could lead to central thromboembolic and pulmonary complications. Less invasive options for decompression of the left ventricle, such as an atrial septostomy, were considered but excluded. Other venting options included percutaneous VADs, such as Impella (Abiomed, Aachen, Germany) or TandemHeart (CardiacAssist, Inc., Pittsburgh, PA, USA), but these were not available.

Based on a presumptive diagnosis of acute myocarditis and potential for recovery, his MCS configuration was changed to a temporary biventricular assist device (BiVAD) configuration using two ECMO circuits and centrifugal pumps (CentriMag, Levitronix LLC, Waltham, MA). A Quadrox D Oxygenator (Maquet, Rastatt, Germany) was included in the right ventricular assist device (RVAD) circuit to facilitate gas exchange and temperature control in the early postoperative period. The surgical cannulation strategy employed (transfemoral right atrial [RA] drainage → allograft to pulmonary artery [PA] return; and left ventricular [LV] apex drainage to aorta return) allowed for awakening, mobilization and exercise in bed on BiVAD support. This was necessary to allow physical conditioning and urgent listing for a heart transplant if cardiac recovery failed to occur. Cardiac tissue at the time of LV apical cannulation demonstrated fulminant giant cell myocarditis raising concerns about cardiac recovery.

After hemostasis had been achieved, the oxygenator was removed from the circuit on postoperative day 2 and a tracheostomy was performed to allow weaning from sedation and ventilation. Over the next 2 weeks, the patient was liberated from mechanical ventilation and the tracheostomy removed, with the patient remaining stable on the BiVAD, with some physical recovery, but no cardiac recovery. He was urgently listed for a heart transplant after confirming eligibility. No organ became available for transplant in the following two weeks whilst on temporary BiVAD. Given the patient had a less favorable blood group and a more ambulatory support strategy was needed to move forward, the temporary LVAD was converted to a left side long-term implantable rotary VAD (HVAD, HeartWare, Framingham, MA). Support from the temporary RVAD was continued due to concerns of RV failure post-LVAD implantation.

The early post-VAD insertion was complicated by bleeding requiring reopening but over the next few days a tracheotomy was again performed and rehabilitation was recommenced. Over the next 10 days, the RVAD was removed and the patient was weaned off ventilation and was eventually discharged from the ICU on LVAD support. He received inotropes for RV support in the ward for another 2 weeks. He was relisted for heart transplant a few weeks later. Three months later he received a heart transplant and was discharged to the ward after 1 week in the ICU and subsequently discharged home after a prolonged rehabilitation.

This case illustrates how a spectrum of MCS strategies was used to successfully bridge a young patient with acute heart failure to heart transplantation. Equally this case demonstrates the resources, forward-planning and multidisciplinary inputs that are required to provide such a level of care. Although there are understandable concerns regarding the costs associated with these therapies, they are likely to become more widely used, and with appropriate usage, their costs will drop, as with all new technology.

This article will discuss the bridging options in more detail in the sections below to reflect the advancements in MCS and to reinforce the importance of choosing the 'right perfusion strategy for the right patient at the right time'. The intensivist will be a key contributor to MCS – both in terms of patient selection, and in determining and enacting at least the initial percutaneous strategies – either pre- or post-retrieval from peripheral centers to an advanced MCS center. This article will focus mainly on principles of various MCS strategies and will refer the readers elsewhere for more information on the technicalities of the devices used. Equally, this article discusses more commonly used devices only and is by no means a comprehensive review of all MCS devices in clinical use or development.

Mechanical Circulatory Support Strategies

Intra-aortic Balloon Pumps

Despite the controversies around their efficacy in the setting of cardiogenic shock [8], IABPs can be seen as a bridge between conventional medical therapy and MCS. IABPs are more widely available than other MCS systems, lower risk, less invasive, easy to institute and may be a useful first-line MCS option while we await definitive evidence for their use in various clinical settings that may lead to cardiogenic shock. More detailed reviews of IABPs and a summary of evidence can be found elsewhere [9]. However, the IABP remains a useful adjunct and it should be noted that while it may improve native cardiac performance by reducing afterload and myocardial oxygen demand, it cannot partially or completely replace cardiopulmonary function. More advanced MCS options need to be considered and an early referral to a MCS center should be considered in a young patient with presumed reversible acute cardiomyopathy or in whom there are no overt contraindications for heart transplantation in the absence of cardiac recovery. Current data suggest that IABPs may assist aortic valve opening in patients requiring peripheral VA-ECMO and they should not necessarily be removed prior to VA-ECMO support.

Venoarterial ECMO

There has been a significant uptake of ECMO technology in adults since the 2009 H1N1 Influenza pandemic. This pandemic not only led to many new ECMO centers but also created greater awareness of the process of ECMO. Success achieved with venovenous (VV) ECMO during the pandemic with contemporary technology has certainly encouraged clinicians to apply ECMO technology to provide cardiorespiratory support in a variety of clinical settings. Providing tailored temporary MCS to patients with acute refractory cardiac failure using ECMO technology is a rapidly evolving area where intervention may be time-critical and mortality is higher than for isolated respiratory failure [10, 11].

The indications listed in the Extracorporeal Life Support Organization (ELSO) guidelines for ECMO for cardiac failure in adults are shown in Box 1 [12]. The use of ECMO in the setting of CPR is discussed elsewhere [13, 14]. International Society for Heart and Lung Transplantation guidelines [15] for MCS provide evidence-based recommendations for long-term MCS options for patients with cardiac failure. These guidelines strongly recommend consideration of the use of temporary MCS in patients with multiorgan failure, sepsis, or on mechanical ventilation, to allow successful optimization of clinical status and neurologic assessment prior to placement of a long-term MCS device. The severity of non-cardiac organ system failures may be used to identify suitable patients and a sequential organ failure assessment (SOFA) score > 15 has been considered a contraindication to VV-ECMO [16]; similar criteria may be applicable for VA-ECMO or for the use of an ECMO circuit as a temporary VAD.

Box 1. Extracorporeal Life Support Organization (ELSO) Recommended Indications for ECMO in Adult Patients with Cardiac Failure [12].
- Inadequate tissue perfusion manifested as hypotension and low cardiac output despite adequate intravascular volume.
- Shock persisting despite volume administration, inotropes and vasoconstrictors, and intra-aortic balloon counter-pulsation if appropriate.
- Typical causes: Acute myocardial infarction, myocarditis, peripartum cardiomyopathy, decompensated chronic heart failure, post cardiotomy shock.
- Septic shock is an indication in some centers.

The underlying cause of cardiac dysfunction and projected time course of recovery, severity of pulmonary dysfunction and projected time course of recovery, functional reserve of each ventricle, the presence and severity of valvular pathology, risk of arterial access and size of vessels, severity of coagulopathy and risk of sternotomy, planned future surgery such as long term VAD or transplant may all have to be considered prior to finalizing an individualized MCS strategy [3].

For patients with predominant cardiac failure and preserved pulmonary function, several MCS strategies may be considered. Central VA-ECMO has traditionally been applied as a bridge to recovery in patients who fail to wean from cardiopulmonary bypass (CPB) after cardiac surgery (Fig. 1a). Central VA-ECMO outside this setting in adults is uncommon. Femoral VA-ECMO (Fig. 1b) is the more commonly used MCS modality in adults requiring urgent cardiac support as it can be initiated rapidly and a sternotomy with its concomitant bleeding is avoided. One of the major limitations of peripheral femoro-femoral VA-ECMO is LV afterload mismatch and inadequate LV decompression. Patients with very low native cardiac output states and severe mitral valve regurgitation are at a greater risk of developing hydrostatic pulmonary edema and further reduction of myocardial oxygenation by the distended LV cavity compressing the intracoronary circulation. Although, some centers use an IABP in conjunction with peripheral VA-ECMO to reduce LV afterload and pulmonary congestion, no definitive data exist to support its routine use. Femoral VA-ECMO is also limited by femoral arterial size and thus cannula size and the requirement for distal limb perfusion. Although use of smaller arterial return cannulae may minimize the need for routine back-flow cannula insertion for distal limb perfusion, early insertion of these cannulae should be considered in all these cases until more supportive evidence becomes available.

LV and aortic root stasis from lack of cardiac ejection and failure of aortic valve opening may result in catastrophic intra-cardiac and aortic root thrombosis. Increased intensity of anticoagulation to minimize this risk may precipitate bleeding. Less invasive strategies, such as percutaneous trans-septal left atrial decompression [17] and subxiphoid surgical approaches to drain the left ventricle [18], have been described to reduce LV distension. The residual atrial defect may require surgical correction once the patient has been weaned from the MCS. Use of a pVAD to decompress the distended left ventricle has also been reported in this setting [19] alleviating the need for a high risk septostomy or surgical venting.

Given its less invasive nature (compared to central MCS strategies) peripheral VA-ECMO, with attention to optimal LV afterload, minimizing LV distension with optimal fluid and inotrope therapy, anticoagulation and pulmonary management remains a viable first-line option for patients with isolated acute cardiac failure refractory to conventional management.

Fig. 1 Cannulation sites for venoarterial extracorporeal membrane oxygenation (VA-ECMO). VA-ECMO can be instituted **a** centrally by cannulating the right atrium/inferior vena cava and the aorta, or peripherally using **b** femoral vein and femoral artery (*dark blue arrow* arterial return cannula, *light blue arrow* back flow cannula for distal limb perfusion), or **c** axillary/subclavian artery. The choice is often guided by the clinical setting, expected duration of support and pulmonary function. From [3] with permission

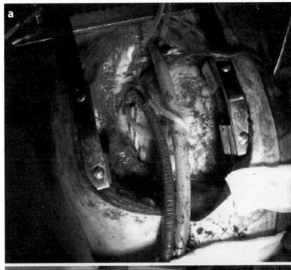

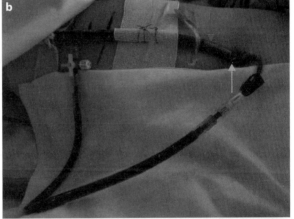

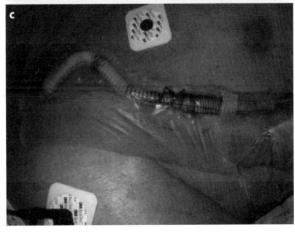

Other Temporary Mechanical Circulatory Support Configurations

Configurations Based on the ECMO Circuit

The limitations of peripheral VA-ECMO have prompted the use of ECMO devices [20] to facilitate ventricular unloading by changing to a temporary left or right VAD or a BiVAD configuration. Any perfusion strategy that creates a right-to-left shunt requires an oxygenator in the circuit. Oxygenators may additionally facilitate temperature management. This strategy effectively provides biventricular support and gas exchange through a double (Fig. 2a) or single (Fig. 2b) pump configuration with the ability to cease RV support when not required and thereafter to discontinue the oxygenator. However, this configuration requires a sternotomy and cannulation of the left ventricle (or left atrium), aorta and /or pulmonary arteries. A reoperation (sternotomy or thoracotomy) is then required for explantation of the cannula from the left ventricle or left atrium upon cardiac recovery or for implantation of a long-term mechanical assist device.

RV support for up to several months can be provided with a CentriMag ECMO system through percutaneous femoral venous access to the right atrium and return to the pulmonary artery via a cannulated exteriorized Dacron graft. Alternatively, venous drainage can also be achieved through a centrally placed right atrial cannula. This strategy is described for temporary support of the right ventricle with insertion of a long term LVAD but is applicable to other causes of severe isolated RV dysfunction, such as post-massive pulmonary embolism. Inclusion of an oxygenator into the circuit at this stage ensures adequate oxygenation, CO_2 removal and temperature regulation whilst facilitating protective ventilation. Upon RV recovery, the pulmonary artery graft can be ligated and buried upon decannulation without re-sternotomy.

Percutaneous VADs

Percutaneously inserted LVADs, such as TandemHeart and Impella [9], are potential options for short-term MCS in the acute setting (Fig. 3). However, there is a paucity of supportive evidence [21] for their use and the complications with arterial access, such as bleeding and limb ischemia, cannot be understated. They may also be viable options to vent the distending left ventricle during peripheral VA-ECMO support. These devices in many ways are likely to form a significant part of our armamentarium whilst providing individualized MCS to a patient with acute cardiac failure.

The TandemHeart uses a centrifugal pump to drain the left atrial blood from a catheter placed transeptally via the femoral vein and returns it to the femoral artery. The Impella uses an axial pump that is inserted retrogradely across the aortic valve via the femoral artery. These devices provide some LV support but lack the ability to provide extracorporeal respiratory support if required. However, there are case reports pertaining to their successful use as RV assist and or biventricular assist devices [23, 24]. Similarly, minimally invasive percutaneous right VADs have been developed (Impella RP system, Abiomed and TandemHeart, CardiacAssist) and may be significant additions to the spectrum of available MCS therapies in the future.

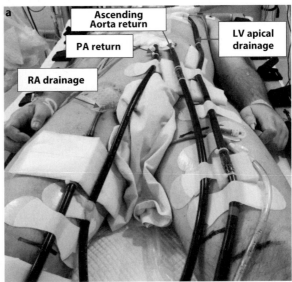

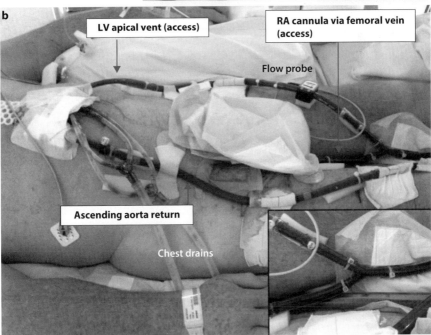

Fig. 2 Temporary biventricular support strategies. **a** Biventricular assist and oxygenation support using two centrifugal pumps. Cannulation details: transfemoral right atrium (RA) drainage → allograft to pulmonary artery (PA) for returning oxygenated blood; and left ventricle (LV) apex drainage to aorta return. An oxygenator was included in the right ventricular assist device circuit. **b** Biventricular and oxygenation support provided using a single centrifugal pump. Dual drainage cannulas positioned in the LV apically and right atrium transfemorally. Oxygenated blood was returned to the ascending aorta through central cannulation. Insert demonstrates how the two drainage tubes were merged using a Y-connector to enable usage of a single pump

Fig. 3 Schematic represen-
tation of two commercially
available percutaneous ven-
tricular assist devices. **a** the
TandemHeart pVAD (Cardiac
Assist Inc., Pittsburgh, PA,
USA), **b** the Impella pVAD
(AbioMed Europe, Aachen,
Germany). From [22] with
permission

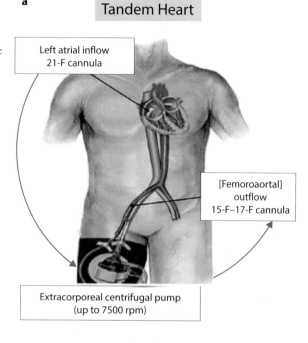

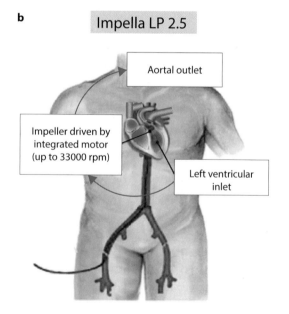

There has been a radical shift in VAD technology and new generation implantable rotary blood pumps are now a viable bridge to destination or heart transplant [25, 26]. The shortage of appropriate donor organs and the expanding pool of patients waiting for heart transplantation have led to growing interest in alternative strategies, particularly in longer term MCS.

Long-Term Implantable VADs

Indications for Support
Eligible patients with progressive, non-reversible, chronic heart failure may be placed on these devices as bridge to destination or heart transplant. Meticulous patient selection and timely insertion of the device/s is the key to positive outcomes [6, 25]. The temporary MCS bridging strategies described above in many ways may eliminate the need for placement of these very expensive devices in critically ill patients. This is important, as urgency of VAD placement has also been shown to play a factor in survival. Patients receiving emergent LVADs have a lower rate of survival than patients who are less unwell when the LVAD is implanted [27].

There are several risk models to predict the survival of heart failure patients [28, 29]. These may be used to identify high-risk patients for potential LVAD therapy. The identified preoperative risk factors for mortality based on the results of the Interagency Registry for Mechanically Assisted Circulatory Support (INTERMACS) indicate that older age, ascites, increased bilirubin, and cardiogenic shock (INTERMACS level 1) are highly associated with post-implant mortality [30]. While it is increasingly obvious that implanting a VAD in these patients is associated with poor survival, refinements in devices and surgical techniques raise an important question: when is it too soon to implant a VAD in a patient with progressive, non-reversible, chronic heart failure? The following sections will briefly discuss the available VAD options and common early complications that intensivists may encounter following VAD implantation.

Devices
Improved results and the increased applicability and durability of LVADs have enhanced this treatment option for end-stage heart failure patients. Results using non-pulsatile continuous flow pumps as a bridge to transplant or destination subsequent to the landmark Randomized Evaluation of Mechanical Assistance for the Treatment of Congestive Heart Failure (REMATCH) Trial [31] are very promising and significantly better when compared with pulsatile LVADs [32]. In 2006, 78 of the 98 implanted devices recorded on the INTERMACS registry were pulsatile, intracorporeal devices [30], whereas in 2013, 2420 of the 2506 implanted devices recorded on the INTERMACS registry were continuous flow intracorporeal devices [30]. Therefore, this section focuses solely on the continuous flow VADs which are commonly used in the clinical setting and does not report on devices no longer clinically available or those under development. A summary of the technical as-

Table 1 Technical summary of clinically available, long-term implantable rotary blood pumps

Device	Size (mm)	Weight (g)	Speed (RPM)	Flow rates (l/min)
Axial Flow				
Thoratec, HeartMate II	$60 \times \phi\,40$	375	6,000–15,000	≥ 10
Reliant Heart, Heart Assist 5	$71 \times \phi\,30$	92	7,500–12,500	≥ 10
Jarvik Inc, Jarvik 2000	$55 \times \phi\,25$	85	8,000–12,000	≥ 7
FlowMaker				
Berlin Heart, INCOR	$120 \times \phi\,30$	200	5,000–10,000	≥ 7
Centrifugal Flow				
HeartWare, HVAD	$57^* \times \phi\,50$	160	1,800–4,000	≥ 10
Terumo, DuraHeart	$45 \times \phi\,72$	540	1,200–2,600	≥ 10
Thoratec, HeartMate III	$30 \times \phi\,69$	474	2,000–5,500$^+$	≥ 10
Mixed Flow				
CircuLite, Synergy	$50 \times \phi\,12$	25	20,000–28,000	≥ 3.5
HeartWare, MVAD	$50 \times \phi\,21$	58	16,000–28,000	≥ 10

RPM: revolutions per minute; ϕ: diameter.
* This value indicates the HeartWare HVAD height including the 32 mm long inflow cannula.
$^+$ This value is taken from minimum and maximum pump speeds shown on the pressure head versus volume flow rate curve in [33].

pects of the devices in this review is provided in Table 1. We briefly discuss the two commonly used rotary blood pump-based VADs in this article.

The HeartMate II (Thoratec Corporation, Pleasanton, CA) is the most widely implanted rotary blood pump (Fig. 4a), with a second-generation design that relies on a pivot bearing; however minimal wear is reported [34]. To date, over 20,000 HeartMate II devices have been implanted with support duration exceeding 8 years [35]. The HeartMate II received Food and Drug Administration (FDA) approval for bridge to transplant in 2008 and for destination therapy in 2010 [36]. In 2014, Thoratec started clinical trials for the HeartMate 3, a third-generation centrifugal flow design with a magnetically levitated impeller to increase blood flow gaps and reduce blood trauma. The HeartMate 3 includes a small artificial pulse to enhance pump washout and textured blood-contacting surfaces to encourage tissue integration. The HeartWare HVAD (Fig. 4b) is a centrifugal, third generation device with passive magnetic and hydrodynamic forces levitating the impeller and two axial flux motors for redundancy in case one fails. The HVAD has also been used for RV support [37], although CE or FDA approval for this purpose has not been obtained. In 2015, HeartWare started clinical trials of the miniaturized MVAD, an axial flow pump approximately one-third the size of the HVAD with similar impeller levitation principles and capable of less-invasive implantation due to its smaller size [38].

Apart from early postoperative hemostatic complications, a major issue in the early postoperative course is that of RV failure. While controversy remains around pre-emptive mechanical RV support using a temporary RVAD based on ECMO circuitry or an implantable LVAD on the right (there is no customized, long-term rotary RVAD at this stage), it should be noted that re-operation to institute mechanical RV

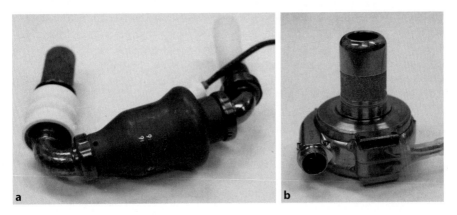

Fig. 4 Two commonly used rotary ventricular assist devices (VADs). **a** Thoratec HeartMate II, **b** HeartWare HVAD

support once RV failure sets in adds to mortality and morbidity in these patients [39]. A high index of suspicion preoperatively and vigilance and prompt escalation of pharmacological and mechanical RV support intra- and postoperatively is the key. We refer the readers elsewhere for a more detailed summary of outcomes and complications [40].

Total Artificial Hearts

Compared to the dramatic increase in continuous intracorporeal pump implants over the last decade, clinical use of total artificial hearts has been much slower. In 2007, the INTERMACS database reported 22 pulsatile intracorporeal total artificial heart implants, which had increased only to 66 by 2013 [30]. The lack of a long-term, low-wear device with small wearable components, as seen in the latest generation of VADs, may have contributed to the slow uptake of total artificial hearts. Meanwhile, the 'safety net' provided with a VAD, where remnant ventricular contractility may sustain life until emergency intervention, could also explain why total artificial hearts are only used when absolutely necessary.

Although several total artificial hearts, such as the Liotta-Cooley, Akutsu III and the AbioCor devices, have been used to support patients [7], these devices are no longer used clinically. The Carmat (Vélizy Villacoublay, France) total artificial heart is currently in clinical use, however very few patients have been supported since the first implant in December 2013. Meanwhile, the use of a dual LVAD configuration for total artificial heart support has been reported using dual Heart-Mate II [41, 42] or HeartWare HVAD [43] devices; however clinical experience with this technique is limited. The only total artificial heart currently available to fully support the circulation for which there is substantial clinical experience is the SynCardia total artificial heart (SynCardia, Tucson, AZ).

Initially developed as the Jarvik 7 and renamed as the Symbion, Cardiowest and now SynCardia total artificial heart, this pulsatile first generation device consists of two pneumatically operated chambers which provide total systemic and pulmonary flow. A pneumatic driver, for which a 6.1 kg portable version now exists, supplies pulses of compressed air through percutaneous leads to the left and right chambers to deliver almost 70 ml/beat. The beat rate can be changed to deliver flow rates up to 9.5 l/min from the device, which weighs 160 g. Unidirectional flow is achieved with four tilting valves, which have reportedly never failed, while the pumping diaphragms have a failure rate of less than 1% [44]. Although the SynCardia total artificial heart has been in clinical use for several decades with CE and FDA approval for bridge-to-transplant (1999 and 2004 respectively) and FDA investigational device exemption for destination therapy (2015), widespread clinical use has been slow with over 1440 implants to date [44]. The longest duration of support with the SynCardia total artificial heart currently stands at 1374 days [44]; however typical support duration is closer to 15–90 days at different centers [7]. Meanwhile, SynCardia have recently had FDA investigational device exemption approval for a smaller total artificial heart version with 50 ml pneumatic chambers.

The quest for a durable, safe, practical and affordable total artificial heart continues and rotary blood pump technology has the potential to deliver the same. In the meantime, the temporary and long term MCS options discussed thus far will have to be used in an individualized, tailored fashion so that positive patient outcomes may be achieved whist making the most of available technology.

Quality Assurance, Governance and Benchmarking

Whilst MCS devices appear to be attractive technologies, the multidisciplinary teamwork required is substantial – and one key to success is a smooth decision-making paradigm including all the relevant players, where all the options discussed are considered, but acted upon in a timely fashion, thus delaying any further physiological deterioration of the patient. Currently, clinicians working with MCS must deal with a developing technology still with substantial risks. To optimize outcome in patients requiring MCS, clearly defined work unit guidelines and protocols are needed that can minimize the risks associated with the currently imperfect technology. The risk/benefit ratio of MCS will be improved further if the multiple stakeholders in this field collaborate in a silo free research environment – bringing together fields as disparate but inextricably linked as engineering, science, medical, surgical, intensive care and allied health. Governance, quality assurance and benchmarking of MCS practices are also essential to determine optimal team make-up and volume of cases/types of case to be undertaken in each advanced center to maintain adequate skills and knowledge base. Centers that are proficient in the full array of MCS options discussed in this chapter may serve as a 'hub' for several peripheral centers that can initiate timely temporary MCS (typically peripheral VA-ECMO). Case volume and outcome relationships are very likely to exist in such specialized areas of care and maintaining staff training and individual/institutional accreditation also needs to be considered. Similarly, patient referral patterns to these advanced MCS centers from other centers will change, creating pressure on transfer capabilities, intensive care and hospital resources. As the field evolves, data from ELSO, INTERMACS and other local and international registries will allow clinicians to audit and improve upon their clinical practice. Governance and organizational issues must be addressed at a number of levels, and this discussion will require health economists and policy makers to be involved *ab initio*.

Resource and Ethical Issues

The resource intensive nature of MCS therapies is a major barrier for their global uptake. Equally, developing, validating and clinically testing is a resource intense exercise as well. Industry, clinicians, researchers and policy makers will all have to work together in delivering these MCS devices, which can radically change the way we deal with a leading cause of death worldwide, i.e., cardiovascular disease. One of the most important ethical dilemmas faced by clinicians who are so invested in evidence-based medicine is the individual centric nature of MCS, in which 'one size doesn't fit all' and there will be a learning curve where patients will have to be offered these extraordinary therapies (especially the temporary MCS options as bridge to decision/recovery/device/transplant) outside the comfort zone of compelling favorable evidence from a randomized controlled trial. Equally it may be emotionally challenging for the staff involved to see their patients not get a positive outcome despite spending long periods of time in intensive care/hospital on various bridging MCS options and then not reach their ultimate goal of destination device or heart transplantation. Thus, MCS can raise significant ethical issues [45–47] in a world that is diverse from social, cultural and financial points of view. None of these factors should be a deterrent towards an ultimate goal of delivering temporary and longer term MCS devices.

Research Priorities and Advancing the Field of Mechanical Circulatory Support

Despite an ongoing debate on the merits and demerits of a non-pulsatile circulation, which results in the setting of many of these MCS strategies based on rotary blood pumps, short-term clinical results are encouraging. Equally, more research is needed in the area of microcirculatory alterations in the presence of a non-pulsatile circulation. When it comes to MCS, the simplicity of rotary blood pumps results in less shear forces on blood cells and biotrauma as compared to displacement pumps.

Temporary Acute Mechanical Circulatory Support

Peripheral VA-ECMO is an imperfect but viable tool in patients with cardiac failure. Improvement in cannula design for ease of insertion eliminating the need for backflow cannulation will improve its risk/benefit ratio. Technological solutions to minimize the afterload increases imposed on the native heart and timed afterload reduction if possible to promote aortic valve opening and minimize LV distension may alleviate the need for invasive central strategies. Development of minimally invasive LV venting strategies is also desirable. Similarly, an advanced understanding of the biological burden of adding an extracorporeal circuit with vast surface area is poorly understood and basic science research to advance our understanding of the pathophysiology of ECMO is the first step towards optimization of hematological, inflammatory, infectious and pharmacokinetic issues that add to the morbidity of ECMO. Clinical research currently must focus on establishing best practice guidelines for use of ECMO in the clinical setting of cardiogenic shock or severe cardiorespiratory failure. Paracorporeal short-term VADs are an attractive but underutilized option for acute MCS and further research should focus on improving the durability of these devices [48], minimizing morbidity especially ischemic limb complications and generating much needed evidence for their use.

Long-term Mechanical Circulatory Support-VADs and Total Artificial Hearts

With durable and miniaturized pumps that have proven clinical success, and the upcoming evolution to even smaller devices, future development of MCS should focus on developing the system around the pump to reduce postoperative complications. The two most frequent adverse events identified in the sixth INTERMACS report [30] were bleeding and infection. Bleeding is partly due to the anticoagulation regime following VAD implantation and acquired von Willebrand syndrome [49, 50]. Research will simultaneously focus on improving implantation techniques, through development of less-invasive procedures off-CPB, whilst developing a more complete understanding of the complex blood-VAD interaction. The relative lack of pulsatility seen with rotary VADs is known to at least contribute to gastrointestinal bleeding, arteriovenous malformations, hemolysis and pump thrombosis [51]. Interest in pulsing rotary blood pumps (i.e., speed modulation) has therefore increased and should be further explored, with the potential added benefits of increased aortic valve opening, coronary perfusion, baroreflex sensitivity and ventricular washout.

Early percutaneous driveline infections are a feared and catastrophic complication [52], while late-onset driveline infections are the equal highest cause of death in VAD patients after 4 years of support [30]. Therefore, improved driveline development and implantation techniques along with clinically approved transcutaneous energy transfer systems are required. Meanwhile, right heart failure is a frequent and potentially fatal complication following LVAD implantation [53, 54] and is associated with worse outcomes [30]. Further research and clinical experience with dual LVAD biventricular support configurations must be carried out, while the continued development of RVAD-specific devices and rotary total artificial heart technology should be completed in parallel to source an optimal solution. The low preload and high afterload sensitivities of these rotary VADs can result in venous congestion and ventricular suction events [55]. Physiological control systems, which actively change pump speed based on hemodynamic feedback variables, have been developed but not clinically accepted. Further research should focus on progression into clinical practice; however, this may depend on the development of a reliable, implantable sensor (pressure and/or flow) for hemodynamic feedback.

Global Databases and Registries

The diversity of MCS techniques, especially in the acute setting, adds to the challenges of performing meaningful clinical studies in the area. Preliminary understanding of global MCS practices and inherent heterogeneity in practice is a key pre-requisite. Similar to INTERMACS, establishment of a broader acute MCS registry collecting data in the acute setting using ECMO or pVAD based strategies may be an important step forward. The ELSO registry, over time, has become an invaluable tool; however, current data collection does not involve advanced temporary MCS strategies discussed in this article and some modifications to reporting structure may have to be made to ensure that all MCS runs based on an ECMO circuit are reported. It should be noted that most reporting to these global databases remains optional.

Global Trial Networks

Without global engagement, it will be impossible to drive the high quality randomized trials necessary for the safe development of these therapies. In the last few years, ELSO has developed strong regional representations with most geographical regions having their own active chapters that promote training, education and research. Networks such as the International ECMO Network (ECMONet), and the International Society for Rotary Blood Pumps have been formed to foster further research and development of best practice guidelines in the field of MCS. These existing platforms can be effectively used to design and conduct high quality MCS trials. Responsible and ethically-sound industry engagement is also paramount when designing such trials.

Conclusion

This review highlights the spectrum of available therapies for acute and chronic heart failure patients and circulatory shock in general. The flexible nature of MCS configurations allows for an individualized approach driven by the ultimate goal of achieving organ recovery or bridging to long-term options. Intensivists, when faced with severe cardiac failure, especially in younger patients, may have to consider MCS as a viable option and initiate timely referrals. Similarly in patients with chronic heart failure, timely insertion of long-term VADs prior to development of irreversible end-organ dysfunction will minimize postoperative morbidity and eliminate the need for short-term temporary bridging mechanical support. Some patients will need short-term mechanical right heart support with a temporary RVAD and in others a long-term BiVAD may be inevitable and customized implantable RVADs may become a reality in future. Both VAD and total artificial heart technology will see many more refinements with time and it is difficult to predict which of these devices will prove to be a perfect bridge to heart transplant or destination. Whilst these technologies may seem excessively complex and expensive, this was once said of dialysis. In the current era, in an appropriately resourced setting, no eligible patient should die on maximal medical therapy without MCS being considered

Acknowledgements

Ms Lynette Munck for administrative support and proof reading the manuscript. John Fraser currently holds a Health Research Fellowship awarded by the Office of Health and Medical Research, Queensland, Australia. The authors would like to recognize the financial assistance provided by the National Health and Medical Research Council (APP1079421). The contents are solely the responsibility of the authors and do not reflect the views of the NHMRC.

References

1. Beurtheret S, Mordant P, Paoletti X et al (2013) Emergency circulatory support in refractory cardiogenic shock patients in remote institutions: a pilot study (the cardiac-RESCUE program). Eur Heart J 34:112–120
2. Reynolds HR, Hochman JS (2008) Cardiogenic shock: current concepts and improving outcomes. Circulation 117:686–697
3. Shekar K, Mullany DV, Thomson B, Ziegenfuss M, Platts DG, Fraser JF (2014) Extracorporeal life support devices and strategies for management of acute cardiorespiratory failure in adult patients: a comprehensive review. Crit Care 18:219
4. Abrams D, Combes A, Brodie D (2014) Extracorporeal membrane oxygenation in cardiopulmonary disease in adults. J Am Coll Cardiol 63:2769–2778
5. Stub D, Bernard S, Pellegrino V et al (2015) Refractory cardiac arrest treated with mechanical CPR, hypothermia, ECMO and early reperfusion (the CHEER trial). Resuscitation 86:88–94
6. Pinney SP (2015) Left ventricular assist devices: The adolescence of a disruptive technology. J Card Fail 21:824–834

7. Cohn WE, Timms DL, Frazier OH (2015) Total artificial hearts: past, present, and future. Nat Rev Cardiol 12:609–617
8. Thiele H, Zeymer U, Neumann FJ et al (2012) Intraaortic balloon support for myocardial infarction with cardiogenic shock. N Engl J Med 367:1287–1296
9. Cove ME, MacLaren G (2010) Clinical review: mechanical circulatory support for cardiogenic shock complicating acute myocardial infarction. Crit Care 14:235
10. Combes A, Leprince P, Luyt CE et al (2008) Outcomes and long-term quality-of-life of patients supported by extracorporeal membrane oxygenation for refractory cardiogenic shock. Crit Care Med 36:1404–1411
11. Extracorporeal Life Support Organization (2015) ECLS Registry Report International Summary. https://www.elso.org/Registry/Statistics/InternationalSummary.aspx. Accessed Nov 2015
12. ELSO (2013) Guidelines for Adult Cardiac Failure Supplement Version 1.3. https://www.elso.org/Portals/0/IGD/Archive/FileManager/e76ef78eabcusersshyerdocumentselsoguidelinesforadultcardiacfailure1.3.pdf. Accessed Nov 2015
13. Chen YS, Lin JW, Yu HY et al (2008) Cardiopulmonary resuscitation with assisted extracorporeal life-support versus conventional cardiopulmonary resuscitation in adults with in-hospital cardiac arrest: an observational study and propensity analysis. Lancet 372:554–561
14. Thiagarajan RR (2011) Extracorporeal membrane oxygenation to support cardiopulmonary resuscitation: Useful, but for whom? Crit Care Med 39:190–191
15. Feldman D, Pamboukian SV, Teuteberg JJ et al (2013) The 2013 International Society for Heart and Lung Transplantation Guidelines for mechanical circulatory support: Executive summary. J Heart Lung Transplant 32:157–187
16. Combes A, Bacchetta M, Brodie D, Muller T, Pellegrino V (2012) Extracorporeal membrane oxygenation for respiratory failure in adults. Curr Opin Crit Care 18:99–104
17. Aiyagari RM, Rocchini AP, Remenapp RT, Graziano JN (2006) Decompression of the left atrium during extracorporeal membrane oxygenation using a transseptal cannula incorporated into the circuit. Crit Care Med 34:2603–2066
18. Guirgis M, Kumar K, Menkis AH, Freed DH (2010) Minimally invasive left-heart decompression during venoarterial extracorporeal membrane oxygenation: an alternative to a percutaneous approach. Interact Cardiovasc Thorac Surg 10:672–674
19. Vlasselaers D, Desmet M, Desmet L, Meyns B, Dens J (2006) Ventricular unloading with a miniature axial flow pump in combination with extracorporeal membrane oxygenation. Intensive Care Med 32:3293
20. Aggarwal A, Modi S, Kumar S et al (2013) Use of a single-circuit CentriMag(R) for biventricular support in postpartum cardiomyopathy. Perfusion 28:156–159
21. Massetti M, Gaudino M, Saplacan V, Farina P (2013) From extracorporeal membrane oxygenation to ventricular assist device oxygenation without sternotomy. J Heart Lung Transplant 32:138–139
22. Arroyo D, Cook S (2011) Percutaneous ventricular assist devices: new deus ex machina? Minim Invasive Surg 2011:604397
23. Prutkin JM, Strote JA, Stout KK (2008) Percutaneous right ventricular assist device as support for cardiogenic shock due to right ventricular infarction. J Invasive Cardiol 20:E215–216
24. Rajagopal V, Steahr G, Wilmer CI, Raval NY (2010) A novel percutaneous mechanical biventricular bridge to recovery in severe cardiac allograft rejection. J Heart Lung Transplant 29:93–95
25. Garbade J, Bittner HB, Barten MJ, Mohr FW (2011) Current trends in implantable left ventricular assist devices. Cardiol Res Pract 2011:290561
26. Stewart GC, Givertz MM (2012) Mechanical circulatory support for advanced heart failure: patients and technology in evolution. Circulation 125:1304–1315
27. Drakos SG, Janicki L, Horne BD et al (2010) Risk factors predictive of right ventricular failure after left ventricular assist device implantation. Am J Cardiol 105:1030–1035

28. Cowger J, Sundareswaran K, Rogers JG et al (2013) Predicting survival in patients receiving continuous flow left ventricular assist devices: the HeartMate II risk score. J Am Coll Cardiol 61:313–321
29. Teuteberg JJ, Ewald GA, Adamson RM et al (2012) Risk assessment for continuous flow left ventricular assist devices: does the destination therapy risk score work? An analysis of over 1,000 patients. J Am Coll Cardiol 60:44–51
30. Kirklin JK, Naftel DC, Pagani FD et al (2014) Sixth INTERMACS annual report: A 10,000-patient database. J Heart Lung Transplant 33:555–564
31. Rose EA, Gelijns AC, Moskowitz AJ et al (2001) Long-term use of a left ventricular assist device for end-stage heart failure. N Engl J Med 345:1435–1443
32. Slaughter MS, Rogers JG, Milano CA et al (2009) Advanced heart failure treated with continuous-flow left ventricular assist device. N Engl J Med 361:2241–2251
33. Bourque K, Gernes DB, Loree HM 2nd (2001) HeartMate III: pump design for a centrifugal LVAD with a magnetically levitated rotor. ASAIO J 47:401–405
34. Sundareswaran KS, Reichenbach SH, Masterson KB, Butler KC, Farrar DJ (2013) Low bearing wear in explanted HeartMate II left ventricular assist devices after chronic clinical support. ASAIO J 59:41–45
35. Thoratec Corporation. HeartMate II Clinical Outcomes. http://www.thoratec.com/vad-trials-outcomes/clinical-outcomes/hm2-ce-phase1.aspx. Accessed November 2015
36. Timms D (2011) A review of clinical ventricular assist devices. Med Eng Phys 33:1041–1047
37. Krabatsch T, Potapov E, Stepanenko A et al (2011) Biventricular circulatory support with two miniaturized implantable assist devices. Circulation 124:179–186
38. Slaughter MS, Sobieski MA, Tamcz D et al (2009) HeartWare miniature axial-flow ventricular assist device: design and initial feasibility test. Texas Heart Inst J 36:12–16
39. Fitzpatrick JR, Frederick JR, Hiesinger W et al (2009) Early planned institution of biventricular mechanical circulatory support results in improved outcomes compared with delayed conversion of a left ventricular assist device to a biventricular assist device. J Thorac Cardiovasc Surg 137:971–977
40. Milano CA, Simeone AA (2013) Mechanical circulatory support: devices, outcomes and complications. Heart Fail Rev 18:35–53
41. Frazier OH, Cohn WE (2012) Continuous-flow total heart replacement device implanted in a 55-year-old man with end-stage heart failure and severe amyloidosis. Texas Heart Inst J 39:542–546
42. Pirk J, Maly J, Szarszoi O et al (2013) Total artificial heart support with two continuous-flow ventricular assist devices in a patient with an infiltrating cardiac sarcoma. ASAIO J 59:178–180
43. Strueber M, Schmitto JD, Kutschka I, Haverich A (2012) Placement of 2 implantable centrifugal pumps to serve as a total artificial heart after cardiectomy. J Thorac Cardiovasc Surg 143:507–509
44. SynCardia Systems Inc. Total Artificial Heart Facts. http://www.syncardia.com/total-facts/total-artificial-heart-facts.html. Accessed November 2015
45. Abrams DC, Prager K, Blinderman CD, Burkart KM, Brodie D (2014) Ethical dilemmas encountered with the use of extracorporeal membrane oxygenation in adults. Chest 145:876–882
46. Rizzieri AG, Verheijde JL, Rady MY, McGregor JL (2008) Ethical challenges with the left ventricular assist device as a destination therapy. Philos Ethics Humanit Med 3:20
47. Bruce CR (2013) A review of ethical considerations for ventricular assist device placement in older adults. Aging Dis 4:100–112
48. Kar B, Basra SS, Shah NR, Loyalka P (2012) Percutaneous circulatory support in cardiogenic shock: interventional bridge to recovery. Circulation 125:1809–1817
49. Uriel N, Pak SW, Jorde UP et al (2010) Acquired von Willebrand syndrome after continuous-flow mechanical device support contributes to a high prevalence of bleeding during long-term support and at the time of transplantation. J Am Coll Cardiol 56:1207–1213

50. Geisen U, Heilmann C, Beyersdorf F et al (2008) Non-surgical bleeding in patients with ventricular assist devices could be explained by acquired von Willebrand disease. Eur J Cardiothorac Surg 33:679–684
51. Cheng A, Williamitis CA, Slaughter MS (2014) Comparison of continuous-flow and pulsatile-flow left ventricular assist devices: is there an advantage to pulsatility? Ann Cardiothorac Surg 3:573–581
52. Holman WL, Kirklin JK, Naftel DC et al (2010) Infection after implantation of pulsatile mechanical circulatory support devices. J Thorac Cardiovasc Surg 139:1632–1636
53. Aissaoui N, Morshuis M, Schoenbrodt M et al (2013) Temporary right ventricular mechanical circulatory support for the management of right ventricular failure in critically ill patients. J Thorac Cardiovasc Surg 146:186–191
54. Drakos SG, Janicki L, Horne BD et al (2010) Risk factors predictive of right ventricular failure after left ventricular assist device implantation. Am J Cardiol 105:1030–1035
55. Salamonsen RF, Mason DG, Ayre PJ (2011) Response of rotary blood pumps to changes in preload and afterload at a fixed speed setting are unphysiological when compared with the natural heart. Artif Organs 35:E47–E53

Part VII
Cardiac Arrest

Cardiac Arrest in the Elderly: Epidemiology and Outcome

C. Sandroni, S. D'Arrigo, and M. Antonelli

Introduction

As a result of the combined effect of decreasing fertility and increasing life expectancy, the world's population is ageing rapidly, and the process has accelerated in the last three decades. For the first time since the beginning of recorded history, elderly people are outnumbering young children [1]. By 2050, the numbers of people aged 60 years and over will have more than doubled, increasing from 901 million in 2015 to 2.1 billion [2]. The numbers of people aged 80 years and over will more than triple, increasing from 125 million in 2015 to 464 million in 2050. Although Europe has currently the highest percentage (24%) of people older than 60 years of age, the fastest growth in this age group is occurring in Asia, Africa and Latin America, so that relevant ageing will affect the whole world population in the next 30 years [2].

Consistently with a progressive ageing of the world population, the number of cardiac arrests in older people is expected to increase in the next decades. This will raise a series of social, ethical, and economic concerns. Given the inherent frailty of aged patients and the high rates of death or persistent disability associated with cardiac arrest, resuscitation of many aged patients may be seen as inappropriate. To assist with decisions on providing resuscitation in these patients, healthcare providers will need to predict as accurately as possible the likelihood of survival with an acceptable quality of life.

C. Sandroni (✉) · S. D'Arrigo · M. Antonelli
Department of Anesthesiology and Intensive Care, Catholic University School of Medicine
Rome, Italy
email: sandroni@rm.unicatt.it

© Springer International Publishing Switzerland 2016

219

J.-L. Vincent (ed.), *Annual Update in Intensive Care and Emergency Medicine 2016*,
DOI 10.1007/978-3-319-27349-5_18

Epidemiology of Cardiac Arrest in the Elderly

There are only a few large prospective observational studies specifically focused on the older age population resuscitated from cardiac arrest. Epidemiological studies are hampered by the lack of a consistent definition of the term 'elderly' [3, 4]. Different cut-off values have been used to divide younger from older adults: 65 years, 70 years, 75 years, or even 80 years (Table 1). Taking as a reference the median age of retirement of the 37 most developed countries in the world reported by the Organization for Economic Co-operation and Development [5], elderly people can be arbitrarily defined as those aged 65 years and over. Among 31,689 patients with out-of-hospital cardiac arrest (OHCA) included in the CARES registry, 16,160 (51%) were above that threshold [6]. Similar results have been reported in other studies on OHCA conducted in Europe and Australia [7, 8] and in Asia ([9, 10]; Table 1). According to these data and to the definition given above, the elderly therefore already represent the majority of patients resuscitated from OHCA. As far as in-hospital cardiac arrest is concerned, among 14,720 adults included in the American NRCPR registry, 50% were above 70 years of age [11].

The proportion of elderly patients undergoing cardiac arrest is expected to increase in the years to come not only because of the increased proportion of aged people in the World population, but also because higher age is associated with a proportionally higher risk of cardiac arrest. In an observational study including 269,956 consecutive hospital admissions [12] the incidence of in-hospital cardiac arrest in patients older than 65 years of age was more than twice as high as that of the younger patient population (2.2 vs. 1.0 per 1000 patient admissions; $p < 0.01$). In males, the incidence of OHCA at 80 years of age is about seven times greater than at 40 years of age [13]. In females older than 70 years of age the incidence of OHCA is more than 40 times greater than in women less than 45 years of age.

Sex-related differences in the incidence of cardiac arrest in the elderly are only partially known. While the risk of cardiac arrest in general is slightly higher in men [14], the proportion of women among elderly patients resuscitated from OHCA seems to progressively increase with age [7]. This may be partly due to the higher age expectancy of women as compared to men.

Causes of Cardiac Arrest

Aging is associated with a progressive increase in the incidence of both coronary heart disease and chronic heart failure. This results in an increased incidence of cardiac disease as a cause of death among elderly people [15]. However, the proportion of cardiac deaths that are sudden (i.e., due to ventricular fibrillation [VF] or pulseless ventricular tachycardia [pVT]) decreases with age, due to a parallel increase in the proportion of other cardiovascular causes of death [3]. In an observational study including 1277 OHCA patients, the incidence of pulseless electrical activity (PEA) as the first recorded rhythm increased significantly with age [16], as also reported in earlier studies [15]. Among patients older than 70 years of age who were re-

Table 1 Studies comparing the outcome of older vs. younger patients resuscitated from cardiac arrest

Author, year [reference]	In-hospital CA/OHCA	Country	Data collection period	Threshold age, years	N° of patients	Elderly, n (%)	Male, n (%)	Witnessed n (%)	VF/pVT, n (%)	Overall survival, n (%)	Survival, elderly n (%)
Ahn, 2010 [9]	OHCA	Korea	2006–2007	≥ 65	14,739	7,962 (54)	9,925 (67.3)	8,236 (43.2)	829 (6.3)	513 (3.5)	163 (2.0)
Chien, 2008 [10]	OHCA	Taiwan	2005	≥ 65	299	198 (66.2)	179 (59.8)	193 (64.5)	32 (10.7)	22 (7.4)	12 (6.1)
Deasy, 2011 [7]	OHCA	Australia	2008–2009	≥ 65	30,006	17,609 (58.7)	19,654 (65.5)	9,492 (31.6)	4,485 (15)	1,105 (3.7)	511 (2.9)
Hagiwara, 2015 [19]	OHCA	Japan	2013–2014	≥ 80	103	48 (46.6)	55 (53.3)	25 (24.2)	1 (0.9)	2 (1.9)	0 (0.0)
Kim, 2000 [20]	OHCA	USA	1996–1997	≥ 80	5,882	1,310 (22.3)	4,086 (69.4)	3,234 (54.9)	2,792 (47.4)	999 (17)	112 (8.5)
McNally, 2011 [6]	OHCA	USA	2005–2010	≥ 65	31,609	16,150 (51.1)	21,386 (67.6)	17,381 (55)	9,539 (30.1)	3,037 (9.6)	1,169 (7.2)
Pleskot, 2011 [21]	OHCA	Czech Republic	2002–2004	≥ 70	560	253 (45.2)	415 (74.1)	495 (88.3)	238 (42.5)	64 (11.4)	14 (5.5)
Schwenzer, 1993 [22]	In-hospital	USA	1987–1988	≥ 70	573	160 (27.9)	N/A	N/A	N/A	140 (24.4)	32 (20.0)
Seder, 2014 [23]	Mixed	USA	2006–2011	> 75	754	129 (17.1)	513 (68)	615 (81.5)	435 (57.7)	324 (43.0)	42 (32.6)
Snyder, 2010 [24]	In-hospital	USA	2005–2008	≥ 70	691	318 (46)	N/A	N/A	N/A	173 (25.0)	64 (20.1)
Swor, 2000 [25]	OHCA	USA	1989–1993	≥ 70	2,608	1,213 (46.5)	1,650 (63.2)	1,283 (49.2)	1,302 (49.9)	192 (7.4)	69 (5.7)
Winther-Jensen, 2015 [8]	OHCA	Europe – Australia	2010–2012	> 65	939	485 (51.7)	761 (81)	838 (89.2)	729 (77.6)	340 (36.2)	103 (21.2)

VF/pVT: Ventricular fibrillation/pulseless ventricular tachycardia; *CA*: cardiac arrest; *OHCA*: out-of-hospital cardiac arrest; *N/A*: not available. Survival is reported to hospital discharge in all studies except [21] (30 days).

suscitated from OHCA and randomized in the Targeted Temperature Management (TTM) trial, the incidence of VF/pVT as a cause of arrest decreased progressively and significantly with increasing age. The same occurred with the incidence of ST segment elevation on the electrocardiogram (EKG) at admission [8].

Outcome

Older age is associated with increased mortality after cardiac arrest [7, 17, 18]. A comparison between the crude mortality rates reported in 11 observational studies [6, 7, 9, 10, 19–25] on cardiac arrest (both in and out-of-hospital) and in one sub-study [8] of a clinical trial shows a consistently higher likelihood of death in elderly vs. younger age groups (pooled odds ratio [OR] 2.08, 95% confidence interval [CI] 1.75–2.47, p < 0.001; Fig. 1). In an Australian registry [7] of 17,609 OHCA patients older than 65 years of age, the rates of survival to discharge for those aged 65–79 years, 80–89 years and ≥ 90 years were 8%, 4% and 2%, respectively. In a study on OHCA patients who underwent targeted temperature management [8], the adjusted hazard ratio for 30-day mortality increased progressively with age (1.04 [1.03–1.06] per year; p < 0.001). This study also showed that in older patients death after an initially successful resuscitation was more frequently due to a cardiovascular cause or multiorgan failure and the incidence of cerebral causes decreased in older age groups.

Similar results have been documented for in-hospital cardiac arrest. An analysis of the National Cardiac Arrest Audit database in the UK, including 22,628 patients, showed a steady decrease in survival to discharge in those aged 50 years or older (Fig. 2) [26]. Another cohort study [27] conducted in 433,985 elderly patients resuscitated from in-hospital cardiac arrest in North America showed that survival to discharge decreased consistently by 2% every 5 years of age over 65.

Age affects long-term survival as well. In a large observational study [17] on patients aged ≥ 65 years who were discharged from the hospital after surviving an in-hospital cardiac arrest, the risk-adjusted rates of 1-year survival were 63.7%, 58.6%, and 49.7% among patients 65 to 74, 75 to 84, and ≥ 85 years of age, respectively (p < 0.001). In contrast to younger subjects, patients ≥ 65 years of age discharged from hospital after successful resuscitation from cardiac arrest due to VF/VT had a significantly lower long-term survival than age- and sex-matched controls [28].

Despite these results, the nature of the association between age and survival after cardiopulmonary resuscitation (CPR) is still debated. While some investigators have reported that increasing age is an independent factor for mortality after cardiac arrest [29] others have not [30]. In general, age seems to be less important in determining final outcome than event variables like initial cardiac rhythm, witnessed status or the interval between cardiac arrest and resuscitation interventions [31, 32]. Moreover, separating the effect on outcome of age from that of comorbidities that are naturally associated with ageing is difficult and this point has been only rarely investigated [18]. Finally, the lower survival rates observed in older victims of cardiac arrest may be due to a higher incidence of withdrawal of life-

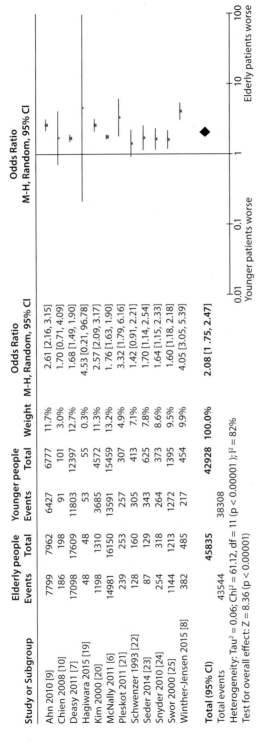

| Study or Subgroup | Elderly people | | Younger people | | | Odds Ratio | Odds Ratio |
	Events	Total	Events	Total	Weight	M-H, Random, 95% CI	M-H, Random, 95% CI
Ahn 2010 [9]	7799	7962	6427	6777	11.7%	2.61 [2.16, 3.15]	
Chien 2008 [10]	186	198	91	101	3.0%	1.70 [0.71, 4.09]	
Deasy 2011 [7]	17098	17609	11803	12397	12.7%	1.68 [1.49, 1.90]	
Hagiwara 2015 [19]	48	48	53	55	0.3%	4.53 [0.21, 96.78]	
Kim 2000 [20]	1198	1310	3685	4572	11.3%	2.57 [2.09, 3.17]	
McNally 2011 [6]	14981	16150	13591	15459	13.2%	1.76 [1.63, 1.90]	
Pleskot 2011 [21]	239	253	257	307	4.9%	3.32 [1.79, 6.16]	
Schwenzer 1993 [22]	128	160	305	413	7.1%	1.42 [0.91, 2.21]	
Seder 2014 [23]	87	129	343	625	7.8%	1.70 [1.14, 2.54]	
Snyder 2010 [24]	254	318	264	373	8.6%	1.64 [1.15, 2.33]	
Swor 2000 [25]	1144	1213	1272	1395	9.5%	1.60 [1.18, 2.18]	
Winther-Jensen 2015 [8]	382	485	217	454	9.9%	4.05 [3.05, 5.39]	
Total (95% CI)		45835		42928	100.0%	2.08 [1.75, 2.47]	
Total events	43544		38308				

Heterogeneity: Tau² = 0.06; Chi² = 61.12, df = 11 (p < 0.00001); I² = 82%
Test for overall effect: Z = 8.36 (p < 0.00001)

Fig. 1 Odds ratio (OR) for mortality in older patients resuscitated from cardiac arrest compared with younger patients. Pooled analysis of twelve studies (total 88,763 patients) according to the Mantel-Haenszel (M-H) method, random effect model

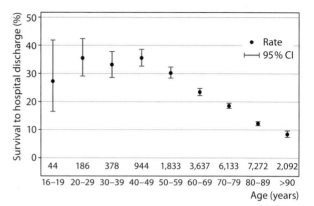

Fig. 2 Survival to discharge by age in a UK cohort of 22,628 patients resuscitated from in-hospital cardiac arrest. From [26] with permission

sustaining therapies due to perception of poor long-term outcome in this category of patients [33]. In a retrospective evaluation of recent registry data from six regional percutaneous coronary intervention (PCI) centers in the United States [23], cardiac arrest survivors aged > 75 years were more likely to have do-not-resuscitate (DNR) orders (65.9% vs. 48.2%, p < 0.001) and to undergo withdrawal of life-sustaining therapies (61.2% vs. 47.5%, p = 0.005) than younger patients with similar arrest characteristics. Age > 75 years was independently associated with poor outcome but this association disappeared when DNR status was added to a multivariate logistic regression analysis model.

Survival Trends

There is evidence that the outcome of aged patients resuscitated from cardiac arrest has improved in the last few years. Results from a large registry in Japan [34] showed a five-fold increase in survival with good neurological outcome after witnessed OHCA of cardiac origin among patients aged ≥ 65 years resuscitated between 1999 and 2011. Another cohort study [7] showed a significant increase in survival to hospital discharge between 2000 and 2009 after OHCA in patients ≥ 65 years of age, but only among those with a shockable rhythm.

Neurological Outcome and Quality of Life

In a recent registry study [32] on older (≥ 75 years) survivors of cardiac arrest, 95% of patients evaluated at discharge from the intensive care unit (ICU) and 100% of those evaluated at 5-year follow-up had a good neurological outcome (cerebral performance category [CPC] 1 or 2). Despite a progressive increase in the mean age of resuscitated patients across the study period (from 79.5 to 82 years) the proportion of patients with a good outcome remained stable over time. However, only 10% of the patients who were initially admitted to ICU after resuscitation were alive at a mean of 28.4 months after the event. After adjustment for covariates, an initial shockable rhythm, a short no flow-time and low lactate levels on admission were independent predictors of good short- or long-term outcome, while age < 79.5 years was not.

In a large retrospective study [17] including 6972 patients aged ≥ 65 years who were discharged to the hospital after having been resuscitated from in-hospital cardiac arrest, 82.4% had good neurological status (CPC 1–2) at discharge. One year later, however, 65.6% had been readmitted to the hospital. Neurological disability was a major predictor of increased risk of readmission.

Prevention of In-Hospital Cardiac Arrest in the Elderly

Given the high mortality rate of cardiac arrest, prevention is paramount. Early identification and treatment of deteriorating patients in hospital wards by rapid response systems has been demonstrated to reduce in-hospital mortality [35]. Unfortunately, deterioration of vital signs leading to cardiac arrest is detected less accurately in elderly patients compared with younger patients [36]. Clinical history may be less reliable due to cognitive impairment [37]. In a registry study [12] including 422 ward cardiac arrests (65% occurring in patients >65 years of age), elderly patients had significantly lower mean heart rate (88 vs 99 beats/min, p < 0.001), shock index (0.82 vs 0.93, p < 0.001), and Modified Early Warning Score (MEWS) (mean 2.6 vs 3.3, p < 0.001) within 4 h of cardiac arrest than non-elderly patients. The area under the receiver operating characteristic curves for all vital signs and the MEWS was also smaller for elderly vs. non-elderly patients (0.71 [95% CI 0.68–0.75] vs. 0.85 [95% CI 0.82–0.88], p < 0.001).

Decision to Resuscitate

Elderly cardiac arrest patients are significantly less likely to receive CPR than younger patients [22, 33]. Reasons for withholding CPR from elderly patients include an increased risk of short-term mortality, a higher rate of associated co-morbidities and a reduced long-term life expectancy. Nevertheless, age has not been officially included as a criterion in the most diffuse validated termination-of-resuscitation rules [38–40].

Apart from age itself, very little is known about the specific pre-arrest predictors of survival in this category of patients [18]. One observational study [41] found a significant association between female sex, heart failure, hypertension and lower survival to discharge after witnessed cardiac arrest in the elderly; however, that study did not correct for major confounders.

Intra-arrest factors are better documented. In particular, bystander CPR, longer response times of emergency medical system and non-VF/pVT as initial rhythm have been demonstrated to be independently associated with a significantly lower survival, as occurs in younger age groups [7, 32, 34, 42].

Age has been used as a criterion for treatment limitation after resuscitation. In a recent multicenter study conducted in the United States [23], DNR was ordered significantly more frequently in cardiac arrest survivors aged >75 years than in younger patients with similar arrest characteristics. Interestingly, among 385/754 (51%) patients for whom a DNR order was placed after resuscitation from cardiac arrest, 28 (8%) survived to hospital discharge and 9 (2%) had a good outcome at 6-month follow up. In patients resuscitated from cardiac arrest, treatment limitations are usually based on prognostication of poor neurological outcome [43, 44]. However, most predictors of neurological outcome after cardiac arrest have recently been demonstrated to be much less accurate than previously believed [45–47].

Age alone should not be the only criterion to consider when deciding to resuscitate elderly patients and other more established criteria, such as witnessed status, resuscitation times and first recorded rhythm, should be used. In addition, other pre-arrest factors, such as the degree of autonomy, quality of life, mental status and presence of major comorbidities, can be considered. However, collecting this information accurately may be difficult when resuscitation is ongoing. Whenever possible, decision on resuscitation should be discussed in advance with the patient and his/her family.

Conclusion

More than half of the patients resuscitated from cardiac arrest are aged 65 years or older, and this proportion is expected to increase in the near future, due to the progressive ageing of the world population. In comparison with younger age groups, cardiac arrest in the elderly is more frequently due to cardiac causes but it is less frequently associated with shockable rhythms (VF/pVT). Advancing age is associated with progressively lower survival rates after cardiac arrest, although the role of age as an independent predictor of survival is debated. A relatively good quality of life can be achieved by elderly patients surviving to hospital discharge. Decisions about resuscitation in the elderly should not be based on age alone, but should take into account the pre-arrest quality of life and autonomy, along with the patient's previously documented preferences.

References

1. US Department of Health and Human Services – National Institute on Aging (2015) Global health and aging. https://www.nia.nih.gov/research/publication/global-health-and-aging/assessing-costs-aging-and-health-care. Accessed October 2015
2. United Nations – Department of Economic and Social Affairs – Population Division (2015) World Population Prospects – The 2015 Revision. Working Paper No ESA/P/WP241. http://esa.un.org/unpd/wpp/. Accessed October 2015
3. Tung P, Albert CM (2013) Causes and prevention of sudden cardiac death in the elderly. Nat Rev Cardiol 10:135–142

4. Sandroni C, Nolan J, Cavallaro F, Antonelli M (2007) In-hospital cardiac arrest: incidence, prognosis and possible measures to improve survival. Intensive Care Med 33:237–245
5. Organisation for Economic Co-operation and Development (2012) Ageing and Employment Policies – Statistics on average effective age of retirement. http://www.oecd.org/els/emp/ageingandemploymentpolicies-statisticsonaverageeffectiveageofretirement.htm. Accessed October 2015
6. McNally B, Robb R, Mehta M et al (2011) Out-of-hospital cardiac arrest surveillance – Cardiac Arrest Registry to Enhance Survival (CARES), United States, October 1, 2005 – December 31, 2010. MMWR Surveill Summ 60:1–19
7. Deasy C, Bray JE, Smith K, Harriss LR, Bernard SA, Cameron P (2011) Out-of-hospital cardiac arrests in the older age groups in Melbourne. Australia Resuscitation 82:398–403
8. Winther-Jensen M, Pellis T, Kuiper M et al (2015) Mortality and neurological outcome in the elderly after target temperature management for out-of-hospital cardiac arrest. Resuscitation 91:92–98
9. Ahn KO, Shin SD, Suh GJ et al (2010) Epidemiology and outcomes from non-traumatic out-of-hospital cardiac arrest in Korea: A nationwide observational study. Resuscitation 81:974–981
10. Chien DK, Chang WH, Tsai SH, Chang KS, Chen CC, Su YJ (2008) Outcome of non-traumatic out-of-hospital cardiac arrest in the elderly. International Journal of Gerontology 2:60–66
11. Peberdy MA, Kaye W, Ornato JP et al (2003) Cardiopulmonary resuscitation of adults in the hospital: a report of 14720 cardiac arrests from the National Registry of Cardiopulmonary Resuscitation. Resuscitation 58:297–308
12. Churpek MM, Yuen TC, Winslow C, Hall J, Edelson DP (2014) Differences in vital signs between elderly and nonelderly patients prior to ward cardiac arrest. Crit Care Med 43:816–822
13. Chugh SS, Jui J, Gunson K, Stecker EC et al (2004) Current burden of sudden cardiac death: multiple source surveillance versus retrospective death certificate-based review in a large U.S. community. J Am Coll Cardiol 44:1268–1275
14. George J, Rapsomaniki E, Pujades-Rodriguez M et al (2015) How does cardiovascular disease first present in women and men? Incidence of 12 cardiovascular diseases in a contemporary cohort of 1,937,360 people. Circulation 132:1320–1328
15. Van Hoeyweghen RJ, Bossaert LL, Mullie A et al (1992) Survival after out-of-hospital cardiac arrest in elderly patients. Belgian Cerebral Resuscitation Study Group. Ann Emerg Med 21:1179–1184
16. Teodorescu C, Reinier K, Dervan C et al (2010) Factors associated with pulseless electric activity versus ventricular fibrillation: the Oregon sudden unexpected death study. Circulation 122:2116–2122
17. Chan PS, Nallamothu BK, Krumholz HM et al (2013) Long-term outcomes in elderly survivors of in-hospital cardiac arrest. N Engl J Med 368:1019–1026
18. Van De Glind EM, Van Munster BC, Van De Wetering FT, Van Delden JJ, Scholten RJ, Hooft L (2013) Pre-arrest predictors of survival after resuscitation from out-of-hospital cardiac arrest in the elderly a systematic review. BMC Geriatrics 13:68
19. Hagiwara S, Kaneko M, Murata M et al (2015) Study on the effectiveness of cardiopulmonary resuscitation in elderly patients presenting with cardiopulmonary arrest on arrival. Intern Med 54:1859–1863
20. Kim C, Becker L, Eisenberg MS (2000) Out-of-hospital cardiac arrest in octogenarians and nonagenarians. Arch Intern Med 160:3439–3443
21. Pleskot M, Hazukova R, Stritecka H, Cermakova E (2011) Five-year survival of patients after out-of-hospital cardiac arrest depending on age. Arch Gerontol Geriatr 53:e88–e92
22. Schwenzer KJ, Smith WT, Durbin CG Jr (1993) Selective application of cardiopulmonary resuscitation improves survival rates. Anesth Analg 76:478–484

23. Seder DB, Patel N, McPherson J et al (2014) Geriatric experience following cardiac arrest at Six Interventional Cardiology Centers in the United States 2006–2011: Interplay of age, do-not-resuscitate order, and outcomes. Crit Care Med 42:289–295
24. Snyder JE, Loschner AL, Kepley HO (2010) The effect of patient age on perceived resuscitation outcomes by practitioners. N C Med J 71:199–205
25. Swor RA, Jackson RE, Tintinalli JE, Pirrallo RG (2000) Does advanced age matter in outcomes after out-of-hospital cardiac arrest in community-dwelling adults? Acad Emerg Med 7:762–768
26. Nolan JP, Soar J, Smith GB et al (2014) Incidence and outcome of in-hospital cardiac arrest in the United Kingdom National Cardiac Arrest Audit. Resuscitation 85:987–992
27. Ehlenbach WJ, Barnato AE, Curtis JR et al (2009) Epidemiologic study of in-hospital cardiopulmonary resuscitation in the elderly. N Engl J Med 361:22–31
28. Bunch TJ, White RD, Khan AH, Packer DL (2004) Impact of age on long-term survival and quality of life following out-of-hospital cardiac arrest. Crit Care Med 32:963–967
29. Cooper S, Cade J (1997) Predicting survival, in-hospital cardiac arrests: resuscitation survival variables and training effectiveness. Resuscitation 35:17–22
30. Di Bari M, Chiarlone M, Fumagalli S et al (2000) Cardiopulmonary resuscitation of older, inhospital patients: immediate efficacy and long-term outcome. Crit Care Med 28:2320–2325
31. Wuerz RC, Holliman CJ, Meador SA, Swope GE, Balogh R (1995) Effect of age on prehospital cardiac resuscitation outcome. Am J Emerg Med 13:389–391
32. Grimaldi D, Dumas F, Perier MC et al (2014) Short- and long-term outcome in elderly patients after out-of-hospital cardiac arrest: a cohort study. Crit Care Med 42:2350–2357
33. Boyd K, Teres D, Rapoport J, Lemeshow S (1996) The relationship between age and the use of DNR orders in critical care patients. Evidence for age discrimination. Arch Intern Med 156:1821–1826
34. Kitamura T, Morita S, Kiyohara K et al (2014) Trends in survival among elderly patients with out-of-hospital cardiac arrest: A prospective, population-based observation from 1999 to 2011 in Osaka. Resuscitation 85:1432–1438
35. Sandroni C, D'Arrigo S, Antonelli M (2015) Rapid response systems: are they really effective? Crit Care 19:104
36. Lamantia MA, Stewart PW, Platts-Mills TF et al (2013) Predictive value of initial triage vital signs for critically ill older adults. West J Emerg Med 14:453–460
37. Nasa P, Juneja D, Singh O (2012) Severe sepsis and septic shock in the elderly: An overview. World J Crit Care Med 1:23–30
38. Morrison LJ, Verbeek PR, Zhan C, Kiss A, Allan KS (2009) Validation of a universal prehospital termination of resuscitation clinical prediction rule for advanced and basic life support providers. Resuscitation 80:324–328
39. Morrison LJ, Visentin LM, Kiss A et al (2006) Validation of a rule for termination of resuscitation in out-of-hospital cardiac arrest. N Engl J Med 355:478–487
40. Richman PB, Vadeboncoeur TF, Chikani V, Clark L, Bobrow BJ (2008) Independent evaluation of an out-of-hospital termination of resuscitation (TOR) clinical decision rule. Acad Emerg Med 15:517–521
41. Fabbri A, Marchesini G, Spada M, Iervese T, Dente M, Galvani M (2006) Monitoring intervention programmes for out-of-hospital cardiac arrest in a mixed urban and rural setting. Resuscitation 71:180–187
42. Sandroni C, Dell'Anna AM (2014) Cardiopulmonary resuscitation above 75 years: is it worthwhile? Crit Care Med 42:2446–2447
43. Geocadin RG, Buitrago MM, Torbey MT, Chandra-Strobos N, Williams MA, Kaplan PW (2006) Neurologic prognosis and withdrawal of life support after resuscitation from cardiac arrest. Neurology 67:105–108
44. Dragancea I, Rundgren M, Englund E, Friberg H, Cronberg T (2013) The influence of induced hypothermia and delayed prognostication on the mode of death after cardiac arrest. Resuscitation 84:337–342

45. Sandroni C, Cariou A, Cavallaro F et al (2014) Prognostication in comatose survivors of cardiac arrest: An advisory statement from the European Resuscitation Council and the European Society of Intensive Care Medicine. Resuscitation 85:1779–1789
46. Sandroni C, Cavallaro F, Callaway CW et al (2013) Predictors of poor neurological outcome in adult comatose survivors of cardiac arrest: a systematic review and meta-analysis. Part 2: Patients treated with therapeutic hypothermia. Resuscitation 84:1324–1338
47. Sandroni C, Cavallaro F, Callaway CW et al (2013) Predictors of poor neurological outcome in adult comatose survivors of cardiac arrest: a systematic review and meta-analysis. Part 1: patients not treated with therapeutic hypothermia. Resuscitation 84:1310–1323

Regional Systems of Care: The Final Link in the "Chain of Survival" Concept for Out-of-Hospital Cardiac Arrest

T. Tagami, H. Yasunaga, and H. Yokota

Introduction

Out-of-hospital cardiac arrest (OHCA) affects approximately 300,000 people in the United States [1], 280,000 in Europe [2], and 100,000 in Japan [3] each year, with a high mortality. To overcome this time-sensitive condition with a low survival rate, the four links of the "chain of survival" concept were first introduced by Newman [4] in the 1980s as follows: (1) early access to emergency medical care; (2) early cardiopulmonary resuscitation (CPR); (3) early defibrillation; and (4) early advanced cardiac life support. The American Heart Association (AHA) adopted this concept in its 1992 guidelines [5], and the International Liaison Committee on Resuscitation (ILCOR) subsequently echoed this concept. Although the chain of survival was subtly updated and differed among associations/councils globally, a similar concept was implemented until the 2005 guidelines [6–8].

In 2005, the European Resuscitation Council (ERC) revised the final link in the chain of survival concept to a provision for "post-resuscitation care" from "early advanced cardiac life support" [8]. In the 2005 ERC guidelines, the final link is

T. Tagami (✉)
Department of Emergency and Critical Care Medicine, Nippon Medical School Tama Nagayama Hospital
Tama-shi, Japan
Graduate School of Medicine, Department of Clinical Epidemiology and Health Economics, School of Public Health, The University of Tokyo
Bunkyo-ku, Japan
email: t-tagami@nms.ac.jp

H. Yasunaga
Graduate School of Medicine, Department of Clinical Epidemiology and Health Economics, School of Public Health, The University of Tokyo
Bunkyo-ku, Japan

H. Yokota
Department of Emergency and Critical Care Medicine, Nippon Medical School Hospital
Bunkyo-ku, Japan

© Springer International Publishing Switzerland 2016
J.-L. Vincent (ed.), *Annual Update in Intensive Care and Emergency Medicine 2016*,
DOI 10.1007/978-3-319-27349-5_19

targeted at preserving function, particularly of the brain and heart, and recognizes the importance of restoring quality of life to the cardiac arrest survivor [8]. In 2010, the AHA guidelines implemented a "fifth link", namely "post-cardiac arrest care", in addition to the previous four links, as another critical link in the chain of survival concept [9]. In all guidelines, the links before the final link of the "chain of survival" have been simplified with each revision. For example, in the AHA guidelines between 2000 and 2010, the focus is now more on recognition of cardiac arrest for the first link. For the second link, hands-only CPR without rescue breathing is recommended, which is much simpler than conventional CPR. In addition, "Look, Listen, and Feel" has been removed from the algorithm for layperson CPR. For the third link, the defibrillation sequence has been reduced from three stacked shocks to a single shock. For the fourth link, whereas several kinds of medication were recommended in the 2000 guidelines (i.e., epinephrine, atropine, several antiarrhythmic drugs and sodium bicarbonate), these have been greatly reduced in the 2010 guidelines (i.e., only epinephrine and amiodarone). However, the final link, "post-cardiac arrest care", cannot be simplified, and there is a need for a different, additional, integrated approach to counteract post-cardiac arrest syndrome [8–10].

According to the ILCOR consensus statement for post-cardiac arrest syndrome published in 2008 [10] and the 2010 AHA guidelines [9], one of the main objectives of post-cardiac arrest care after OHCA is to transport the patient to an appropriate hospital with a comprehensive post-cardiac arrest treatment system of care that includes acute coronary intervention, neurological care, goal-directed critical care, and therapeutic hypothermia. At that time, however, limited evidence existed to support the implementation of regional systems of care for post-cardiac arrest patients [9, 10]. In this chapter, we review the recent evidence for providing regional systems of care for post-cardiac arrest care in the final link of the "chain of survival" concept for OHCA.

Rationale for Regional Systems of Care for Post-Cardiac Arrest Care

The in-hospital mortality rate for post-cardiac arrest patients is very high worldwide [9–14]. Even after spontaneous circulation is restored, most patients die within two days after admission [10]. Post-cardiac arrest syndrome is a severe medical condition caused by prolonged complete whole-body ischemia and reperfusion, which was first reported by Negovsky [15] more than 40 years ago. Although the ILCOR consensus statement of post-cardiac arrest syndrome suggests the importance of providing post-resuscitation care [10], the management of patients with post-cardiac arrest syndrome is challenging. Early arterial hypotension is common and is associated with increased in-hospital mortality [15, 16]. In addition to hemodynamic instability, pulmonary dysfunction is also common after cardiac arrest [10]. During this critical condition, several treatments are available and required to improve the outcome following cardiac arrest, including therapeutic hypothermia [17, 18], percutaneous coronary intervention (PCI) [19, 20], and other advanced interventions [10]. However, several studies suggest that large inter-hospital variations exist in the provision of post-resuscitation treatments and outcomes after cardiac arrest [21, 22]. Thus, it is difficult for non-tertiary-care hospitals to deliver all the necessary treatments for post-cardiac arrest syndrome and improve outcome. In contrast, implementation of regional systems of care has improved outcomes in similarly severe conditions such as severe trauma [23] and acute myocardial infarction [24]. In addition, several studies suggest that transporting resuscitated cardiac arrest patients to a tertiary-care facility is a feasible approach [25–27]. Therefore, many resuscitation experts have previously suggested the development and implementation of regional systems of care for OHCA [10, 28, 29].

Provision of Post-Resuscitation Care and Outcome

The last decade has witnessed improvement in survival following OHCA worldwide [30–32]. Several large nationwide studies have suggested that the improvement in outcomes may be related to the provision of post-resuscitation care [12, 31, 33, 34] in addition to the improvement of the actions of bystanders and treatments before the return of spontaneous circulation (ROSC) [3, 32, 35]. Fugate et al. [31] reported the annual in-hospital mortality rate of the American National Inpatient Sample database from 2001 to 2009. They found that the in-hospital mortality rate of patients hospitalized with cardiac arrest in the United States decreased by 11.8% from 2001 to 2009 [31]. Van der Wal et al. [33] reported the results of a retrospective observational survey from the Netherlands. They found that implementation of mild therapeutic hypothermia was associated with a 20% relative reduction of hospital mortality in cardiac arrest patients in Dutch intensive care units (ICUs) [33]. Kim et al. [12] reported a nationwide retrospective study from Korea. They found that active post-resuscitation care resulted in a significant improvement in patient outcome in propensity score-matched cohort analyses [12]. In addition, they recommended the systematic inclusion of the fifth link to improve patient outcome [12]. We recently reported results from a Japanese nationwide study of 3413 adult patients from 385 hospitals with cardiogenic OHCA related to ventricular fibrillation (VF) [34]. We found that the provision of therapeutic hypothermia and/or PCI increased over the period from 2008 to 2012 in Japan. In contrast, in-hospital mortality decreased significantly over these 5 years. The results of logistic regression using multiple propensity score analyses suggested that the decrease in mortality could be explained by the increase in the provision of both therapeutic hypothermia and PCI [34].

Hospital Case-Volumes and the Level-of-Care

Several retrospective studies have suggested that hospital factors affect the outcome of post-resuscitation patients. These hospital factors include case-volume (i.e., high vs. low volume centers) and level-of-care of the institution (i.e., tertiary-care, level 1, vs. non- tertiary-care, level 2 or 3, centers).

Two recent studies from Korea reported a positive volume-outcome relationship in OHCA [36, 37]. Cha et al. [36] reported a higher rate of survival when patients were transported to high-volume rather than low-volume centers in both urban and rural areas. The rate of survival remained significantly higher in the high-volume centers even when the transportation time to the center was longer compared with that of low-volume centers [36]. Lee et al. [37] performed a propensity-score analysis of the Korean Hypothermia Network Registry database. In 24 hospitals, a higher case volume of patients treated with targeted temperature management (TTM) was associated with early initiation of TTM and a lower incidence of adverse events [37].

Several region-wide retrospective database studies have compared the effects of level-of-care of the institution [22, 38–40]. Kajino et al. [38] found that the survival of patients after OHCA with presumed cardiac etiology without field ROSC who were transported to critical care medical centers (i.e., tertiary-care centers in Japan) was better than the survival of those transported to non-critical care center (i.e., non-tertiary-care centers) in the Osaka area, Japan. Similar studies were recently reported from the Copenhagen area in Denmark [39, 40]. In addition, Stub et al. [22] previously reported that a hospital factor significantly associated with survival was treatment at hospitals with 24 h cardiac interventional services. Moreover, Schober et al. [14] evaluated the association between patient-related factors, comorbidities, intensive care measures, and their impact on outcome for patients treated after cardiac arrest in 87 Austrian ICUs. Patients treated in ICUs with a high frequency of post-resuscitation care generally had a high severity of illness. However, ICUs with a higher frequency of care showed improved risk-adjusted mortality. Thus, the authors concluded that a high frequency of post-cardiac arrest care in an ICU seemed to be associated with improved outcome of cardiac-arrest patients [14]. These studies suggest that admission to high level-of-care centers and intensive care admission after OHCA is associated with a significantly higher survival rate even after adjustment for prognostic factors including pre-arrest comorbidity [14, 22, 38–40].

Interventional Programs to Improve the Provision of Post-Resuscitation Care

Several region-wide programs and campaigns have been reported to increase provision of post-resuscitation care (Table 1). The Cool It protocol [41] enables rapid, coordinated, and consistent delivery of therapeutic hypothermia. The authors of this study [41] found that a comprehensive therapeutic hypothermia protocol could be integrated into a regional ST-segment elevation myocardial infarction (STEMI) network and achieve broad dispersion of this essential therapy for OHCA (no control group study).

Take Heart America [42] was a public health approach project (before-after study) that not only focused on the final link in the chain of survival, but on all links. The project increased public awareness and trained laypeople to perform

Table 1 Studies of interventional regional systems-of-care programs/campaigns to improve the provision of post-resuscitation care

	Lick et al. [42]	Tagami et al. [11]	Spaite et al. [44]	Hwang et al. [43]
Published year	2011	2012	2014	2015
Study period	Nov 2005 to June 2009	Jan 2006 to Dec 2010	Dec 2007 to Dec 2010	Jan 2009 to Dec 2013
Country	USA	Japan	USA	Korea
Area	Anoka County and greater St. Cloud	Aizu region	Arizona state	Sungbuk county
Area population (approximately)	440,000	300,000	6,400,000	500,000
Strengthened link in chain of survival	All links	Final link	Final link	All links
Change in survival to hospital discharge	8.5% (9/106) to 19% (48/247)	2.3% (18/770) to 4.2% (30/712)	8.9% (39/440) to 14.4% (250/1734)	8.8% (16/182) to 18.1% (51/282)
Change in favorable neurologic outcome	NA	0.5% (4/770) to 3.0% (21/712)	5.9% (26/439) to 8.9% (153/1727)	3.3% (6/182) to 8.8% (24/282)

NA: not available

CPR. Moreover, this project also trained emergency medical services (EMS) personnel to deliver effective CPR. In addition, the project encouraged the treatment of cardiac arrest patients in cardiac arrest centers for therapeutic hypothermia, coronary artery evaluation and treatment, and all other treatments for post-cardiac arrest syndrome. This program resulted in a significant increase in the use of hypothermia and catheterization. The Take Heart America program doubled cardiac arrest survival when compared with historical controls [42]. Recently, a similar study was reported from Korea [43]. In this before-after design study, compression-only CPR for citizens, a state-wide standard dispatcher-assisted CPR protocol, medical control for regional EMS, provision of high-quality advanced cardiac life support with capnography and extracorporeal CPR (ECPR), and a standard post-cardiac arrest care protocol were implemented in a system-wide CPR program [43]. This system-wide CPR program was associated with enhancements in CPR performance at both the pre-hospital and hospital levels [43]. However, although these two before-after studies [42, 43] showed improved patient outcome after implementation of the program, they did so by strengthening not only the final link, but also the initial links in the chain of survival.

To our knowledge, two studies have focused on strengthening the final link in the chain of survival. We performed a region-wide multicenter prospective study, the Aizu Chain of Survival Concept Campaign, to evaluate the effect of the fifth link in the chain of survival, which was defined as multidisciplinary post-resuscitation care [11]. The Aizu region (Fukushima, Japan) is a suburban/rural area with

300,000 residents. All 12 emergency hospitals (one tertiary care and 11 non-tertiary care hospitals) in the region participated in the study. After patients with OHCA achieved ROSC at each hospital, they were concentrated in one tertiary care hospital and treated aggressively to focus on the fifth link [11]. After implementation of the fifth link, the proportion of survivors with a favorable neurological outcome increased significantly, and the fifth link was found to be an independent factor for a favorable neurologic outcome [11]. Although the 2010 AHA guidelines recommended a new chain of survival concept including the fifth link [9], we entered our study in a clinical trials registry and initiated the study approximately two years before the release of the guidelines [11]. A similar concept with a larger study was reported by Spaite et al. [44] in Arizona, United States. They performed a state-wide prospective observational study comparing patients admitted to 31 cardiac receiving centers before implementation of the interventions ("before") versus those admitted after ("after"). The interventions in the study included implementation of post-arrest care at cardiac-receiving centers focused on providing therapeutic hypothermia and coronary angiography or PCI; and implementation of EMS bypass triage protocols [44]. They found that implementation of a state-wide system of cardiac receiving centers and EMS bypass were independently associated with increased overall survival and a favorable neurologic outcome [29, 44].

Even for Elderly Patients?

OHCA occurs more frequently among the elderly than the younger generation, and patient age may significantly confound both treatment (i.e., as a confounder by indication of both pre- and post-resuscitation care) and outcome of these patents [45, 46]. Thus, determining who should receive aggressive treatment is a very important medical and ethical issue. Although this issue remains unresolved, important evidence has recently been reported. We recently determined that one-month survival with a favorable neurological outcome improved significantly among elderly OHCA patients (age > 65) during the last 10 years in the Kanto area of Japan [47]. Our results were consistent with those of two previous studies that evaluated the changes in outcome among elderly OHCA patients [48, 49]. The results of the two logistic regression analyses in our study suggested that this increase in favorable neurological outcome was associated with an increase in the provision of advanced in-hospital treatments [47].

The Links in the "Chain of Survival" Are a Relay Baton from Layperson to Pre-Hospital and In-Hospital Specialists

Each link in the 'chain of survival' could be represented as a relay baton. There is no doubt from recent evidence that the initial links before achieving ROSC are critical; the final link is initiated after the previous links in the chain [50]. Therefore, the baton should not be dropped before the final runner. However, if the baton is passed to the final runner, that specialist should perform to the best of their ability in order to achieve the goal of treatment. The goal is not only to achieve spontaneous circulation but also to restore the patient's previous quality of life. The true goal occurs after completion of the final link. Thus, an emergency room doctor must start the final link immediately after the patient achieves ROSC. Intensivists, cardiologists, neurocritical care physicians, nurses, medical engineers, and all providers working in the ICU have the responsibility to complete the final chain in the survival link.

Limitations

Although the development and implementation of regional care centers might be considered a health improvement initiative, there are not yet any results of randomized trials to support this idea. In addition, not all regions in the world can provide intensive care nor do they have regional high-quality centers for managing post-cardiac arrest syndrome.

Conclusion

Although randomized trials have not yet been performed, providing regional systems of care for post-cardiac arrest care is a reasonable approach. Several large nationwide studies have suggested that the recent improvements in outcome in OHCA patients are associated with the provision of post-resuscitation care. In addition, admission to high level-of-care centers and administration of intensive care after OHCA was associated with a significantly higher survival rate even after adjusting for prognostic factors including pre-arrest comorbidity. Moreover, several region-wide programs and campaigns have been reported to increase the provision of post-resuscitation care and are related to an improvement in patient outcome. Therefore, implementation of the fifth link in the chain of survival in regional systems of care can be associated with significant and important improvements in survival and a favorable neurologic outcome.

References

1. Nichol G, Thomas E, Callaway CW et al (2008) Regional variation in out-of-hospital cardiac arrest incidence and outcome. JAMA 300:1423–1431
2. Atwood C, Eisenberg MS, Herlitz J, Rea TD (2005) Incidence of EMS-treated out-of-hospital cardiac arrest in Europe. Resuscitation 67:75–80
3. Kitamura T, Iwami T, Kawamura T et al (2010) Nationwide public-access defibrillation in Japan. N Engl J Med 362:994–1004
4. Newman M (1989) The chain of survival concept takes hold. J Emerg Med Serve 14:11–13
5. Emergency Cardiac Care Committee and Subcommittees, American Heart Association (1992) Guidelines for cardiopulmonary resuscitation and emergency cardiac care. Part I. Introduction JAMA 268:2171–2183

6. The American Heart Association in collaboration with the International Liaison Committee on Resuscitation (2000) Guidelines 2000 for Cardiopulmonary Resuscitation and Emergency Cardiovascular Care. Part 3: adult basic life support. Circulation 102:I22–59

7. Ecc Committee, Subcommittees and Task Forces of the American Heart Association (2005) American Heart Association Guidelines for cardiopulmonary resuscitation and emergency cardiovascular care. Circulation 112:IV1–203

8. Nolan J, European Resuscitation Council (2005) European Resuscitation Council guidelines for resuscitation 2005. Section 1. Introduction. Resuscitation 67(Suppl 1):S3–S6

9. Peberdy MA, Callaway CW, Neumar RW et al (2010) Part 9: post-cardiac arrest care: 2010 American Heart Association Guidelines for Cardiopulmonary Resuscitation and Emergency Cardiovascular Care. Circulation 122:S768–S786

10. Neumar RW, Nolan JP, Adrie C et al (2008) Post-cardiac arrest syndrome: epidemiology, pathophysiology, treatment, and prognostication. A consensus statement from the International Liaison Committee on Resuscitation (American Heart Association, Australian and New Zealand Council on Resuscitation, European Resuscitation Council, Heart and Stroke Foundation of Canada, InterAmerican Heart Foundation, Resuscitation Council of Asia, and the Resuscitation Council of Southern Africa); the American Heart Association Emergency Cardiovascular Care Committee; the Council on Cardiovascular Surgery and Anesthesia; the Council on Cardiopulmonary, Perioperative, and Critical Care; the Council on Clinical Cardiology; and the Stroke Council. Circulation 118:2452–2483

11. Tagami T, Hirata K, Takeshige T et al (2012) Implementation of the fifth link of the chain of survival concept for out-of-hospital cardiac arrest. Circulation 126:589–597

12. Kim JY, Shin SD, Ro YS et al (2013) Post-resuscitation care and outcomes of out-of-hospital cardiac arrest: a nationwide propensity score-matching analysis. Resuscitation 84:1068–1077

13. Bosson N, Kaji AH, Niemann JT et al (2014) Survival and neurologic outcome after out-of-hospital cardiac arrest: results one year after regionalization of post-cardiac arrest care in a large metropolitan area. Prehosp Emerg Care 18:217–223

14. Schober A, Holzer M, Hochrieser H, Posch M, Schmutz R, Metnitz P (2014) Effect of intensive care after cardiac arrest on patient outcome: a database analysis. Crit Care 18:R84

15. Negovsky VA (1972) The second step in resuscitation – the treatment of the 'post-resuscitation disease'. Resuscitation 1:1–7

16. Chang WT, Ma MH, Chien KL et al (2007) Postresuscitation myocardial dysfunction: correlated factors and prognostic implications. Intensive Care Med 33:88–95

17. Hypothermia after Cardiac Arrest Study (2002) Mild therapeutic hypothermia to improve the neurologic outcome after cardiac arrest. N Engl J Med 346:549–556

18. Bernard SA, Gray TW, Buist MD et al (2002) Treatment of comatose survivors of out-of-hospital cardiac arrest with induced hypothermia. N Engl J Med 346:557–563

19. Spaulding CM, Joly LM, Rosenberg A et al (1997) Immediate coronary angiography in survivors of out-of-hospital cardiac arrest. N Engl J Med 336:1629–1633

20. Zanuttini D, Armellini I, Nucifora G et al (2012) Impact of emergency coronary angiography on in-hospital outcome of unconscious survivors after out-of-hospital cardiac arrest. Am J Cardiol 110:1723–1728

21. Carr BG, Kahn JM, Merchant RM, Kramer AA, Neumar RW (2009) Inter-hospital variability in post-cardiac arrest mortality. Resuscitation 80:30–34

22. Stub D, Smith K, Bray JE, Bernard S, Duffy SJ, Kaye DM (2011) Hospital characteristics are associated with patient outcomes following out-of-hospital cardiac arrest. Heart 97:1489–1494

23. MacKenzie EJ, Rivara FP, Jurkovich GJ et al (2006) A national evaluation of the effect of trauma-center care on mortality. N Engl J Med 354:366–378

24. Henry TD, Sharkey SW, Burke MN et al (2007) A regional system to provide timely access to percutaneous coronary intervention for ST-elevation myocardial infarction. Circulation 116:721–728

25. Davis DP, Fisher R, Aguilar S et al (2007) The feasibility of a regional cardiac arrest receiving system. Resuscitation 74:44–51

26. Hartke A, Mumma BE, Rittenberger JC, Callaway CW, Guyette FX (2010) Incidence of re-arrest and critical events during prolonged transport of post-cardiac arrest patients. Resuscitation 81:938–942

27. Spaite DW, Stiell IG, Bobrow BJ et al (2009) Effect of transport interval on out-of-hospital cardiac arrest survival in the OPALS study: implications for triaging patients to specialized cardiac arrest centers. Ann Emerg Med 54:248–255

28. Nichol G, Aufderheide TP, Eigel B et al (2010) Regional systems of care for out-of-hospital cardiac arrest: A policy statement from the American Heart Association. Circulation 121:709–729

29. Kern KB (2015) Usefulness of cardiac arrest centers – extending lifesaving post-resuscitation therapies: the Arizona experience. Circ J 79:1156–1163

30. SOS-KANTO 2012 study group (2015) Changes in pre- and in-hospital management and outcomes for out-of-hospital cardiac arrest between 2002 and 2012 in Kanto, Japan: the SOS-KANTO 2012 Study. Acute Medicine & Surgery 2:225–233

31. Fugate JE, Brinjikji W, Mandrekar JN et al (2012) Post-cardiac arrest mortality is declining: a study of the US National Inpatient Sample 2001 to 2009. Circulation 126:546–550

32. Wissenberg M, Lippert FK, Folke F et al (2013) Association of national initiatives to improve cardiac arrest management with rates of bystander intervention and patient survival after out-of-hospital cardiac arrest. JAMA 310:1377–1384

33. van der Wal G, Brinkman S, Bisschops LL et al (2011) Influence of mild therapeutic hypothermia after cardiac arrest on hospital mortality. Crit Care Med 39:84–88

34. Tagami T, Matsui H, Fushimi K, Yasunaga H (2016) Changes in therapeutic hypothermia and coronary intervention provision and in-hospital mortality of patients with out-of-hospital cardiac arrest: A nationwide-database study. Crit Care Med (in press)

35. Kitamura T, Iwami T, Kawamura T et al (2012) Nationwide improvements in survival from out-of-hospital cardiac arrest in Japan. Circulation 126:2834–2843

36. Cha WC, Lee SC, Shin SD, Song KJ, Sung AJ, Hwang SS (2012) Regionalisation of out-of-hospital cardiac arrest care for patients without prehospital return of spontaneous circulation. Resuscitation 83:1338–1342

37. Lee SJ, Jeung KW, Lee BK et al (2015) Impact of case volume on outcome and performance of targeted temperature management in out-of-hospital cardiac arrest survivors. Am J Emerg Med 33:31–36

38. Kajino K, Iwami T, Daya M et al (2010) Impact of transport to critical care medical centers on outcomes after out-of-hospital cardiac arrest. Resuscitation 81:549–554

39. Soholm H, Kjaergaard J, Bro-Jeppesen J et al (2015) Prognostic implications of level-of-care at tertiary heart centers compared with other hospitals after resuscitation from out-of-hospital cardiac arrest. Circ Cardiovasc Qual Outcomes 8:268–276

40. Soholm H, Wachtell K, Nielsen SL et al (2013) Tertiary centres have improved survival compared to other hospitals in the Copenhagen area after out-of-hospital cardiac arrest. Resuscitation 84:162–167

41. Mooney MR, Unger BT, Boland LL et al (2011) Therapeutic hypothermia after out-of-hospital cardiac arrest: evaluation of a regional system to increase access to cooling. Circulation 124:206–214

42. Lick CJ, Aufderheide TP, Niskanen RA et al (2011) Take Heart America: A comprehensive, community-wide, systems-based approach to the treatment of cardiac arrest. Crit Care Med 39:26–33

43. Hwang WS, Park JS, Kim SJ, Hong YS, Moon SW, Lee SW (2015) A system-wide approach from the community to the hospital for improving neurologic outcomes in out-of-hospital cardiac arrest patients. Eur J Emerg Med (in press)

44. Spaite DW, Bobrow BJ, Stolz U et al (2014) Statewide regionalization of postarrest care for out-of-hospital cardiac arrest: association with survival and neurologic outcome. Ann Emerg Med 64:496–506

45. Terman SW, Shields TA, Hume B, Silbergleit R (2015) The influence of age and chronic medi-cal conditions on neurological outcomes in out of hospital cardiac arrest. Resuscitation 89:169–176

46. Winther-Jensen M, Pellis T, Kuiper M et al (2015) Mortality and neurological outcome in the elderly after target temperature management for out-of-hospital cardiac arrest. Resuscitation 91:92–98

47. SOS-KANTO 2012 Study Group (2015) Changes in treatments and outcomes among elderly patients with out-of-hospital cardiac arrest between 2002 and 2012: a post-hoc analysis of the SOS-KANTO 2002 and 2012. Resuscitation 97:76–82

48. Deasy C, Bray JE, Smith K et al (2011) Out-of-hospital cardiac arrests in the older age groups in Melbourne. Australia Resuscitation 82:398–403

49. Kitamura T, Morita S, Kiyohara K et al (2014) Trends in survival among elderly patients with out-of-hospital cardiac arrest: a prospective, population-based observation from 1999 to 2011 in Osaka. Resuscitation 85:1432–1438

50. Tagami T, Yokota H, Hirata K et al (2013) Response to Letter Regarding Article, "Imple-mentation of the fifth link of the chain of survival concept for out-of-hospital cardiac arrest". Circulation 127:e567–e567

Cardiac Arrest Centers

E. L. Riley, M. Thomas, and J. P. Nolan

Introduction

Cardiac arrest accounts for considerable mortality and morbidity in the developed world. In the United States, it is estimated that the emergency medical services (EMS) assess out-of-hospital cardiac arrest (OHCA) in 103 per 100,000 inhabitants each year (a total of 326,000); approximately 56% of these are treated and 5.6% survive to hospital discharge [1]. United Kingdom ambulance services initiate resuscitation on about 28,000 people who sustain an OHCA each year (52 cases per 100,000 inhabitants) and approximately 8% survive to leave hospital [2]. Recent evidence suggests improved patient outcomes when care for certain conditions is centralized to nominated healthcare centers [3–6]. Conditions that appear to benefit from this structured approach are those with high acuity requiring time-sensitive specialist interventions, such as ST segment elevation myocardial infarction (STEMI), major trauma and acute stroke. It seems feasible that patients with OHCA might also benefit from regionalization of their care.

In 2010, the American Heart Association (AHA) [7] published a policy statement outlining the evidence and goals for regionalization of OHCA care services, based on the concept of cardiac arrest centers. Recently, efforts have been made to define

E. L. Riley (✉)
Department of Anaesthesia, Royal United Hospital
Bath, UK
email: emmariley1@nhs.net

M. Thomas
Intensive Care Unit, University Hospitals
Bristol, UK

J. P. Nolan
School of Clinical Sciences, University of Bristol
Bristol, UK
Department of Anaesthesia and Intensive Care Medicine, Royal United Hospital
Bath, UK

© Springer International Publishing Switzerland 2016
J.-L. Vincent (ed.), *Annual Update in Intensive Care and Emergency Medicine 2016*,
DOI 10.1007/978-3-319-27349-5_20

regionalization of cardiac arrest care and, in particular, the services that a cardiac arrest center should provide. Observational studies have documented the impact of such regionalization on patient outcome.

Lessons from Existing Regionalization of Non-Cardiac Care

In the USA, regionalized trauma care has improved outcomes for patients with major trauma transported directly to trauma centers [3]. In-hospital mortality from major trauma has decreased from 9.5 to 7.6% (relative risk [RR] 0.80, 95% confidence interval [CI] 0.66–0.98). Since the introduction of Trauma Networks in the UK, the survival rate from major trauma has increased by 19% and variation in mortality between centers has been reduced [4]. Following centralization of stroke services in London in 2010 [5], there has been a 1.1% (95% CI −2.1 to −0.1) reduction in mortality among patients presenting with acute stroke. Eight designated hyperacute stroke units were created which provide 24/7 specialist stroke medical teams and facilities for immediate brain imaging and thrombolysis. Given the high incidence of stroke in an ageing population, this modest improvement in survival rate represents a large number of lives saved· 168 (95% CI 19–316) lives saved at 90-days post-stroke.

Possible explanations for improved outcomes include the volume of cases managed by individual hospitals and the characteristics of those hospitals. There is evidence to suggest that a volume-outcome relationship exists for surgery [8], whereby outcomes are improved for patients operated on in centers undertaking a high volume of cases. In some operations, the volume of cases undertaken by the individual surgeon has the strongest effect on patient outcome; for example, after aortic valve replacement surgery. In other surgical procedures such as hernia operations, the volume-outcome effect is related to the organization of care and the whole team rather than just the surgeon.

Clinical decision-making and acquired skills may improve with the number of cases treated; however, case volume is unlikely to be the sole reason for the effects of regionalization. Clinical conditions that require time-sensitive interventions may benefit most from regionalization. Models of care in designated centers involve well-coordinated multidisciplinary teams led by senior clinicians as well as 24-h on site access to specialist services. These resources may not be available in all hospitals, and so this possibly contributes to the variation in patient outcomes.

OHCA and Emergency Cardiac Intervention

Cardiac Disease and OHCA

About two thirds of OHCAs have a cardiac cause [9]. Of 714 patients presenting with OHCA in Paris, 39% had an obvious extra-cardiac cause [10]; of the remaining 435 patients, 134 (31%) had evidence of a STEMI, 96% of whom had at least one significant coronary lesion at angiography. There were 301 patients without STEMI who went on to undergo coronary angiography. Of these, 176 (58%) had at least one significant lesion, with just over a quarter undergoing successful percutaneous coronary intervention (PCI). This study identified that it is important to consider the evidence supporting the current recommendations for care of patients presenting with OHCA caused by underlying cardiac pathology, specifically STEMI and non-STEMI.

ST-Elevation Myocardial Infarction

Early Reperfusion Therapy

Early coronary reperfusion is integral to the management of patients presenting with STEMI. This is achieved via pharmacological thrombolysis or primary PCI. The most recent European guidelines [11] recommend primary PCI as the method of reperfusion that is supported by Class I Level A evidence. Direct transport to a primary PCI capable healthcare facility should occur for all patients with STEMI unless the time from first medical contact (FMC)-to-device is estimated to be > 90 min. For patients who have already arrived at a non-PCI capable facility, this period is extended to 120 min to facilitate secondary transfer. For all other patients, and in the absence of contraindications, thrombolysis should be administered within 30 min of hospital arrival.

Urgent transfer to a primary PCI capable facility is also recommended for STEMI patients who develop complications, such as failed reperfusion or re-occlusion following fibrinolytic therapy. Patients who develop acute severe heart failure or cardiogenic shock should be transferred immediately to a PCI capable facility. These guidelines [11] also include recommendations on the use of temporary pacing, intra-aortic balloon counter pulsation and the consideration of patients for urgent coronary artery bypass grafting (CABG). These advanced cardiac interventions are usually available 24 h a day, 7 days a week, only in specialist cardiac centers. Many centers do not have cardiac surgery services at all. In the context of the cardiac arrest center debate, the lack of these services in smaller hospitals would support the argument for regionalization.

Regionalization

Many of the recommended services and time frames for STEMI management are difficult to achieve 24 h a day 7 days a week in every acute hospital. For this reason PCI services in many countries have been extensively regionalized. In some healthcare systems, smaller hospitals tend to provide emergency PCI services during working hours, with larger centers providing 24 hours a day 7 days a week cover for a larger geographical area. Regionalization of emergency angioplasty services has improved outcomes for these patients and there does not appear to be a negative effect of increased transport times [12].

OHCA Survivors with STEMI

Patients who present with cardiac arrest *and* STEMI are distinct from those with STEMI but without cardiac arrest. Resuscitated OHCA patients whose initial electrocardiogram (EKG) shows STEMI should undergo immediate angiography and PCI [13]. Data published from the US National Cardiovascular Data Registry [14], which includes the "Cath PCI Registry" from > 1300 sites in the USA, compared the characteristics of these two groups. Of almost 600,000 patients undergoing PCI, 114,768 had STEMI and of these 8.2% had been in cardiac arrest. Mortality was 24.9% in this group, versus 3.1% in the remaining 91.8% who had not been in cardiac arrest before the PCI. Patients resuscitated from cardiac arrest were significantly more likely to have more complex coronary artery lesions and to have cardiogenic shock within 24 h of PCI. Intra-aortic balloon pump (IABP) usage was higher in the cardiac arrest group, as were several post-procedural complications, such as kidney injury, stroke and bleeding events. These patients require treatment by highly skilled healthcare personnel and such individuals will not be available 24/7 in all hospitals, which implies the need for regionalization.

OHCA Survivors Without STEMI

Despite the lack of randomized controlled trial data, there is consensus for urgent PCI following cardiac arrest in patients with STEMI. With reproducible data [10, 15] demonstrating that up to 90% of post-cardiac arrest patients with STEMI will have one or more acute thrombotic lesions on angiography, there are clear potential benefits for urgent PCI [16, 17]. There is conflicting evidence from retrospective studies and meta-analyses about whether all patients, and not just those with STEMI, can benefit from urgent PCI following OHCA of likely cardiac cause. A retrospective study in Sweden of 638 cardiac arrest patients (451, 88% OHCA) found the rate of acute coronary occlusion to be 37% in patients without STEMI [15]. A recent meta-analysis included 50 studies of patients who did and did not undergo angiography following OHCA [18]. The analysis included patients with and without STEMI. Survival with good neurological outcome occurred in 58% in the angiography group versus 35.8% in the non-angiography group. A *post hoc* analysis from the targeted temperature management (TTM) trial documented that out of 544 patients without STEMI following OHCA, 46% received early (within 6 h) coronary angiography [19]. Mortality was 48% in this group compared with 54% in those who did not undergo early coronary angiogram. After secondary analysis, the adjusted hazard ratio (HR) for death in the group who underwent early coronary angiography compared with the group who did not undergo coronary angiography during their hospital stay was 0.77 (95% CI 0.59–1.0; p = 0.05). A selective approach to urgent angiography should probably be taken for those OHCA patients without STEMI. Factors to be considered would include the presence of shockable rhythms, EKG evidence suggesting ischemia, and age.

The 2015 European Society of Cardiology (ESC) guidelines [20] for the treatment of patients presenting with non-STEMI recommends that patients with one 'very high risk' criterion undergo an immediate invasive strategy (within 2 h). Cardiac arrest is classed as a very high risk criterion. A recent consensus statement from the European Association for Percutaneous Cardiovascular Interventions (EAPCI) and Stent for Life (SFL) groups recommends a management plan for comatose survivors of OHCA without EKG evidence of STEMI based on an analysis of the most recent research [17]. The authors recommend a short "emergency department or intensive care unit stop" to exclude non-coronary causes. This would include pulmonary embolism, aortic dissection and stroke. Once appropriate investigations, such as computed tomography (CT) angiogram, echocardiogram or CT head are complete, urgent coronary angiogram is performed. Ideally, this is done within 2 h according to the same guidelines as for high-risk non-STEMI acute coronary syndromes (ACS) without cardiac arrest. The American College of Cardiology Foundation (ACCF) also advocates early angiography +/− PCI in OHCA patients without STEMI when they are deemed 'suitable' after consultation with interventional cardiologists and intensivists [21]. The expectation is that this would involve direct discussion with, and patient assessment by, senior experienced clinicians. This is likely to be available 24/7 only at larger hospitals, thus implying the need to regionalize such services.

Post-Resuscitation Critical Care Management

The model of care for patients with OHCA is summarized in the Chain of Survival (Fig. 1). This has 4 key links: 1) early recognition, 2) early CPR, 3) early defibrillation and 4) post-resuscitation care [22].

These patients require high-quality, coordinated critical care focused on maximizing both cardiac and neurological recovery. Several other specialized critical care interventions, such as temperature control, emerging therapies for advanced management of cardiogenic shock, followed by delayed neurological prognostication can improve patient outcome following OHCA [13].

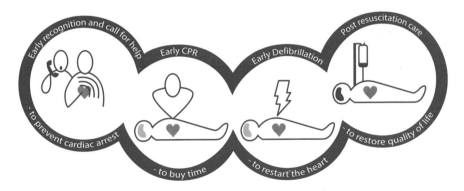

Fig. 1 The Chain of Survival. From [22] with permission

Temperature Control

Post-cardiac arrest hyperthermia is associated with worse neurological outcome. Landmark studies of therapeutic hypothermia led to the widespread introduction of active cooling for OHCA patients in an effort to improve neurological recovery [23, 24]. Subsequently, the term TTM has been adopted because this reflects a wider range of possible target temperatures up to and including 36 °C [25]. Control of temperature for at least 24 h following OHCA is now recommended by the International Liaison Committee on Resuscitation (ILCOR) [26]. Automated temperature management devices will enable tighter control of temperature although there is no evidence that they improve neurological outcome in comparison with basic techniques [27]. In a secondary analysis of data from North America, which included almost 4000 patients arriving at hospital following OHCA, the rate of survival with a favorable functional outcome was 25.3%, but among a subgroup of patients who received both early coronary intervention and induced hypothermia it was 53.0% [28]. These interventions were more likely to be undertaken in hospitals that admitted more OHCAs per year thus suggesting a potential beneficial volume effect.

Emerging Therapies for Cardiac Support

Several specialist interventions for patients with OHCA have evolved in recent years. Such therapies include intra-arrest PCI, mechanical cardiopulmonary resuscitation (mCPR) and the use of extracorporeal membrane oxygenation (ECMO) [29].

A case series of 86 patients [30] with either in-hospital or out-of-hospital cardiac arrest were treated with veno-arterial ECMO before return of spontaneous circulation (ROSC) (extracorporeal CPR [ECPR]), intra-arrest angiography, and PCI when indicated. OHCA patients represented just over 40% of the cohort. ROSC was achieved in 88%; 30-day overall survival was 29% and survival with a favorable neurological outcome was 24%. Those patients who underwent PCI (71%) had significantly improved outcomes at all endpoints. A shorter time interval from collapse to initiation of ECPR was associated with a higher survival rate and all survivors had had an IABP inserted. Echocardiography was performed during the cardiac arrest period to rule out pericardial effusion and observe for return of spontaneous heartbeat.

In Australia, the CHEER study investigators implemented an ECPR protocol for patients with refractory in and out-of hospital ventricular fibrillation (VF) cardiac arrest [31]. This consisted of mechanical chest compressions, intra-arrest therapeutic hypothermia and percutaneous cannulation for veno-arterial ECMO. If the patient was suspected of having a coronary artery occlusion as the cause for the cardiac arrest they underwent immediate PCI. In a cohort of 26 patients, survival was 54%. All survivors had a good neurological outcome (Cerebral Performance Category [CPC] score 1–2). This small but important study demonstrates that regionalization of services around a tertiary center enables multiple interventions to be implemented consistently. Most, if not all, of these interventions are not routinely available in hospitals across the developed world and in many cases it is unlikely that resources would enable development beyond tertiary centers.

Neurological Prognostication

Following the worldwide adoption of guidelines for therapeutic hypothermia, the time frame after which prognostication of neurological recovery should occur has lengthened. There has also been considerable development in the predictors recommended for use by clinicians and these are summarized in the most recent advisory statement from the European Resuscitation Council and European Society of Intensive Care Medicine [32].

Cooling is recommended for the first 24 h post-ROSC and then rewarming is undertaken slowly at 0.5 °C/h [13]. Normothermia is then normally maintained for 72 h [25]. Common practice is for sedation to be withheld once rewarming is complete. For comatose survivors of cardiac arrest, prognostication is not recommended before 72 h post-ROSC or within 12 h of sedative withdrawal [32].

There is increasing evidence that signs previously regarded as reliable predictors of poor outcome (e.g., myoclonus within 24 h following ROSC), cannot be used in isolation for prognostication. Use of multiple modalities, in conjunction with repeated clinical examination, is now considered the gold-standard [13, 32]. These modalities include electrophysiology (electroencephalogram [EEG], somatosensory evoked potentials [SSEP]); biomarkers (e.g., neuron specific enolase [NSE]) and imaging (CT and magnetic resonance imaging [MRI]). These investigations need to be reported and interpreted by experienced teams. An algorithm summarizes this approach to prognostication (Fig. 2).

The availability of these modalities varies among hospitals and the neurophysiological tests, in particular, require a high level of skills and experience for interpretation. It may not be possible for these tests to be immediately available in hospitals treating few OHCA patients.

High-Volume Centers Versus Low-Volume Centers

The effect of the volume of OHCA admissions on mortality is unclear. An Australian study of 2700 OHCA patients admitted to hospital over an 8-year period (2003–2010) found no effect of volume of admissions on mortality [33]. This study did find that other hospital characteristics, such as availability of a 24-h cardiac interventional service, were associated with better survival rates. An Austrian study compared low (< 18 OHCAs per year), medium (18–25) and high (> 25) treatment-frequency ICUs and found no significant differences in crude mortality [34]. Patients admitted to the high-frequency ICUs had higher organ dysfunction scores and, when controlled for this, there was significantly higher survival in high-volume ICUs. Both of these studies stratified hospitals based on the number of OHCA

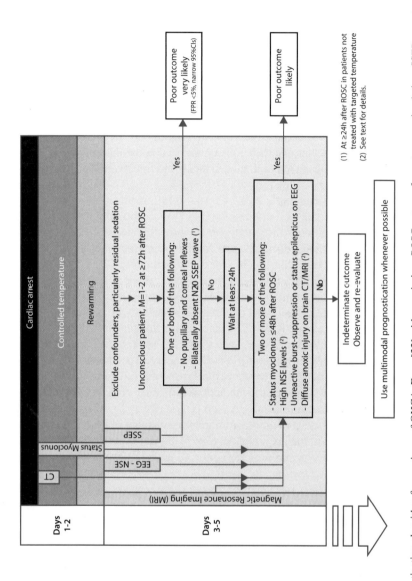

Fig. 2 Suggested prognostication algorithm for survivors of OHCA. From [32] with permission. *ROSC*: return of spontaneous circulation; *SSEP*: somatosensory evoked potential; *FPR*: false positive rate; *CT*: computed tomography; *EEG*: electroencephalogram; *NSE*: neuron specific enolase; *M*: Glasgow Motor Score

cases admitted annually. One difficulty with the studies is that the differences in the range of annual admissions may not be clinically significant. The difference between 18 and 25 admissions is small and probably insignificant compared with larger tertiary cardiac centers that exist in other countries. For example, unpublished data from the southwest UK shows that 140 OHCA patients were admitted to the ICU in the regional cardiac center in 2014.

One observational study from the USA showed increased survival rates for patients admitted to ICUs with a higher annual OHCA caseload [35]. After risk-adjustment using APACHE IV scores, survival rates were significantly higher in those ICUs admitting >50 patients with OHCA per annum (adjusted odds ratio [OR] 0.62; 95% CI 0.45–0.86; p = 0.01). However, in another study from the USA, there was no reduction in mortality in hospitals admitting >50 OHCA patients annually compared with those admitting < 19 [36]. Thus, hospital OHCA case volume alone may not influence outcome.

Tertiary Cardiac Centers Versus Non-Tertiary Centers

The characteristics of the hospital, such as availability of specialist teams and interventions, rather than volume of admissions alone, may have more effect on mortality rates. In the Australian study cited above, transport of patients to a cardiac center and admission between 09:00 and 17:00 were associated with increased risk-adjusted odds of survival [33].

An observational study of over > 10,000 OHCA cases from Japan documented a better rate of neurologically favorable survival (6.7% versus 2.8%, p < 0.001), in patients transported to a "critical care medical center" compared with those transported elsewhere [37]. A Danish study of 1218 patients over 8 years demonstrated increased 30-day and long-term survival in patients admitted to tertiary cardiac centers following OHCA when compared to the 6 non-tertiary centers [38]. Importantly, these investigators excluded patients with STEMI, who were already being directed to the regional center during the study time period. There was a 30% increase in mortality among those admitted to a non-tertiary cardiac center compared with those admitted to a tertiary center. This was after controlling for confounders such as patient age, presenting cardiac arrest rhythm, underlying etiology and pre-hospital factors (such as witnessed arrest, time to resuscitation efforts, bystander CPR). This implies that the better results obtained by tertiary centers does not simply reflect selection bias, i.e., patients with favorable presenting factors, such as shockable rhythm and younger age, being selectively admitted to the tertiary cardiac center.

Existing Models of Regionalized Cardiac Arrest Care

Centralization of post-cardiac arrest care has already been implemented in many areas in the USA and Europe. In the UK, several tertiary centers have been designated 'cardiac arrest centers' or 'heart attack centers' [39]. In some of these areas, not all OHCA patients are automatically transported to the regional center; for example, some accept only those patients with ST-elevation on their EKG.

Trends in Survival Rates Following OHCA

Data from the London Ambulance Service (LAS) Cardiac Arrest Annual Report show that the survival rate to hospital discharge of patients following a witnessed OHCA with VF increased from 5% in 2001/2002 to 32.4% in 2013/2014 [40]. More detailed analysis of the data [41] from 2007–2012 showed that the characteristics of the patients did not differ over this period. The increase in survival rate may be associated with designation in 2010 of eight heart attack centers in London. Since 2010, patients with ROSC following OHCA with EKG evidence of ST-elevation have been conveyed directly to one of these centers. Analysis of a one-year period (2010/2011) of LAS data [42] documented that 131 (66%) of 206 OHCA STEMI patients conveyed directly to a heart attack center survived to hospital discharge and 97% of these patients were alive at 1 year.

It is not possible to directly compare the survival rates from the latter study with those of unselected OHCA cohorts. Those patients with witnessed VF OHCA with STEMI as the underlying pathology clearly have a better outcome compared with other OHCA patients [39]. These studies also do not address directly whether the implementation of heart attack centers has improved outcomes because there are no data comparing pre- and post-implementation.

Effects of Current Models of Regionalization on Outcome Following OHCA

Patient outcomes following OHCA have been compared before and after regionalization of cardiac arrest care. In Arizona [43], a state-wide initiative of regionalization of post-arrest care created designated cardiac receiving centers, where patients would be directly transported following OHCA; here they could undergo urgent coronary angiography, receive primary PCI and therapeutic hypothermia. Before implementation, none of the hospitals provided therapeutic hypothermia; 44% of patients received this therapy after implementation. There was a 60% increase in the rate of patients being transported to the cardiac receiving centers in the 18 months after implementation compared with 6 months pre-implementation. Survival to hospital discharge for the 2000 OHCA patients increased from 8.9 to 14.4% (OR 2.2; 95% CI 1.47–3.34). The main increase in survival occurred among those with a witnessed OHCA and initial shockable cardiac arrest rhythm (VF/VT) (OR 2.96;

95% CI 1.63–5.38). A limitation of this study is that there are no data for patients who were admitted to the non-cardiac receiving centers. The intervention being tested was possibly more akin to a post-arrest care bundle.

In Los Angeles, since 2010, all patients with ROSC following OHCA secondary to presumed cardiac cause are transported directly to so-called STEMI receiving centers [44]. The rate of survival to hospital discharge with good neurological outcome for patients transported to STEMI receiving centers following OHCA with an initial shockable rhythm increased from 6% in 2001 to 40% in 2012. However, these are observational data with numerous confounders – regionalization is not the only change in cardiac arrest care that has occurred in Los Angeles during this time period.

A regionalization protocol campaign for OHCA was introduced in a region of Japan in 2009 [45]. After implementation, OHCA patients were admitted to the tertiary center and received a bundle of post-resuscitation care including PCI, ECMO, therapeutic hypothermia, IABP and ionotropic support where indicated. Patients admitted initially to the non-tertiary center were stabilized and transferred to the tertiary center once ROSC was achieved if ongoing care was deemed appropriate by the admitting clinician. Approximately 700 patients were studied before (28 months) and 700 after (24 months) protocol implementation. The rate of survival with good neurological outcome increased from 0.5 to 3% (p = < 0.001). This study reflects the effects of regionalization pre- and post-implementation more reliably than most studies because there was a clear cohort group to compare with and characteristics of both groups were well documented.

Alternative Models of Regionalization

An interesting concept has been developed by the Carolinas Medical Center in the USA [46]. In contrast to most other models of regionalization, direct transport to the STEMI-receiving hospital is not the key component of the treatment pathway for cardiac arrest. A post-cardiac arrest bundle developed by a multidisciplinary team of experts, which incorporates the most up-to-date evidence-based interventions has been implemented. The hub cardiac resuscitation center coordinates the treatment pathway. It has focused efforts on disseminating the information to all local hospitals in the region and has supported and encouraged clinicians to use the pathway consistently. Of 222 patients studied between 2007 and 2011, just over half received their initial care at the tertiary center: 43% of patients survived with good neurological outcome and there was no statistically significant difference in survival based on initial site of post-arrest care. The authors propose this system as an interim framework in the progression to complete regionalization of cardiac arrest care.

Conclusion

The evidence for regionalization of OHCA care is of low quality, comprising predominantly observational studies. Outcomes vary widely among hospitals and there is indirect evidence of improved outcomes at tertiary cardiac institutions. The logistics of conducting a randomized controlled trial of cardiac centers versus non-cardiac centers are challenging. In London, the ARREST trial (International Standard Randomized Controlled Trial Number [ISRCTN] 96585404) is being undertaken. OHCA patients without ST-elevation on their EKG are being randomized to either direct transfer to a heart attack center and immediate coronary angiography or standard care. The provision of comprehensive post-resuscitation care includes 24-h access to a cardiac catheterization laboratory with PCI capability and a critical care team providing advanced management of shock, temperature control and resources for multi-modal neurological prognostication. In many countries there is already progression towards regionalization of post-resuscitation care following OHCA and this is reflected by recent international recommendations [47]. Several unanswered questions remain, including the specific treatments that a cardiac arrest center should provide, the effects of journey times on outcome, the role of secondary transport to cardiac arrest centers, and precisely which patients should be taken to a cardiac arrest center.

References

1. Mozaffarian D, Benjamin EJ, Go AS et al (2014) Heart Disease and Stroke Statistics – 2015 Update: A Report From the American Heart Association. Circulation 131:e29–e322
2. Perkins GD, Lockey AS, de Belder MA (2016) National initiatives to improve outcomes from out of hospital cardiac arrest in England. Emerg Med J (in press)
3. MacKenzie EJ, Rivara FP, Jurkovich GJ et al (2006) A national evaluation of the effect of trauma-center care on mortality. N Engl J Med 354:366–378
4. McCullough AL, Haycock JC, Forward DP, Moran CG (2014) II. Major trauma networks in England. Br J Anaesth 113:202–206
5. Morris S, Hunter RM, Ramsay AIG et al (2014) Impact of centralising acute stroke services in English metropolitan areas on mortality and length of hospital stay: difference-in-differences analysis. BMJ 349:g4757–g4767
6. Jollis JG, Roettig ML, Aluko AO et al (2007) Implementation of a statewide system for coronary reperfusion for st-segment elevation myocardial infarction. JAMA 298:2371–2380
7. Nichol G, Aufderheide TP, Eigel B et al (2010) Regional systems of care for out-of-hospital cardiac arrest: A policy statement From the American Heart Association. Circulation 121:709–729
8. Birkmeyer JD, Siewers AE, Stukel TA et al (2002) Hospital volume and surgical mortality in the United States. N Engl J Med 346:1128–1137
9. Bougouin W, Lamhaut L, Marijon E et al (2014) Characteristics and prognosis of sudden cardiac death in Greater Paris. Intensive Care Med 40:846–854
10. Dumas F, Cariou A, Manzo-Silberman S et al (2010) Immediate percutaneous coronary intervention is associated with better survival after out-of-hospital cardiac arrest: Insights From the PROCAT (Parisian Region Out of Hospital Cardiac Arrest) Registry. Circ Cardiovasc Interv 3:200–207

11. Members AF, Steg PG, James SK et al (2012) ESC Guidelines for the management of acute myocardial infarction in patients presenting with ST-segment elevation: The Task Force on the management of ST-segment elevation acute myocardial infarction of the European Society of Cardiology (ESC). Eur Heart J 33:2569–2619

12. Dalby M (2003) Transfer for primary angioplasty versus immediate thrombolysis in acute myocardial infarction: a meta-analysis. Circulation 108:1809–1814

13. Nolan JP, Soar J, Cariou A (2015) European Resuscitation Council and European Society of Intensive Care Medicine Guidelines for Resuscitation 2015 Section 5 Post Resuscitation Care. Resuscitation 95:201–221

14. Gupta N, Kontos MC, Gupta A et al (2014) Characteristics and outcomes in patients undergoing percutaneous coronary intervention following cardiac arrest (from the NCDR). Am J Cardiol 113:1087–1092

15. Redfors B, Råmunddal T, Angerås O et al (2015) Angiographic findings and survival in patients undergoing coronary angiography due to sudden cardiac arrest in Western Sweden. Resuscitation 90:13–20

16. O'Gara PT, Kushner FG, Ascheim DD et al (2013) ACCF/AHA Guideline. Circulation 127:529–555

17. Noc M, Fajadet J, Lassen JF et al (2014) Invasive coronary treatment strategies for out-of-hospital cardiac arrest: a consensus statement from the European Association for Percutaneous Cardiovascular Interventions (EAPCI)/Stent for Life (SFL) groups. EuroIntervention 10:31–37

18. Camuglia AC, Randhawa VK, Lavi S, Walters DL (2014) Cardiac catheterization is associated with superior outcomes for survivors of out of hospital cardiac arrest: Review and meta-analysis. Resuscitation 85:1533–1540

19. Dankiewicz J, Nielsen N, Annborn M et al (2015) Survival in patients without acute ST elevation after cardiac arrest and association with early coronary angiography: a post hoc analysis from the TTM trial. Intensive Care Med 41:856–864

20. Roffi M, Patrono C, Collet J, Mueller C et al (2016) 2015 ESC Guidelines for the management of acute coronary syndromes in patients presenting without persistent ST-segment elevation. Eur Heart J (in press)

21. Rab T, Kern KB, Tamis JE (2015) Cardiac arrest: a treatment algorithm for emergent invasive cardiac procedures in the resuscitated comatose patient. J Am Coll Cardiol 66:62–73

22. Nolan J, Soar J, Eikeland H (2006) The chain of survival. Resuscitation 71:270

23. Holzer M, Cerchiari E, Martens P et al (2002) Mild Therapeutic hypothermia to improve the neurologic outcome after cardiac arrest. N Engl J Med 346:549–556

24. Bernard SA, Gray TW, Buist MD et al (2002) Treatment of comatose survivors of out-of-hospital cardiac arrest with induced hypothermia. N Engl J Med 346:557–563

25. Nielsen N, Wetterslev J, Cronberg T et al (2013) Targeted temperature management at 33 °C versus 36 °C after cardiac arrest. N Engl J Med 369:2197–2206

26. Soar J, Callaway CW, Aibiki M (2015) 2015 International consensus on cardiopulmonary resuscitation and emergency cardiovascular care science with treatment recommendations: Part 4: Advanced life support. Resuscitation 95:e71–e122

27. Deye N, Cariou A, Girardie P et al (2015) Endovascular versus external targeted temperature management for patients with out-of-hospital cardiac arrest. Circulation 132:182–193

28. Callaway CW, Schmicker RH, Brown SP et al (2014) Early coronary angiography and induced hypothermia are associated with survival and functional recovery after out-of-hospital cardiac arrest. Resuscitation 85:657–663

29. Fagnoul D, Combes A, De Backer D (2014) Extracorporeal cardiopulmonary resuscitation. Curr Opin Crit Care 20:259–265

30. Kagawa E, Dote K, Kato M et al (2012) Should we emergently revascularize occluded coronaries for cardiac arrest?: rapid-response extracorporeal membrane oxygenation and intra-arrest percutaneous coronary intervention. Circulation 126:1605–1613

31. Stub D, Bernard S, Pellegrino V et al (2015) Refractory cardiac arrest treated with mechanical CPR, hypothermia, ECMO and early reperfusion (the CHEER trial). Resuscitation 86:88–94
32. Sandroni C, Cariou A, Cavallaro F et al (2014) Prognostication in comatose survivors of cardiac arrest: An advisory statement from the European Resuscitation Council and the European Society of Intensive Care Medicine. Resuscitation 85:1779–1789
33. Stub D, Smith K, Bray JE et al (2011) Hospital characteristics are associated with patient outcomes following out-of-hospital cardiac arrest. Heart 97:1489–1495
34. Schober A, Holzer M, Hochrieser H et al (2014) Effect of intensive care after cardiac arrest on patient outcome: a database analysis. Critical Care 18:R84–R90
35. Carr BG, Kahn JM, Merchant RM et al (2009) Inter-hospital variability in post-cardiac arrest mortality. Resuscitation 80:30–34
36. Cudnik MT, Sasson C, Rea TD et al (2012) Increasing hospital volume is not associated with improved survival in out of hospital cardiac arrest of cardiac etiology. Resuscitation 83:862–868
37. Kajino K, Iwami T, Daya M et al (2010) Impact of transport to critical care medical centers on outcomes after out-of-hospital cardiac arrest. Resuscitation 81:549–554
38. Søholm H, Wachtell K, Nielsen SL et al (2013) Tertiary centers have improved survival compared to other hospitals in the Copenhagen area after out-of-hospital cardiac arrest. Resuscitation 84:162–167
39. Iqbal MB, Al-Hussaini A, Rosser G et al (2015) Predictors of survival and favorable functional outcomes after an out-of-hospital cardiac arrest in patients systematically brought to a dedicated heart attack center (from the Harefield Cardiac Arrest Study). Am J Cardiol 115:730–737
40. London Ambulance Service Cardiac Arrest Annual Report 2014. Available at: http://www.londonambulance.nhs.uk/about_us/publications.aspx#clinicalaudit
41. Fothergill RT, Watson LR, Chamberlain D et al (2013) Increases in survival from out-of-hospital cardiac arrest: A five year study. Resuscitation 84:1089–1092
42. Fothergill RT, Watson LR, Virdi GK et al (2014) Survival of resuscitated cardiac arrest patients with ST-elevation myocardial infarction (STEMI) conveyed directly to a Heart Attack Center by ambulance clinicians. Resuscitation 85:96–98
43. Spaite DW, Bobrow BJ, Stolz U et al (2014) Statewide regionalization of postarrest care for out-of-hospital cardiac arrest: association with survival and neurologic outcome. Ann Emerg Med 64:496–506
44. Bosson N, Kaji AH, Niemann JT et al (2014) Survival and neurologic outcome after out-of-hospital cardiac arrest: results one year after regionalization of post-cardiac arrest care in a large metropolitan area. Prehosp Emerg Care 18:217–223
45. Tagami T, Tosa R, Omura M et al (2012) Implementation of the fifth link of the Chain of Survival concept for out-of-hospital cardiac arrest. Circulation 126:589–597
46. Heffner AC, Pearson DA, Nussbaum ML, Jones AE (2012) Regionalization of post-cardiac arrest care: Implementation of a cardiac resuscitation center. Am Heart J 164:493–501
47. Finn J, Bhanji F, Bigham B (2015) 2015 International Consensus on Cardiopulmonary Resuscitation and Emergency Cardiovascular Care Science with Treatment Recommendations: Part 8: Education, implementation and teams. Resuscitation 95:e205–e227

Part VIII
Oxygenation and Respiratory Failure

High-Flow Nasal Cannula Oxygen Therapy: Physiological Effects and Clinical Data

D. Chiumello, M. Gotti, and C. Chiurazzi

Introduction

In patients with mild to moderate acute respiratory failure the commonly used techniques to ameliorate gas exchange are oxygen therapy and non-invasive ventilation (NIV). However due to mask intolerance, hypercapnia, respiratory acidosis, muscle fatigue and hypoxemia, intubation and invasive mechanical ventilation are frequently required. High-flow nasal cannulas, originally developed to improve gas exchange in neonatal and pediatric settings, have recently been evaluated in various groups of adult critically ill patients. High-flow nasal cannulas deliver a high humidified air/oxygen gas flow (up to 60 l/min) via a nasal cannula. The main advantages of high-flow nasal cannulas are the ability to deliver a very high flow of humidified gas, exceeding, in the majority of patients, the peak inspiratory flow, with a constant oxygen fraction and the use, as interface, of a nasal cannula which can insure patient comfort. Several studies have shown that use of high-flow nasal cannulas was able to improve gas exchange and reduce the respiratory rate and, in selected patients, also to improve outcomes.

D. Chiumello (✉)
Dipartimento di Anestesia, Rianimazione (Intensiva e Subintensiva) e Terapia del Dolore,
Fondazione IRCCS Ca' Granda – Ospedale Maggiore Policlinico
Milan, Italy
Dipartimento di Fisiopatologia Medico-Chirurgica e dei Trapianti, Università degli Studi di
Milano
Milan, Italy
email: chiumello@libero.it

M. Gotti · C. Chiurazzi
Dipartimento di Fisiopatologia Medico-Chirurgica e dei Trapianti, Università degli Studi di
Milano
Milan, Italy

© Springer International Publishing Switzerland 2016
J.-L. Vincent (ed.), *Annual Update in Intensive Care and Emergency Medicine 2016*,
DOI 10.1007/978-3-319-27349-5_21

Main Mechanisms of Action

The principle physiological advantages of the high gas flow rate delivered by high-flow nasal cannulas can be summarized as:

- provision of distending pressure and the increase in end-expiratory lung volume;
- reduction in the work of breathing;
- washout of nasopharyngeal dead space.

In Table 1, we show the principle mechanisms of action of high-flow nasal cannulas reported in clinical settings.

Provision of Distending Pressure and Increase in End-Expiratory Lung Volume

The first evidence on the provision of distending pressure with high-flow nasal cannulas came from studies in preterm infants. In this population, when using a nasal cannula with an outer diameter of 0.3 cm there was a significant direct relationship between the pressure generated and the applied gas flow rate [1]. In a population of a similar age, equal positive distending pressures, evaluated by esophageal pressure excursion, have been reported with nasal continuous positive airways pressure (CPAP) set at 6 cmH$_2$O and high-flow nasal cannulas [2]; the flow required with high-flow nasal cannulas to obtain the same distending pressure was significantly related to infant body weight. Similarly, Spence et al. evaluated the intrapharyngeal pressure generated in infants for gas flow rates ranging between 1 to 5 l/min [3]. Intrapharyngeal pressure can be assumed to be a surrogate of airway pressure when the mouth of the patient is closed. For gas flow rates from 1 up to 5 l/min, the intrapharyngeal pressure increased from 1.7 ± 0.3 to 4.8 ± 0.5 cmH$_2$O, respectively. The high-flow nasal cannulas did not generate a clinical increase in intrapharyngeal pressure until 3 l/min of gas flow was reached, above which the intrapharyngeal pressure increased linearly with flow rate with huge differences among subjects. The direct relationship between expiratory intrapharyngeal pressure and flow rate in preterm infants was also confirmed by Collins et al. some years later [4]. The average end-expiratory esophageal pressure was less than 2 cmH$_2$O for gas flow rates less than 6 l/min [5]. However, large variations in the end-expiratory esophageal pressure were recorded for the same gas flow rate applied by the high-flow nasal cannulas.

The high-flow nasal cannula effect was also studied in infants affected by viral bronchiolitis, where the gold standard for respiratory support is nasal CPAP [6]. A linear relationship was found between mean pharyngeal pressure and flow rate ($r = 0.65$, $p < 0.0001$), but only flow rates greater than 6 l/min generated increases in pharyngeal pressure resulting in positive pressure values during both inspiration and expiration. At each flow rate, end-expiratory pharyngeal pressure was positive.

Table 1 Studies reporting mechanisms of action

Author, year [ref]	Age	Number of patients	Type of patient	Main results
Provision of distending pressure				
Locke, 1993 [1]	Infants	13	Preterm	Esophageal pressure variations ↑ when flow rate ↑
Sreenan, 2001 [2]	Infants	40	Preterm	End-expiratory esophageal pressure variations ↑ when flow rate ↑
Spence, 2007 [3]	Infants	6	Preterm	Intrapharyngeal pressure ↑ when flow rate ↑
Collins, 2013 [4]	Infants	9	Preterm	Expiratory intrapharyngeal pressure ↑ when flow rate ↑
Lampland, 2009 [5]	Infants	15	Preterm	Expiratory esophageal pressure ↑ when flow rate ↑, but a large variability exists
Milesi, 2013 [6]	Infants	21	Bronchiolitis	Expiratory pharyngeal pressure is higher at each flow rate
Groves, 2007 [7]	Adults	8	Healthy volunteers	Expiratory pharyngeal pressure ↑ when flow rate ↑, both with mouth open and closed
Ritchie, 2011 [8]	Adults	10	Healthy volunteers	Intrapharyngeal pressure ↑ when flow rate ↑
McGinley, 2007 [9]	Adults	11	COPD	Expiratory intrapharyngeal pressure ↑, airways obstruction ↓, ventilatory drive ↓
Parke, 2009 [10]	Adults	15	Post-cardiac surgery	Intrapharyngeal pressure higher with HFNC than with standard face mask
Corley, 2011 [11]	Adults	20	Post-cardiac surgery	Intrapharyngeal pressure ↑, end-expiratory lung impedance ↑
Riera, 2013 [12]	Adults	20	Healthy volunteers	End-expiratory lung impedance ↑ both in prone and supine position
Reduction in work of breathing				
Saslow, 2006 [13]	Infants	18	Preterm	Thoraco-abdominal synchrony higher with HFNC than nasal CPAP
Itagaki, 2014 [14]	Adults	40	Mild to moderate respiratory failure	Thoraco-abdominal synchrony higher with HFNC than with low-flow device
Washout of nasopharyngeal dead space				
Mundel, 2013 [15]	Adults	10	Healthy volunteers	Dead space ↓ because tidal volume ↑

HFNC: high-flow nasal cannula; *CPAP*: continuous positive end-expiratory pressure; *COPD*: chronic obstructive pulmonary disease

In healthy adult subjects, the increase in gas flow rates by high-flow nasal cannulas significantly increased both the expiratory and inspiratory pharyngeal pressures [7]. The expiratory pressures were higher with the mouth closed compared to the mouth open, while the inspiratory pharyngeal pressures were not different with the mouth open or closed. These data were also confirmed by Ritchie et al. in a group of healthy subjects in which a high-flow nasal cannula, with the mouth closed, delivered a clinically relevant positive airway pressure proportional to the delivered gas flow rate. For a gas flow of 30 l/min, the mean pharyngeal pressure was about 3 cmH$_2$O, at 40 l/min it was approximately 4 cmH$_2$O, and at 50 l/min approximately 5 cmH$_2$O [8]. In a group of patients with chronic obstructive pulmonary disease (COPD), a gas flow rate of 20 l/min by high-flow nasal cannula significantly increased end-expiratory pharyngeal pressure from atmospheric to 1.8 ± 0.1 cmH$_2$O [9]. Parke et al., in cardiac surgery patients, showed that high-flow nasal cannulas provided a larger amount of distending pressure, measured as pharyngeal pressure, compared to standard face mask [10]. However, the positive effects of the increase in the pharyngeal pressure should be associated to changes in lung volumes. In 20 adult patients, Corley et al. found a good relationship between changes in pharyngeal pressure and end-expiratory lung impedance, suggesting an increase in end-expiratory lung volume [11]. Interestingly, the increase in end-expiratory lung impedance was significantly higher in patients with a higher body mass index (BMI). These data were subsequently confirmed by Riera et al. in supine and prone positions. Prone positioning was related to a more homogeneous distribution

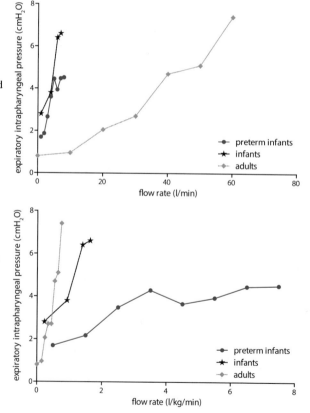

Fig. 1 Flow rates and end-expiratory pharyngeal pressure in literature. Plotted data are calculated (mean) from data published in the following studies: Preterm infants – Spence et al. [3] and Collins et al. [4]; infants – Milesi et al. [6]; adults – McGinley et al. [9], Groves et al. [7], Parke et al. [10] and Ritchie et al. [8]. *Upper Panel*: end-expiratory pharyngeal pressure (cmH$_2$O) plotted as a function of flow rate (l/min). *Lower Panel*: end-expiratory pharyngeal pressure (cmH$_2$O) plotted as a function of flow rate adjusted by patient body weight (l/kg/min)

of end-expiratory lung impedance variations, whereas in the supine position, end-expiratory lung impedance variation was higher in the ventral lung regions [12].

In adults, a higher flow rate is needed to obtain the same pharyngeal pressure as in pediatric or neonatal patients (Fig. 1). Interestingly, plotting end-expiratory pharyngeal pressure as a function of flow rate, adjusted for body weight, high-flow nasal cannulas were more efficient in producing end-expiratory pharyngeal pressure in adults than in pediatric and neonatal patients.

Reduction in Work of Breathing

In 2006, Saslow et al. [13] compared the work of breathing in a group of premature infants treated with high-flow nasal cannulas and those managed with nasal CPAP. Chest wall and abdominal movements were studied using respiratory inductance plethysmography bands placed around the infant's rib cage and abdomen to measure volume variation, and measurements of tidal esophageal pressure were used to estimate pleural pressures. No differences in work of breathing, tidal volume or respiratory rate were found when comparing nasal CPAP ($6\,cmH_2O$) to high-flow nasal cannulas at flow rates of 3, 4 and 5 l/min. However, better thoraco-abdominal synchrony was seen with high-flow nasal cannulas than with nasal CPAP [13].

In adult critically ill patients, Itagaki et al. reported better thoraco-abdominal synchrony, measured using respiratory inductance plethysmography, in patients with mild to moderate respiratory failure when comparing high-flow nasal cannulas to standard oxygen therapy [14].

Washout of Nasopharyngeal Dead Space

At the present time, there are no data on a direct effect of high-flow nasal cannulas on dead space. By contrast, there are several studies that showed a beneficial effect of high-flow nasal cannulas on respiratory rate and tidal volume in infants and in adult patients [11, 12, 14]. Thus a dead space washout remains an interesting hypothesis. Mundel et al. demonstrated that high-flow nasal cannulas increased tidal volume during ventilation when awake. As a consequence, the proportion of dead space volume decreased, thus breathing efficiency improved, as defined by the ratio of dead space volume to tidal volume. The decrease in dead space by high-flow nasal cannulas during wakefulness was more likely largely due to a significant increase in tidal volume rather than a washout effect of the nasal cavity [15].

Clinical Trials in Adults

Several recent trials have been published on the use of high-flow nasal cannulas in adult patients (Table 2).

Table 2 Clinical trials in adults

Authors, year [ref]	Study design	Number of patients	Type of patient	Groups	Main outcomes
Hypoxemic respiratory failure					
Frat, 2015 [16]	Randomized controlled trial	310	Acute respiratory failure	– Standard O_2 therapy (n = 94) – HFNC (n = 106) – NIV (n = 110)	– Intubation rate: HFNC lower than NIV/standard O_2 therapy – Ventilator-free days at 28: HFNC higher than NIV/standard O_2 therapy – Survival rate: HFNC higher than NIV/standard O_2 therapy – Oxygenation ↑
Sztrymf, 2011 [17]	Prospective single center study	38	Acute respiratory failure	HFNC	– Well-tolerated – Respiratory rate as early predictor of HFNC failure – HFNC failed in 45% patients
Rello, 2012 [18]	Single center *post hoc* analysis	20	Acute respiratory failure due to H1N1	HFNC	– Predictors of failure: refractory shock, low PaO_2/FiO_2 – Patient comfort: HFNC higher than face mask
Roca, 2010 [19]	Prospective comparative sequential study	20	Acute respiratory failure	Face mask HFNC	– Respiratory rate: HFNC lower than face mask with a similar $PaCO_2$ – Oxygenation: HFNC higher than face mask
Messika, 2015 [20]	Observational single center study	45	ARDS patients	HFNC	– HFNC failed in 40% patients – Predictors of failure: low SAPS II, low PaO_2/FiO_2, refractory shock

Table 2 (Continued)

Authors, year [ref]	Study design	Number of patients	Type of patient	Groups	Main outcomes
Post-extubation					
Maggiore, 2014 [21]	Randomized controlled trial	105	Extubation after respiratory failure	– HFNC (n = 53) – Venturi mask (n = 52)	– PaO$_2$/FiO$_2$: HFNC higher than Venturi mask – Discomfort: HFNC lower than Venturi mask – Re-intubation: HFNC lower than Venturi mask
Tiruvoipati, 2010 [22]	Randomized cross over trial	50	Extubation after respiratory failure	– HFNC – Non re-breathing mask	– No differences in gas exchange, respiratory rate, heart rate, blood pressure – Comfort: HFNC higher than/equal non re-breathing mask
Stephan, 2015 [23]	Randomized controlled trial	830	Extubation after cardiothoracic surgery	– HFNC (n = 414) – BiPAP (n = 416)	– No differences in preventing respiratory failure, dyspnea and mortality – Respiratory rate: HFNC lower than BiPAP with similar PaCO$_2$ – Oxygenation: HFNC higher than BiPAP
Pre-intubation oxygenation					
Miguel-Montanes, 2015 [24]	Prospective before-after study	101	ICU patients	– HFNC (n = 51) – Non re-breathing mask (n = 50)	– Oxygenation: HFNC higher than non re-breathing mask

HFNC: high-flow nasal cannula; *NIV*: non-invasive ventilation; *ICU*: intensive care unit; *BiPAP*: bilevel positive airway pressure

Hypoxemic Respiratory Failure

Although several approaches for providing supplemental oxygen have been suggested, the best option for patients with acute respiratory failure remains unclear. In a recent study published by Frat et al. [16], 310 patients with respiratory insufficiency were randomized to receive high-flow nasal cannula oxygen, NIV or low-flow oxygen. In the low-flow oxygen group, oxygen was delivered through a non-rebreathing mask in order to reach a saturation of 92%. Similarly patients in the high-flow nasal cannula group received a baseline oxygen flow of 50 l/min, which was subsequently titrated to reach an arterial saturation of 92%. The NIV group was supported with a face mask, setting the pressure support in order to reach a tidal volume of 7–10 ml/kg and a positive end-expiratory pressure (PEEP) between 2 and 10 cmH$_2$O. The intubation rate was similar in the three groups: 38% vs 47% vs 50% for the high-flow nasal cannula, low flow oxygen and NIV groups, respectively. The hazard ratio for death at 90 days was 2.01 with low flow oxygen versus high-flow nasal cannula (p = 0.046) and 2.50 with NIV versus high-flow nasal cannula (p = 0.006). Despite a main limitation of low power to detect a significant between group difference in the intubation rate, this study shows a clear clinical benefit of high-flow nasal cannula oxygen therapy [16].

Before this large prospective trial, high-flow nasal cannulas had been studied as a possible alternative to non-rebreathing masks to treat respiratory failure. In a prospective monocenter observational trial, Sztrymf et al. evaluated high-flow nasal cannulas (mean flow rate of 49 ± 9 l/min) compared to low-flow oxygen therapy. High-flow nasal cannulas were associated with significant reductions in respiratory rate and thoraco-abdominal asynchrony and a significant improvement in arterial oxygen saturation. Furthermore, an early lack of decrease in respiratory rate and the persistence of thoraco-abdominal asynchrony were identified as early indicators of high-flow nasal cannula failure [17]. In a small trial, Rello et al. evaluated high-flow nasal cannulas in 35 patients with hypoxemic respiratory failure due to influenza A/H1N1. The presence of shock, high sequential organ failure assessment (SOFA) and APACHE II scores, the persistence of elevated respiratory rate and hypoxemia after 6 h of high-flow nasal cannula treatment, were associated factors for high-flow nasal cannula failure. All patients with successful high-flow nasal cannula support survived, whereas high-flow nasal cannula failure was associated with an intensive care unit (ICU) mortality of 27.3% [18].

Roca et al. [19] compared the comfort of high-flow nasal cannulas versus conventional oxygen therapy in patients with acute respiratory failure. This was a prospective comparative study of sequential intervention in which patients received 30 min of humidified oxygen through a face mask and then 30 min of oxygen through a high-flow nasal cannula at an initial flow rate of 20–30 l/min, which could be increased at the discretion of the physician in charge. Better patient comfort, a reduction in respiratory rate with a similar arterial carbon dioxide and a higher oxygenation were reported during high-flow nasal cannula support. Interestingly some patients reported a sensation of cervical-thoracic discomfort that appeared during the initial period of increasing flow rate and immediately disappeared when the flow rate was decreased [19].

One observational single center study has evaluated the effect of high-flow nasal cannula oxygen in patients with acute respiratory distress syndrome (ARDS). Over a one-year period, 560 patients were admitted to intensive care for acute respiratory failure; high-flow nasal cannulas were used in 87 subjects, 45 of whom had ARDS. Considering only these patients, 26 were successfully treated with high-flow nasal cannulas, one needed NIV and 18 failed and needed intubation. The failure of high-flow nasal cannula therapy was associated with a lower PaO_2/FiO_2, worse hemodynamic impairment and a higher SAPS II score at admission [20].

In summary, we can conclude that a large amount of literature has shown a role of high-flow nasal cannulas in the treatment of acute respiratory failure, but further, larger studies are needed to confirm the specific role of this relatively new device.

Post-Extubation

As re-intubation is associated with an increase in ICU length of stay and mortality, high-flow nasal cannulas could be used as a post-extubation device, similar to NIV, to reduce the requirement of re-intubation and invasive mechanical ventilation. Maggiore et al. [21] compared the effects of high-flow nasal cannulas and Venturi masks in post-extubated patients. One hundred and five patients with a $PaO_2/FiO_2 < 300$ were enrolled. After 24 h, the PaO_2/FiO_2 was significantly higher in the high-flow nasal cannula group (287 ± 74 vs 247 ± 81, $p = 0.03$) with a lower arterial carbon dioxide and respiratory rate. The rate of re-intubation was lower and comfort was higher in the high-flow nasal cannula group [21]. Tirovuipati et al. evaluated the effects of high-flow nasal cannulas and non-rebreathing masks in post-extubated patients in a small crossover study. The gas exchange and respiratory rate were similar among the two groups with better comfort in the high-flow nasal cannula group [22]. In contrast to the two previous studies [21, 22] in which mask oxygen therapy was tested, the effect of bilevel positive airway pressure (BiPAP) was compared to high-flow nasal cannula therapy in a large multicenter study. A total of 830 patients who developed acute respiratory failure or were at risk of development because of pre-existing risk factors after cardiothoracic surgery were enrolled. Patients were randomly assigned to receive high-flow nasal cannula oxygen or BiPAP through a full face mask for at least 4 h per day. High-flow nasal cannula oxygen was non-inferior to BiPAP in the treatment of postoperative hypoxemia; treatment failure occurred in 91 out of 416 patients during BiPAP (21.9%) compared to 87 out of 414 patients with high-flow nasal cannulas (21%). Re-intubation was performed in 57 (13.7%) patients with BiPAP and 58 (14%) with high-flow nasal cannulas ($p = 0.99$). The ICU mortality was similar in the two groups (5.5% with BiPAP vs 6.8% with high-flow nasal cannula, $p = 0.66$) [23].

From the available literature, we can conclude that high-flow nasal cannula oxygen seems to be a useful device to solve post-extubation hypoxemia.

Pre-Intubation Oxygenation

Although tracheal intubation is routinely performed in critically ill patients, it can be associated with severe morbidity and mortality. To reduce the risk of hypoxemia during the maneuver, pre-oxygenation using a non-rebreathing face mask is usually performed. High-flow nasal cannulas could be used as an alternative to a non-rebreathing mask. Miguel-Montanes et al. evaluated the arterial saturation during intubation in a prospective quasi experimental before-after study (pre-oxygenation with a non-rebreathing face mask compared to high-flow nasal cannulas). High-flow nasal cannula oxygen was associated with a higher arterial saturation compared to face mask (100% vs 94%, $p < 0.0001$). Moreover, patients with the high-flow nasal cannulas had significantly fewer episodes of severe hypoxemia (2% vs 14%, $p = 0.03$) [24].

As life-threatening hypoxemia is the most frequently complication of intubation in the ICU, this study clearly showed that high-flow nasal cannula oxygen could be considered as the best device to reach a good pre-oxygenation level.

Clinical Trials in Children

A summary of the main published findings of clinical trials using high-flow nasal cannula in children is given in Table 3.

Respiratory Failure

Bronchiolitis is one of the most common causes of lower respiratory tract infection during the first year of life. Although the role of high-flow nasal cannulas in infants with bronchiolitis could therefore be of particular interest, there are limited prospective data. In a small pilot study, 19 infants with bronchiolitis were randomized to head-box oxygen or high-flow nasal cannula oxygen for at least 24 h (started at 4 l/min and increased to 8 l/min if tolerated). Median oxygen saturation was higher in infants with high-flow nasal cannulas at 8 and 12 h after randomization, but duration of oxygen therapy, time to feed and total length of stay were similar in the two groups; no infant required further respiratory support [25].

Another retrospective observational trial compared high-flow nasal cannula oxygen to nasal CPAP (gold-standard therapy) to treat children with bronchiolitis [26]. Thirty-four patients were enrolled and analyzed and no differences in ICU length of stay and oxygenation were found between the groups. Oxygen weaning occurred over the same time period for the two groups and there were no differences in respiratory rate or gas exchange evolution. Based on their findings, the authors concluded that there were no differences between nasal CPAP and high-flow nasal cannula oxygen in the treatment of bronchiolitis [26].

A recent prospective randomized controlled trial tested high-flow nasal cannula oxygen (2 l/kg/min), bubble CPAP (starting with a PEEP of 5 cmH$_2$O) and low-

Table 3 Clinical trials in children

Authors, year [ref]	Study design	No of patients	Type of patient	Groups	Main outcomes
Respiratory failure					
Hilliard, 2012 [25]	Prospective randomized trial	19	Bronchiolitis	– HFNC (n = 11) – Head box oxygen (n = 8)	– SpO$_2$: HFNC higher than head box oxygen – No differences in oxygen therapy duration, time to feed and LOS
Chisti, 2015 [27]	Randomized controlled trial	225	Pneumonia	– HFNC (n = 79) – Bubble CPAP (n = 79) – Low flow oxygen (n = 67)	– No differences in outcome and time to resolution of hypoxemia between HFNC and bubble CPAP – ↑ mortality in low flow oxygen group
Metge, 2014 [26]	Retrospective observational study	34	Bronchiolitis	– HFNC (n = 15) – Nasal CPAP (n = 19)	– No differences in LOS, oxygenation, weaning, respiratory rate, heart rate, FiO$_2$ and PaCO$_2$
Post-extubation support					
Testa, 2014 [28]	Randomized controlled trial	89	Extubation after cardiothoracic surgery	– HFNC (n = 43) – Standard O$_2$ therapy (n = 46)	– Treatment failure: HFNC lower than standard O$_2$ therapy – Intubation rate: HFNC lower than standard O$_2$ therapy – No differences in atelectasis and LOS

HFNC: high-flow nasal cannula; *LOS*: length of stay; *CPAP*: continuous positive airway pressure; *SpO$_2$*: pulse oximetry oxygen saturation

flow oxygen therapy at 2 l/min in children with severe pneumonia [27]. A total of 225 patients were recruited. There were no differences in treatment failure and time to resolution of hypoxemia between bubble CPAP and high-flow nasal cannula oxygen. However, the trial was stopped early because of a higher mortality in the low-flow oxygen group, so further study is needed to determine eventual differences between high-flow nasal cannula oxygen and bubble CPAP.

Postoperative Support

After cardiothoracic surgery, acute respiratory failure, due to fluid accumulation or edema, increased vascular resistance, muscular weakness and diaphragm fatigue, is frequently observed, and NIV or CPAP are frequently required. Hence, high-flow nasal cannula oxygen could have a role after extubation. Testa et al. [28], in a randomized controlled trial enrolling 89 cardiac surgical patients, compared high-flow nasal cannula and conventional oxygen delivery in the first 48 h after postoperative extubation. The PaO_2/FiO_2 improved similarly in the two groups without any difference in arterial carbon dioxide. As there was no difference in the rate of re-intubation in the two groups, the authors concluded that the use of high-flow nasal cannula appeared to be safe and could improve oxygenation in pediatric cardiac surgical patients [28].

Conclusion

Because of the absence of continuous respiratory monitoring in terms of respiratory rate, tidal volume and the requirement of active muscle efforts, high-flow nasal cannula oxygen should not be applied in every patient. Possible contraindications are patients with hemodynamic instability, respiratory arrest and coma. Moreover in patients with severe respiratory failure, high-flow nasal cannula oxygen should not be used because it is impossible to estimate the applied level of PEEP.

Although several aspects of high-flow nasal cannula oxygen remain to be elucidated, such as the timing of application, the duration, the amount of oxygen flow, and contraindications, high-flow nasal cannula should be used as an alternative tool to NIV or low-flow oxygen therapy in patients with mild to moderate forms of acute respiratory failure. Furthermore, high-flow nasal cannulas are an innovative support that can be applied outside the ICU thus improving the care of hypoxemic patients.

References

1. Locke RG, Wolfson MR, Shaffer TH, Rubenstein SD, Greenspan JS (1993) Inadvertent administration of positive end-distending pressure during nasal cannula flow. Pediatrics 91:135–138
2. Sreenan C, Lemke RP, Hudson-Mason A, Osiovich H (2001) High-flow nasal cannulae in the management of apnea of prematurity: a comparison with conventional nasal continuous positive airway pressure. Pediatrics 107:1081–1083

3. Spence KL, Murphy D, Kilian C, McGonigle R, Kilani RA (2007) High-flow nasal cannula as a device to provide continuous positive airway pressure in infants. J Perinatol 27:772–775

4. Collins CL, Barfield C, Horne RS, Davis PG (2014) A comparison of nasal trauma in preterm infants extubated to either heated humidified high-flow nasal cannulae or nasal continuous positive airway pressure. Eur J Pediatr 173:181–186

5. Lampland AL, Plumm B, Meyers PA, Worwa CT, Mammel MC (2009) Observational study of humidified high-flow nasal cannula compared with nasal continuous positive airway pressure. J Pediatr 154:177–182

6. Milesi C, Baleine J, Matecki S et al (2013) Is treatment with a high flow nasal cannula effective in acute viral bronchiolitis? A physiologic study. Intensive Care Med 39:1088–1094

7. Groves N, Tobin A (2007) High flow nasal oxygen generates positive airway pressure in adult volunteers. Aust Crit Care 20:126–131

8. Ritchie JE, Williams AB, Gerard C, Hockey H (2011) Evaluation of a humidified nasal high-flow oxygen system, using oxygraphy, capnography and measurement of upper airway pressures. Anaesth Intensive Care 39:1103–1110

9. McGinley BM, Patil SP, Kirkness JP, Smith PL, Schwartz AR, Schneider H (2007) A nasal cannula can be used to treat obstructive sleep apnea. Am J Respir Crit Care Med 176:194–200

10. Parke R, McGuinness S, Eccleston M (2009) Nasal high-flow therapy delivers low level positive airway pressure. Br J Anaesth 103:886–890

11. Corley A, Caruana LR, Barnett AG, Tronstad O, Fraser JF (2011) Oxygen delivery through high-flow nasal cannulae increase end-expiratory lung volume and reduce respiratory rate in post-cardiac surgical patients. Br J Anaesth 107:998–1004

12. Riera J, Perez P, Cortes J, Roca O, Masclans JR, Rello J (2013) Effect of high-flow nasal cannula and body position on end-expiratory lung volume: a cohort study using electrical impedance tomography. Respir Care 58:589–596

13. Saslow JG, Aghai ZH, Nakhla TA et al (2006) Work of breathing using high-flow nasal cannula in preterm infants. J Perinatol 26:476–480

14. Itagaki T, Okuda N, Tsunano Y et al (2014) Effect of high-flow nasal cannula on thoraco-abdominal synchrony in adult critically ill patients. Respir Care 59:70–74

15. Mundel T, Feng S, Tatkov S, Schneider H (1985) Mechanisms of nasal high flow on ventilation during wakefulness and sleep. J Appl Physiol 114:1058–1065

16. Frat JP, Thille AW, Mercat A et al (2015) High-flow oxygen through nasal cannula in acute hypoxemic respiratory failure. N Engl J Med 372:2185–2196

17. Sztrymf B, Messika J, Bertrand F et al (2011) Beneficial effects of humidified high flow nasal oxygen in critical care patients: a prospective pilot study. Intensive Care Med 37:1780–1786

18. Rello J, Perez M, Roca O et al (2012) High-flow nasal therapy in adults with severe acute respiratory infection: a cohort study in patients with 2009 influenza A/H1N1v. J Crit Care 27:434–439

19. Roca O, Riera J, Torres F, Masclans JR (2010) High-flow oxygen therapy in acute respiratory failure. Respir Care 55:408–413

20. Messika J, Ben Ahmed K, Gaudry S et al (2015) Use of high-flow nasal cannula oxygen therapy in subjects with ARDS: A 1-year observational study. Respir Care 60:162–169

21. Maggiore SM, Idone FA, Vaschetto R et al (2014) Nasal high-flow versus Venturi mask oxygen therapy after extubation. Effects on oxygenation, comfort, and clinical outcome. Am J Respir Crit Care Med 190:282–288

22. Tiruvoipati R, Lewis D, Haji K, Botha J (2010) High-flow nasal oxygen vs high-flow face mask: a randomized crossover trial in extubated patients. J Crit Care 25:463–468

23. Stephan F, Barrucand B, Petit P et al (2015) High-flow nasal oxygen vs noninvasive positive airway pressure in hypoxemic patients after cardiothoracic surgery: A randomized clinical trial. JAMA 313:2331–2339

24. Miguel-Montanes R, Hajage D, Messika J et al (2015) Use of high-flow nasal cannula oxygen therapy to prevent desaturation during tracheal intubation of intensive care patients with mild-to-moderate hypoxemia. Crit Care Med 43:574–583

25. Hilliard TN, Archer N, Laura H et al (2012) Pilot study of vapotherm oxygen delivery in moderately severe bronchiolitis. Arch Dis Child 97:182–183
26. Metge P, Grimaldi C, Hassid S et al (2014) Comparison of a high-flow humidified nasal cannula to nasal continuous positive airway pressure in children with acute bronchiolitis: experience in a pediatric intensive care unit. Eur J Pediatr 173:953–958
27. Chisti MJ, Salam MA, Smith JH et al (2015) Bubble continuous positive airway pressure for children with severe pneumonia and hypoxaemia in Bangladesh: an open, randomised controlled trial. Lancet 386:1057–1068
28. Testa G, Iodice F, Ricci Z et al (2014) Comparative evaluation of high-flow nasal cannula and conventional oxygen therapy in paediatric cardiac surgical patients: a randomized controlled trial. Interact Cardiovasc Thorac Surg 19:456–461

The Potential Value of Monitoring the Oxygen Reserve Index in Patients Receiving Oxygen

A. Perel

Introduction

Early detection of hypoxemia followed by a prompt and appropriate intervention is one of the cornerstones of caring for acutely ill patients. This life-saving process has been greatly facilitated by the introduction of pulse oximetry and its adoption as a standard monitoring tool. However, one of the major limitations of pulse oximetry (SpO_2) is that it cannot reflect the oxygenation status beyond the point of maximal hemoglobin oxygen saturation, when the oxygen dissociation flattens out. This limitation is of special significance in patients who receive supplemental oxygen, as the level of oxygenation in this "hyperoxic" range may reflect severity of disease as well as the presence of a potentially detrimental high concentration of inspired oxygen (FiO_2).

The oxygen reserve index (ORI) is a new feature of multiple wavelength pulse oximetry that reflects, in real-time, the oxygenation status in the moderate hyperoxic range (PaO_2 of approximately 100 to 200 mmHg) (Fig. 1). This new parameter may make pre-oxygenation 'visible', may provide an early alarm when oxygenation deteriorates well before SpO_2 decreases, may facilitate FiO_2 titration and prevent unintended hyperoxia, and may reflect the immediate response to positive end-expiratory pressure (PEEP) and to recruitment maneuvers, spontaneous improvement in acute respiratory distress syndrome (ARDS), etc. Because of the significant clinical potential of the ORI, and despite the lack of data because of its newness, a theoretical exploration of its possible value in patients who receive O_2 seems warranted even at this early phase. As the ORI should serve as a complement to SpO_2 in assessing oxygenation, I will start by reviewing the clinical value and the limitations of monitoring SpO_2 alone.

A. Perel (✉)
Department of Anesthesiology and Intensive Care, Sheba Medical Center, Tel Aviv University
Tel Aviv, Israel
email: perelao@shani.net

© Springer International Publishing Switzerland 2016
J.-L. Vincent (ed.), *Annual Update in Intensive Care and Emergency Medicine 2016*,
DOI 10.1007/978-3-319-27349-5_22

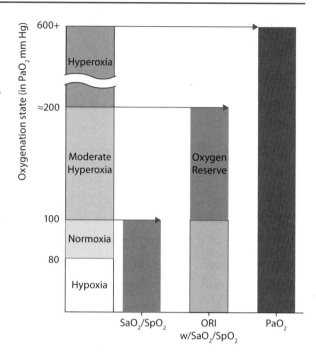

Fig. 1 The oxygen reserve index (ORI) reflects the moderate hyperoxic range ($PaO_2 > 100$ and $< \approx 200$ mmHg) which is defined as the patient's 'oxygen reserve'. Figure kindly provided by Masimo Corp., Irvine, CA, USA

The Clinical Value of Monitoring O$_2$ Saturation (SpO$_2$)

Benefits

Pulse oximetry has become a mandatory monitoring modality in anesthesia and intensive care [1, 2] despite lack of robust evidence regarding its ability to improve outcomes [3, 4]. This has happened because the technology is non-invasive and can be easily applied, and because of the frequent repeated observations by clinicians of its potential life-saving impact. Indeed the routine monitoring of SpO$_2$ has greatly improved patient safety, as evidenced by the marked decrease in the proportion of malpractice claims due to respiratory events during anesthesia [5].

However, despite advances in monitoring technology, hypoxemia continues to occur commonly in the operating room [6] and in the post-anesthesia care unit (PACU) [7]. Hypoxemia has also been found to be prevalent in patients during transport to the PACU, although it could be identified clinically in only a few of these patients [8]. Nevertheless, considering the uncertainty about the deleterious effects of transient short-lasting hypoxemia, Aust et al. suggest that pulse oximetry be used routinely for patient transfer to the PACU [8]. Older age, higher BMI, lower preoperative SpO$_2$, longer surgery and absence of supplemental O$_2$ were found to be among the predictors of a decline in SpO$_2$ during transport to the PACU [9]. These authors concluded that given the protective effect of oxygen supplementation in limiting hypoxemia, it should be considered after every general anesthetic, especially in higher risk patients [9].

In the intensive care unit (ICU), pulse oximetry is often used to titrate FiO_2 and an SpO_2 value of 92% is considered reasonable for ensuring satisfactory oxygenation in patients requiring mechanical ventilation [2]. SpO_2 has also been suggested to be useful in defining ARDS. In pediatric patients, it was suggested that pulse oximetry-based criteria be used when PaO_2 is unavailable, and that the oxygen saturation index (SpO_2/FiO_2) replace the PaO_2/FiO_2 ratio [10]. In adults it was recently suggested that the PaO_2/FiO_2 ratio should be calculated under standardized ventilator settings of PEEP (10 mmHg) and FiO_2 (0.5), unless the SpO_2 is < 88% [11]. In under-resourced settings where arterial blood gas testing and chest radiography are not readily available, pulse oximetry and pulmonary ultrasound have been found to be useful tools to screen for, or rule out, impaired oxygenation or lung abnormalities consistent with ARDS [12]. Obviously a robust SpO_2 monitor is needed in such circumstances, which may often be associated with decreased perfusion [2].

The use of pulse oximetry is slowly expanding to high-risk patients in the general, less-acute areas in the hospital. A change in breathing and a decrease in SpO_2 are considered by nurses to be the most important indicators of patient deterioration on the general ward and the main reason for 'worry' calls to rapid-response teams [13]. An earlier study did not, however, find that the use of pulse oximetry affected the rate of transfer from the post-cardiothoracic surgery care floor to the ICU, although it did alter the reasons for such transfers [14]. A more recent study found that introduction of a pulse oximetry and respiratory rate-based patient surveillance system (SafetyNet, Masimo, Irvine, USA) with nursing alarm notification via a wireless pager in a 36-bed orthopedic unit, resulted in a significant decrease in rescue events and in ICU transfers [15]. The monitoring of pulse oximetry in the general ward may be especially warranted in high-risk patients. The recent Prospective Evaluation of a RIsk Score for Postoperative Pulmonary COmPlications in Europe (PERISCOPE) study showed that about 4.2% of surgical patients develop postoperative respiratory failure, carrying an in-hospital mortality of 10.3% (versus 0.4% in the rest of the patients), and defined risk factors for development of postoperative respiratory failure [16]. Susceptible high-risk surgical patients may benefit from earlier detection of postoperative respiratory failure and postoperative monitoring with a pulse oximeter should be considered. The SpO_2 should also be routinely measured in patients following bariatric surgery, in whom severe and prolonged episodes of hypoxemia have been described as a consistent finding [17]. We can therefore expect that in the future the monitoring of SpO_2 will become more prevalent in the general wards of acute care hospitals.

Limitations

The main limitation of SpO_2 monitoring is its inability to reflect the oxygenation status when the hemoglobin is fully saturated with O_2 as may often be the case in patients who are administered supplemental oxygen. As a result, pulse oximetry is an inadequate, and at times misleading, tool to assess ventilation abnormalities in the presence of supplemental inspired oxygen. For example, if severe hypoventilation occurs when the inspired FiO_2 is 0.3, the partial pressures of CO_2 ($PaCO_2$) and O_2 (PaO_2) may be around 100 mmHg each, with an SpO_2 value close to 100% [18]. This limitation may have important safety consequences in patients who are recovering from anesthesia, undergoing procedural sedation or receiving potent opioids. In a recent review of 357 acute pain claims from the Anesthesia Closed Claims Project database, 92 cases involved likely opioid-related respiratory depression [19]. The vast majority of these injuries occurred within 24 h of surgery, resulted in death or severe brain damage, and was judged as preventable with better monitoring and response. Thirty-three percent of these patients were monitored with pulse oximeters and 15% were receiving oxygen [19]. It is obvious that a more effective means of ventilatory monitoring, such as capnography or the monitoring of respiratory rate [20], should be used more frequently in all patients who are susceptible to develop respiratory depression, especially when they are being administered supplemental oxygen.

The inability of pulse oximetry to reflect oxygenation once the oxygen dissociation curve starts to flatten ($PaO_2 > 100$ mmHg) also presents a serious limitation to monitoring the oxygenation status of mechanically ventilated patients who have, or may develop, respiratory failure. It is only the PaO_2 that can be used to assess oxygenation in the 'hyperoxic' range. However, PaO_2 measurement is intermittent, frequently delayed, and necessitates the withdrawal of arterial blood samples for gas analysis through direct puncture or an arterial cannula. Hence, in the range where SpO_2 is no longer informative, unexpected relative hypoxia or unintended hyperoxia may go unnoticed in-between arterial blood gas analyses. The introduction of the ORI may partially fill this gap.

The Oxygen Reserve Index

The ORI is a new feature of pulse oximetry that provides continuous real-time visibility of oxygenation status in the moderate hyperoxic range (PaO_2 of approximately 100 to 200 mmHg) (Fig. 1). Measurement of the ORI has become possible through the utilization of more than 7 wavelengths of light in the new generation of pulse oximetry sensors (Rainbow® sensor, Masimo, Irvine, CA, USA). The use of multiple wavelength pulse oximetry enables the monitoring of multiple blood constituent data based on light absorption, including the changes in the venous oxygen saturation (SvO_2) when the PaO_2 is in the range of 100 mmHg and roughly 200 mmHg (beyond which such changes are less discernable). Utilizing this information, in addition to the noted proportionality relationship between SvO_2 and PaO_2 (through the combination of the Fick and Oxygen Content equations), it was possible to develop the ORI, which is a relative indicator of changes in PaO_2 in the moderate hyperoxic range. Given that the ORI is a relative indicator of PaO_2 and not a measured value, it is provided as an 'index' parameter with a unitless scale between 0.0 and 1.0 that can be trended and has optional alarms.

Preliminary internal validation studies have shown that an ORI value of 0.3 provides $> 85\%$ sensitivity and $> 80\%$ specificity for $PaO_2 > 150$ mmHg. In a recent trial in 103 anesthetized adult patients, ORI could be calculated $\sim 91.5\%$ of monitored time, and was positively correlated with PaO_2 values ≤ 240 mmHg but not with $PaO_2 > 240$ mmHg. PaO_2 was ≥ 150 mmHg in 96.5% of ORI > 0.54, and was > 100 mmHg for all ORI > 0.24 [21]. It seems therefore that, when utilized in conjunction with SpO_2 monitoring, the ORI may extend the visibility of a patient's oxygen status into ranges previously unmonitored in this fashion. The ORI may make pre-oxygenation visible, may provide early warning when oxygenation deteriorates (Fig. 2), may facilitate a more precise setting of the required FiO_2 level and may prevent unintended hyperoxemia.

Making Pre-Oxygenation Visible

The administration of high levels of inspired O_2 before tracheal intubation (pre-oxygenation) is considered to be routine practice because oxygen reserves are not always sufficient to prevent hypoxia during the duration of intubation [22, 23]. Effective pre-oxygenation in patients with normal lung function can be achieved by 3 min of spontaneous breathing or 8 deep breaths within 60 s at $FiO_2 = 1$, or by the addition of positive pressure ventilation with 100% O_2 before intubation [22]. Considering the three main physiological O_2 reserves, namely the lungs, the hemoglobin and the plasma, the total O_2 reserve is about 1450 ml when breathing in ambient air. This reserve increases to approximately 3700 ml when breathing 100% oxygen during the pre-oxygenation process. In turn, the increased O_2 reserve may extend the 'tolerable apnea time', defined as the time until the SpO_2 reaches 90%, to almost 10 min [22], and hence provide valuable additional time to secure the airway and make induction of anesthesia and tracheal intubation safer.

However, inadequate pre-oxygenation, defined as an expired oxygen fraction (FeO_2) $\geq 90\%$ despite 3-min tidal volume breathing, seems to be a common occurrence in the clinical setting. For example, inadequate pre-oxygenation was found to occur in 56% of 1050 consecutive patients undergoing general anesthesia [24]. The independent risk factors for inadequate pre-oxygenation included the presence of a beard, male sex, American Society of Anesthesiologists (ASA) score of 4, lack of teeth and age > 55 years, and were similar to those previously identified for difficult mask ventilation [24]. Monitoring the effectiveness of the pre-oxygenation process cannot be achieved by pulse oximetry as, normally, the hemoglobin immediately becomes 100% saturated once the process starts. Possible indicators of the completeness of pre-oxygenation are end-tidal nitrogen fraction ($FetN_2$) or end-tidal oxygen fraction ($FetO_2$), although the $FetO_2$ value alone cannot accurately predict the duration of apnea without desaturation [23]. In addition, the accuracy of these end-tidal gas values is greatly decreased in the presence of gas-leaks due to an ill-fitting mask, which is frequently the case in clinical practice.

Monitoring of the ORI during pre-oxygenation may make this process visible, ensuring that the PaO_2 is indeed increasing in the presence of a constant maxi-

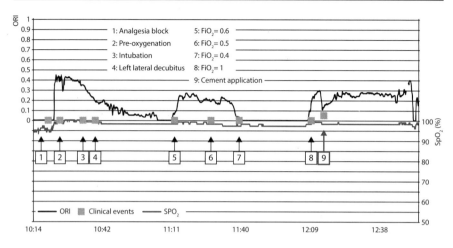

Fig. 2 Oxygen reserve index (ORI) and SpO_2 trends during acetabular replacement in a 77-year old, ASA 1, female patient (see text for further details). Figure and data kindly provided by Dr Antoine Brandely and Prof Emmanuel Futier, CHU Gabriel Montpied, Clermont Ferrand, France

mal SpO_2 level. This is nicely demonstrated in Fig. 2. During the performance of the nerve block at the beginning of the case (point 1), the patient did not receive any oxygen, the SpO_2 was around 95% and the ORI was naturally invisible. Once oxygen was administered before induction of general anesthesia (point 2), the SpO_2 increased to 100% following which the ORI increased sharply to a value of 0.4 and endotracheal intubation was performed. Monitoring the ORI in such a manner may be especially important in the presence of predictive risk factors for inadequate pre-oxygenation, and in patients in whom the duration of apnea without desaturation is characteristically decreased, namely, obese patients, pregnant women, and patients with increased metabolism [23]. Other clinical scenarios where the ORI may be of benefit in ensuring adequate pre-oxygenation include suctioning of hypoxemic patients [25], emergency rapid sequence induction (RSI) [26], during intubation in the ICU [27], and in hypoxic patients who may require non-invasive ventilation (NIV) before intubation [28].

Early Warning of Impending Hypoxemia

The ORI may provide early warning of deteriorating oxygenation before any changes in SpO_2 occur. This is nicely demonstrated in Fig. 2, in which the ORI started to decrease following intubation (point 3) and lateral decubitus positioning (point 4), prompting an increase in FiO_2 (point 5) although the SpO_2 remained unchanged. A more dramatic example of the value of the ORI can be seen later in the operation. Following the application of bone cement there was a sharp decline in the ORI (Fig. 2, point 9) even though the FiO_2 was increased to 1.0 a few minutes earlier (point 8) and in the absence of any change in SpO_2. This transient hypoxemia, which reminds us of the severe adverse effects that can occur following bone cement application, could not have been identified without the ORI.

The ability of the ORI to provide early warning of deteriorating oxygenation was recently demonstrated in a study in anesthetized pediatric patients [29]. In this patient population, which is characteristically more prone to develop hypoxemia, the mean time ($\pm$ SD) from the start of the ORI alarm to a decrease in SpO_2 below 98% was 40 ± 523 s, while the time from SpO_2 98 to 90% was 52 ± 44 s. The authors concluded that the ORI alarm provides an increased warning time for avoiding potential hypoxia and could help in optimizing oxygenation before and during prolonged intubation. The early warning that the ORI may provide may give the clinician precious time for earlier institution of timely remedial measures. It is important to note that the ORI is intended to supplement and not replace PaO_2 measurements and that it reflects PaO_2 changes only in the 100–200 mmHg range.

Preventing Unintended Hyperoxemia

Oxygen is considered a life-saving drug during urgent care because it helps minimize cellular hypoxia. This is the reason that oxygen is one of the most widely used drugs in anesthesia, intensive care and acute hospital care [30]. However, oxygen, especially when given in excess, also has deleterious properties through the formation of reactive oxygen species (ROS), also known as oxygen free radicals, within mitochondria. For example, among patients admitted to the ICU following resuscitation from cardiac arrest, arterial hyperoxia was independently associated with increased in-hospital mortality compared with either hypoxia or normoxia [31]. The risks associated with hyperoxemia have been repeatedly reviewed in the recent anesthesia and critical care literature [30, 32–34].

In order to minimize the possible deleterious effects of hyperoxemia, current guidelines recommend using the lowest FiO_2 possible, and consider an SpO_2 of 92% as a reasonable target for ensuring satisfactory oxygenation [2]. More recently more restrictive approaches, namely 'precise control of arterial oxygenation' and 'permissive hypoxemia', have been recommended in order to achieve an even tighter control of blood oxygen levels [30]. Recently, however, it was proposed that the target range for arterial oxygenation should be reset at higher values (85–110 mmHg) as a potential strategy to improve the long-term outcomes (cognitive and physical impairment) of ARDS survivors [35]. Hyperoxia is considered by others to be beneficial in septic shock and other acute clinical situations [36], as well as during acute anemia, when hyperoxic ventilation establishes a highly available source of O_2 that can be effectively utilized for tissue oxygenation [37].

While the debate about the optimal FiO_2 continues, it seems that very often patients receive more oxygen than is needed to achieve arterial oxygenation goals [34]. Clinicians usually respond quickly when the PaO_2 or SpO_2 decreases below the goal range, but they are slow to respond when arterial oxygenation exceeds the goal range. This may be related to a lack of understanding of oxygen toxicity in humans and a culture that has not highlighted the importance of precise control [34]. Perhaps more importantly, providers focus on avoiding hypoxemia, and therefore feel uncomfortable leaving patients at SpO_2 levels that are too close to the exponential decrease that occurs at 90% (the 'Desaturation Cliff'). Unintended hyperoxia seems to be quite common as well. According to a large Dutch study including 126,778 arterial blood gas samples from 5,498 mechanically ventilated patients, hyperoxia (PaO_2 was > 120 mmHg) was found in 22% of the samples but the FiO_2 was decreased in only 25% of these instances, implying that hyperoxia was accepted without adjustment of ventilator settings if FiO_2 was 0.4 or less [38].

Taking all the above into consideration, it seems that the ORI may facilitate a more accurate control of the FiO_2 in patients receiving O_2 as it may identify and help avoid unwarranted or unintended hyperoxia. Furthermore, the ORI may be able to reflect the immediate effects of increasing PEEP or of a recruitment maneuver on oxygenation, and, when spontaneously increasing, may also be the first sign of pulmonary improvement in patients with respiratory failure.

Conclusion

The ORI is a relative indicator of the PaO_2 in the range of 100–200 mmHg. Its addition to conventional pulse oximetry opens new opportunities in the continuous, non-invasive monitoring of the oxygenation status in patients receiving oxygen. The ORI may potentially allow better control of pre-oxygenation, provide an alarm of decreasing oxygenation well before any decrease in SpO_2, allow a more adequate titration of oxygen therapy, identify unintended hyperoxia, and provide information about changes in the oxygenation status in the PaO_2 range of 100–200 mmHg. Further studies are needed to determine the potential role of the ORI in the management of acutely ill patients who are in need of oxygen supplementation.

References

1. Shah A, Shelley KH (2013) Is pulse oximetry an essential tool or just another distraction? The role of the pulse oximeter in modern anesthesia care. J Clin Monit Comput 27:235–242
2. Jubran A (2015) Pulse oximetry. Crit Care 19:272
3. Moller JT, Johannessen NW, Espersen K et al (1993) Randomized evaluation of pulse oximetry in 20,802 patients: II. Perioperative events and postoperative complications. Anesthesiology 78:445–453
4. Pedersen T, Nicholson A, Hovhannisyan K et al (2014) Pulse oximetry for perioperative monitoring. Cochrane Database Syst Rev 3:CD002013
5. Lee LA, Domino KB (2002) The Closed Claims Project. Has it influenced anesthetic practice and outcome? Anesthesiol Clin North America 2002:485–501
6. Ehrenfeld JM, Funk LM, Van Schalkwyk J, Merry AF, Sandberg WS, Gawande A (2010) The incidence of hypoxemia during surgery: evidence from two institutions. Can J Anaesth 57:888–897
7. Epstein RH, Dexter F, Lopez MG, Ehrenfeld JM (2014) Anesthesiologist staffing considerations consequent to the temporal distribution of hypoxemic episodes in the postanesthesia care unit. Anesth Analg 119:1322–1333

8. Aust H, Kranke P, Eberhart LH et al (2015) Impact of medical training and clinical experience on the assessment of oxygenation and hypoxemia after general anesthesia: an observational study. J Clin Monit Comput 29:415–426

9. Walker M, Farmer RG, Schelew B (2015) Risk factors for oxygen desaturation on arrival in the postanesthesia care unit. Can J Anaesth 62:1019–1020

10. Khemani RG, Rubin S, Belani S et al (2015) Pulse oximetry vs. PaO2 metrics in mechanically ventilated children: Berlin definition of ARDS and mortality risk. Intensive Care Med 41:94–102

11. Villar J, Blanco J, del Campo R et al (2015) Assessment of PaO2/FiO2 for stratification of patients with moderate and severe acute respiratory distress syndrome. BMJ open 5:e006812

12. Bass CM, Sajed DR, Adedipe AA, West TE (2015) Pulmonary ultrasound and pulse oximetry versus chest radiography and arterial blood gas analysis for the diagnosis of acute respiratory distress syndrome: a pilot study. Crit Care 19:282

13. Douw G, Schoonhoven L, Holwerda T et al (2015) Nurses' worry or concern and early recognition of deteriorating patients on general wards in acute care hospitals: a systematic review. Crit Care 19:230

14. Ochroch EA, Russell MW, Hanson WC et al (2006) The impact of continuous pulse oximetry monitoring on intensive care unit admissions from a postsurgical care floor. Anesth Analg 102:868–875

15. Taenzer AH, Pyke JB, McGrath SP, Blike GT (2010) Impact of pulse oximetry surveillance on rescue events and intensive care unit transfers: a before-and-after concurrence study. Anesthesiology 112:282–287

16. Canet J, Sabate S, Mazo V et al (2015) Development and validation of a score to predict postoperative respiratory failure in a multicentre European cohort: A prospective, observational study. Eur J Anaesthesiol 32:458–470

17. Gallagher SF, Haines KL, Osterlund LG, Mullen M, Downs JB (2010) Postoperative hypoxemia: common, undetected, and unsuspected after bariatric surgery. J Surg Research 159:622–626

18. Fu ES, Downs JB, Schweiger JW, Miguel RV, Smith RA (2004) Supplemental oxygen impairs detection of hypoventilation by pulse oximetry. Chest 126:1552–1558

19. Lee LA, Caplan RA, Stephens LS et al (2015) Postoperative opioid-induced respiratory depression: a closed claims analysis. Anesthesiology 122:659–665

20. Kelley SD, Ramsay MA (2014) Respiratory rate monitoring: characterizing performance for emerging technologies. Anesth Analg 119:1246–1248

21. Applegate R, Dorotta I, Applegate P, Andrews G, Olson M, Um MH (2015) Relationship between oxygen reserve index and arterial partial pressure of oxygen during surgery. Anesth Analg 120(suppl 1):S–377 (abst)

22. Bouroche G, Bourgain JL (2015) Pre-oxygenation and general anesthesia: a review. Minerva Anestesiol 81:910–920

23. Tanoubi I, Drolet P, Donati F (2009) Optimizing preoxygenation in adults. Can J Anaesth 56:449–466

24. Baillard C, Depret F, Levy V, Boubaya M, Beloucif S (2014) Incidence and prediction of inadequate preoxygenation before induction of anesthesia. Ann Fr Anesth Reanim 33:e55–e58

25. Day T, Farnell S, Wilson-Barnett J (2002) Suctioning: a review of current research recommendations. Intensive Crit Care Nurs 18:79–89

26. Gebremedhn EG, Mesele D, Aemero D, Alemu E (2014) The incidence of oxygen desaturation during rapid sequence induction and intubation. World J Emerg Med 5:279–285

27. Lapinsky SE (2015) Endotracheal intubation in the ICU. Crit Care 19:258

28. Baillard C, Fosse JP, Sebbane M et al (2006) Noninvasive ventilation improves preoxygenation before intubation of hypoxic patients. Am J Respir Crit Care Med 174:171–177

29. Szmuk P, Steiner JW, Olumu PN, Curuz JD, Sessler D (2014) Oxygen reserve index – a new, noninvasive method of oxygen reserve measurement. Presented at the American Society of Anesthesiologists Annual Meeting, October 14, 2014, New Orleans, BOC12 (abst)

30. Martin DS, Grocott MP (2013) Oxygen therapy in anaesthesia: the yin and yang of O2. Br J Anaesth 111:867–871

31. Kilgannon JH, Jones AE, Shapiro NI et al (2010) Association between arterial hyperoxia following resuscitation from cardiac arrest and in-hospital mortality. JAMA 303:2165–2171

32. Helmerhorst HJ, Schultz MJ, van der Voort PH, de Jonge E, van Westerloo DJ (2015) Bench-to-bedside review: the effects of hyperoxia during critical illness. Crit Care 19:284

33. Branson RD, Robinson BR (2011) Oxygen: when is more the enemy of good? Intensive Care Med 37:1–3

34. Aggarwal NR, Brower RG (2014) Targeting normoxemia in acute respiratory distress syndrome may cause worse short-term outcomes because of oxygen toxicity. Ann Am Thorac Soc 11:1449–1453

35. Mikkelsen ME, Anderson B, Christie JD, Hopkins RO, Lanken PN (2014) Can we optimize long-term outcomes in acute respiratory distress syndrome by targeting normoxemia? Ann Am Thorac Soc 11:613–618

36. Asfar P, Singer M, Radermacher P (2015) Understanding the benefits and harms of oxygen therapy. Intensive Care Med 41:1118–1121

37. Lauscher P, Mirakaj V, Koenig K, Meier J (2013) Why hyperoxia matters during acute anemia. Minerva Anestesiol 79:643–651

38. de Graaff AE, Dongelmans DA, Binnekade JM, de Jonge E (2011) Clinicians' response to hyperoxia in ventilated patients in a Dutch ICU depends on the level of FiO2. Intensive Care Med 37:46–51

Variable Ventilation from Bench to Bedside

R. Huhle, P. Pelosi, and M. G. de Abreu

Introduction

Biological systems constantly adjust their inner condition according to the external environment in order to achieve a steady state that allows their adaptation to the environment. Healthy biological systems are able to quickly adapt to changing environmental conditions and exhibit intrinsic fluctuations in function within each subsystem, for example the cardiovascular [1] and respiratory [2] systems, during steady-state conditions. In diseased biological systems, however, such intrinsic functional fluctuation (variability) is usually reduced. In fact, reduced variability of the heart rate in patients with coronary heart disease [3], of blood pressure during pre-eclampsia [4], of heart rate and blood pressure during pathological sleep [5], and of respiratory rate and tidal volume in patients with chronic obstructive pulmonary disease (COPD) [6] and prolonged weaning [7] have been documented.

Different from most biological systems, the variability of the respiratory system can be easily influenced in an attempt to improve its function. In controlled, as well as in assisted mechanical ventilation, the variability of tidal volume and/or respiratory rate may be modulated externally by the mechanical ventilator to reproduce certain characteristics of spontaneous breathing in healthy subjects. Because mechanical ventilation represents a common intervention in intensive care and emergency medicine, interest in modes that can enhance the variability of the respiratory pattern has increased in recent years.

R. Huhle · M. G. de Abreu
Pulmonary Engineering Group, Department of Anesthesiology and Intensive Care Medicine, University Hospital Carl Gustav Carus, Technische Universität Dresden
Dresden, Germany

P. Pelosi (✉)
Department of Surgical Sciences and Integrated Diagnostics, IRCCS AOU San Martino IST, University of Genoa
Genoa, Italy
email: ppelosi@hotmail.com

© Springer International Publishing Switzerland 2016
J.-L. Vincent (ed.), *Annual Update in Intensive Care and Emergency Medicine 2016*,
DOI 10.1007/978-3-319-27349-5_23

In this article, we will review the rationale and mechanisms of variable ventilation, and provide a comprehensive review of the literature for both controlled and assisted variable mechanical ventilation. We will focus mainly on the translational aspects that may be relevant for the clinical practice of mechanical ventilation.

Respiratory Variability and Rationale

Physiological breathing patterns are usually highly variable and, to some extent, unpredictable. The variability of a pattern is usually quantified by the coefficient of variation, which is approximately $33 \pm 14.9\%$ of the tidal volume in healthy spontaneous breathing at rest [8]. The importance of variability in the respiratory pattern is partially explained by the anatomical structure of the lung. The airways and the pulmonary circulation are branching trees with a typical fractal structure in the sense that lower airway generations closely resemble higher generations, and small branches of the pulmonary circulation are similar to larger ones [9]. Such a fractal structure maximizes the area for gas exchange and supports irregular gas-mixing in the lower branches [10]. Breath-by-breath variation in tidal volume and respiratory rate contribute to sustain fast state transition, while minimizing the ratio between tissue stress and strain [11]. Interestingly, tidal volume variability in the physiological resting awake state is generally higher than in other physiological states, as for example during non-rapid eye movement sleep [5] and in the diseased state. In patients with restrictive lung disease [6] and in patients with COPD [12], the variability in the tidal volume pattern is reduced to $22 \pm 5\%$ and $25.3 \pm 16.3\%$, respectively.

The basic rationale for variable controlled mechanical ventilation is that the use of a physiological variability in the respiratory pattern, as observed in the healthy resting state, may be beneficial to improve function and reduce damage in the diseased lung.

Modes of Variable Ventilation

For the purposes of this review, a system is considered to be variable/have variability when its input/state/output changes over time. Variability can be regular (or deterministic), irregular, or a combination of the two. Deterministic variability occurs when the output changes in a predictable way, while irregular variability is when the variability follows an unpredictable pattern. Regular variability is usually seen when the pattern of output changes is not complex, as for instance in a sinus wave. Conversely, in irregular variability the pattern of change among levels is complex. For example, tidal breathing has a regular component and an irregular component that changes from cycle to cycle.

Variability of a system can be deterministic (i.e., non-random) when it works according to pre-defined rules without random components and the output of the system can be predicted by these rules. Furthermore, systems can show a hybrid

Fig. 1 Distribution of tidal volumes (V_T) according to power-law (*black*) or Gaussian distribution (*blue*)

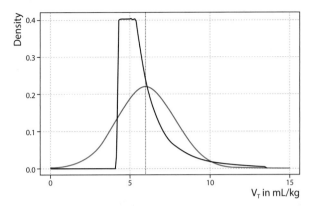

or near-deterministic behavior when both deterministic and stochastic components are present, which is usually the case for biological systems. In respect to variable ventilation, patterns with different distributions have been used: Gaussian distribution being purely stochastic and power-law distributions showing hybrid or near-deterministic behavior (Fig. 1). There have been no direct comparisons of the two patterns in an experimental setting, but both show the same effects when compared to non-variable ventilation.

External variation of tidal volume and/or respiratory rate has been used mainly during controlled mechanical ventilation. Since the first description of variable controlled mechanical ventilation by Lefevre et al. [13], various authors have confirmed that variable controlled mechanical ventilation can improve lung mechanics and arterial oxygenation compared to monotonic, regular controlled ventilation in experimental acute lung injury, although this claim has been challenged. Apart from the benefits in gas exchange, the most striking and common finding during variable controlled mechanical ventilation across different studies is the improvement in lung mechanics. In an experimental model of the acute respiratory distress syndrome (ARDS), variable controlled mechanical ventilation improved lung function compared to the ARDS Network lung protective strategy, as well as the open lung approach [14, 15]. In addition, it has been shown that variable ventilation may also be used during assisted ventilation by means of random variation of pressure support (variable pressure-support ventilation [PSV]) leading to comparable improvements in lung function compared to conventional PSV [16]. Typical signal tracings for flow, volume and airway pressure in variable controlled mechanical ventilation and variable PSV are shown in Fig. 2. Addition of variability to controlled or assisted ventilation modes in general will be referred to as "variable ventilation" throughout this review.

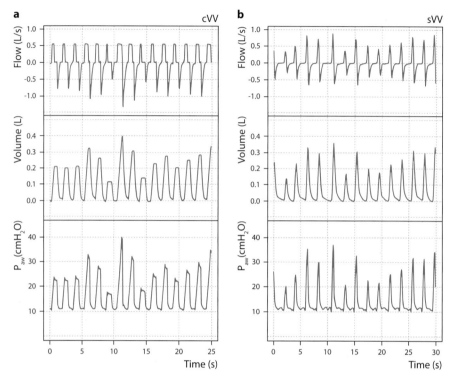

Fig. 2 Signal traces during variable volume controlled ventilation (*cVV*) and variable pressure support ventilation (*sVV*). P_{aw}: airway pressure

Mechanisms of Variable Ventilation

There are two main epiphenomena that underlie improved lung function during variable ventilation:

1. recruitment and stabilization of lung regions contributing to gas exchange; and
2. improvement in ventilation-perfusion matching.

Different macroscopic (respiratory system) and microscopic (alveolar and cell level) mechanisms can explain these epiphenomena (Fig. 3).

Recruitment and Stabilization of Ventilated Lung Regions

One of the most common problems observed in mechanically ventilated lungs is the closure of peripheral airways during expiration. Failure to reopen these airways during inspiration may lead to atelectasis with consequent deterioration of gas exchange and respiratory mechanics. On the other hand, cyclic closing/reopening

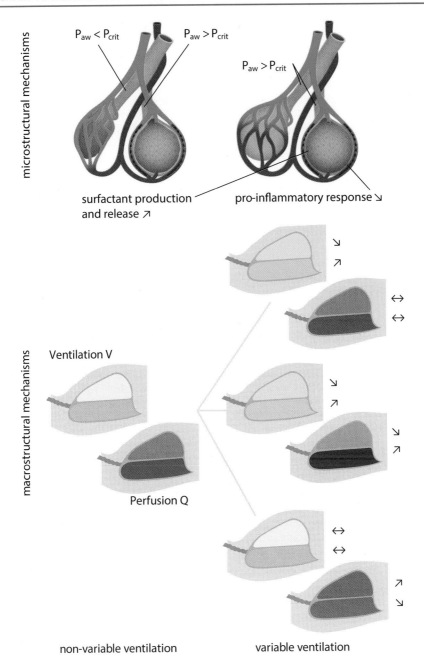

Fig. 3 Microstructural (*top*) and macrostructural (*bottom*) mechanisms of variable ventilation (*right side*) compared to non-variable counter-parts (*left side*), with distribution of perfusion (*red*) and distribution of ventilation (*white*) within the non-dependent (*upper half*) and dependent (*lower half*) parts of the lung; arrows indicate increase ($\nearrow$), decrease ($\searrow$) and unchanged ($\leftrightarrow$) ventilation/perfusion in the respective lung region. P_{aw}: airway pressure; P_{crit}: critical opening pressure. (© Illustration by Peter Ernst)

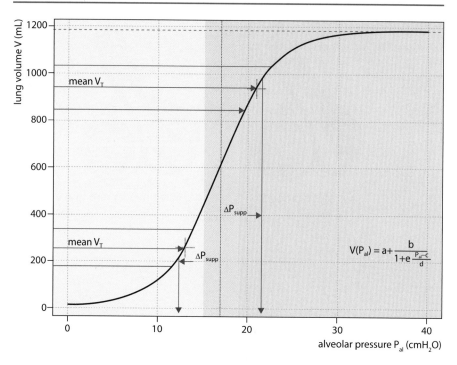

Fig. 4 Advantageous (*blue*) and disadvantageous (*gray*) ranges of alveolar pressure of variable ventilation on a representative static pressure – volume curve described by the Venegas equation with parameters a, b, c and d from [18]. ΔP_{supp}: change in support pressure needed to gain the displayed tidal volume (V_T) in variable ventilation

can increase the shear-stress and trigger the inflammatory response, worsening or leading to lung injury [17].

The beneficial effects of variable ventilation on lung mechanics, especially in acute lung injury, may be explained by the so-called Jensen's theorem [18], which states that on a convex airway pressure versus lung volume relationship (PV curve) the addition of noise to the airway pressure leads to an amplification in the mean tidal volume (also known as Stochastic resonance) [11]. Consequently, during variable ventilation, the driving pressure for a given tidal volume would be theoretically reduced, as shown in Fig. 4. Such a theoretical model, however, also implies that variability could have detrimental effects during mechanical ventilation if high positive end-expiratory pressure (PEEP) is used and/or in more severely injured lungs. In both conditions, ventilation would mainly occur in the zone of the PV curve where variable tidal volumes increase the mean driving pressure. In addition, Jensen's theorem foresees that, in non-injured lungs, variability in tidal volumes would only limit derecruitment, given that no convex portion is present on the PV curve [19].

The amplification of ventilated lung regions is mainly achieved by recruitment of previously collapsed alveoli. Suki et al. [20] showed that once the critical opening pressure (P_{crit}) of collapsed airways/alveoli has been exceeded, all subtended or daughter airways/alveoli with lower P_{crit} will be opened like an avalanche. Since the P_{crit} values of closed airways as well as the time to achieve those values may differ across the lungs, mechanical ventilation patterns that produce different airway pressures and inspiratory times may be advantageous to maximize lung recruitment and stabilization, as compared to regular patterns.

For stabilization of these newly opened lung regions and prevention of collapse during mechanical ventilation of healthy lungs, the production and release of surfactant is crucial [21]. Surfactant release increases exponentially with stretch in alveolar type II cells. Thus, high tidal volume cycles during variable ventilation may stimulate the release of surfactant to a similar or even higher degree than the average increased stretch during conventional mechanical ventilation [22].

Enhanced Ventilation-Perfusion Matching

During variable ventilation, improvement in gas exchange is usually a consequence of enhanced ventilation/perfusion (V/Q) matching, which results either from redistribution of ventilation to perfused areas (reduction of shunt), or redistribution of pulmonary blood flow towards better ventilated lung zones (decreasing dead space). Variable ventilation leads intermittently to airway pressures that exceed the critical opening pressures of single airways in dependent lung zones, resulting in alveolar recruitment in those areas. Following that, aeration and ventilation increase in the dependent lung and, as perfusion shows a prominent gravity-dependent ventral-to-caudal gradient, local and global V/Q matching increase. Perfusion may also accompany the redistribution of ventilation to dependent lung zones, further increasing the V/Q matching.

However, gas exchange may also improve without redistribution of ventilation. It has been suggested that during variable PSV, oxygenation increases despite a lack of improvement of aeration in dependent lung zones. In fact, in experimental models of ARDS, a redistribution of perfusion from dependent to non-dependent lung regions has been observed [23], resulting in enhanced V/Q matching. Therefore, in the presence of preserved hypoxic pulmonary vasoconstriction, a phenomenon of 'capillary recruitment' may occur, shifting perfusion towards the better aerated and ventilated non-dependent lung zones.

Variable Mechanical Ventilation in Experimental Studies (Table 1)

Healthy and Pre-term Lungs

In anesthetized pigs without lung injury, variable controlled mechanical ventilation compared to conventional controlled mechanical ventilation prevented the deterioration in gas exchange that is usually observed during prolonged mechanical ventilation [24].

In pre-term lambs with immature lungs, variable controlled mechanical ventilation compared to conventional controlled mechanical ventilation improved the dynamic respiratory system compliance and reduced the $PaCO_2$ without influencing oxygenation, the protein content in the bronchoalveolar lavage (BAL) fluid, or the gene expression of interleukin (IL)-1β [25].

Similarly, respiratory system elastance increased during conventional mechanical ventilation but to a smaller amount during variable ventilation without significant effects on ventral-dorsal and craniocaudal reduction of aeration or lung tissue cytokine concentrations [26, 27].

Table 1 Effects of variable ventilation compared to conventional ventilation from *in vitro* and *in vivo* experimental models

Endpoint	Effect	Species	Disease model	Type of variable ventilation mode	References
Oxygenation	↗	Porcine/	Healthy	Controlled	[24]
	↗	canine	ARDS (surfactant lavage)	Controlled/ assisted	[15, 16, 28]
	↗		ARDS (oleic acid)	Controlled	[13, 14, 29, 30]
	↗		ARDS (double-hit model[1])	Controlled/ assisted	[31, 32]
	↔		ARDS (oleic acid)	Controlled	[33–35]
	↗	Guinea pig	ARDS (endotoxin induced)	Controlled	[36]
	↗		Healthy	Controlled	[37]
	↔	Rats	Healthy	Controlled	[26]
	↗		ARDS (HCl acid)	Controlled	[27]
	↗	Mice	ARDS (HCl acid)	Controlled	[38]
Aeration	↗	Porcine	ARDS (oleic acid)	Controlled	[33]
	↔		ARDS (surfactant lavage)	Assisted	[39]
Perfusion	↗	Porcine	ARDS (surfactant lavage)	Assisted	[39]
Respiratory system compliance (C_{RS})	↗	Porcine/	Healthy	Controlled	[24]
	↗	canine	ARDS (surfactant lavage)	Controlled/ assisted	[15, 16, 28]
	↗		ARDS (oleic acid)	Controlled	[13, 29, 30, 33, 35]
	↔				[14, 34]
	↗		ARDS (double-hit model[1])	Controlled/ assisted	[31, 32]
	↗	Guinea pig	ARDS (endotoxin induced)	Controlled	[36]
	↔		Healthy		[37]
	↗	Rats	Healthy; ARDS (HCl acid)	Controlled	[26, 27]
	↗	Mice	ARDS (HCl acid)	Controlled	[38]
Surfactant release and production	↗	Guinea pig	None	Controlled	[37]
	↔	Porcine	ARDS (oleic acid)	Controlled	[30]

Table 1 (Continued)

Endpoint	Effect	Species	Disease Model	Type of variable ventilation mode	References
Inflammation	↘	Cell	ARDS (LPS)	Controlled	[40]
	↘	Mice	ARDS (HCl acid)	Controlled	[38]
	↘	Guinea pig	None	Controlled	[37]
	↘	Porcine	ARDS (oleic acid)	Controlled	[14]
	↔		ARDS (oleic acid/surfactant lavage); Bronchospasm	Controlled	[15, 30, 41]
	↔	Lambs	Pre-term	Controlled	[25]
	↔	Porcine	ARDS (surfactant lavage)	Assisted	[23, 32]
Damage (histology)	↘	Porcine	ARDS (surfactant lavage)	Controlled	[15]
	↔		ARDS (oleic acid)		[30]
	↔		ARDS (surfactant lavage)	Assisted	[23, 32]
Resolution of edema	↗↔	Porcine	ARDS (oleic acid)	Controlled	[35]
	↗		ARDS (surfactant lavage)	Assisted	[23, 32]

ARDS: acute respiratory distress syndrome; *LPS*: lipopolysaccharide; *HCl*: hydrochloric

Models of Acute Respiratory Distress Syndrome

Most investigations on variable ventilation have been performed in experimental models of ARDS using different animal species (86% in large animals and 14% in rodents) and injury models (50% oleic acid aspiration, 35% surfactant depletion, 10% hydrochloric (HCl) acid aspiration). However, ARDS models do not reproduce all features of human ARDS. Moreover, the degrees of recruitability, tissue damage and inflammation differ widely among models. Although the saline lung lavage model usually shows the best recruitability and relatively low inflammatory response, HCl acid aspiration typically results in a more heterogeneous injury and less recruitable lung. In this section, the main results of the numerous experimental studies are discussed.

Gas Exchange Effects

Variable controlled mechanical ventilation outperformed conventional controlled mechanical ventilation in terms of arterial oxygenation in 10 out of 12 experimental studies in models of ARDS, including surfactant depletion [15, 28], oleic acid [13, 14, 29, 30, 33] and HCl aspiration [38]. In two studies using oleic acid injury, variable controlled mechanical ventilation did not improve arterial oxygenation compared to conventional controlled mechanical ventilation in mongrel dogs [34] or in pigs [35]. Interestingly, the effects of variable ventilation on arterial oxygenation seem to be dependent on the degree of tidal volume variability. In guinea pigs with lung injury induced by endotoxin, a coefficient of variation of 23–35% in tidal volume maximized arterial oxygenation [36].

Improvements in gas exchange were also shown during variable PSV compared to conventional PSV in pigs with lung injury induced by saline lung lavage [16, 23, 32, 42]. Such effects seem also to depend on the degree of variability of pressure support variability, whereby a coefficient of variation of 30% was associated with the highest levels of arterial oxygenation [42] while for a coefficient of variation > 30% detrimental effects on hemodynamics inhibited a further increase in PaO_2.

Independent of the injury model and also in lung healthy animals, the $PaCO_2$ was reduced during variable ventilation compared to conventional mechanical ventilation when minute ventilation was comparable between groups [23, 24, 28, 37].

Ventilation-Perfusion Matching

In an oleic acid model of ARDS in pigs, total lung volume measured by computed tomography (CT) increased after 4 h of variable ventilation but not with conventional mechanical ventilation [33, 35]. Variable ventilation also resulted in a significant increase in normally aerated, and a decrease in non- and poorly aerated lung tissue. In addition, with variable controlled mechanical ventilation compared to conventional controlled mechanical ventilation, surfactant was simultaneously redistributed towards dorsal regions. Thus, although perfusion was not measured and the regions of recruitment were not reported, an increase in V/Q matching was indicated. Assisted variable ventilation had no effects on recruitment or on redistribution of aeration in a surfactant depletion model when compared to conventional assisted ventilation [16, 39].

In porcine models of lung injury induced by oleic acid [13, 14, 29, 30, 33, 43] and surfactant depletion [15], as well as in healthy lungs [24], variable controlled mechanical ventilation reduced pulmonary shunt. Similarly, venous admixture was reduced in variable PSV but not in conventional PSV [16, 32]. In a model of lung injury induced by oleic acid in pigs [13, 14, 35], variable controlled mechanical ventilation did not importantly influence the dead space, suggesting that shunt reduction is more prominent then reduction of dead space during variable ventilation.

Lung Mechanics

In 10 out of 12 experimental studies [13–15, 27–30, 33–36, 38] in different species and models of ARDS, respiratory system compliance (C_{RS}) was positively influenced by variable controlled mechanical ventilation. There are only two studies, in a porcine oleic acid injury model, in which C_{RS} was not affected positively by variable ventilation [14, 34]. C_{RS} showed a linear dependence on the level of variability, reaching its maximal values at a coefficient of variation = 35% [36]. Respiratory system resistance (R_{RS}) was only improved by variable controlled mechanical ventilation in one [38] of three studies [26, 27, 38] in a rodent acid aspiration model. However, an effect on R_{RS} may only be secondary to recruitment of large portions of the lung (see section on "Mechanisms of variable ventilation" above).

In a porcine surfactant depletion model, variable PSV improved lung mechanics, reducing R_{RS} [32] and increasing C_{RS} [16, 23, 32, 39, 42, 44]. Comparable C_{RS} improved linearly with variability of the support, reaching its maximum at a coefficient of variation of 45% [42].

Surfactant Production and Release

In healthy guinea pigs, variable controlled mechanical ventilation led to an increase in surfactant-associated phospholipid concentration and a decrease in membrane-associated phospholipid concentration compared to conventional controlled mechanical ventilation [37]. In contrast, in oleic acid-injured pigs, variable controlled mechanical ventilation had no positive effects on surfactant surface tension as measured by capillary surfactometry on raw and chloroform/methanol extracted BAL fluid [30].

In non-ARDS lungs, variable controlled mechanical ventilation augmented surfactant secretion, but had no effect on surfactant surface tension in oleic acid injured lungs. Thus, in healthy lungs, but not in injured lungs, surfactant production and release might be an important mechanism to explain the benefits of variable ventilation. However further investigations in different models of experimental ARDS are necessary.

Inflammation and Damage

Inflammation in the lung occurs during ARDS as a consequence of cell injury. Depending on the ventilator strategy, the initial injury may be amplified, mediating pulmonary edema, alveolar disruption and release of cytokines [17]. Thus, a potential means of quantifying the protectiveness of a ventilation mode is the measurement of inflammatory cytokine and mRNA concentrations in BAL fluid and lung tissue, respectively.

In tracheal aspirates from oleic acid-injured pigs, IL-8 concentrations decreased after 5 h of variable controlled mechanical ventilation compared to conventional controlled mechanical ventilation but the investigated pro-inflammatory cytokines, tumor necrosis factor-α (TNF-α) and IL-6, were not measurable in serum or in tracheal aspirates. The concentration of the anti-inflammatory cytokine, IL-10, did not differ between groups in serum or tracheal aspirate samples. In HCl-injured mice, IL-1β levels, as measured by Western Blot Analysis, were significantly higher with conventional controlled mechanical ventilation than in the baseline injury group and with variable ventilation [38]. In guinea pigs after three hours of variable controlled mechanical ventilation, similar results were seen in the concentrations of the pro-inflammatory cytokines TNF-α, IL-6 and monocyte chemoattractant protein-1 (MCP-1) in BAL fluid [37]. TNF-α concentrations were two-fold and ten-fold increased during conventional controlled mechanical ventilation compared with variable controlled mechanical ventilation and unventilated controls, respectively. IL-6 concentrations were increased six-fold and thirty fold in conventional controlled mechanical ventilation compared to variable controlled mechanical ventilation and unventilated controls, respectively, and similarly MCP-1 was increased about three-fold and six-fold in conventional controlled mechanical ventilation compared to variable controlled mechanical ventilation and unventilated controls, respectively.

By contrast, several groups found no differences in the inflammatory response between conventional and variable controlled mechanical ventilation. In an oleic acid injured porcine model, IL-8 concentrations in BAL fluid were similar with conventional and variable controlled mechanical ventilation [30]. In a model of bronchospasm initiated by administration of methacholine aerosol in pigs, there were no differences in the concentrations of IL-6 and IL-10 in BAL fluid with variable compared to conventional controlled mechanical ventilation [41]. In preterm-lambs, there were no differences between conventional and variable controlled mechanical ventilation in total protein content for BAL fluid and mRNA levels of IL1-β or quantitative reverse transcription polymerase chain reaction (qRT-PCR) in lung tissue [25].

In a surfactant depletion model in pigs, gene expression and lung tissue cytokine levels of IL-6, IL-8 and transforming growth factor-β (TGF-β) were not different between variable controlled mechanical ventilation and conventional controlled mechanical ventilation after six hours of therapy [15]. Similarly, in the same injury model, no effects of variable PSV were found on plasma or tissue levels of inflammatory markers compared to PSV [23, 32].

The available literature is not conclusive on the relationship between inflammation and variable controlled mechanical ventilation compared to conventional controlled mechanical ventilation. Although in studies in large animals no differences in pro-inflammatory or anti-inflammatory reactions could be established during ARDS independent of the animal model, studies performed on healthy and HCl-injured rodents suggest a reduced pro-inflammatory response during variable ventilation. However, an *in vitro* study on lipopolysaccharide (LPS)-injured alveolar epithelial L2-cells confirmed a reduction in the inflammatory response, involving the ERK1/2 signaling pathway, suggesting a cellular mechanism, when a variable instead of a constant tidal stretch was applied [40].

There were no differences in lung injury in post-mortem acquired tissue samples of the lung with variable controlled mechanical ventilation compared to conventional controlled mechanical ventilation in oleic acid injury [30], but in a surfactant depletion model variable controlled mechanical ventilation reduced overall tissue damage as assessed by the diffuse alveolar damage (DAD) score when compared to conventional controlled mechanical ventilation [15] and variable controlled mechanical ventilation was also associated with reduced interstitial edema, hemorrhage and epithelial dysfunction in this study. In a porcine oleic acid model, total lung weight and density were reduced with variable controlled mechanical ventilation compared to conventional controlled mechanical ventilation and average alveolar fluid clearance rates were positive compared to negative [35]. However, analysis of corresponding wet:dry ratios of the post-mortem lung showed no effects of variable controlled mechanical ventilation compared to conventional controlled mechanical ventilation in five out of six investigations, independent of the injury model [13, 29, 30, 33, 35, 45]. Consequently, variable controlled mechanical ventilation has only limited effects on edema clearance during ARDS independent of ventilator mode. Comparably, in a surfactant depletion model in pigs, alveolar edema was slightly but significantly reduced in variable PSV compared to conventional PSV [23, 32].

Non-ARDS Models

Variable controlled mechanical ventilation has also been reported to improve lung function in porcine models of severe bronchospasm [41], atelectasis [43] and one-lung ventilation [45]. In each of these models variable controlled mechanical ventilation was associated with increased PaO_2 and C_{RS} and decreased $PaCO_2$ compared to conventional controlled mechanical ventilation. Additionally shunt fraction was reduced by variable controlled mechanical ventilation in the one-lung ventilation and atelectasis models [43, 45], dead space was reduced only in the one-lung ventilation model [45] and R_{RS} only in the asthma model [41]. The results of the study in severe bronchospasm [41] are of special importance as they show that variable controlled mechanical ventilation can improve lung function also in models of secondary atelectasis and can also reduce R_{RS}. This finding can be explained by the excessive critical opening pressures that are potentially even higher in this asthma model than in ARDS models.

Clinical Application of Variable Mechanical Ventilation

Variable ventilation has been studied in only a small number of clinical trials to date, which are summarized below.

Variable Controlled Mechanical Ventilation

Variable controlled mechanical ventilation was first used in a clinical setting by Boker et al. [46] in an open-label, randomized, two-arm, longitudinal perioperative study. Forty-one patients undergoing abdominal aortic aneurysmectomy were ventilated with conventional or variable controlled mechanical ventilation for 6 h during surgery and subsequent recovery. Exclusion criteria were chronic diseases of respiratory and cardiovascular systems, obesity (body mass index [BMI] > 35 kg/m^2), previous thoracic surgery, drug abuse or pregnancy. Anesthesia consisted of propofol, sufentanil and rocuronium, initiated by intravenous bolus doses and infused continuously for six hours with an additional continuous infusion of 0.06 mg/ml bupivacaine and 30 mcg/ml hydromorphone for pain control. Initially ventilator settings were tidal volume 10 ml/kg (ideal body weight), respiratory rate 10 breath/min (adjusted for a $PaCO_2$ target range 35–45 mmHg), zero positive end-inspiratory pressure, I:E ratio of 1:2 and FiO_2 of 0.6. Respiratory mechanics, blood gas and hemodynamics were monitored, analyzed offline and compared. A significant group-time interaction was found for PaO_2 between groups, being increased by approximately 40 mmHg with variable controlled mechanical ventilation at 3, 4 and 5 h of therapy. $PaCO_2$ did not differ between groups as intended by the protocol but the minute ventilation to accomplish this goal was significantly reduced in the variable controlled mechanical ventilation group (8.1 ± 1 vs. 7.7 ± 1.1 l/min). Dead space ventilation was significantly reduced with variable controlled mechanical ventilation compared to conventional controlled mechanical ventilation (group x time effects). Static compliance was significantly increased in the variable ventilation group after three hours (0.54 ± 0.13 vs. 0.62 ± 0.17 ml/cmH$_2$O/kg). This study suggested that variable controlled mechanical ventilation was advantageous for lung function even in healthy lungs during abdominal surgery.

In a pilot cross-over study in eight critically ill patients ventilated for at least 72 h in a postsurgical ICU, oxygen index (PaO$_2$ = 7.1 vs. 11.5 cmH$_2$O/mmHg, p = 0.034) and static lung compliance (0.36 vs. 0.34 ml/cmH$_2$O/kg, p = 0.049) were increased and dead space decreased (0.64 vs. 0.68, p = 0.017) during variable compared with conventional controlled mechanical ventilation. PaCO$_2$ did not differ between the modes of ventilation [47]. Patients had a baseline Horovitz Index of 100–300 mmHg and were randomly selected to begin either with conventional or with variable controlled mechanical ventilation for four hour periods for each mode. Tidal volume was set to 6 ml/kg to comply with the ARDSnet protocol. Respiratory rate and PEEP remained constant. Unfortunately patient anamneses as well as methods to obtain static lung compliance were not reported in detail.

Although the first theoretical framework suggested increased benefits of variable ventilation in damaged lungs with large collapsed and recruitable regions, there are no large study population data available on variable ventilation in a clinical setting in ARDS patients. Clinical studies are currently in progress using variable controlled mechanical ventilation during open-abdominal surgery [48] and in patients with ARDS (ClinicalTrials.gov ID: NCT00202098 and NCT01083277).

Variable Assisted Mechanical Ventilation

In a randomized crossover study performed in 13 ICU patients with acute hypoxemic respiratory failure, variable PSV was not associated with adverse events. Compared to traditional PSV, variable PSV yielded no differences in gas exchange, hemodynamics, or lung mechanics. The reported increase in tidal volume variability ($24.4 \pm 7.8\%$ vs. $13.7 \pm 9.1\%$) during variable PSV was associated with improved patient-ventilator synchrony. The externally increased tidal volume variability mimics the intrinsic healthy variability more closely than can be achieved by the patient through simple on/off triggering during conventional PSV, which may explain the improved patient-ventilator synchrony [49].

Clinical studies using variable PSV during weaning [50], respiratory failure (ClinicalTrials.gov ID: NCT02499276 and NCT01580956) and ARDS (NCT00267241) are being conducted. The results of these investigations will shed further light into the potential applications of this ventilation strategy.

Potential Application of Variable Ventilation

Variable ventilation is probably one of the ventilatory strategies that has undergone most extensive testing in animal models of disease, as well as in small patient series, before being introduced into clinical practice. Such studies have consistently showed that variable controlled mechanical ventilation improves lung function, and reduces or does not worsen lung damage and inflammation compared to non-variable modes. The most promising potential of variable controlled mechanical ventilation is to decrease and prevent deterioration of the mean driving pressure during mechanical ventilation. However, experience with variable controlled mechanical ventilation is so far limited to mild and moderate lung injury, as well as relatively short periods of time. Furthermore, variable controlled mechanical ventilation is not yet commercially available, precluding its clinical use.

In contrast to variable controlled mechanical ventilation, variable PSV is available for clinical use, and preliminary results in small patient series indicate it may improve patient/ventilator synchrony, although its effects on lung function are not as pronounced as those of variable controlled mechanical ventilation. Possible clinical applications of variable PSV include: reduction in the inspiratory work of breathing in patients with increased respiratory drive; improvement in patient/ventilator synchrony in the presence of restrictive lung disease; increase in the variability of the respiratory pattern in patients with reduced intrinsic variability; weaning from the mechanical ventilator.

Conclusion

Variable ventilation enables some aspects of the respiratory pattern of healthy, spontaneously breathing subjects to be mimicked in mechanically ventilated patients. Experimental studies have shown that variable controlled mechanical ventilation improves lung function and reduces damage in mild to moderate lung injury, in the short term. Similar, but less pronounced findings have been reported with variable pressure support ventilation in models of acute lung injury. Initial clinical experience suggests that both variable controlled and variable support ventilation can be safely applied, but not necessarily with improved lung function. Variable PSV is potentially associated with improved patient/ventilator synchrony. Ongoing clinical studies on variable ventilation may contribute to define the role of variable ventilation in the ICU and emergency room.

References

1. Ivanov PC, Amaral LA, Goldberger AL et al (1999) Multifractality in human heartbeat dynamics. Nature 399:461–465
2. Frey U, Silverman M, Barabási AL, Suki B (1998) Irregularities and power law distributions in the breathing pattern in preterm and term infants. J Appl Physiol Bethesda Md 1985(85):789–797
3. Huikuri HV, Mäkikallio TH (2001) Heart rate variability in ischemic heart disease. Auton Neurosci Basic Clin 90:95–101
4. Malberg H, Bauernschmitt R, Voss A et al (2007) Analysis of cardiovascular oscillations: a new approach to the early prediction of pre-eclampsia. Chaos 17:015113

5. Penzel T, Wessel N, Riedl M et al (2007) Cardiovascular and respiratory dynamics during normal and pathological sleep. Chaos 17:015116
6. Brack T, Jubran A, Tobin MJ (2002) Dyspnea and decreased variability of breathing in patients with restrictive lung disease. Am J Respir Crit Care Med 165:1260–1264
7. Wysocki M, Cracco C, Teixeira A et al (2006) Reduced breathing variability as a predictor of unsuccessful patient separation from mechanical ventilation. Crit Care Med 34:2076–2083
8. Tobin MJ, Mador MJ, Guenther SM, Lodato RF, Sackner MA (1988) Variability of resting respiratory drive and timing in healthy subjects. J Appl Physiol 1985(65):309–317
9. Boxt LM, Katz J, Liebovitch LS, Jones R, Esser PD, Reid L (1994) Fractal analysis of pulmonary arteries: the fractal dimension is lower in pulmonary hypertension. J Thorac Imaging 9:8–13
10. Tsuda A, Rogers RA, Hydon PE, Butler JP (2002) Chaotic mixing deep in the lung. Proc Natl Acad Sci USA 99:10173–10178
11. Suki B, Alencar AM, Sujeer MK et al (1998) Life-support system benefits from noise. Nature 393:127–128
12. Loveridge B, West P, Anthonisen NR, Kryger MH (1984) Breathing patterns in patients with chronic obstructive pulmonary disease. Am Rev Respir Dis 130:730–733
13. Lefevre GR, Kowalski SE, Girling LG, Thiessen DB, Mutch WA (1996) Improved arterial oxygenation after oleic acid lung injury in the pig using a computer-controlled mechanical ventilator. Am J Respir Crit Care Med 154:1567–1572
14. Boker A, Graham MR, Walley KR et al (2002) Improved arterial oxygenation with biologically variable or fractal ventilation using low tidal volumes in a porcine model of acute respiratory distress syndrome. Am J Respir Crit Care Med 165:456–462
15. Spieth PM, Carvalho AR, Pelosi P et al (2009) Variable tidal volumes improve lung protective ventilation strategies in experimental lung injury. Am J Respir Crit Care Med 179:684–693
16. de Gama AM, Spieth PM, Pelosi P et al (2008) Noisy pressure support ventilation: a pilot study on a new assisted ventilation mode in experimental lung injury. Crit Care Med 36:818–827
17. Slutsky AS, Ranieri VM (2013) Ventilator-induced lung injury. N Engl J Med 369:2126–2136
18. Venegas JG, Harris RS, Simon BA (1998) A comprehensive equation for the pulmonary pressure-volume curve. J Appl Physiol Bethesda Md 1985(84):389–395
19. Runck H, Schumann S, Tacke S, Haberstroh J, Guttmann J (2012) Time-dependent recruitment effects in ventilated healthy and lung-injured rats: "recruitment-memory". Respir Physiol Neurobiol 184:65–72
20. Suki B, Barabási AL, Hantos Z, Peták F, Stanley HE (1994) Avalanches and power-law behaviour in lung inflation. Nature 368:615–618
21. Lutz D, Gazdhar A, Lopez-Rodriguez E et al (2015) Alveolar derecruitment and collapse induration as crucial mechanisms in lung injury and fibrosis. Am J Respir Cell Mol Biol 52:232–243
22. Wirtz HR, Dobbs LG (1990) Calcium mobilization and exocytosis after one mechanical stretch of lung epithelial cells. Science 250:1266–1269
23. Spieth PM, Carvalho AR, Güldner A et al (2011) Pressure support improves oxygenation and lung protection compared to pressure-controlled ventilation and is further improved by random variation of pressure support. Crit Care Med 39:746–755
24. Mutch WA, Eschun GM, Kowalski SE, Graham MR, Girling LG, Lefevre GR (2000) Biologically variable ventilation prevents deterioration of gas exchange during prolonged anaesthesia. Br J Anaesth 84:197–203
25. Pillow JJ, Musk GC, McLean CM et al (2011) Variable ventilation improves ventilation and lung compliance in preterm lambs. Intensive Care Med 37:1352–1359
26. Camilo LM, Ávila MB, Cruz LFS et al (2014) Positive end-expiratory pressure and variable ventilation in lung-healthy rats under general anesthesia. PLoS ONE 9:e110817

27. Spieth PM, Bluth T, Hegeman MA et al (2013) Mechanical ventilation with variable tidal volumes in a rodent model of acute acid aspiration. Am J Respir Crit care Med Meeting Abstracts 187:A1118 (abst)

28. Bellardine CL, Hoffman AM, Tsai L et al (2006) Comparison of variable and conventional ventilation in a sheep saline lavage lung injury model. Crit Care Med 34:439–445

29. Mutch WA, Harms S, Lefevre GR, Graham MR, Girling LG, Kowalski SE (2000) Biologically variable ventilation increases arterial oxygenation over that seen with positive end-expiratory pressure alone in a porcine model of acute respiratory distress syndrome. Crit Care Med 28:2457–2464

30. Funk DJ, Graham MR, Girling LG et al (2004) A comparison of biologically variable ventilation to recruitment manoeuvres in a porcine model of acute lung injury. Respir Res 5:22

31. Güldner A, Beda A, Kiss T et al (2012) Effects of random and pseudo-random variable ventilation on lung function in experimental lung injury. Am J Respir Crit Care Med 185:A5442 (abst)

32. Spieth PM, Güldner A, Beda A et al (2012) Comparative effects of proportional assist and variable pressure support ventilation on lung function and damage in experimental lung injury. Crit Care Med 40:2654–2661

33. Graham MR, Goertzen AL, Girling LG et al (2011) Quantitative computed tomography in porcine lung injury with variable versus conventional ventilation: recruitment and surfactant replacement. Crit Care Med 39:1721–1730

34. Nam AJ, Brower RG, Fessler HE, Simon BA (2000) Biologic variability in mechanical ventilation rate and tidal volume does not improve oxygenation or lung mechanics in canine oleic acid lung injury. Am J Respir Crit Care Med 161:1797–1804

35. Graham MR, Gulati H, Kha L, Girling LG, Goertzen A, Mutch WAC (2011) Resolution of pulmonary edema with variable mechanical ventilation in a porcine model of acute lung injury. Can J Anaesth 58:740–750

36. Arold SP, Mora R, Lutchen KR, Ingenito EP, Suki B (2002) Variable tidal volume ventilation improves lung mechanics and gas exchange in a rodent model of acute lung injury. Am J Respir Crit Care Med 165:366–371

37. Arold SP, Suki B, Alencar AM, Lutchen KR, Ingenito EP (2003) Variable ventilation induces endogenous surfactant release in normal guinea pigs. Am J Physiol Lung Cell Mol Physiol 285:L370–L375

38. Thammanomai A, Hamakawa H, Bartolák-Suki E, Suki B (2013) Combined effects of ventilation mode and positive end-expiratory pressure on mechanics, gas exchange and the epithelium in mice with acute lung injury. PloS One 8:e53934

39. Carvalho AR, Spieth PM, Güldner A et al (2011) Distribution of regional lung aeration and perfusion during conventional and noisy pressure support ventilation in experimental lung injury. J Appl Physiol 110(1985):1083–1092

40. Rentzsch I, Santos CL, Huhle R et al (2015) Variable cell stretch reduces the release of CXCL-2 by LPS-stimulated L2 cells via the ERK1/2-pathway. Am J Respir Crit Care Med 191:A2042 (abst)

41. Mutch WAC, Buchman TG, Girling LG, Walker EK-Y, McManus BM, Graham MR (2007) Biologically variable ventilation improves gas exchange and respiratory mechanics in a model of severe bronchospasm. Crit Care Med 35:1749–1755

42. Spieth PM, Carvalho AR, Güldner A et al (2009) Effects of different levels of pressure support variability in experimental lung injury. Anesthesiology 110:342–350

43. Mutch WAC, Harms S, Graham RM, Kowalski SE, Girling LG, Lefevre GR (2000) Biologically variable or naturally noisy mechanical ventilation recruits atelectatic lung. Am J Respir Crit Care Med 162:319–323

44. Beda A, Güldner A, Simpson DM et al (2012) Effects of assisted and variable mechanical ventilation on cardiorespiratory interactions in anesthetized pigs. Physiol Meas 33:503–519

45. McMullen MC, Girling LG, Graham MR, Mutch WAC (2006) Biologically variable ventilation improves oxygenation and respiratory mechanics during one-lung ventilation. Anesthesiology 105:91–97
46. Boker A, Haberman CJ, Girling L et al (2004) Variable ventilation improves perioperative lung function in patients undergoing abdominal aortic aneurysmectomy. Anesthesiology 100:608–616
47. Kowalski S, McMullen MC, Girling LG, McCarthy BG (2013) Biologically variable ventilation in patients with acute lung injury: a pilot study. Can J Anaesth 60:502–503
48. Spieth PM, Güldner A, Uhlig C et al (2014) Variable versus conventional lung protective mechanical ventilation during open abdominal surgery: study protocol for a randomized controlled trial. Trials 15:155–155
49. Spieth PM, Güldner A, Huhle R et al (2013) Short-term effects of noisy pressure support ventilation in patients with acute hypoxemic respiratory failure. Crit Care 17:R261
50. Kiss T, Güldner A, Bluth T et al (2013) Rationale and study design of ViPS – variable pressure support for weaning from mechanical ventilation: study protocol for an international multicenter randomized controlled open trial. Trials 14:363–363

Monitoring Respiratory Effort by Means of the Electrical Activity of the Diaphragm

G. Grasselli, M. Pozzi, and G. Bellani

Introduction

During mechanical ventilation, preservation of a patient's spontaneous breathing is allowed by several ventilatory modalities, such as volume or pressure assist-control, synchronized intermittent mandatory ventilation (SIMV), pressure support ventilation (PSV), proportionally-assisted ventilation and neurally-adjusted ventilator assist (NAVA). With these modalities there is a continuous interaction between the patient's respiratory muscles, which generate negative and positive pressures (P_{mus}) and the ventilator, which controls airway pressure and flow [1]. Two main aspects of the interaction between the patient and the ventilator need to be considered: synchrony in the timing of inspiration and expiration, and the division of the work of breathing between the ventilator and the patient. Both asynchrony [2] and inadequate (too high or too low) workload can be detrimental [3]. For example, it is well known that patient-ventilator dyssynchrony is associated with discomfort, sleep disruption, increased duration of mechanical ventilation and prolonged intensive care unit (ICU) length of stay [2, 4]. Patient-ventilator dyssynchrony represents a serious clinical problem: 25% of invasively ventilated patients and more than 40%

G. Grasselli
Department of Emergency Medicine, San Gerardo Hospital
Monza, Italy

M. Pozzi
Department of Emergency Medicine, San Gerardo Hospital
Monza, Italy
School of Medicine and Surgery, University of Milan-Bicocca
Monza, Italy

G. Bellani (✉)
School of Medicine and Surgery, University of Milan-Bicocca
Monza, Italy
Department of Emergency Medicine, San Gerardo Hospital
Monza, Italy
email: giacomo.bellani1@unimib.it

© Springer International Publishing Switzerland 2016
J.-L. Vincent (ed.), *Annual Update in Intensive Care and Emergency Medicine 2016*,
DOI 10.1007/978-3-319-27349-5_24

of those assisted with non-invasive ventilation (NIV) have a high incidence of asynchronies (indicated by an asynchrony index > 10%). In a recent prospective trial in 50 patients, asynchronies were detected in all subjects and those with an asynchrony index ≥ 10% had higher ICU and hospital mortality [5].

Applying correct ventilator settings during an assisted modality of mechanical ventilation represent a real challenge for clinicians: while airway pressure and flow tracings are readily displayed at the bedside, monitoring the patient's activity is less straightforward. The standard technique is to use esophageal pressure (P_{es}), which, mirroring pleural pressure swings, is very sensitive in detecting P_{mus} [6]. Unfortunately this technique is seldom applied in routine clinical practice: although the invasiveness of an esophageal pressure catheter is minimal (particularly in critically ill patients), obtaining reliable P_{es} waveforms and interpreting them at the bedside can be quite demanding. For this reason, several other methods, which circumvent the use of P_{es} have been described [7], the $P_{0.1}$ (i.e., the airway pressure decrease in the first 100 msec against an occluded airway) probably being one of the more robust and widely used [7]. More recently, some investigators have demonstrated the reliability of ultrasound-based evaluation of the diaphragm in quantifying the breathing effort [8].

Electromyography (EMG) of the diaphragm (and of other respiratory muscles) and its tight relationship with the mechanical activity of the muscle has been known about in classical physiology for several decades [9]. Only recently, however, has the availability of diaphragm EMG at the bedside, mainly with the aim of driving the ventilator during NAVA [10], led to a reappraisal of this technique as a routine monitoring tool.

What Is EAdi?

Control of breathing is an extremely complex and tightly regulated process. Briefly, the output of the brainstem breathing centers is transmitted to the diaphragm through the phrenic nerve. Diaphragm contraction generates a negative intrathoracic pressure which, in turn, generates an inspiratory flow of air to the lungs leading to lung inflation. By contrast, expiration is mainly a passive process. Breathing activity is strictly controlled through feedback loops originating from mechanical, chemical and cortical afferent signals and integrated at the level of the brainstem breathing centers [11].

Diaphragm fibers contract in response to an electrical stimulus originating from the respiratory motoneurons: transmission of this signal to the neuromuscular junctions generates an action potential that propagates along the diaphragm myofibers and leads to their contraction. The term diaphragm EMG or diaphragm electrical activity (EAdi) indicates the summation in time and space of action potentials from the recruited diaphragm motor units [12].

It is important to refute a common misconception: EAdi represents the output of the respiratory centers (respiratory drive) and not diaphragm contractility. For this reason, the amplitude of the signal is not indicative of the force generated by diaphragm contraction, but only of the number of muscle fibers recruited to generate a certain amount of force: the higher the EAdi, the higher the number of diaphragm fibers that are contracting in response to the nervous stimulus, but this can translate into very different P_{mus} values, as highlighted below.

In recent years, a simple and reliable method to acquire and monitor the EAdi signal at the bedside has become available for clinical use. It consists of a modified nasogastric tube (EAdi catheter) equipped with several microelectrodes that acquire the electrical activity from a sample of crural diaphragmatic motor units. The signal is then integrated, filtered to remove noise and electrocardiogram (EKG) interference, and displayed on the screen of the ventilator for continuous real-time monitoring of the patient's EAdi.

The catheter is inserted exactly like a standard nasogastric tube and can be used for enteral feeding. Correct positioning of the catheter, which is crucial to obtain a stable and reliable EAdi signal, is controlled through a dedicated window of the ventilator according to the manufacturer's instructions [13]. The signal is expressed in microvolts (μV); in healthy humans, it usually ranges from 0 to 10 μV, but with huge inter- and intra-individual variability [11].

In the last two decades, considerable experimental work has been done in animal models and in humans to confirm the reliability of EAdi monitoring. Some important experiments demonstrated that the electrical activity of the crural portion of the diaphragm was related to global diaphragm activation expressed by the transdiaphragmatic pressure (P_{di}) [14]. This relationship is not artifactually influenced by changes in chest wall configuration, lung volume [14] or inspiratory flow [15] and is also maintained in mechanically ventilated patients with acute respiratory failure [16].

Since global diaphragm activation is an expression of respiratory drive, it follows that recording the EAdi signal may be a sensitive and reliable method to monitor a patient's neural respiratory drive. To this end, it is worth citing the important work by Lourenco et al. who studied the nervous output from the respiratory centers in dogs with obstructed breathing. They recorded phrenic nerve activity and the EAdi (obtained with needles inserted in the muscle fibers and with esophageal electrodes) and observed that during severe inspiratory loading, tidal volume decreased while phrenic nerve and diaphragm activity increased in parallel. They concluded that minute ventilation does not measure the nervous output from respiratory centers, which is instead reliably measured by phrenic nerve activity or EAdi [17]. These findings were confirmed by Sinderby et al., who studied diaphragm EMG and pressure generation during breathing at rest in healthy subjects and in patients with obstructive or restrictive (post-polio infection) respiratory failure: they observed that chronic obstructive pulmonary disease (COPD) and polio patients had significantly increased diaphragm activation compared to healthy subjects [18]. Similarly, Beck et al. showed that in mechanically ventilated patients with acute respiratory failure, increasing the level of pressure support (and consequently decreasing patient effort) was associated with a progressive decrease in EAdi [16].

From this discussion it should be clear that when an increase in EAdi signal amplitude is observed in a patient, one of the following causes should be hypothesized:

(a) increased central respiratory drive (e.g., due to agitation, pain, fever);
(b) increased mechanical load (elastic or resistive) imposed on the respiratory system;
(c) reduced efficiency of diaphragm contraction: paradoxically, a higher EAdi may indicate that the muscle is becoming weaker (i.e., generates less force per unit of electrical activity) and consequently more fibers need to be recruited to generate a certain amount of mechanical work.

Monitoring Patient-Ventilator Interaction and Dynamic Hyperinflation

The use of assisted modes of mechanical ventilation is becoming increasingly popular, not only during weaning from mechanical ventilation but also in the early, acute phases of respiratory failure. As stated, it is of paramount importance to maintain a good interaction between the patient and the ventilator.

It is now widely accepted that EAdi monitoring is a very sensitive and reliable method to assess breathing pattern and detect asynchronies during mechanical ventilation. In 2011, Colombo et al. found that visual inspection of ventilator pressure and flow waveforms significantly underestimated the prevalence of asynchronies and showed that adding EAdi signal examination significantly improved the recognition of asynchronies; in addition, EAdi is superior to other pneumatic signals reflecting patient effort (such as esophageal or transdiaphragmatic pressure) since it is not affected by altered neuromechanical coupling [19]. Moreover, unlike pneumatic signals, EAdi allows a direct and precise assessment of neural inspiratory time, a parameter of crucial importance to study the interaction between the patient and the ventilator [20]. To improve physicians' ability to detect asynchronies, a new automated and standardized index of patient-ventilator interaction (called the NeuroSync index) has recently been proposed that seems to be more sensitive than the standard manual analysis [21].

We recently demonstrated that these concepts can be applied in clinical practice. We evaluated patient-ventilator interaction in 10 patients with acute respiratory distress syndrome (ARDS) with very low respiratory system compliance, undergoing extracorporeal membrane oxygenation (ECMO) and two different modes of assisted mechanical ventilation (PSV and NAVA). EAdi was monitored continuously and an EAdi-based asynchrony index (AI_{EAdi}) was calculated during both ventilatory modes. The AI_{EAdi} index was defined as the number of flow-, pressure- and EAdi-based asynchrony events divided by the patient's EAdi-based neural respiratory rate. Four different asynchronies were identified, namely ineffective triggering, double triggering, auto-triggering and premature cycling; in addition, EAdi monitoring allows measurement of inspiratory trigger delay and cycle off time for detection of expiratory asynchronies (early cycle off). We observed that AI_{EAdi}

was correlated with neural inspiratory time and cycle off time but not with trigger delay; patient ventilator interaction was significantly improved, although suboptimal, during NAVA compared to PSV (mean AI_{EAdi} 20% vs 74%, respectively) [22].

EAdi monitoring allows the easy identification of a frequently unrecognized form of asynchrony called 'reverse triggering', consisting of diaphragmatic contraction triggered by ventilator insufflations (ventilator-triggered muscular efforts). In eight heavily sedated patients with ARDS ventilated with an assist-control mode, Akoumianaki et al. observed a relatively high frequency of reverse-triggered breaths with a varying entrainment ratio and concluded that this phenomenon may have important clinical consequences, including increased respiratory muscle work and generation of excessive tidal volumes and transpulmonary pressure swings during assist-control modes [23].

Finally, a clinically valuable application of EAdi monitoring has recently been proposed by Bellani et al., who demonstrated that EAdi can be used to estimate intrinsic positive end-expiratory pressure (PEEP) during assisted ventilation [24]. Auto-PEEP may substantially increase patient effort and work of breathing and significantly worsen patient-ventilator interaction by reducing the ventilator's efficiency to detect an inspiratory effort. In 10 patients with dynamic hyperinflation, the value of EAdi at the onset of inspiratory flow (called auto-EAdi) was tightly correlated with auto-PEEP measured with P_{es} (i.e., the decrease in esophageal pressure required to generate an inspiratory flow) during both NAVA and PSV. The product of auto-EAdi × P_{mus}/EAdi index (see next paragraph) gave a value of EAdi-based auto-PEEP (auto-$PEEP_{EAdi}$), which was a clinically acceptable estimate of intrinsic PEEP measured with P_{es}. The study demonstrated that monitoring auto-EAdi is a reliable bedside method to detect the presence of auto-PEEP and to quantify it [24].

Monitoring Inspiratory Muscle Pressure and Work of Breathing

As already mentioned, when setting the ventilator it is very important to avoid under-assistance (which is associated with muscular exhaustion and fatigue) and over-assistance (which in turn is associated with a high incidence of missed efforts and disuse atrophy of the diaphragm) [3]. EAdi monitoring may significantly improve our ability to select the appropriate level of assist for each patient. For example, it is not uncommon to observe a complete disappearance of the EAdi signal in patients on very high levels of pressure support: this is indicative of an excessive level of assist with complete suppression of diaphragm activity, exactly the same as during fully controlled modes of ventilation. On the other hand, a progressive increase in EAdi level over time may indicate that the ventilatory support is insufficient, suggesting that the respiratory muscles are not sufficiently unloaded and may be unable to sustain the work of breathing.

A clinical application of these concepts has been presented by Rozé et al., who proposed an EAdi-based method to titrate the level of ventilatory assist during NAVA: in 15 patients, the maximum EAdi was assessed by means of a spontaneous breathing trial (EAdi$_{maxSBT}$) and then the NAVA level was adjusted to obtain an EAdi of about 60% of the EAdi$_{maxSBT}$. The procedure was repeated every day during the weaning phase, allowing a progressive reduction of the NAVA level until extubation [25]. It is important to underline that this method can theoretically be applied during any assisted ventilation mode and not only during NAVA.

EAdi monitoring has also been applied during weaning. Comparison of two groups of patients who failed or succeeded an SBT showed that the first group had a higher EAdi peak and integral at baseline and at any time point during the trial, likely indicating a higher breathing effort [26]. Similar findings were reported by Barwing et al., who found a greater increase in peak inspiratory EAdi in patients failing a SBT, again suggesting the role of EAdi as a reliable monitoring tool for breathing effort [27]. Moreover, Muttini et al. demonstrated that additional information on a patient's ability to sustain a weaning trial can be disclosed from the ratio between the peak EAdi and its integral: in each subject this ratio was constant, independent of the level of assistance, but it clearly differentiated the weaning success and failure groups [28].

Using a different approach, Grasselli et al. used the EAdi signal to calculate the patient-ventilator breath contribution (PVBC) index [29]. The index is obtained by suddenly reducing to zero (i.e., to continuous positive airway pressure [CPAP]) the level of assist for a single breath: if the patient's effort remains unchanged between the unassisted and assisted breath, the ratio of the two tidal volumes should reflect the relative contribution of the patient and the ventilator to the inspiratory volume. Since this is unlikely, the authors divided each tidal volume (V_T) for the respective peak EAdi and calculated the index as follows:

$$PVBC = (V_{Tno\text{-}assist}/EAdi_{no\text{-}assist})/(V_{Tassist}/EAdi_{assist}).$$

A PVBC index close to 1 indicates that the patient is generating the tidal volume almost entirely, whereas a PVBC index close to zero indicates that the ventilator is mostly contributing. This index was evaluated in an animal model, showing a tight correlation with the P_{es} swings [29]; more recently it has also been validated in patients with acute respiratory failure [30].

Our group has presented a method which enables the direct conversion of EAdi into P_{mus}, then allowing the calculation of the derived indexes of work of breathing, such as the pressure-time product [31]. This approach relies on the described linear relationship between EAdi and the pressure generated by the diaphragm. However, this relationship is different in different patients: for example, an EAdi swing of $10\,\mu V$ can correspond to a P_{mus} of $5\,cmH_2O$ in one patient and to a P_{mus} of $20\,cmH_2O$ in another, with obviously different effects on transpulmonary pressure. If a brief expiratory hold is performed, it is possible to measure the airway pressure drop (which, in the absence of flow, will equal P_{mus}) and the corresponding EAdi necessary to generate this P_{mus} (Fig. 1). The ratio between these two entities, $P_{mus}/EAdi$ ($P_{mus}/EAdi$ index or "PEI"), has dimensions of $cmH_2O/\mu V$ and indicates how much pressure (in cmH_2O) the respiratory muscles of the patients are generating for each μV of electrical activity. During the ensuing tidal ventilation, the PEI

Fig. 1 During an expiratory occlusion, hence in the absence of flow, the pressure generated by the inspiratory muscles causes a decrease in airway pressure (P_{aw}), which is then divided by the corresponding electrical activity of the diaphragm (EAdi). This allows calculation of the ratio of inspiratory muscle pressure (P_{mus}) to EAdi, giving the P_{mus}/EAdi index (PEI)

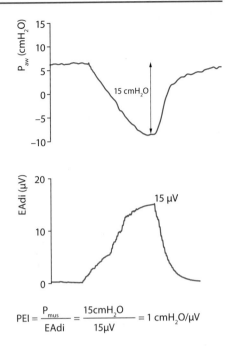

$$PEI = \frac{P_{mus}}{EAdi} = \frac{15 cmH_2O}{15\mu V} = 1 \, cmH_2O/\mu V$$

serves as a conversion factor between μV and cmH_2O (according to the formula $P_{mus} = EAdi * PEI / 1.5$) thus allowing a continuous and reliable estimate of patient P_{mus}. The 1.5 correction is necessary since, in the presence of flow, the diaphragm generates less pressure for the same EAdi than during an occlusion. Since, at variance from EAdi, which monitors only the diaphragm, P_{mus} would be affected by other accessory muscles, one could expect that, for lower levels of assistance, if accessory muscles are recruited, PEI might increase (greater P_{mus} for the same EAdi). However, this was not the case as PEI remained substantially stable across a large spectrum of assistance levels [31].

Monitoring by Surface Electromyography

Despite being the main inspiratory muscle, the diaphragm is not the only muscle activated during breathing. Respiratory activity is distributed among different chest wall and upper airway muscles, with a tempo-spatial pattern (i.e., which muscles are recruited and in which order) that varies according to muscle fatigue, inspiratory load, posture and intrinsic neuromechanical advantage of different muscle groups [32]. Furthermore, passive expiration can become active through the activation of expiratory muscles (such as internal intercostals and the abdominal wall muscles) [33, 34]. EMG with surface electrodes attached to the skin (sEMG) has been proposed as a promising technique to provide a reliable and non-invasive measurement of the electrical activity not only of the diaphragm but also of extradiaphragmatic muscles. Previous studies on respiratory muscle sEMG in healthy volunteers found a correlation between the electrical activity of extradiaphragmatic muscles and the respiratory load [35–38].

As stated above, adequate unloading of respiratory muscles is of paramount importance during assisted ventilation modes and especially during weaning from mechanical ventilation. In this scenario, accessory muscle monitoring can provide useful information to titrate ventilatory support level and to detect respiratory muscle fatigue. Early insights into the response of accessory muscles to ventilatory loading or unloading were provided by Brochard et al. [39], who studied the electrical activity from diaphragm and sternocleidomastoid muscles in a population of long-term ventilated and difficult-to-wean patients. For each subject they identified the "optimal" level of ventilatory support that allowed the patient to breath without developing diaphragmatic "electrical" fatigue, defined with power spectrum EMG criteria. The sternocleidomastoid sEMG signal progressively decreased at increasing support levels until the "optimal" assist level was reached, without any further reduction at higher levels of ventilatory assistance [39]. Recently, similar results were published by Schmidt et al. who studied sEMG inspiratory activity from accessory muscles (alae nasi, scalene and sternocleidomastoid muscles) in 12 intubated patients on assisted ventilation. Accessory muscle activity was significantly lowered by increasing assist level and was strongly correlated with the intensity of

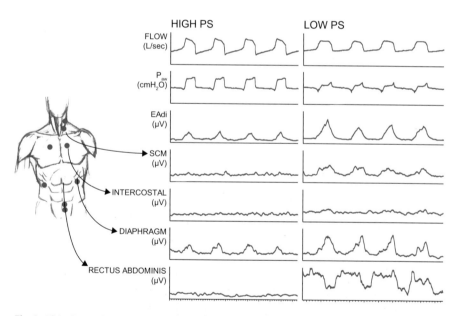

Fig. 2 This figure shows the feasibility of monitoring electrical activity of the diaphragm (EAdi) using surface electromyography (EAdi recorded from nasogastric tube serves as reference). A decrease in assistance by the ventilator leads to an increase in diaphragmatic activity and to the recruitment of accessory muscles. *SCM*: sternocleidomastoid; *PS*: pressure support; P_{aw}: airway pressure

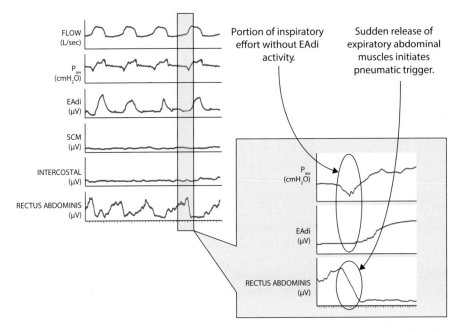

Fig. 3 In this patient, pneumatic trigger of the ventilator occurs earlier than the electrical activity of the diaphragm onset. This finding, consistent over several consecutive breaths, is likely due to the sudden release of expiratory muscles. *SCM*: sternocleidomastoid; P_{aw}: airway pressure

dyspnea experienced by the subjects [40]. In a population of 12 ICU patients on assisted ventilation, Cecchini et al. recently observed comparable effects of NAVA and PSV on reduction of scalene and alae nasi muscle activity. By contrast, for each level of assistance, the ratio between accessory muscle EA and EAdi was significantly lower with NAVA, which probably improved diaphragm efficiency allowing a further unloading of accessory musculature [41].

Looking at sEMG traces can also provide interesting new insight into patient-ventilator interaction as shown in Figs. 2 and 3. For example a decrease in ventilatory assistance can induce a prompt recruitment of accessory muscles (Fig. 2). Furthermore, the possibility to detect activity from expiratory muscles can provide a new point of view into the 'dogma' of normally passive expiration to the point that pneumatic triggering of the ventilator is achieved by the patient by releasing the expiratory muscles (Fig. 3).

It is worth noting that clinical application of respiratory muscle sEMG faces some technical issues. First, we must remember that the ICU environment is very different from that of an EMG lab, with considerable electrical pollution from non-removable devices and poor patient collaboration; in addition, correct electrode placement can be difficult because of surgical dressings or medical devices. Beyond the obvious need to remove movement and EKG artifacts, noise reduction and cross-talk recognition (e.g., an electrical signal coming from a muscle different from the one below the electrodes) require adequate data processing and trace interpretation. In addition, electrode positioning needs standardization and must take into account muscle edges (to limit cross-talk), orientation and anatomy.

Conclusion

Growing interest in the role of spontaneous breathing and assisted ventilatory modes during the treatment of patients with acute respiratory failure [42] has dramatically highlighted the need for instruments to monitor breathing effort. Although P_{es} represents the standard technique, recent technological advances have led to the introduction in the clinical arena of other tools, including EMG of the diaphragm (and of accessory muscles), from the surface. This signal allows continuous 'qualitative' monitoring of patient-ventilator synchrony, but can also be converted to pressure units, enabling the absolute value of P_{mus} to be quantitated. While robust literature data demonstrate that reduction in asynchronies improves patient outcome, more clinical research is needed to understand better what part of the work of breathing the patient should bear, while the remaining part is relieved by the ventilator.

References

1. Grinnan DC, Truwit JD (2005) Clinical review: respiratory mechanics in spontaneous and assisted ventilation. Crit Care 9:472–484
2. Gilstrap D, MacIntyre N (2013) Patient-ventilator interactions. Implications for clinical management. Am J Respir Crit Care Med 188:1058–1068
3. Saddy F, Sutherasan Y, Rocco PR, Pelosi P (2014) Ventilator-associated lung injury during assisted mechanical ventilation. Semin Respir Crit Care Med 35:409–417
4. Thille AW, Rodriguez P, Cabello B, Lellouche F, Brochard L (2006) Patient-ventilator asynchrony during assisted mechanical ventilation. Intensive Care Med 32:1515–1522
5. Blanch L, Villagra A, Sales B et al (2015) Asynchronies during mechanical ventilation are associated with mortality. Intensive Care Med 41:633–641
6. Akoumianaki E, Maggiore SM, Valenza F et al (2014) The application of esophageal pressure measurement in patients with respiratory failure. Am J Respir Crit Care Med 189:520–531
7. Bellani G, Pesenti A (2014) Assessing effort and work of breathing. Curr Opin Crit Care 20:352–358
8. Vivier E, Mekontso DA, Dimassi S et al (2012) Diaphragm ultrasonography to estimate the work of breathing during non-invasive ventilation. Intensive Care Med 38:796–803
9. Eldridge FL (1975) Relationship between respiratory nerve and muscle activity and muscle force output. J Appl Physiol 39:567–574
10. Terzi N, Piquilloud L, Roze H et al (2012) Clinical review: Update on neurally adjusted ventilatory assist – report of a round-table conference. Crit Care 16:225
11. Sinderby C, Beck J (2008) Proportional assist ventilation and neurally adjusted ventilatory assist – better approaches to patient ventilator synchrony? Clin Chest Med 29:329–342
12. Sinderby C, Navalesi P, Beck J et al (1999) Neural control of mechanical ventilation in respiratory failure. Nature Med 5:1433–1436

13. Barwing J, Ambold M, Linden N, Quintel M, Moerer O (2009) Evaluation of the catheter positioning for neurally adjusted ventilatory assist. Intensive Care Med 35:1809–1814
14. Beck J, Sinderby C, Lindstrom L, Grassino A (1998) Effects of lung volume on diaphragm EMG signal strength during voluntary contractions. J Appl Physiol (1985) 85:1123–1134
15. Beck J, Sinderby C, Lindstrom L, Grassino A (1998) Crural diaphragm activation during dynamic contractions at various inspiratory flow rates. J Appl Physiol (1985) 85:451–458
16. Beck J, Gottfried SB, Navalesi P et al (2001) Electrical activity of the diaphragm during pressure support ventilation in acute respiratory failure. Am J Respir Crit Care Med 164:419–424
17. Lourenco RV, Cherniack NS, Malm JR, Fishman AP (1966) Nervous output from the respiratory center during obstructed breathing. J Appl Physiol 21:527–533
18. Sinderby C, Beck J, Spahija J, Weinberg J, Grassino A (1998) Voluntary activation of the human diaphragm in health and disease. J Appl Physiol (1985) 85:2146–2158
19. Colombo D, Cammarota G, Alemani M et al (2011) Efficacy of ventilator waveforms observation in detecting patient-ventilator asynchrony. Crit Care Med 39:2452–2457
20. Parthasarathy S, Jubran A, Tobin MJ (2000) Assessment of neural inspiratory time in ventilator-supported patients. Am J Respir Crit Care Med 162:546–552
21. Sinderby C, Liu S, Colombo D et al (2013) An automated and standardized neural index to quantify patient-ventilator interaction. Crit Care 17:R239
22. Mauri T, Bellani G, Grasselli G et al (2013) Patient-ventilator interaction in ARDS patients with extremely low compliance undergoing ECMO: a novel approach based on diaphragm electrical activity. Intensive Care Med 39:282–291
23. Akoumianaki E, Lyazidi A, Rey N et al (2013) Mechanical ventilation-induced reverse-triggered breaths: a frequently unrecognized form of neuromechanical coupling. Chest 143:927–938
24. Bellani G, Coppadoro A, Patroniti N et al (2014) Clinical assessment of auto-positive end-expiratory pressure by diaphragmatic electrical activity during pressure support and neurally adjusted ventilatory assist. Anesthesiology 121:563–571
25. Roze H, Lafrikh A, Perrier V et al (2011) Daily titration of neurally adjusted ventilatory assist using the diaphragm electrical activity. Intensive Care Med 37:1087–1094
26. Dres M, Schmidt M, Ferre A, Mayaux J, Similowski T, Demoule A (2012) Diaphragm electromyographic activity as a predictor of weaning failure. Intensive Care Med 38:2017–2025
27. Barwing J, Pedroni C, Olgemoller U, Quintel M, Moerer O (2013) Electrical activity of the diaphragm (EAdi) as a monitoring parameter in difficult weaning from respirator: a pilot study. Crit Care 17:R182
28. Muttini S, Villani PG, Trimarco R, Bellani G, Grasselli G, Patroniti N (2015) Relation between peak and integral of the diaphragm electromyographic activity at different levels of support during weaning from mechanical ventilation: a physiologic study. J Crit Care 30:7–12
29. Grasselli G, Beck J, Mirabella L, Pesenti A, Slutsky AS, Sinderby C (2012) Assessment of patient-ventilator breath contribution during neurally adjusted ventilatory assist. Intensive Care Med 38:1224–1232
30. Liu L, Xia F, Yang Y et al (2015) Neural versus pneumatic control of pressure support in patients with chronic obstructive pulmonary diseases at different levels of positive end expiratory pressure: a physiological study. Crit Care 19:244
31. Bellani G, Mauri T, Coppadoro A et al (2013) Estimation of patient's inspiratory effort from the electrical activity of the diaphragm. Crit Care Med 41:1483–1491
32. Butler JE (2007) Drive to the human respiratory muscles. Respir Physiol Neurobiol 159:115–126
33. Smith CA, Ainsworth DM, Henderson KS, Dempsey JA (1989) Differential responses of expiratory muscles to chemical stimuli in awake dogs. J Appl Physiol (1985) 66:384–391
34. Fregosi RF, Hwang JC, Bartlett D Jr, St John WM (1992) Activity of abdominal muscle motoneurons during hypercapnia. Respir Physiol 89:179–194
35. Mezzanotte WS, Tangel DJ, White DP (1992) Mechanisms of control of alae nasi muscle activity. J Appl Physiol (1985) 72:925–933

36. Chiti L, Biondi G, Morelot-Panzini C, Raux M, Similowski T, Hug F (2008) Scalene muscle activity during progressive inspiratory loading under pressure support ventilation in normal humans. Respir Physiol Neurobiol 164:441–448
37. Hug F, Raux M, Morelot-Panzini C, Similowski T (2011) Surface EMG to assess and quantify upper airway dilators activity during non-invasive ventilation. Respir Physiol Neurobiol 178:341–345
38. Parthasarathy S, Jubran A, Laghi F, Tobin MJ (2007) Sternomastoid, rib cage, and expiratory muscle activity during weaning failure. J Appl Physiol (1985) 103:140–147
39. Brochard L, Harf A, Lorino H, Lemaire F (1989) Inspiratory pressure support prevents diaphragmatic fatigue during weaning from mechanical ventilation. Am Rev Respir Dis 139:513–521
40. Schmidt M, Kindler F, Gottfried SB et al (2013) Dyspnea and surface inspiratory electromyograms in mechanically ventilated patients. Intensive Care Med 39:1368–1376
41. Cecchini J, Schmidt M, Demoule A, Similowski T (2014) Increased diaphragmatic contribution to inspiratory effort during neurally adjusted ventilatory assistance versus pressure support: an electromyographic study. Anesthesiology 121:1028–1036
42. Guldner A, Pelosi P, de Gama AM (2014) Spontaneous breathing in mild and moderate versus severe acute respiratory distress syndrome. Curr Opin Crit Care 20:69–76

Dissipated Energy is a Key Mediator of VILI: Rationale for Using Low Driving Pressures

A. Serpa Neto, M. B. P. Amato, and M. J. Schultz

Introduction

Positive pressure ventilation should never be seen as a simple and safe intervention, either in patients under general anesthesia for surgery in whom ventilation usually lasts minutes to hours, or in critically ill patients who generally need invasive ventilation for days to weeks. Indeed, positive pressure ventilation is increasingly recognized as a potentially harmful intervention, with ventilator-induced lung injury (VILI) as one of its most important adverse-effects [1]. So-called 'lung-protective' ventilation strategies, i.e., ventilation strategies aiming at prevention of VILI, have a strong potential to benefit patients with acute respiratory distress syndrome (ARDS) as well as patients with uninjured lungs [2].

What is the best way to protect the lungs during positive pressure ventilation? Should 'lung-protective' mechanical ventilation always include the use of low tidal volumes, because clinical studies showed that tidal volume restriction improved outcome of ARDS patients [3, 4] and suggested benefit in patients with uninjured lungs [5–7]? And should it always include higher levels of positive end-expiratory pressure (PEEP), because PEEP up-titration has been shown to improve outcome of ARDS patients [8]?

A. Serpa Neto
Department of Critical Care Medicine, Hospital Israelita Albert Einstein
São Paulo, Brazil

M. B. P. Amato
Faculdade de Medicina, Universidade de São Paulo
São Paulo, Brazil

M. J. Schultz (✉)
Department of Intensive Care, Academic Medical Center
Amsterdam, Netherlands
Mahidol Oxford Research Unit, Mahidol University
Bangkok, Thailand
email: marcus.j.schultz@gmail.com

© Springer International Publishing Switzerland 2016
J.-L. Vincent (ed.), *Annual Update in Intensive Care and Emergency Medicine 2016*,
DOI 10.1007/978-3-319-27349-5_25

Recently, another ventilator setting has been suggested that could reduce harm from positive pressure ventilation. In a large cohort of patients with ARDS the "driving pressure", defined as the plateau pressure or its equivalent minus the level of PEEP, appeared to be strongly and independently associated with mortality [9]. This review focuses on the interaction between energy dissipated in the lung during positive pressure ventilation as a rationale for aiming for the lowest driving pressure by manipulating tidal volume size and the level of PEEP in individual patients.

History of Ventilator-Induced Lung Injury

Barotrauma Versus Volutrauma

Shortly after its introduction, several investigators raised concerns that inflation of the lung with positive pressure ventilation could potentially damage the lungs and produce air leaks [10]. These lesions, termed 'barotrauma', were for several years believed to be the most relevant in the pathogenesis of VILI. Dreyfuss et al. [11] explored whether it was the high airway pressure *per se* or the resulting tidal volume that led to VILI. The key finding of their landmark preclinical study in which animals were ventilated with various tidal volumes at similar airway pressures was that high tidal volumes, and not high airway pressures, produced VILI [12]. This was called 'volutrauma' and from then on researchers considered this more important than barotrauma [13]. Interestingly, the lungs of healthy animals without preceding lung injury also seemed sensitive to ventilation with high tidal volumes [14] suggesting that volutrauma could not only be an entity in ARDS patients, but also in patients with uninjured lungs.

Atelectotrauma and Biotrauma

Meanwhile, investigators started to be interested in the beneficial effects of PEEP in the prevention of lung injury. Use of too low levels of PEEP, or no PEEP, was associated with lung injury and lung dysfunction [12, 15]. This effect was thought to result from repetitive opening and closing of lung tissue that collapses at the end of expiration, a phenomenon called 'atelectrauma' [13]. Positive pressure ventilation was also found to increase pulmonary and systemic levels of inflammatory mediators, responsible for local injury through inflammation and multisystem organ failure [16, 17], a phenomenon called 'biotrauma'.

Clinical Evidence for Benefit of Tidal Volume Reduction and Up-Titration of PEEP

Tidal Volume Restriction

The harmful effects of high tidal volumes in patients with ARDS continued to be considered as unimportant until a series of randomized controlled trials (RCTs) showed mortality reduction with the use of low tidal volumes [3, 4]. Recent clinical studies have shown that tidal volume restriction also prevents pulmonary complications in critically ill patients with uninjured lungs [5–7] and in surgical patients who receive short-lasting ventilation during general anesthesia [18, 19].

Up-Titration of PEEP

Although individual RCTs in patients with ARDS showed no benefit from ventilation using higher levels of PEEP, one meta-analysis that used the individual patient data from these trials showed that up-titration of PEEP was associated with improved survival, though only in patients with severe forms of ARDS [8]. The best-protective level of PEEP in critically ill patients with uninjured lungs has never been determined, although physicians have tended to use higher levels of PEEP in recent years. Recent studies suggest that PEEP does not protect against postoperative pulmonary complications in surgical patients ventilated during general anesthesia [18, 19].

A New Concept: Energy Transferred from the Ventilator to the Lung

Stretch and Strain

Preclinical studies have shown that damage of lung cells or lung strips is closely related to the amplitude of cyclic stretch, rather than to the maximal or sustained level of maximum stretch [20–25]. This seems related to the fact that lung cells can slowly adapt and expand their size, especially the size of their external cell membrane (anchored to the extracellular matrix), provided that the imposed stretch is performed in a slow or sustained manner. This process involves exocytosis and active traffic of lipids from the inner cell vesicles to the outer membrane. The inner vesicles rapidly fuse into a large 'lipid patch', in close vicinity to the newly formed gaps, resulting in the sealing of the membrane, with decreased wall tension [26, 27]. Extrapolation of these findings to the three-dimensional lung parenchyma predicts that a high, but sustained lung stretch is not necessarily deleterious, with epithelial lung cells preserving their integrity if the cyclic stretch is kept low, or if occurring at a slow pace.

The Driving Pressure

Translating these findings to the pressure domain, we should consider that a high plateau pressure or its equivalent does not necessarily represent an increased risk of cell damage, except if accompanied by a high cyclic driving pressure. Corroborating this concept, most of the *in vivo* experiments demonstrating the occurrence of VILI or the deleterious effects of cyclic alveolar recruitment consistently used high driving pressures [28–31]. Similarly, some recent studies trying to prove the major role of absolute lung strain as a key factor for VILI had to conclude that the cyclic strain was, indeed, the most important factor [20, 21]. Moreover, studies in which high inspiratory pressures were associated with lower levels of PEEP, either at equivalent levels of inspiratory lung strain or equivalent levels of plateau pressure, were consistently deleterious, with all of them presenting extremely high levels of driving pressure, the difference between plateau pressure or its equivalent, and the level of PEEP [20, 21, 32, 33].

'Energytrauma'

From a physical perspective, the VILI process must be related to the energy transfer from the ventilator to the fragile lung. At each breath, the ventilator transfers some energy to the respiratory system, which must equal the integral of the proximal airway pressure (at the Y connection between the ventilator and the artificial airway) over the volume delivered. This energy is basically spent in four processes: 1) elastic storage of energy (stored in the lung tissue and chest wall); 2) airway resistive losses (energy wasted to move the tidal volume through the upper and lower airways); 3) acceleration of air molecules and masses involved in lung and chest wall deformation (a negligible component during low frequency ventilation); and 4) parenchymal losses, comprising a mixture of phenomena such as plastic tissue deformation, recruitment and derecruitment of new lung units during the breath, viscous movements within liquid filled airways, stress relaxation of the lung scaffold, and dynamic changes in the surface tension forces due to the complex behavior of the surfactant system. All these latter phenomena are partially responsible for lung hysteresis, i.e., the phenomenon in which the lung conserves energy during one respiratory cycle, with the elastic recoil of the lung always returning less energy during exhalation than that absorbed during inspiration. In other words, there is considerable dissipation of energy, probably resulting in heat and lung tissue damage during each breath. In physical terms, the hysteresis area represents precisely this energy dissipated across the parenchyma (after discounting the energy loss along the airways) and should bear some correlation with VILI.

Interestingly, classical physiological studies have demonstrated that, provided the tidal volume does not vary too much, there is a strong, linear relationship between the hysteresis area and driving pressure, regardless of volume history and regardless of the end-expiratory lung volume [34–36]. Typically, the hysteresis area represents 10–13% of the total energy transferred from the ventilator to the lung, irrespective of the lung condition. It is also interesting to note that, for a patient in whom the respiratory system compliance (C_{RS}) is known, the total energy transfer is proportional to (driving pressure)$^2 \times C_{RS}$. Therefore, the hysteresis area and the total energy transferred are strongly determined by the driving pressure [34–36].

Clinical Evidence for Benefit of Low Driving Pressure

Several studies have considered the impact of driving pressure on clinical outcomes (Table 1). In a landmark study in patients with ARDS in Brazil, Amato et al. showed that a protective strategy of ventilation with low tidal volume and high levels of PEEP with recruitment maneuvers decreased 28-day mortality compared to conventional ventilation with high tidal volume and low levels of PEEP without recruitment maneuvers [37]. Since the effect of the protective strategy was observed in the context of many concomitant maneuvers the authors conducted an analysis to determine the key combination of ventilatory variables responsible for the ventilatory treatment effect on mortality. They found that the driving pressure during the first 36 h was independently associated with high mortality [37]. This was the first time that a possible relationship between high driving pressure and worse outcomes had been found.

This finding was confirmed in an Argentinian study in patients with ARDS, in which a higher driving pressure was independently associated with in-hospital mortality [38]. In a cohort of patients in which lung recruitability was studied using computed tomography, de Matos et al. showed that the only ventilatory parameter associated with higher in-hospital mortality was the driving pressure [39]. By contrast, in a retrospective analysis of an RCT comparing ventilation with low tidal volumes versus high tidal volumes, Boussarsar et al. did not find an association between driving pressure and development of barotrauma [40], although this was rather a small study.

The recent individual patient data meta-analysis by Amato et al. using data from several RCTs testing various strategies of positive pressure ventilation in patients with ARDS showed that, irrespective of the plateau pressure, tidal volume size and level of PEEP, the driving pressure was the key ventilatory parameter associated with mortality [9]. This was confirmed in a causal mediation analysis, showing that although driving pressure was not an explicit target of the ventilation strategy tested, survival benefits were proportional to reductions in driving pressure driven by treatment group assignments rather than to reductions in tidal volume or increments in PEEP.

In a study focusing on the incidence of cor pulmonale in patients with ARDS undergoing lung-protective ventilation, Boissier et al. found that higher driving pressure was associated with development of cor pulmonale as well as increased 28-day mortality [41]; these findings were, however, not confirmed in another study [42]. More recently, in a subgroup of patients with severe ARDS treated with extracorporeal membrane oxygenation (ECMO) because of refractory hypoxemia, Schmidt et al. showed that non-survivors had higher driving pressure before and in

Table 1 Studies describing the impact of driving pressure on clinical outcome

First author, year [ref]	Design	Number of patients	Comparison	Primary outcome	Findings on driving pressure
Amato, 1998 [37]	RCT	53	Protective vs. conventional ventilation	28-day mortality	Driving pressure associated with high mortality in patients with ARDS (Cox proportional-hazard model)
Estenssoro, 2002 [38]	Cohort	235	None	In-hospital mortality	Higher driving pressure associated with mortality in patients with ARDS (multivariate analysis)
Boussarsar, 2002 [40]	Retrospective	116	None	Barotrauma	Driving pressure was not associated with the incidence of barotrauma in patients with ARDS (direct comparison)
de Matos, 2012 [39]	Cohort	51	None	Lung recruitability	Higher driving pressure associated with higher mortality in patients with ARDS (multivariate logistic regression)
Boissier, 2013 [41]	Cohort	226	None	Cor pulmonale	Higher driving pressure associated with cor pulmonale and 28-day mortality in patients with ARDS (multivariate logistic regression)
Amato, 2015 [9]	IPD	3562	None	60-day mortality	Higher driving pressure associated with mortality in patients with ARDS (causal mediation analysis)
Schmidt, 2015 [43]	Cohort	168	None	ICU mortality	Higher driving pressure associated with mortality in patients with ARDS treated with ECMO (direct comparison)
Goligher, 2015 [44]	Cohort	107	None	Diaphragm thickness	Higher driving pressure associated with decreased contractile activity and decrease in diaphragm thickness in patients under mechanical ventilation
Legras, 2015 [42]	Cohort	195	None	Acute cor pulmonale and patent foramen ovale	No effect of driving pressure on cor pulmonale or patent foramen ovale in patients with ARDS

RCT: randomized controlled trial; *IPD*: individual patient data meta-analysis; *ICU*: intensive care unit; *ARDS*: acute respiratory distress syndrome; *ECMO*: extracorporeal membrane oxygenation

the first three days of ECMO compared to survivors [43]. Finally, Goligher et al. showed that a higher driving pressure was associated with a decrease in contractile activity and decrease in diaphragm thickness in critically ill patients receiving positive pressure ventilation [44].

How to Limit the Driving Pressure?

It remains uncertain how to achieve a low driving pressure in an individual patient. One strategy that certainly makes sense is to aim for low tidal volumes, as this usually results in low driving pressures. On the other hand, in some patients, tidal volumes remain high, or become higher during the course of ventilation even at a low driving pressure. This suggests that a low tidal volume is not the sole key of protective ventilation.

Another strategy concerns a more adequate up- (or down-) titration of PEEP and the use of recruitment maneuvers. While PEEP up-titration, with or without the use of recruitment maneuvers usually focuses on the impact on oxygenation this may be, at least in part, wrong. For example, if PEEP up-titration, with or without the use of recruitment maneuvers, results in better oxygenation at the price of a higher driving pressure, it could be that the intervention not only resulted in recruitment of lung tissue, but also overdistension of other parts of the lung. Or if PEEP up-titration, with or without the use of recruitment maneuvers, does not affect oxygenation at all but results in a higher driving pressure, the intervention did recruit lung tissue but only caused overdistension. The best response to an up-titration of PEEP, with or without the use of recruitment maneuvers, is a decrease in the driving pressure, meaning that the intervention resulted in recruitment of lung tissue without causing overdistension. As such, energy delivered by or transferred from the ventilator to the lungs decreases, while there is sufficient gas-exchange. Thus PEEP up-titration, with or without recruitment maneuvers, should not be seen as a goal in itself, but as a way to achieve the lowest driving pressure. Of note, it is uncertain what the effects on driving pressures are of other interventions that could lead to recruitment of lung tissue, such as proning.

Limitations of Aiming at Low Driving Pressures

It is well established that VILI results from non-physiological lung stress (transpulmonary pressure) and strain (inflated volume to functional residual capacity ratio) [45], and that transpulmonary pressure (the pressure difference from airway opening to pleural space) is the relevant distending pressure for the lung. This concept is often overlooked when practitioners focus on the plateau pressure without considering the effect of the chest wall in determining lung expansion and stress. The same plateau pressure produced largely variable transpulmonary pressure due to the variability of the lung elastance to respiratory system elastance ratio [46]. This suggests that the plateau pressure is an inadequate surrogate for transpulmonary pressure and driving pressure could suffer from this limitation. Nevertheless, because lung compliance in patients with ARDS is much more affected than chest wall compliance [47, 48], approximately 80% of the driving pressure is typically attributable to the lung during inspiration, making it a reasonable surrogate for transpulmonary driving pressure. Moreover, although elevated pleural pressures occur frequently in critically ill patients, especially in the obese or those with large pleural effusions, they are seldom associated with changes in chest wall compliance. Commonly, there is an offset in pleural pressures, causing proportional increases in inspiratory and expiratory pleural pressures, thus not affecting the driving pressure [9]. Finally, patients with spontaneous breathing activity have pleural pressure decreases during inspiration as a result of their own efforts to breathe, which result in high transpulmonary pressures without the possibility to control the driving pressure [48].

Because driving pressure is the tidal increase in static respiratory pressure, it is proportional to tidal volume, with respiratory system elastance being the constant of proportionality. Thus, the ability of driving pressure to predict outcome could be attributable to the fact that variables that define it are known to predict or affect mortality in ARDS [48]. Finally, the studies reported above were not designed to assess driving pressure as an independent variable, and thus the findings should be considered hypothesis-generating: is it possible to aim for the lowest driving pressure during positive pressure ventilation, and if so, does this strategy truly benefit ventilated patients?

Conclusion

A high driving pressure results in more 'energytrauma', and as such is a key mediator of VILI in positive pressure ventilation. We are in need of clinical studies that show the best way to limit driving pressures and RCTs that test whether strategies aiming for low driving pressures truly affect the outcome of patients with ARDS, and maybe even those with uninjured lungs.

References

1. Slutsky AS, Ranieri VM (2013) Ventilator-induced lung injury. N Engl J Med 369:2126–2136
2. Serpa NA, Nagtzaam L, Schultz MJ (2014) Ventilation with lower tidal volumes for critically ill patients without the acute respiratory distress syndrome: a systematic translational review and metaanalysis. Curr Opin Crit Care 20:25–32
3. Putensen C, Theuerkauf N, Zinserling J, Wrigge H, Pelosi P (2009) Meta-analysis: ventilation strategies and outcomes of the acute respiratory distress syndrome and acute lung injury. Ann Intern Med 151:566–576
4. Burns KE, Adhikari NK, Slutsky AS et al (2011) Pressure and volume limited ventilation for the ventilatory management of patients with acute lung injury: a systematic review and meta-analysis. PLoS One 6:e14623
5. Serpa NA, Simonis FD, Barbas CS et al (2014) Association between tidal volume size, duration of ventilation, and sedation needs in patients without acute respiratory distress syndrome: an individual patient data meta-analysis. Intensive Care Med 40:950–957

6. Serpa NA, Cardoso SO, Manetta JA et al (2012) Association between use of lung-protective ventilation with lower tidal volumes and clinical outcomes among patients without acute respiratory distress syndrome: a meta-analysis. JAMA 308:1651–1659

7. Serpa NA, Simonis FD, Barbas CS et al (2015) Lung-protective ventilation with low tidal volumes and the occurrence of pulmonary complications in patients without acute respiratory distress syndrome: a systematic review and individual patient data analysis. Crit Care Med 43:2155–2163

8. Briel M, Meade M, Mercat A et al (2010) Higher vs lower positive end-expiratory pressure in patients with acute lung injury and acute respiratory distress syndrome: systematic review and meta-analysis. JAMA 303:865–873

9. Amato MB, Meade MO, Slutsky AS et al (2015) Driving pressure and survival in the acute respiratory distress syndrome. N Engl J Med 372:747–755

10. Baker AB (1971) Artificial respiration, the history of an idea. Med Hist 15:336–351

11. Dreyfuss D, Soler P, Basset G, Saumon G (1988) High inflation pressure pulmonary edema. Respective effects of high airway pressure, high tidal volume, and positive end-expiratory pressure. Am Rev Respir Dis 137:1159–1164

12. Dreyfuss D, Saumon G (1998) Ventilator-induced lung injury: lessons from experimental studies. Am J Respir Crit Care Med 157:294–323

13. Slutsky AS (1999) Lung injury caused by mechanical ventilation. Chest 116:9S–15S

14. Wolthuis EK, Vlaar AP, Choi G, Roelofs JJ, Juffermans NP, Schultz MJ (2009) Mechanical ventilation using non-injurious ventilation settings causes lung injury in the absence of pre-existing lung injury in healthy mice. Crit Care 13:R1

15. Trembley LN, Slutsky AS (2006) Ventilator-induced lung injury: from the bench to the bedside. Intensive Care Med 32:24–33

16. Tremblay LN, Slutsky AS (1998) Ventilator-induced injury: from barotrauma to biotrauma. Proc Assoc Am Physicians 110:482–438

17. Imai Y, Parodo J, Kajikawa O et al (2003) Injurious mechanical ventilation and end-organ epithelial cell apoptosis and organ dysfunction in an experimental model of acute respiratory distress syndrome. JAMA 289:2104–2112

18. Serpa NA, Hemmes SNT, Barbas CSV et al (2015) Protective versus conventional ventilation for surgery: a systematic review and individual patient data meta-analysis. Anesthesiology 123:66–78

19. Güldner A, Kiss T, Serpa NA, Hemmes SN et al (2015) Intraoperative protective mechanical ventilation for prevention of postoperative pulmonary complications: a comprehensive review of the role of tidal volume, positive end-expiratory pressure, and lung recruitment maneuvers. Anesthesiology 123:692–713

20. Protti A, Votta E, Gattinoni L (2014) Which is the most important strain in the pathogenesis of ventilator-induced lung injury: dynamic or static? Curr Opin Crit Care 20:33–38

21. Protti A, Andreis DT, Monti M et al (2013) Lung stress and strain during mechanical ventilation: any difference between statics and dynamics? Crit Care Med 41:1046–1055

22. Tschumperlin DJ, Oswari J, Margulies AS (2000) Deformation-induced injury of alveolar epithelial cells. Effect of frequency, duration, and amplitude. Am J Respir Crit Care Med 162:357–362

23. Birukov KG, Jacobson JR, Flores AA et al (2003) Magnitude-dependent regulation of pulmonary endothelial cell barrier function by cyclic stretch. Am J Physiol Lung Cell Mol Physiol 285:L785–L797

24. Ye H, Zhan Q, Ren Y, Liu X, Yang C, Wang C (2012) Cyclic deformation-induced injury and differentiation of rat alveolar epithelial type II cells. Respir Physiol Neurobiol 180:237–246

25. Garcia CS, Rocco PR, Facchinetti LD et al (2004) What increases type III procollagen mRNA levels in lung tissue: stress induced by changes in force or amplitude? Respir Physiol Neurobiol 144:59–70

26. Vlahakis NE, Schroeder MA, Pagano RE, Hubmayr RD (2001) Deformation-induced lipid trafficking in alveolar epithelial cells. Am J Physiol Lung Cell Mol Physiol 280:L938–L946

27. Vlahakis NE, Schroeder MA, Pagano RE, Hubmayr RD (2002) Role of deformation-induced lipid trafficking in the prevention of plasma membrane stress failure. Am J Respir Crit Care Med 166:1282–1289
28. Dreyfuss D, Saumon G (1993) Role of tidal volume, FRC, and end-inspiratory volume in the development of pulmonary edema following mechanical ventilation. Am Rev Respir Dis 148:1194–1203
29. Tremblay L, Valenza F, Ribeiro SP, Li J, Slutsky AS (1997) Injurious ventilatory strategies increase cytokines and c-fos m-RNA expression in an isolated rat lung model. J Clin Invest 99:944–952
30. Caironi P, Cressoni M, Chiumello D et al (2010) Lung opening and closing during ventilation of acute respiratory distress syndrome. Am J Respir Crit Care Med 181:578–586
31. Muscedere JG, Mullen JB, Gan K, Slutsky AS (1994) Tidal ventilation at low airway pressures can augment lung injury. Am J Respir Crit Care Med 149:1327–1334
32. Webb HH, Tierney DF (1974) Experimental pulmonary edema due to intermittent positive pressure ventilation with high inflation pressures. Protection by positive end-expiratory pressure. Am Rev Respir Dis 110:556–565
33. Verbrugge SJ, Sorm V, van't Veen A, Mouton JW, Gommers D, Lachmann B (1998) Lung overinflation without positive end-expiratory pressure promotes bacteremia after experimental Klebsiella pneumoniae inoculation. Intensive Care Med 24:172–177
34. Bachofen H (1968) Lung tissue resistance and pulmonary hysteresis. J Appl Physiol 24:296–301
35. Bachofen H, Hildebrandt J (1971) Area analysis of pressure-volume hysteresis in mammalian lungs. J Appl Physiol 30:493–497
36. Horie T, Hildebrandt J (1973) Dependence of lung hysteresis area on tidal volume, duration of ventilation, and history. J Appl Physiol 35:596–600
37. Amato MB, Barbas CS, Medeiros DM et al (1998) Effect of a protective-ventilation strategy on mortality in the acute respiratory distress syndrome. N Engl J Med 338:347–354
38. Estenssoro E, Dubin A, Laffaire E et al (2002) Incidence, clinical course, and outcome in 217 patients with acute respiratory distress syndrome. Crit Care Med 30:2450–2456
39. de Matos GF, Stanzani F, Passos RH et al (2012) How large is the lung recruitability in early acute respiratory distress syndrome: a prospective case series of patients monitored by computed tomography. Crit Care 16:R4
40. Boussarsar M, Thierry G, Jaber S, Roudot-Thoraval F, Lemaire F, Brochard L (2002) Relationship between ventilatory settings and barotrauma in the acute respiratory distress syndrome. Intensive Care Med 28:406–413
41. Boissier F, Katsahian S, Razazi K et al (2013) Prevalence and prognosis of cor pulmonale during protective ventilation for acute respiratory distress syndrome. Intensive Care Med 39:1725–1733
42. Legras A, Caille A, Begot E et al (2015) Acute respiratory distress syndrome (ARDS)-associated acute cor pulmonale and patent foramen ovale: a multicenter noninvasive hemodynamic study. Crit Care 19:174
43. Schmidt M, Stewart C, Bailey M et al (2015) Mechanical ventilation management during extracorporeal membrane oxygenation for acute respiratory distress syndrome: a retrospective international multicenter study. Crit Care Med 43:654–664
44. Goligher EC, Fan E, Herridge MS et al (2015) Evolution of diaphragm thickness during mechanical ventilation: impact of inspiratory effort. Am J Respir Crit Care Med 192:1080–1088
45. Chiumello D, Carlesso E, Cadringher P et al (2008) Lung stress and strain during mechanical ventilation for acute respiratory distress syndrome. Am J Respir Crit Care Med 178:346–355
46. Loring SH, Malhotra A (2015) Driving pressure and respiratory mechanics in ARDS. N Engl J Med 372:776–777

47. Talmor D, Sarge T, Malhotra A et al (2008) Mechanical ventilation guided by esophageal pressure in acute lung injury. N Engl J Med 359:2095–2104
48. Albaiceta GM, Taboada F, Parra D, Blanco A, Escudero D, Otero J (2003) Differences in the deflation limb of the pressure-volume curves in acute respiratory distress syndrome from pulmonary and extrapulmonary origin. Intensive Care Med 29:1943–1949

Corticosteroids as Adjunctive Therapy in Severe Community-Acquired Pneumonia

C. Cillóniz, A. San José, and A. Torres

Introduction

Mortality in community acquired pneumonia (CAP) has not decreased in the intensive care unit (ICU), despite progress in antimicrobial therapy [1, 2]. Approximately 10% of patients hospitalized with CAP are admitted to the ICU [3]. In a multicenter study by Mongardon et al. in patients with severe pneumococcal CAP admitted to the ICU, the mortality rate was 29%, with high proportions of patients in septic shock and needing mechanical ventilation [4]. Severe CAP is a progressive disease and patients may die despite early and adequate antibiotic treatment. The host local and systemic inflammatory immune response in patients with severe CAP is exacerbated and disproportionate and this is probably the main cause for the high mortality in this specific population, as it contributes to impaired alveolar gas exchange, sepsis and end-organ dysfunction [5]. In this specific population of patients with severe CAP, adjuvant treatments, such as corticosteroids, may be beneficial.

C. Cillóniz · A. San José · A. Torres (✉)
Department of Pneumology, Institut Clinic del Tórax, Hospital Clinic
Barcelona, Spain
Institut d'Investigacions Biomèdiques August Pi i Sunyer (IDIBAPS), University of Barcelona (UB)
Barcelona, Spain
Ciber de Enfermedades Respiratorias (Ciberes)
www.ciberes.org
email: atorres@clinic.ub.es

© Springer International Publishing Switzerland 2016
J.-L. Vincent (ed.), *Annual Update in Intensive Care and Emergency Medicine 2016*,
DOI 10.1007/978-3-319-27349-5_26

Systemic Adjunctive Corticosteroid Therapy in Severe CAP

The principle action of corticosteroids is the inhibition of the expression and action of several cytokines involved in the immune inflammatory response to pneumonia [6]. It is known that, in CAP patients, the use of systemic adjunctive corticosteroid therapy attenuates the local and systemic inflammatory response [7], and may potentially reduce the development of acute respiratory distress syndrome (ARDS), sepsis and mortality. Sibila et al. [8], in a study of *Pseudomonas aeruginosa* pneumonia in mechanically ventilated piglets, observed a lower lung bacterial burden and less severe histological pneumonia in piglets treated with corticosteroids plus antibiotics compared to antibiotics alone.

Several randomized controlled trials (RCT) have been performed in humans, the majority of which included hospitalized patients with non-severe CAP. The results of these trials have been negative [9], or have demonstrated a reduction in length of stay [10] or time to clinical stability [11]. To date, four studies have been performed in patients with severe CAP [12–15]. A meta-analysis published by Nie et al. [16] showed that in a subgroup of patients with severe CAP, steroids reduced mortality. More recently, a meta-analysis [17] showed that the use of systemic corticosteroids in CAP was associated with a moderate reduction in the need for mechanical ventilation, development of ARDS and, with high certainty, a reduction in time to clinical stability and duration of hospitalization. This study also showed a possible reduction in mortality, but this effect was seen mainly in the subgroup of patients with severe pneumonia.

However, most of these RCTs had important limitations: a) the inclusion of many patients with low severity without ICU admission, which makes it difficult to demonstrate differences in clinical outcomes, such as treatment failure and mortality, because of the rates of these outcomes; and b) the inclusion of patients regardless of the initial level of inflammation. To date, this latter variable has not been taken into account in the any of the RCTs. CAP patients with a marked inflammatory response have high levels of C-reactive protein (CRP), higher rates of treatment failure [18] and worse mortality rates [19]. Furthermore, there are marked differences in variables in the majority of RCTs, regardless of dosages, type and length of steroid treatment, which makes it very difficult to compare results. The primary end-points are different between studies, and some of them, such as length of stay or even time to clinical stability, are 'soft' endpoints: length of stay depends on other variables and clinical stability is driven by the persistence of fever which is, in fact, down-regulated by corticosteroids.

More recently, Torres et al. [20] performed an RCT comparing methylprednisolone (0.5 mg/kg every 12 h for 5 days) vs. placebo, with important specific characteristics: a) the authors included only patients with severe CAP with major or minor modified criteria of the American Thoracic Society, or with a Pneumonia Severity Index (PSI) risk class V; b) they chose patients with a large systemic inflammatory response, with a threshold for serum levels of CRP of 15 mg/dl; c) treatment failure was defined as early (clinical deterioration indicated by the development of shock, need for invasive mechanical ventilation, not present at baseline, or death, within 72 h) or late (radiographic progression or persistence of respiratory failure, development of shock, need for invasive mechanical ventilation not present at baseline, or death, between 72 and 120 h after treatment initiation), and was the primary end-point, rather than mortality. In addition, it is known that treatment failure in CAP is associated with higher mortality, as previously shown in the study by Menendez et al. [21].

The principal results showed a decrease in the treatment failure rate from 31 to 13% (p = 0.02). Corticosteroids reduced the risk of treatment failure with an odds ratio of 0.34. Mortality did not differ significantly between groups, but the study was not designed to find differences in mortality (10% in the methylprednisolone arm *vs.* 15% in the placebo arm, p = 0.37). The reduction in treatment failure was more evident in late treatment failure (3% vs. 25%, p = 0.001), and especially in radiographic progression, which was one of the variables included in the composite definition of late treatment failure (2% vs. 15%, p = 0.007). The rates of adverse effects were small and similar between arms. A limitation of this study was the long recruitment period (8 years) and the use of methylprednisolone for 5 days only, with an abrupt interruption of the treatment.

The results of this study, which found fewer treatment failures, particularly late treatment failure, and less radiographic progression, may be explained by stopping of the progression to ARDS or a potential blocking of the Jarisch-Herxheimer reaction, which is thought to be due to high concentrations of cytokines released after the initiation of antibiotics, possibly through the release of endotoxins or other bacterial mediators in patients with a high bacterial burden, as occurs in meningococcal disease [22].

Corticosteroids in Patients with Severe CAP with Marked Inflammation and Non-Influenza Pneumonia

In patients with severe CAP, treatment with corticosteroids should be considered in clinical practice. It is important to select patients with severe CAP with a marked inflammatory response measured by CRP. Another important point is to exclude patients with influenza pneumonia, as growing evidence suggests that corticosteroids increase mortality in patients with influenza pneumonia [23]. Little information is available on the possible effect of corticosteroids on other viral pneumonias caused by adenovirus, rhinovirus, respiratory syncytial virus, or others. However, high serum levels of CRP indicate that pure viral pneumonia is unlikely. We propose an algorithm for the administration of corticosteroids as an adjunctive treatment for CAP (Fig. 1).

There is another CAP population in which corticosteroids may have a role to play. Shindo et al. [24] described the risk factors for 30-day mortality in patients with pneumonia who received appropriate initial antibiotics. They found that blood levels of albumin, pH < 7.35, respiratory rate > 30 breaths per minute, and blood urea nitrogen of at least 7.14 mmol/l were independent risk factors for mortality. In

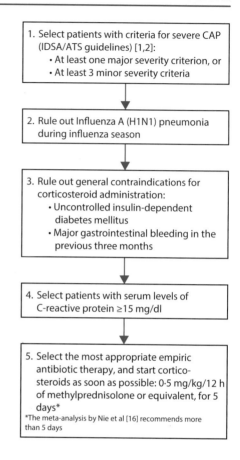

Fig. 1 Proposed algorithm for administration of corticosteroids in severe community-acquired pneumonia (CAP)

1. Select patients with criteria for severe CAP (IDSA/ATS guidelines) [1,2]:
   • At least one major severity criterion, or
   • At least 3 minor severity criteria

2. Rule out Influenza A (H1N1) pneumonia during influenza season

3. Rule out general contraindications for corticosteroid administration:
   • Uncontrolled insulin-dependent diabetes mellitus
   • Major gastrointestinal bleeding in the previous three months

4. Select patients with serum levels of C-reactive protein ≥15 mg/dl

5. Select the most appropriate empiric antibiotic therapy, and start corticosteroids as soon as possible: 0·5 mg/kg/12 h of methylprednisolone or equivalent, for 5 days*
   *The meta-analysis by Nie et al [16] recommends more than 5 days

the accompanying editorial [25], it was pointed out that these results would make it possible to develop a predictive score for use in clinical trials of immunomodulatory drugs. This indication needs new RCTs.

Future studies should include the following research steps:

(a) Investigation of the potential synergies between macrolides and corticosteroids. Such investigations can be performed in animal models of pneumonia. An animal study of *Mycoplasma pneumoniae* pneumonia [26] showed histological benefits of combined clarithromycin and dexamethasone treatment compared to either treatment alone.

(b) A meta-analysis, using individual data with a particular focus on severe CAP, which can provide useful clinical information.

(c) Randomized trials in other CAP populations, such as patients with a high risk of mortality despite appropriate antibiotics.

Conclusion

Mortality rates in severe CAP remain high [27, 28]. Corticosteroids are the most effective and widely used anti-inflammatory drugs. Corticosteroids are useful in patients with severe CAP with a high degree of systemic inflammatory response and in whom influenza pneumonia has been ruled out, and can help to decrease treatment failure and probably mortality in these patients.

References

1. Mandell LA, Wunderink RG, Anzueto A et al (2007) Infectious Diseases Society of America/American Thoracic Society consensus guidelines on the management of community-acquired pneumonia in adults. Clin Infect Dis 44(Suppl 2):S27–S72
2. Restrepo MI, Anzueto A (2009) Severe community-acquired pneumonia. Infect Dis Clin North Am 23:503–520
3. Ewig S, Woodhead M, Torres A (2011) Towards a sensible comprehension of severe community-acquired pneumonia. Intensive Care Med 37:214–223
4. Mongardon N, Max A, Bougle A et al (2012) Epidemiology and outcome of severe pneumococcal pneumonia admitted to intensive care unit: a multicenter study. Crit Care 16:R155
5. Rittirsch D, Flierl MA, Ward PA (2008) Harmful molecular mechanisms in sepsis. Nat Rev Immunol 8:776–787
6. Rhen T, Cidlowski JA (2005) Antiinflammatory action of glucocorticoids – new mechanisms for old drugs. N Engl J Med 353:1711–1723
7. Monton C, Ewig S, Torres A et al (1999) Role of glucocorticoids on inflammatory response in nonimmunosuppressed patients with pneumonia: a pilot study. Eur Respir J 14:218–220
8. Sibila O, Luna CM, Agusti C et al (2008) Effects of glucocorticoids in ventilated piglets with severe pneumonia. Eur Respir J 32:1037–1046
9. Snijders D, Daniels JM, de Graaff CS, van der Werf TS, Boersma WG (2010) Efficacy of corticosteroids in community-acquired pneumonia: a randomized double-blinded clinical trial. Am J Respir Crit Care Med 181:975–982
10. Meijvis SC, Hardeman H, Remmelts HH et al (2011) Dexamethasone and length of hospital stay in patients with community-acquired pneumonia: a randomised, double-blind, placebo-controlled trial. Lancet 377:2023–2030
11. Blum CA, Nigro N, Briel M et al (2015) Adjunct prednisone therapy for patients with community-acquired pneumonia: a multicentre, double-blind, randomised, placebo-controlled trial. Lancet 385:1511–1518
12. Confalonieri M, Urbino R, Potena A et al (2005) Hydrocortisone infusion for severe community-acquired pneumonia: a preliminary randomized study. Am J Respir Crit Care Med 171:242–248
13. Nafae RM, Ragab MI, Amany FM, Rashed SB (2013) Adjuvant role of corticosteroids in the treatment of community-acquired pneumonia. Egyptian Journal of Chest Diseases and Tuberculosis 62:439–445
14. Sabry N, Omar E (2011) Corticosteroids and ICU course of community acquired pneumonia in Egyptian settings. Pharmacology & Pharmacy 2:73–81
15. Marik P, Kraus P, Sribante J, Havlik I, Lipman J, Johnson DW (1993) Hydrocortisone and tumor necrosis factor in severe community-acquired pneumonia. A randomized controlled study. Chest 104:389–392
16. Nie W, Zhang Y, Cheng J, Xiu Q (2012) Corticosteroids in the treatment of community-acquired pneumonia in adults: a meta-analysis. PLoS One 7:e47926

17. Siemieniuk RA, Meade MO, Alonso-Coello P et al (2015) Corticosteroid therapy for patients hospitalized with community-acquired pneumonia: a systematic review and meta-analysis. Ann Intern Med 163:519–528

18. Menendez R, Martinez R, al Reyes Set (2009) Biomarkers improve mortality prediction by prognostic scales in community-acquired pneumonia. Thorax 64:587–591

19. Chalmers JD, Smith MP, McHugh BJ, Doherty C, Govan JR, Hill AT (2012) Short- and long-term antibiotic treatment reduces airway and systemic inflammation in non-cystic fibrosis bronchiectasis. Am J Respir Crit Care Med 186:657–665

20. Torres A, Sibila O, Ferrer M et al (2015) Effect of corticosteroids on treatment failure among hospitalized patients with severe community-acquired pneumonia and high inflammatory response: a randomized clinical trial. JAMA 313:677–686

21. Menendez R, Torres A, Zalacain R et al (2004) Risk factors of treatment failure in community acquired pneumonia: implications for disease outcome. Thorax 59:960–965

22. Darton T, Guiver M, Naylor S, Jack DL, Kaczmarski EB, Borrow R, Read RC (2009) Severity of meningococcal disease associated with genomic bacterial load. Clin Infect Dis 48:587–594

23. Lee N, Leo YS, Cao B et al (2015) Neuraminidase inhibitors, superinfection and corticosteroids affect survival of influenza patients. Eur Respir J 45:1642–1652

24. Shindo Y, Ito R, Kobayashi D et al (2015) Risk factors for 30-day mortality in patients with pneumonia who receive appropriate initial antibiotics: an observational cohort study. Lancet Infect Dis 15:1055–1065

25. Wunderink RG (2015) Corticosteroids for severe community-acquired pneumonia: not for everyone. JAMA 313:673–674

26. Tagliabue C, Salvatore CM, Techasaensiri C et al (2008) The impact of steroids given with macrolide therapy on experimental Mycoplasma pneumoniae respiratory infection. J Infect Dis 198:1180–1188

27. Restrepo MI, Mortensen EM, Velez JA, Frei C, Anzueto A (2008) A comparative study of community-acquired pneumonia patients admitted to the ward and the ICU. Chest 133:610–617

28. Alvarez-Lerma F, Torres A (2004) Severe community-acquired pneumonia. Curr Opin Crit Care 10:369–374

Part IX
Abdominal Issues

The Neglected Role of Abdominal Compliance in Organ-Organ Interactions

M. L. N. G. Malbrain, Y. Peeters, and R. Wise

Introduction

Over the last few decades, increasing attention has been given to understanding the pathophysiology, etiology, prognosis, and treatment of elevated intra-abdominal pressure (IAP) in trauma, surgical, and medical patients. However, there is still a relatively poor understanding of intra-abdominal volume (IAV) and the relationship between IAV and IAP (i.e., abdominal compliance [C_{ab}]). According to the consensus definitions proposed by the World Society on Abdominal Compartment Syndrome (WSACS), C_{ab} is defined as a measure of the ease of abdominal expansion, determined by the elasticity of the abdominal wall and diaphragm [1]. C_{ab} should be expressed as the change in IAV per change in IAP (expressed in ml/mmHg). C_{ab} is one of the most neglected parameters in critically ill patients, despite playing a key-role in understanding the deleterious effects of unadapted IAV on IAP, organ-organ interactions and end-organ perfusion [2, 3]. Although there are some papers related to C_{ab} in surgical patients, only a few papers have been published addressing this issue in critically ill patients [2–4].

M. L. N. G. Malbrain (✉) · Y. Peeters
Intensive Care Unit and High Care Burn Unit, Ziekenhuis Netwerk Antwerpen, ZNA Stuivenberg
Antwerp, Belgium
email: manu.malbrain@skynet.be

R. Wise
Edendale Hospital, Perioperative Research Group, Discipline of Anesthesia and Critical Care,
Univeristy of Kwazulu Natal
Pietermaritzburg, South Africa

© Springer International Publishing Switzerland 2016
J.-L. Vincent (ed.), *Annual Update in Intensive Care and Emergency Medicine 2016*,
DOI 10.1007/978-3-319-27349-5_27

Definitions

The Abdominal Compartment

The abdominal compartment is a technical masterpiece as this small human cavity houses 8.5 m of intestine. Analogous to the skull, the abdomen can be considered as a relatively closed box with an anchorage above (costal arch) and rigid (spine and pelvis) or partially flexible walls (abdominal wall and diaphragm) filled with solid organs and hollow viscera [2]. The size and/or volume of the abdomen may be affected by the varying location of the diaphragm, the shifting position of the costal arch, the contractions of the abdominal wall, and the contents contained within the intestines.

The Abdominal Wall

The abdominal wall represents the boundaries of the abdominal cavity between the xyphoid bone and costal margins cranially and the iliac and pubic bones of the pelvis caudally. C_{ab} is mainly defined by the elasticity of the different muscle layers of the abdominal wall (anterior and lateral parts) and to a lesser extent the diaphragm muscle.

Intra-Abdominal Pressure and Abdominal Hypertension

Intra-abdominal pressure The IAP is the steady-state pressure concealed within the abdominal cavity. The reference standard for intermittent IAP measurements is via the bladder. IAP should be expressed in mmHg and measured at the end of exhalation in the supine position after ensuring that abdominal muscle contractions are absent and with the transducer zeroed at the level where the midaxillary line crosses the iliac crest [1].

Baseline IAP Also called resting, starting, static or opening IAP during laparoscopy, the baseline IAP is the IAP obtained at normal resting conditions [2]. Normal IAP is considered as 5–7 mmHg in healthy individuals, and approximately 10 mmHg in critically ill adults [5].

Intra-abdominal hypertension (IAH) IAH is defined as a sustained or repeated pathological elevation in IAP $\geq$ 12 mmHg. IAH is graded as follows: Grade I, IAP 12–15 mmHg; Grade II, IAP 16–20 mmHg; Grade III, IAP 21–25 mmHg; and Grade IV, IAP > 25 mmHg [1].

Abdominal compartment syndrome (ACS) ACS is defined as a sustained IAP > 20 mmHg (with or without an abdominal perfusion pressure [APP]

<60 mmHg) that is associated with new organ dysfunction/failure. In contrast to IAH, ACS is an all-or-nothing phenomenon [1].

Delta IAP ΔIAP is calculated as the difference between the end-inspiratory (IAP_{ei}) and the end-expiratory (IAP_{ee}) IAP value. The higher the ΔIAP, the lower the C_{ab}.

$$\Delta IAP = IAP_{ei} - IAP_{ee}$$

Abdominal pressure variation (APV) APV is calculated as the difference between the IAP_{ei} and the IAP_{ee} value, or ΔIAP, divided by the mean IAP and is expressed as a percentage. The higher the APV, the lower the C_{ab}.

$$APV = \frac{\Delta IAP}{\text{mean IAP}} = \frac{IAP_{ei} - IAP_{ee}}{\text{mean IAP}}$$

Intra-Abdominal Volume

Baseline IAV Also called resting, starting or static IAV, the baseline IAV is the IAV at baseline conditions without additional pathologic volume increase or C_{ab} decrease, with corresponding baseline IAP. The baseline IAV in healthy individuals is around 13 l [2].

Abdominal distension This is defined as a sagittal abdominal diameter (approximately at the level of the umbilicus) higher than the virtual line between the xiphoid and symphysis pubis.

Abdominal workspace This is the additional IAV that can be added to the baseline IAV when IAP is limited to a certain pressure (e.g., 14 mmHg during laparoscopic surgery). The normal workspace during laparoscopy ranges between 3 and 6 l.

Maximal stretched volume The maximal volume is calculated as the baseline IAV + the maximal workspace resulting in maximal stretch of the abdominal cavity (from ellipse to sphere on a transverse plane). The maximal stretched volume depends on baseline IAP and C_{ab}.

Abdominal Compliance

Abdominal compliance C_{ab} is defined as the ease with which abdominal expansion can occur, and is determined by the elasticity of the abdominal wall and diaphragm. Increased compliance indicates a loss of elastic recoil of the abdominal wall. Decreased compliance means that the same change in IAV will result in a greater change in IAP. It should be expressed as the change in IAV per change in IAP (ml/mmHg) [1]. Normal C_{ab} is around 250 to 450 ml/mmHg.

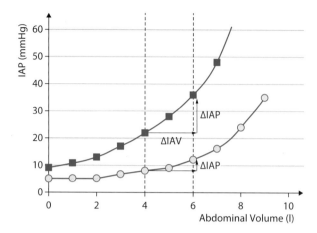

Fig. 1 Pressure-volume curve in the abdominal compartment. Abdominal pressure-volume curves in a patient with low abdominal compliance (*squares*) and normal compliance (*circles*). At a baseline IAV of 4 l, the same 2 l increase in IAV will only lead to a small increase in IAP (5 mmHg) in a patient with good abdominal compliance versus a high increase in IAP (15 mmHg) in the case of a stiff abdominal wall and diaphragm. The compliance is 133 ml/mmHg [2000/(37 − 22)] versus 400 ml/mmHg [2000/(12 − 7)] for the same change in IAV from 4 to 6 l. Adapted from [2] with permission

Abdominal PV relationship Importantly, C_{ab} is measured differently than IAP, it is only a part of the total abdominal pressure-volume (PV) relationship.

$$\text{Compliance (C)} = \frac{\Delta V}{\Delta P} \text{ or thus } C_{ab} = \frac{\Delta IAV}{\Delta IAP}$$

$$\text{Elastance (E)} = \frac{\Delta P}{\Delta V} = \frac{1}{C} \text{ or thus } E_{ab} = \frac{\Delta IAP}{\Delta IAV}$$

The relationship between IAV and IAP is curvilinear with an initial linear part followed by an exponential increase once a critical volume is reached (Fig. 1).

Pathophysiology

Accommodation of the Abdominal Cavity

In contrast to the intracranial compartment that is confined within a rigid bony structure, the abdominal compartment can change shape during increasing IAV. During the initial phase of increasing IAV (e.g., laparoscopic insufflation), IAP only rises minimally (linear 'reshaping phase' from spherical to circular shape). This is followed by a 'stretching phase' of the rectus abdominis muscle (curvilinear phase) and finally, when further IAV is added, only small increases in IAV will result in dramatic increase in IAP (exponential 'pressurization phase') (Fig. 2) [6, 7]. During the stretching phase, the shape of the abdomen will change from elliptical to

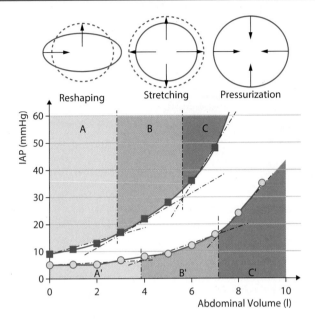

Fig. 2 Accommodation of the abdominal cavity. Schematic representation of different phases during increasing intraabdominal volume (IAV) in two patients undergoing laparoscopy (CO_2-insufflation). Shaded areas represent the reshaping phase (*light blue* – A and A'), the stretching phase (*medium blue* – B and B') and the pressurization phase (*dark blue* – C and C'). The apostrophe (') indicates the patient with good abdominal compliance. In the patient with poor compliance, the reshaping phase went from an IAV of 0 to 2.8 l (vs 0 to 3.8 l when compliance was normal), the stretching phase from IAV of 2.8 to 5.6 l (vs 3.8 to 7.2 l) and the pressurization phase from > 5.6 l vs 7.2 l in the patient with normal compliance. Adapted from [2] with permission

spherical. This change in shape is mainly due to an increase in the antero-posterior diameter and a decrease in the transverse diameter (transverse plane) of the internal abdominal perimeter [8–12].

Predictors for Stretching and Reshaping Capacity

Factors determining the reshaping properties of the abdominal wall and diaphragm are not well understood but the mechanical properties are related to C_{ab}. The stretching capacity is influenced by body anthropomorphy (weight, height, body mass index [BMI]), age, sex and visceral versus subcutaneous fat distribution [11]. Comorbidities like chronic obstructive lung disease (COPD) with emphysema (flatting of diaphragm), fluid overload (tissue and interstitial edema) or burn injury (with circular eschars) all have negative effects on stretching capacity. Android obesity usually results in increased visceral fat and a sphere-like baseline shape of the abdominal cavity with poor stretching capacity, whereas gynoid obesity presents with more subcutaneous fat for the same BMI or abdominal perimeter (Fig. 3). In gy-

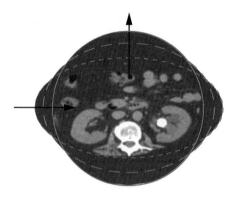

---- Baseline IAV at baseline IAP
Long/short axis: 42/26 cm
Internal perimeter: 108 cm
Surface area: 858 cm²

— — Streched IAV at IAP of 15 mmHg
Long/short axis: 40/31 cm
Internal perimeter: 112 cm
Surface area: 974 cm²

——— Maximal streched IAV (IAP 25 mmHg)
Long/short axis: 38/36 cm
Internal perimeter: 116 cm
Surface area: 1074 cm²

Fig. 3 Evolution of internal abdominal cavity perimeter during increase in volume. In case of gynoid obesity, the internal abdominal perimeter is shaped as an ellipse. Patients with an ellipse-shaped internal perimeter have a huge stretching capacity (and thus very good abdominal compliance); this is illustrated with the progression of the shape from ellipse (*dotted line*) at baseline to a sphere (*solid line*) at very high intra-abdominal pressures (IAP) obtained during laparoscopy. The arrows show the centripetal movement of the lateral edges of the ellipse and a centrifugal movement of the cranio-caudal edges. During increase in intra-abdominal volume (IAV) from baseline to stretched and maximal stretched IAV, the difference between the long and short axes of the ellipse decreases, while the internal perimeter and surface area increase. At maximal stretch, the external and internal abdominal perimeter are equal. Patients with android obesity do not have this reshaping and stretching capability. Adapted from [2] with permission

noid obesity, the internal abdominal perimeter is elliptical. Patients with an ellipse-shaped internal perimeter have a much greater stretching capacity (and thus very good C_{ab}).

Abdominal Pressure-Volume Relationship

A linear abdominal PV relationship has been described previously. However, this was mainly in studies where the observed IAP values were < 15 mmHg. During laparoscopy with limitation of insufflation pressures at 12 to 15 mmHg, the IAV did not reach a critical point at which an exponential increase in IAP occured [13]. As discussed above, the initial phase of the PV curve may indeed be linear (as observed during laparoscopy) but the remaining part is curvilinear or rather exponential [13–15]. Because of this exponential relationship, it is important to know both the shape and the position on the curve, as the actual position will determine the corresponding C_{ab}. In patients with IAH a small increase in IAV may push them into ACS (especially if C_{ab} is low) and, *vice versa*, in patients with ACS a small decrease in IAV (with paracentesis) may result in a dramatic improvement in IAP.

Measurement

Intra-Abdominal Pressure

Because of the fluid-like nature of the abdomen, following Pascal's law, the IAP can be measured in nearly every part of it. Rectal, uterine, inferior vena cava, bladder and gastric pressure measurements have all been described [16]. The use of direct intraperitoneal pressure measurement cannot be advocated in patients because of the complication risks, such as bleeding or infection. Bladder pressure measurements have been forwarded as the gold standard with the technique suggested in the WSACS consensus guidelines [1].

Intra-Abdominal Volume

The abdominal volume is more difficult to measure. However, it can be estimated by anthropomorphic indices and imaging techniques. Anthropomorphic-based indices for estimation of IAV have been described in obesity [17]. However, BMI does not correlate with C_{ab} but does correlate with IAP at the resting volume. This only applies in healthy individuals and sometimes in critically ill patients. The external abdominal perimeter (or circumference), although often used in the past, correlates reasonably with IAV, but poorly with IAP [18]. Changes in external abdominal perimeter over time on the other hand may correlate well with changes in IAP [18]. Another useful parameter is the waist-to-hip ratio. The waist is the smallest horizontal girth between the rib cage and iliac crest and the hip is the largest horizontal girth between waist and thigh. The waist-to-hip ratio correlates with IAP in men only [17]. A promising index is the abdominal volume index (AVI). A formula developed for calculating AVI estimates the overall abdominal volume between the symphysis pubis and the xiphoid process. This measure theoretically includes intra-abdominal fat and adipose volumes, with the waist and the hip dimensions. Although this index is superior to BMI, waist-to-hip ratio, and waist circumference, it has not yet been correlated to IAP [19]. Recently, techniques for estimating abdominal volume via three-dimensional (3D) ultrasound, water-suppressed breath hold magnetic resonance imaging (MRI), and computed tomography (CT) have been described. These techniques have not yet gained entrance to the intensive care unit (ICU). Although 3D ultrasound cannot measure IAV *in toto*, it estimates the volumes of separate intra-abdominal organs. MRI and CT techniques calculate the visceral and subcutaneous fat volume or thus the volume of the adipose tissue. Quantitative CT analysis assessing volume, density and weight of abdominal organs may be a promising tool for the future [9, 10, 20, 21].

Abdominal Compliance

Qualitative Measurement of Abdominal Wall Tension During Palpation

The grade of indentation at the site where the downward force is applied can be measured during palpation of the abdomen. Palpation examines intra-abdominal tension, passive and active muscle tension. However, it is not able to quantify C_{ab} properly nor has it been validated in the clinical setting. The use of an abdominal tensiometer has also been described; however, this technique is only in its infancy [22].

PV Relationship During Laparoscopy with CO_2 Pneumoperitoneum

It has been observed that the compliance of the abdominal cavity decreases when additional volume is added [23]. The linear abdominal PV curve changed to a rather exponential shape when a pressure of 15 mmHg was achieved by insufflation of CO_2 [13, 14]. In studies, the initial C_{ab} at the beginning of the CO_2 inflation varied between 333 and 400 ml/mmHg and at higher IAV (with corresponding IAP > 15 mmHg), the C_{ab} decreased to 60 and 90 ml/mmHg [3]. Similar relationships have been described with addition or removal of gastric contents [3].

PV Relationship During Drainage or Addition of Abdominal Free Fluid

Measurements of C_{ab} have been performed in humans by IAP assessment with at least two corresponding IAV values by addition of abdominal fluid during peritoneal dialysis or by drainage of intra-abdominal fluid (ascites in liver cirrhosis, peripancreatic fluid or pseudocyst, serous fluid collections in trauma or burns) [2–4].

Interactions Between Different Compartments

Polycompartment Model

Being linked and bound by the diaphragm, the thoracic and abdominal compartments cannot be treated in isolation. Applied airway pressure (P_{aw}) by mechanical ventilation will be transmitted to the lungs, pleural (P_{pl}) and abdominal spaces (IAP). In a simplified model, the lung and thorax are in series and coupled to the diaphragm and abdomen in series. Changes in IAP are paralleled by changes in P_{pl}. Changes in thoracic compliance will be reflected by changes in abdominal compliance and *vice versa*; as a consequence, increased IAP will result in reduced chest wall compliance. The interactions between different compartments have been referred to as the polycompartment model and syndrome [24, 25]. For example, transmission of airway pressures to the abdomen results from interactions between the thoracic and abdominal compartment and the percentage of pressure transmission is called the thoraco-abdominal index (TAI) of transmission. This occurs in patients receiving positive pressure ventilation, application of positive end-expiratory pressure (PEEP), presence of intrinsic or auto-PEEP or a tension pneumothorax. Conversely, transmission of pressure from the abdomen to the thorax is called the abdomino-thoracic index (ATI) and occurs in any physiologic (pregnancy) or pathologic condition associated with increased IAP; the ATI ranges from 20 to 80% and is on average 50% [26, 27]. The effects of increased IAP on end-organ function are numerous: neurologic, respiratory, cardiovascular and renal adverse effects have all been described in patients with IAH and ACS. Increased IAP leads to diminished venous return, necessitating more fluid loading, causing mesenteric vein compression and venous hypertension, finally triggering a vicious cycle.

Estimation of Abdominal Compliance During Low Flow Pressure Volume Loop

C_{ab} can be estimated by analysis of the dynamic changes caused by mechanical ventilation on IAP. During a low flow PV loop to determine the best PEEP, one can observe the change in mean IAP. The compliance obtained by this maneuver can be calculated as follows:

$$C_{abPV} = \Delta V_T / \Delta \text{ mean IAP}$$

with ΔV_T the insufflated tidal volume and ΔIAP the difference between meanIAP at the end and start of the PV loop.

Estimation of Abdominal Compliance During Mechanical Ventilation

Whilst looking at the effects of tidal volume excursions on IAP and by calculating the difference between IAP_{ei} and IAP_{ee}, one can also obtain an idea of C_{ab} [28]:

$$C_{abV_T} = V_T / \Delta IAP$$

The higher the respiratory excursions seen in a continuous IAP tracing, the lower the C_{ab} (for the same tidal volume). Alternatively, the higher the IAP, the higher the ΔIAP or the lower the C_{ab}.

Calculation of Abdominal Pressure Variation

As discussed previously, the higher the APV for any given IAP, the lower the C_{ab} and *vice versa*, the lower the C_{ab}, the higher the APV; hence APV can be used as a non-invasive and continuous estimation of C_{ab}.

Respiratory Abdominal Variation Test (RAVT)

A final non-invasive method for estimation of C_{ab} can be done by performing a respiratory abdominal variation test (RAVT) (Fig. 4). The C_{ab} obtained with RAVT correlates with the C_{ab} obtained from ΔIAP during mechanical ventilation; increasing tidal volume increases IAP_{ei} while increasing PEEP increases IAP_{ee}.

$$C_{abRAVT} = \Delta V_T / \Delta IAP_{ei}$$

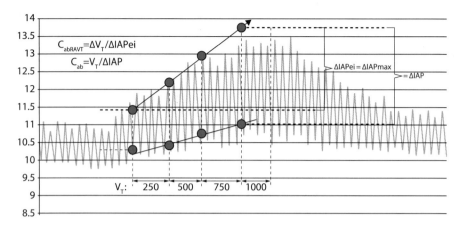

Fig. 4 Estimation of abdominal compliance (C_{ab}) during the respiratory abdominal variation test (RAVT) in intermittent positive pressure ventilation (IPPV)-mode. The graph shows the smoothed average of a continuous intra-abdominal pressure (IAP) tracing (CiMON, Pulsion Medical System, Munich, Germany) obtained during the RAVT in IPPV mode. The tidal volume (V_T) was increased stepwise from 250 to 1000 ml with increments of 250 ml. At each V_T, the following parameters were recorded: end-expiratory IAP (IAP_{ee}), end-inspiratory IAP (IAP_{ei}), IAP and ΔIAP. With increasing V_T mainly the IAP_{ei} increases whereas IAP_{ee} remains relatively unchanged. During the RAVT, the diaphragm is displaced caudally and an additional volume is added to the abdominal cavity. The ΔIAV is probably correlated to the ΔV_T observed between the start and the end of the RAVT (= 750 ml). The slope of the curve connecting the IAP_{ei} at each V_T can be used to estimate the C_{ab}. The C_{abRAVT} in the sample shown can be calculated as follows: $C_{abRAVT} = \Delta V_T / \Delta IAP_{ei} = 750/(13.6 - 11.5) = 357.1$ ml/mmHg and this correlates well with the C_{abVT}: $C_{abVT} = V_T / \Delta IAP = 1000/(13.6 - 11) = 384.6$ ml/mmHg. Adapted from [3] with permission

Prognostic and Predictive Factors Related to Abdominal Compliance

Theoretically, C_{ab} allows prediction of complications during laparoscopy and mechanical ventilation, identification of patients who would benefit from delayed abdominal closure, those in whom to monitor IAP, and those at risk during prone ventilation, etc. ... Therefore, prediction of poor or high C_{ab} can be clinically important.

Conditions Associated with Decreased Abdominal Compliance

Aside from risk factors for IAH, patients should also be screened for risk factors for decreased C_{ab}. These are listed in Box 1 and can be divided into those related to body habitus and anthropomorphy; those related to comorbidities and/or increased non-compressible IAV; and those related to the abdominal wall and diaphragm [3].

Box 1. Factors Associated with Decreased Abdominal Compliance. Adapted from [2] with Permission

1) Related to anthropomorphy and demographics
- Android composition (sphere, apple shape)
- Increased visceral fat
- Waist-to-hip ratio > 1
- Short stature
- Male sex
- Young age (increased elastic recoil)
- Obesity (weight, BMI)

2) Related to comorbidities and/or increased non-compressible intra-abdominal volume (IAV)
- Fluid overload
- Abdominal fluid collections, pseudocyst, abscess
- Sepsis, burns, trauma and bleeding (coagulopathy)
- Bowels filled with fluid
- Stomach filled with fluid
- Tense ascites
- Hepatomegaly
- Splenomegaly

3) Related to abdominal wall and diaphragm
- Interstitial and anasarca edema (skin, abdominal wall)
- Abdominal burn eschars (circular)
- Thoracic burn eschars (circular)
- Tight closure after abdominal surgery
- Abdominal Velcro belt or adhesive drapes
- Prone positioning
- Head-of-bed > 45°
- Umbilical hernia repair
- Muscle contractions (pain)
- Body builders ('6-pack')
- Pneumoperitoneum
- Pneumatic anti-shock garments
- Abdominal wall bleeding
- Rectus sheath hematoma
- Correction of large hernias
- Gastroschisis
- Omphalocele
- Mechanical ventilation (positive pressure)
- Fighting with the ventilator

- Use of accessory muscles
- Use of positive end-expiratory pressure (PEEP)
- Presence of auto-PEEP (tension pneumothorax)
- Chronic obstructive pulmonary disease (COPD) emphysema (diaphragm flattening)
- Basal pleuropneumonia

Morbidly obese patients have a higher baseline IAP around 12–14 mmHg, and this is mainly related to the presence of central obesity [17, 29–32]. Morbidly obese patients with an android (mainly visceral and sphere shaped) fat distribution have a limited reserve to accommodate excess IAV than those patients who, for a similar BMI or abdominal perimeter, have a gynoid (mainly subcutaneous and ellipse shaped) fat distribution [17, 29]. On the other hand, subcutaneous fat accumulation may have a negative effect on the elastic properties of the abdominal wall, although the thin muscle layer may have a beneficial effect. Therefore, it is not possible to predict C_{ab} in obese patients; in general C_{ab} is decreased because of the increased baseline IAV.

Conditions Associated with Increased Abdominal Compliance

These are listed in Box 2 and can be divided into those related to body habitus and anthropomorphy; those related to absence of comorbidities and/or increased compressible IAV; and those related to abdominal wall and diaphragm. Chronic conditions will have higher C_{ab} for the same change in IAV as illustrated in Fig. 5.

> **Box 2. Factors Associated with Increased Abdominal Compliance. Adapted from [2] with Permission**
>
> **1) Related to anthropomorphy and demographics**
> - Gynoid composition (ellipse, pear-shaped)
> - Waist-to-hip ratio < 0.8
> - Peripheral obesity
> - Preferentially subcutaneous fat
> - Height (tall stature)
> - Old age (loss of elastic recoil)
> - Female sex
> - Lean and slim body
> - Normal BMI
>
> **2) Related to absence of comorbidities and/or increased compressible intra-abdominal volume (IAV)**
> - Absence of deadly triad: normothermia, normal pH, normal coagulation
> - Bowels filled with air
> - Stomach filled with air
> - Absence of fluid overload (second or third space fluid accumulation)
>
> **3) Related to abdominal wall and diaphragm**
> - Previous pregnancy
> - Previous laparoscopy
> - Previous abdominal surgery
> - Abdominal wall lift
> - Weight loss
> - Chronic intra-abdominal hypertension (IAH)
> - Umbilical hernia (before repair)
> - Burn escharotomy (thorax and/or abdomen)
> - Avoidance of tight closure
> - Open abdomen with temporary abdominal closure
> - Beach chair positioning
> - Sedation and analgesia
> - Muscle relaxation
> - Bronchodilation
> - Lung protective ventilation
> - Pre-stretching of fascia (cirrhosis with ascites, peritoneal dialysis when fluid is drained from abdomen)

Previous stretching of the abdominal fascia increases C_{ab}. This can be explained by a gradual prestretching of the internal abdominal cavity perimeter during acute or progressive increased IAV (as is the case during laparoscopy, with pregnancy,

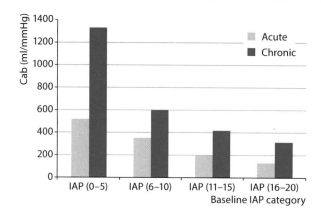

Fig. 5 Abdominal compliance (C_{ab}) in relation to baseline intra-abdominal pressure (IAP). Bar graph showing mean values of C_{ab} (ml/mmHg) per baseline IAP category (mmHg) in acute (*light blue bars*) and chronic (*dark blue bars*) conditions. Acute conditions are laparoscopy and evacuation of ascites, collections or hematomas in acutely ill patients, whereas chronic condition refers to peritoneal dialysis. Adapted from [3] with permission

peritoneal dialysis, cirrhotic ascites) [7–9, 33, 34], which leads to increased reshaping capacity. Prestretching or overdistension may indeed result in tissue damage and fibrosis of the abdominal wall structure with lengthened muscle fibers and diminished elastic retraction capacity. History of a previous laparotomy may lead to scarring of the abdominal wall, which in combination with adhesions may cause decreased elasticity [33]. The C_{ab} may be decreased or increased and the effect of previous laparotomy on baseline IAV and IAP is unpredictable. The use of external bandages (drapings, Velcro belt, etc.) or tight surgical closure causes a mechanical limitation; these should be avoided in high-risk patients and IAP should be measured during their use. In case of capillary leak, fluid overload and fluid collections, IAV and IAP will both increase while reshaping capacity and wall compliance will decrease.

Treatment

How to Decrease Baseline IAP?

In simple terms, in order to reduce IAP, either (additional) IAV has to be removed intra-luminally or intra-abdominally (e.g., weight loss, fluid removal via dialysis, ascites drainage, gastric suctioning, evacuation of abscess or hematoma, etc.), or the C_{ab} has to be improved by increasing the internal abdominal cavity perimeter and surface area (pre-stretching, open abdomen treatment) [35, 36]. Weight loss and the resulting decrease in BMI will decrease IAP [37].

How to Reduce IAV?

The evacuation of intra-luminal and intra-abdominal contents can be done, for example, via placement of a nasogastric tube with suctioning with or without gastro-prokinetics (cisapride, metoclopramide or erythromycin). Paracentesis with evacuation of ascites and the placement of a rectal tube in conjunction with enemas and colonoprokinetics (prostygmin) may also reduce IAV [38]. Colonic pseudo-obstruction or Ogilvie's syndrome may be treated with endoscopic decompression of large bowel or a surgical colostomy or ileostomy together with colonoprokinetics. When in doubt, imaging should be performed and ultrasound or CT guided drainage should be attempted in case of hematoma, abscess, fluid collections, etc. The correction of capillary leak and avoiding a positive fluid balance will eventually lead to a decreased IAV by decreasing organ and bowel edema [39]. This can be achieved with (hypertonic) albumin in combination with diuretics (furosemide), correction of capillary leak (antibiotics, source control, ...), the use of colloids instead of crystalloids and eventually dialysis or continuous veno-venous hemofiltration (CVVH) with ultrafiltration [40]. Targeted APP with the use of vasopressors will reduce venocongestion and this will lower IAV (in analogy to the effect of norepinephrine on intracranial pressure and cerebral perfusion pressure) and dobutamine (but not dopamine) will improve splanchnic perfusion. Ascorbinic acid has been associated with a reduced incidence of secondary ACS in burn patients, although its routine use has yet to be validated.

How to Improve C_{ab}?

Improvement in C_{ab} should be performed in a stepwise approach as suggested by the WSACS consensus recommendations [1, 3].

First Step: Ensure Adequate Sedation and Analgesia
Fentanyl should not be used as it may increase abdominal muscle tone while dexmedetomedine has superior effects over propofol. Thoracic epidural anesthesia has been shown to reduce IAP via an increase in C_{ab} [41].

Second Step: Remove Constrictive Bandages and Eschars
Any tight abdominal closure, like a Velcro belt to prevent incisional hernia in a patient with abdominal hypertension and end-organ dysfunction, should be removed immediately. Likewise, escharotomies (abdominal but also thoracic) will increase C_{ab} while sternotomy will increase not only thoracic wall compliance but also C_{ab} [42–44]. Placing a chest tube in case of a tension pneumothorax or pleural effusion will also increase C_{ab}.

Third Step: Avoid Prone and Head of Bed > 30°and Consider Reverse Trendelenburg Position

Body positioning, such as the Trendelenburg position, may lower bladder pressure; however, it may also compromise respiratory function [29]. The use of head-of-bed elevation > 30° may on the other hand increase bladder pressure and the head-of-bed 45° position will increase IAP by 5 to 15 mmHg [29]. Therefore, in patients with respiratory insufficiency who are mechanically ventilated, the anti-Trendelenburg position may be best to allow lung recruitment, oxygenation and ventilation [16]. During prone positioning there is merit in unloading the abdomen (abdominal suspension) as this will result in a decrease in chest wall compliance, while the effect of gravity will improve C_{ab} and decrease IAP. During laparoscopy, body position can also help to optimize the laparoscopic workspace IAV. The Trendelenburg position with head-of-bed at 20° provides the optimal workspace in lower abdominal laparoscopic surgery, while during upper abdominal laparoscopic surgery in obese patients, the beach-chair position (flexing the legs in reverse Trendelenburg) is optimal [45]. Laparoscopic insufflation pressures should at all times be limited to 15 mmHg. Higher working pressures cannot be routinely recommended in obese patients with high baseline IAP and in morbidly obese patients, open surgery seems the best option because of the high complication risk associated with pneumoperitoneum [31].

Fourth Step: Lose Weight and Avoid Fluid Overload

Similar to weight loss, avoiding a positive cumulative fluid balance and obtaining a negative fluid balance with the use of diuretics in combination or not with hypertonic solutions (albumin 20%) [40, 46] will decrease interstitial edema of the abdominal wall and increase C_{ab}. Fluid resuscitation should be guided by volumetric (and not barometric) preload indicators and, if central venous pressure (CVP) is used, transmural pressures should be calculated:

$$CVP_{tm} = CVP_{ee} - IAP/2.$$

In case diuretics do not have a sufficient effect, renal replacement therapy with hemodialysis or CVVH can be used [1, 3].

Fifth Step: Use Neuromuscular Blockers

Theoretically, the use of neuromuscular blockade should not only lower baseline IAP but also improve C_{ab} [1, 3]. However, some studies showed no additional increase in C_{ab} after full block of abdominal muscle contractions (guided by train of four) [7].

Sixth Step: Less Invasive Surgery

Recently a less invasive percutaneous endoscopic abdominal wall component separation (EACS) technique has been described [47]. With this technique, the abdominal capacity (maximal stretched volume) increased by 1 l while IAP decreased from 15.9 ± 2.1 to 11 ± 1.5 mmHg (p < 0.001) [47]. Another alternative for midline laparotomy is subcutaneous linea alba fasciotomy (SLAF), which seems a promising approach especially in secondary IAH and ACS [48].

When all the above listed treatment options fail to provide a sufficient decrease in IAP and IAV, the only definite solution is to perform a decompressive laparotomy that will assist with IAP, IAV and C_{ab} [49].

Conclusion

C_{ab} is a measure of the ease of abdominal expansion, determined by the elasticity of the abdominal wall and diaphragm. It is expressed as the change in IAV per change in IAP (ml/mmHg). The C_{ab} baseline in 'resting conditions' is determined by the baseline IAP and IAV, the external and internal abdominal cavity perimeter and surface area and shape, the additional and maximal stretched volume, the presence of predisposing conditions and comorbidities as well as tissue properties of the fascia, abdominal wall and diaphragm. As such, C_{ab} should be viewed separately from the abdominal wall and diaphragm compliance with its own specific elastic properties. C_{ab} can be estimated based on demographic and anthropomorphic data and can be assessed by PV relationship analysis of the observed changes in IAP (mirroring induced changes in IAV). The abdominal PV relationship is believed to be linear up to pressures of 12–15 mmHg and increases exponentially thereafter. C_{ab} can also be estimated non-invasively by examining the interactions between pressure variations in the thorax and abdominal compartment during positive pressure ventilation. C_{ab} is one of the most neglected parameters in critically ill patients, although it plays a key-role in understanding organ-organ interactions and the deleterious effects of unadapted IAV on IAP and end-organ perfusion. A large overlap exists between the treatment of patients with IAH and those with low C_{ab}, but when we identify the latter, we should potentially be able to anticipate and select the most appropriate medical or surgical treatment to avoid complications related to IAH or ACS.

References

1. Kirkpatrick AW, Roberts DJ, De Waele J et al (2013) Intra-abdominal hypertension and the abdominal compartment syndrome: updated consensus definitions and clinical practice guidelines from the World Society of the Abdominal Compartment Syndrome. Intensive Care Med 39:1190–1206
2. Malbrain MLNG, Roberts DJ, De laet I (2014) The role of abdominal compliance, the neglected parameter in critically ill patients – a consensus review of 16. Part 1: Definitions and pathophysiology. Anaesthesiol Intensive Ther 46:392–405
3. Malbrain MLNG, De laet I, De Waele J (2014) The role of abdominal compliance, the neglected parameter in critically ill patients – a consensus review of 16. Part 2: Measurement techniques and management recommendations. Anaesthesiol Intensive Ther 46:406–432
4. Blaser AR, Bjorck M, De Keulenaer B, Regli A (2015) Abdominal compliance: A bench-to-bedside review. J Trauma Acute Care Surg 78:1044–1053

5. Malbrain ML, Chiumello D, Pelosi P et al (2005) Incidence and prognosis of intraabdominal hypertension in a mixed population of critically ill patients: a multiple-center epidemiological study. Crit Care Med 33:315–322

6. Mulier JP, Dillemans B, Heremans L (2007) Determinants of the abdominal pressure volume relation in non ACS patients. Acta Clin Belg Suppl 62:289

7. Mulier J, Dillemans B, Crombach M, Missant C, Sels A (2008) On the abdominal pressure volume relationship. The Internet Journal of Anesthesiology 21:1

8. Song C, Alijani A, Frank T, Hanna GB, Cuschieri A (2006) Mechanical properties of the human abdominal wall measured in vivo during insufflation for laparoscopic surgery. Surg Endosc 20:987–990

9. Vlot J, Wijnen R, Stolker RJ, Bax KN (2014) Optimizing working space in laparoscopy: CT measurement of the effect of pre-stretching of the abdominal wall in a porcine model. Surg Endosc 28:841–846

10. Accarino A, Perez F, Azpiroz F, Quiroga S, Malagelada JR (2009) Abdominal distention results from caudo-ventral redistribution of contents. Gastroenterology 136:1544–1551

11. Mulier JP, Coenegrachts K, Van de Moortele K (2008) CT analysis of the elastic deformation and elongation of the abdominal wall during colon insufflation for virtual coloscopy. Eur J Anesth 25(S44):42 (abst)

12. Villoria A, Azpiroz F, Soldevilla A, Perez F, Malagelada JR (2008) Abdominal accommodation: a coordinated adaptation of the abdominal wall to its content. Am J Gastroenterol 103:2807–2815

13. Abu-Rafea B, Vilos GA, Vilos AG, Hollett-Caines J, Al-Omran M (2006) Effect of body habitus and parity on insufflated CO2 volume at various intraabdominal pressures during laparoscopic access in women. J Minim Invasive Gynecol 13:205–210

14. McDougall EM, Figenshau RS, Clayman RV, Monk TG, Smith DS (1994) Laparoscopic pneumoperitoneum: impact of body habitus. J Laparoendosc Surg 4:385–391

15. Fischbach M, Terzic J, Laugel V, Escande B, Dangelser C, Helmstetter A (2003) Measurement of hydrostatic intraperitoneal pressure: a useful tool for the improvement of dialysis dose prescription. Pediatr Nephrol 18:976–980

16. Malbrain ML (2004) Different techniques to measure intra-abdominal pressure (IAP): time for a critical re-appraisal. Intensive Care Med 30:357–371

17. Sugerman H, Windsor A, Bessos M, Wolfe L (1997) Intra-abdominal pressure, sagittal abdominal diameter and obesity comorbidity. J Intern Med 241:71–79

18. Malbrain ML, De laet I, Van Regenmortel N, Schoonheydt K, Dits H (2009) Can the abdominal perimeter be used as an accurate estimation of intra-abdominal pressure? Crit Care Med 37:316–319

19. Guerrero-Romero F, Rodriguez-Moran M (2003) Abdominal volume index. An anthropometry-based index for estimation of obesity is strongly related to impaired glucose tolerance and type 2 diabetes mellitus. Arch Med Res 34:428–432

20. Kirkpatrick AW, Colistro R, Laupland KB et al (2007) Renal arterial resistive index response to intraabdominal hypertension in a porcine model. Crit Care Med 35:207–213

21. Forstemann T, Trzewik J, Holste J et al (2011) Forces and deformations of the abdominal wall – a mechanical and geometrical approach to the linea alba. J Biomech 44:600–606

22. van Ramshorst GH, Salih M, Hop WC et al (2011) Noninvasive assessment of intra-abdominal pressure by measurement of abdominal wall tension. J Surg Res 171:240–244

23. Gilroy RJ Jr, Lavietes MH, Loring SH, Mangura BT, Mead J (1985) Respiratory mechanical effects of abdominal distension. J Appl Physiol 58:1997–2003 (1985)

24. Malbrain ML, Wilmer A (2007) The polycompartment syndrome: towards an understanding of the interactions between different compartments! Intensive Care Med 33:1869–1872

25. Malbrain MLNG, Roberts DJ, Sugrue M et al (2014) The polycompartment syndrome: a concise state-of-the-art review. Anaesthesiol Intensive Ther 46:433–450

26. Wauters J, Wilmer A, Valenza F (2007) Abdomino-thoracic transmission during ACS: facts and figures. Acta Clin Belg Suppl 62:200–205

27. Wauters J, Claus P, Brosens N et al (2012) Relationship between abdominal pressure, pulmonary compliance, and cardiac preload in a porcine model. Crit Care Res Pract 2012:763181
28. Sturini E, Saporito A, Sugrue M, Parr MJ, Bishop G, Braschi A (2008) Respiratory variation of intra-abdominal pressure: indirect indicator of abdominal compliance? Intensive Care Med 34:1632–1637
29. De Keulenaer BL, De Waele JJ, Powell B, Malbrain ML (2009) What is normal intra-abdominal pressure and how is it affected by positioning, body mass and positive end-expiratory pressure? Intensive Care Med 35:969–976
30. Lambert DM, Marceau S, Forse RA (2005) Intra-abdominal pressure in the morbidly obese. Obes Surg 15:1225–1232
31. Nguyen NT, Wolfe BM (2005) The physiologic effects of pneumoperitoneum in the morbidly obese. Ann Surg 241:219–226
32. Sugerman HJ (1998) Increased intra-abdominal pressure in obesity. Int J Obes Relat Metab Disord 22:1138
33. Verbeke K, Casier I, Van Acker B, Dillemans B, Mulier J (2010) Impact of laparoscopy on the abdominal compliance is determined by the duration of the pneumoperitoneum the number of gravidity and the existence of a previous laparoscopy or laparotomy. Eur J Anesth 27:29–30
34. Becker V, Schmid RM, Umgelter A (2009) Comparison of a new device for the continuous intra-gastric measurement of intra-abdominal pressure (CiMon) with direct intra-peritoneal measurements in cirrhotic patients during paracentesis. Intensive Care Med 35:948–952
35. Cheatham ML, Malbrain ML, Kirkpatrick A et al (2007) Results from the International Conference of Experts on Intra-abdominal Hypertension and Abdominal Compartment Syndrome. II. Recommendations. Intensive Care Med 33:951–962
36. De laet I, Malbrain ML (2007) ICU management of the patient with intra-abdominal hypertension: what to do, when and to whom? Acta Clin Belg 62(Suppl):190–199
37. Sugerman H, Windsor A, Bessos M, Kellum J, Reines H, DeMaria E (1998) Effects of surgically induced weight loss on urinary bladder pressure, sagittal abdominal diameter and obesity co-morbidity. Int J Obes Relat Metab Disord 22:230–235
38. Cheatham ML, Safcsak K (2011) Percutaneous catheter decompression in the treatment of elevated intraabdominal pressure. Chest 140:1428–1435
39. Cordemans C, De laet I, Van Regenmortel N et al (2012) Fluid management in critically ill patients: The role of extravascular lung water, abdominal hypertension, capillary leak and fluid balance. Ann Intensive Care 2(Suppl 1):S1
40. Cordemans C, De Laet I, Van Regenmortel N et al (2012) Aiming for a negative fluid balance in patients with acute lung injury and increased intra-abdominal pressure: a pilot study looking at the effects of PAL-treatment. Ann Intensive Care 2(Suppl 1):15
41. Hakobyan RV, Mkhoyan GG (2008) Epidural analgesia decreases intraabdominal pressure in postoperative patients with primary intra-abdominal hypertension. Acta Clin Belg 63:86–92
42. Tsoutsos D, Rodopoulou S, Keramidas E, Lagios M, Stamatopoulos K, Ioannovich J (2003) Early escharotomy as a measure to reduce intraabdominal hypertension in full-thickness burns of the thoracic and abdominal area. World J Surg 27:1323–1328
43. Oda J, Ueyama M, Yamashita K et al (2005) Effects of escharotomy as abdominal decompression on cardiopulmonary function and visceral perfusion in abdominal compartment syndrome with burn patients. J Trauma 59:369–374
44. Bloomfield GL, Ridings PC, Blocher CR, Marmarou A, Sugerman HJ (1997) A proposed relationship between increased intra-abdominal, intrathoracic, and intracranial pressure. Crit Care Med 25:496–503
45. Mulier JP, Dillemans B, Van Cauwenberge S (2010) Impact of the patient's body position on the intraabdominal workspace during laparoscopic surgery. Surg Endosc 24:1398–1402
46. Malbrain ML, Marik PE, Witters I et al (2014) Fluid overload, de-resuscitation, and outcomes in critically ill or injured patients: a systematic review with suggestions for clinical practice. Anaesthesiol Intensive Ther 46:361–380

47. Voss M, Pinheiro J, Reynolds J et al (2003) Endoscopic components separation for abdominal compartment syndrome. Am J Surg 186:158–163
48. Leppaniemi A, Hienonen P, Mentula P, Kemppainen E (2011) Subcutaneous linea alba fasciotomy, does it really work? Am Surg 77:99–102
49. De Waele JJ, Hoste EA, Malbrain ML (2006) Decompressive laparotomy for abdominal compartment syndrome – a critical analysis. Crit Care 10:R51

Part X

Metabolic Support

Metabonomics and Intensive Care

D. Antcliffe and A. C. Gordon

Introduction

Metabonomics is "the quantitative measurement over time of the metabolic responses of an individual or population to drug treatment or other intervention" [1], such as a disease process, and provides a 'top-down' integrated overview of the biochemistry in a complex system. The metabolic profile is determined by both host genetic and environmental factors [2]. As such, metabonomics has great potential for intensive care medicine, where patients are complex and understanding the relationship of host factors, disease and treatment effects is key to improving care. Approaches that focus on single or small sets of biomarkers may fail to capture this complexity, so metabonomics may have advantages for both understanding diseases and improving diagnostics and treatment monitoring.

Spectroscopic techniques, including nuclear magnetic resonance (NMR) spectroscopy and mass spectrometry, have been used to determine the global metabolic profiles of numerous types of biological samples. Most commonly, blood and urine are analyzed but any biological specimens, including tissue, cerebrospinal fluid or exhaled breath condensate, can be used [3–6]. Metabonomic methods have been used to evaluate numerous clinically-significant conditions including trauma [7, 8], acute kidney injury (AKI) and monitoring of dialysis [9–11], subarachnoid hemorrhage [12], and acute lung injury (ALI) [13].

The two broad analytical platforms, NMR and mass spectrometry, each have their own strengths and weaknesses and together give complementary information. Data can be acquired that either provides non-targeted global metabolic information, which is useful for initial biomarker discovery, or can be targeted to obtain detailed information on a specific class of metabolites or metabolic processes.

D. Antcliffe · A. C. Gordon (✉)
Section of Anaesthetics, Pain Medicine & Intensive Care, Department of Surgery & Cancer,
Charing Cross Hospital / Imperial College London
London, UK
email: anthony.gordon@imperial.ac.uk

© Springer International Publishing Switzerland 2016
J.-L. Vincent (ed.), *Annual Update in Intensive Care and Emergency Medicine 2016*,
DOI 10.1007/978-3-319-27349-5_28

Nuclear Magnetic Resonance Spectroscopy

NMR spectroscopy harnesses the magnetic properties of certain nuclei that possess spin, for example ^1H and ^{13}C. Commonly in metabonomics, ^1H or proton NMR is used. NMR spectrometers use superconductors to generate a strong magnetic field (Fig. 1). A spinning charge placed in such a magnetic field produces two spin states: one up, aligned with the magnetic field; and one down, aligned against the magnetic field. The energy difference between the two spin states is influenced by the local electron environment, which acts to shield the nucleus. When a sample containing these nuclei is excited with a radio frequency pulse, those nuclei in the lower energy spin state excite into the higher energy state and the subtle differences in the resonances generated can be used to give information regarding chemical structure. Resonances are reported in relation to a reference signal, such as 3-(trimethyl-silyl) propionic acid (TSP) or tetramethylsilane (TMS), and in order to account for magnetic fields of different strengths these values are given as chemical shifts in parts per million (ppm).

Chemical shifts are predictable based on the local electron shielding and give information about the structure of the molecule. The magnitude or intensity of

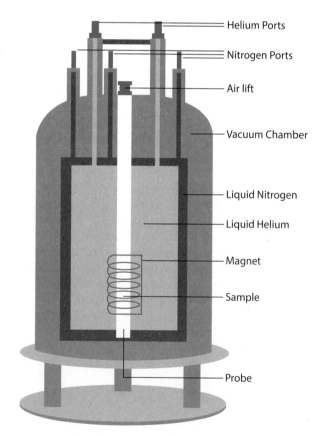

Fig. 1 Schematic diagram detailing the main components of a nuclear magnetic resonance (NMR) spectrometer

Helium Ports

Nitrogen Ports

Air lift

Vacuum Chamber

Liquid Nitrogen

Liquid Helium

Magnet

Sample

Probe

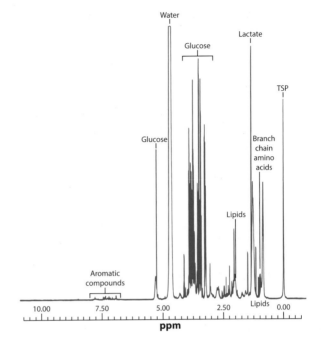

Fig. 2 Example of a ^{1}H nuclear magnetic resonance Carr-Purcell-Meiboom-Gill (NMR CPMG) spectrum of human serum. TSP: 3-(trimethyl-silyl) propionic acid

NMR resonance signals is displayed along the vertical axis of a spectrum, and is proportional to the concentration of the sample.

Typically, ^{1}H NMR spectra of urine contain thousands of narrow, low molecular weight metabolites, whereas those from serum and plasma contain a mixture of low and high molecular weight compounds (Fig. 2). Experimental pulse sequences can be chosen to selectively suppress particular spectral features; for example, the Carr-Purcell-Meiboom-Gill (CPMG) sequence will suppress large molecular weight metabolites revealing those of a smaller weight. Common to all experiments is the need to suppress the large water peak and this is achieved with a solvent suppression pulse sequence.

For the purposes of metabonomics, ^{1}H NMR has several strengths. Little sample preparation is required, and the technique is relatively non-destructive, quantitative, and non-invasive. Data obtained from NMR experiments are reproducible [14] and robust. Concentrations of metabolites are detectable down to micromole/l concentrations and analysis is relatively quick, taking as little as 3–4 min per sample.

Mass Spectrometry

Mass spectrometry is a technique that aims to identify metabolites within a sample based on the detection of the mass-charge ratio (m/z) of ions produced by the ionization of chemical compounds. Molecules in a sample are vaporized before being

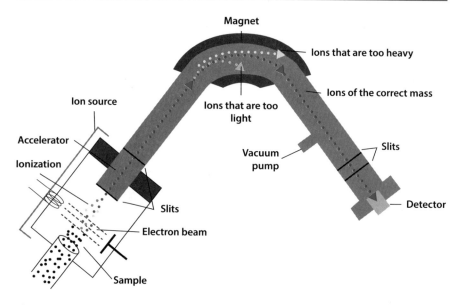

Fig. 3 A schematic diagram of the component parts of a mass spectrometer

ionized by bombardment with either electrons or other ions. The molecule is thus broken into charged fragments which can be sorted based on their m/z ratio and de- tected by a device capable of detecting charged particles. Several techniques exist to separate and detect molecular fragments; an example is separation by accelerat- ing ions and subjecting them to an electric or magnetic field (Fig. 3). The recorded data can be displayed as a spectrum of the relative abundances of the various ions with the same m/z ratios.

In order to improve mass separation, mass spectrometry is often coupled to chromatographic techniques. Such techniques include gas chromatography-mass spectrometry (GC-MS), where a gas chromatogram is used to separate molecules in gaseous phase before they are fed into the ion source. Liquid chromatography- mass spectrometry (LC-MS) and high performance liquid chromatography-mass spectrometry (HPLC-MS) similarly separate molecules in a sample in a liquid mo- bile phase using a liquid chromatogram with a combination of organic solvents prior to ionization.

Mass spectrometry-based platforms have the advantage of greater sensitivity compared to NMR; however, some substances, such as sugars and amino acids, are difficult to analyze with this method due to their polarity and lack of volatil- ity [15]. Mass spectrometry requires reasonably extensive sample preparation and, with long chromatographic times, can take longer to process than NMR. Also, be- cause of the need to vaporize and ionize the sample, mass spectrometry is a more destructive analytical technique than NMR.

Data Analysis

Analytical techniques used in metabonomics generate data sets that are unlike those produced in many other scientific fields. Whereas there would often be many more subjects than variables, metabonomics generally produces thousands of variables, several of which may correlate, and many may not be normally distributed. These features pose problems for regular statistical methods so analysis is generally performed using multivariate statistics. Broadly speaking multivariate methods can be split into unsupervised tests, where no class information is supplied to the model, and supervised tests, designed to look for group separation based on class information. Unsupervised tests are good at finding natural clustering within the data sets and at identifying outliers. Supervised tests, on the other hand, look for variation between predefined groups or classes and are able to build predictive models.

Principal Component Analysis

Principal component analysis (PCA) is a common method of unsupervised multivariate analysis used in metabonomics. It is used to elucidate the covariance structure of the data set by representing the data along new axes based on the direction of the maximum variation, the principal components. The first principal component is the direction of greatest variation and the second principal component is that with the second largest value that is orthogonal to the first (Fig. 4). This method of analysis allows data reduction. Some components will contain very little variation and those with low magnitudes, which contain little information, are discarded. The data can then be re-displayed using the principal components as a new set of axes, giving a PCA scores plot (Fig. 4).

An approximation to the Student's t-test, called the Hotelling's ellipse, can be projected onto the scores plot. This gives an indication of a 95% confidence interval within which 95% of observations should fall. Data points lying outside of this ellipse can be considered as outliers and can be examined in more detail.

Supervised Analysis

Supervised multivariate analysis is aimed at finding the variation in the data matrix that explains predefined classifications. One of the underlying methods of supervised analysis is the partial least squares analysis (PLS). PLS determines the underlying relationship between two data matrices, one that contains the sample data and a second containing class information. This method finds the fewest variables that account for the differences in the class matrix. Overall, the goal is to predict cases and controls from metabolic data. Extensions of the PLS occur with orthogonal partial least squares (OPLS), which works in a similar fashion to PLS. However, in this method the variation in the data is divided into that which explains class separation and that which is orthogonal to it and does not explain class. For

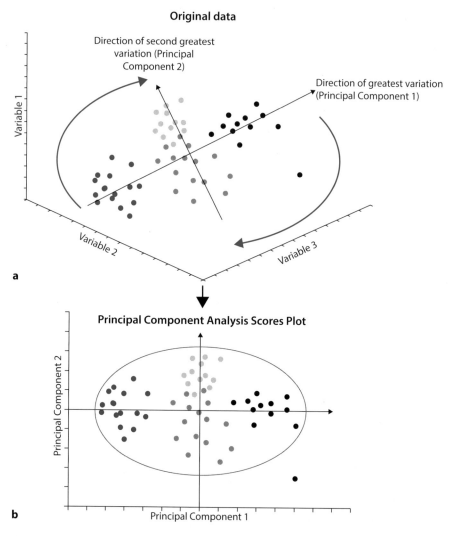

Fig. 4 Demonstration of how a multivariate set of data (**a**) is converted into a principal component analysis (PCA) scores plot (**b**) by detecting the directions of greatest variation and converting these into a new set of axes. The *circle* represents Hotelling's ellipse

clinical studies, supervised analysis allows large metabonomic data sets to be reduced to variables that are important in separating cases and controls without losing predictive power.

To assess the predictive capacity of a model, cross validation can be carried out. A number of methods exist to do this but a commonly utilized approach is to leave out every n^{th} row in the data matrix and build a model based on the remaining data. The remaining data can then be predicted by the model and the results compared to the expected outcome. This process can then be repeated until all of the data has been left out once. After cross validation it is possible to derive two descriptive metrics for the models. The first is known as the R^2 and explains the amount of variation between the classification groups that is explained by the model. This value ranges from 0 to 1.0 with values approaching 1.0 explaining almost all of the variation in the model and lower values suggesting that much of the variation in the data is irrelevant or noise. The second value is the Q^2, which represents the predictive capacity of the model, again ranging from 0 to 1.0. The expected values of both R^2 and Q^2 are dependent on the type of data being analyzed but in general should ideally be no more than 0.2 apart; for biological systems a Q^2 of 0.4 represents a reasonable predictive accuracy. However, the ideal way to test a model is to challenge it with a completely new set of data from a validation cohort of samples that have not been used to generate the model in the first instance.

Metabonomics and Intensive Care

Metabonomics work relevant to critical care has mainly focused on sepsis and infection. A range of studies has been carried out attempting to use metabonomic techniques to explore infection. Cells, animals and human subjects have been used, with both NMR and mass spectroscopy, allowing over 500 metabolites and pathways to be implicated in infective processes.

Several animal models have been used, testing different biofluids including blood [16–20], broncheoalveolar (BAL) fluid [16] and lymph [18] as well as tissue, such as lung [16, 17], liver [17, 21], kidney [22] and spleen [17, 22]. Infections as diffuse as cerebral malaria [22], influenza [23], tuberculosis [17], peritonitis [16, 18, 24] and *Escherichia coli* sepsis [20] have been investigated. Metabolites including amino acids, those involved in energy and carbohydrate metabolism, fatty acids and those associated with mitochondrial dysfunction have all been identified in these models.

In human subjects, several clinical infections have been subject to metabonomic investigation. A number of studies has been carried out examining urinary tract infection using NMR of urine samples [25–29] with an attempt to identify specific causative organisms, potentially allowing for rapid diagnosis and targeted treatment. Other specific infections investigated with metabonomics have included cerebrospinal fluid analysis to distinguish various forms of meningitis and ventriculitis [30] and sepsis from various causes in both adults [31–34] and children [35, 36].

Pneumonia remains a common cause for admission to critical care units and a small amount of work has been carried out investigating this condition using metabonomics. Animal studies have found elevated lipoproteins, triglycerides, unsaturated and polyunsaturated fatty acids, ω-3 fatty acids, lactate, 3-hydroxybutyrate and creatinine and reduced glucose, choline, phosphocholine and glycerophosphocholine levels in the plasma of rats infected with *Klebsiella pneumoniae* compared to controls [37]. Mice with pneumonia caused by *Staphylococcus aureus* or *Streptococcus pneumoniae* have been separated from control animals based on urine metabolic profiles [38].

Human studies have focused on community-acquired pneumonia (CAP). A study using mass spectroscopy analysis of plasma from children in Gambia with pneumonia found elevated uric acid, hypoxanthine and glutamic acid and reduced tryptophan and adenosine diphosphate levels in infected individuals [39]. Another study looking specifically at patients with *S. pneumoniae* pneumonia found 33 urinary metabolites used to separate cases from controls including citrate, succinate, 1-methylnicotinamide, several amino acids, glucose, lactate, acetone, carnitine, acetylcarnitine, hypoxanthine and acetate, most of which were increased in those with infection [40]. This study also aimed to address several potential confounding factors associated with this type of investigation by comparing cases to several control groups, such as those with other types of lung disease, those with other types of pneumonia and those with other acute illnesses. In almost all cases, metabolic profiling was able to distinguish cases of pneumonia from controls.

Work specifically within critical care has focused on the outcomes of patients with CAP and sepsis [41]. Analysis of plasma found higher levels of bile acids, steroid hormone metabolites, markers of oxidative stress and nucleic acid metabolites in non-survivors; however, the statistical models based on these differences had only modest sensitivity with an area under the receiver operating curve of 0.67. Other work in ICU patients has looked at predisposition to sepsis following trauma. Using NMR of plasma samples from 21 trauma patients, valine, citrate, aspartate, allantoin and hydroxybutyrate were identified as associated with the future development of sepsis [42]. Looking at adults with established sepsis on the intensive care unit (ICU), glycerophospholipids and acetylcarnitines were elevated in 33 septic patients when compared to 30 others with non-infective systemic inflammation [34]. In other investigations, metabonomic techniques have been used to try to predict mortality in 37 ICU patients with sepsis [33] and have looked at sepsis in 137 children from different age groups admitted to critical care [36]. In an attempt to explore mortality in adult ICU patients [43], plasma was analyzed with mass spectroscopy and the results showed that 31 metabolites were associated with mortality, most of which were elevated in those who died. As with the other studies, these covered a range of metabolites including lipids, carbohydrates and amino acids. Only six metabolites were greater in those who survived and these were all involved in the lipid metabolism pathway. A metabonomic study in sepsis-induced lung injury [13] compared 13 patients with ALI or acute respiratory distress syndrome (ARDS) to six healthy controls and found differences in plasma levels of glutathione, adenosine, phosphatidylserine and sphingomyelin. In another study using LC-MS of BAL fluid, several lipid metabolites and amino acids were increased and a component of surfactant decreased in those with ARDS compared to healthy controls [44].

The studies outlined above demonstrate that, although only a small number of studies have been conducted in intensive care patients to date, common to all are the finding that a large number of metabolites and metabolic pathways are deranged in critical illness. These range from energy and lipid metabolism to amino acid and steroid hormone synthesis, most of which are not currently routinely measured.

Not only are a range of pathways involved in critical illness but specific elements of these may be up- or down-regulated in different contexts, even within different individuals with similar diseases. At present, it is still too early to draw firm conclusions regarding the role of metabonomics in diagnosis, prognostication or monitoring of treatment effect within ICU patients. However, from the limited work done already, the ability of metabonomics to monitor such a diverse range of markers makes it an attractive approach for biomarker discovery and for understanding the subgroups or phenotypes of patients admitted to critical care. The ability of metabonomics to simultaneously measure several metabolites from a range of metabolic processes allows some understanding to be gained, not only about the impact of critical illness on individual pathways, but the interaction of many metabolic processes during illness. A further understanding of these complex interactions may aid in the identification of phenotypes of patients that are currently not clinically apparent and that may respond to treatments differently, previously termed stratified medicine but now referred to as precision medicine. Further metabonomic research within critical care should focus on addressing current challenges, such as monitoring treatment effect with the early identification of non-responders, identifying phenotypes of sepsis and ARDS that may respond differently to treatment or ventilation strategies and assisting in making challenging diagnoses such as early identification of ventilator-associated pneumonia (VAP).

Conclusion

Metabonomics is a relatively new scientific discipline that aims to explore the changes in global metabolic profiles in response to exogenous influences such as disease states or treatments as well as host factors. Broadly two analytical methods are employed, NMR and mass spectroscopy, to measure a vast array of metabolites that require specialist multivariate statistics for analysis. So far only a limited amount of work has been carried out in intensive care patients. However, from these studies, perturbation in a number of metabolic pathways has been implicated in critical illness. The ability to explore several metabolic processes simultaneously, and their interactions, is an exciting prospect for intensive care medicine. The complexity of this group of patients and the growing understanding that subgroups of patients may require tailored treatments suggests that metabolic profiling or phenotyping may help to improve diagnostics or target treatment strategies in clinical trials and clinical practice.

References

1. Holmes E, Wilson ID, Nicholson JK (2008) Metabolic phenotyping in health and disease. Cell 134:714–717
2. Nicholson JK, Lindon JC (2008) Systems biology: Metabonomics. Nature 455:1054–1056
3. Nicholson JK, Connelly J, Lindon JC, Holmes E (2002) Metabonomics: a platform for studying drug toxicity and gene function. Nat Rev Drug Discov 1:153–161

4. Nicholson JK, Lindon JC (2008) Systems biology – Metabonomics. Nature 455:1054–1056
5. Beckonert O, Keun HC, Ebbels TM et al (2007) Metabolic profiling, metabolomic and metabonomic procedures for NMR spectroscopy of urine, plasma, serum and tissue extracts. Nat Protoc 2:2692–2703
6. Sofia M, Maniscalco M, de Laurentiis G, Paris D, Melck D, Motta A (2011) Exploring airway diseases by NMR-based metabonomics: a review of application to exhaled breath condensate. J Biomed Biotechnol 2011:403260
7. Cohen MJ, Serkova NJ, Wiener-Kronish J, Pittet JF, Niemann CU (2010) 1H-NMR-based metabolic signatures of clinical outcomes in trauma patients – beyond lactate and base deficit. The Journal of trauma 69:31–40
8. Mao H, Wang H, Wang B et al (2009) Systemic metabolic changes of traumatic critically ill patients revealed by an NMR-based metabonomic approach. J Proteome Res 8:5423–5430
9. Sato E, Kohno M, Yamamoto M, Fujisawa T, Fujiwara K, Tanaka N (2011) Metabolomic analysis of human plasma from haemodialysis patients. Eur J Clin Invest 41:241–255
10. Beger RD, Holland RD, Sun J et al (2008) Metabonomics of acute kidney injury in children after cardiac surgery. Pediatr Nephrol 23:977–984
11. Al-Ismaili Z, Palijan A, Zappitelli M (2011) Biomarkers of acute kidney injury in children: discovery, evaluation, and clinical application. Pediatr Nephrol 26:29–40
12. Dunne VG, Bhattachayya S, Besser M, Rae C, Griffin JL (2005) Metabolites from cerebrospinal fluid in aneurysmal subarachnoid haemorrhage correlate with vasospasm and clinical outcome: a pattern-recognition 1H NMR study. NMR Biomed 18:24–33
13. Stringer KA, Serkova NJ, Karnovsky A, Guire K, Paine R, Standiford TJ (2011) Metabolic consequences of sepsis-induced acute lung injury revealed by plasma (1)H-nuclear magnetic resonance quantitative metabolomics and computational analysis. Am J Physiol Lung Cell Mol Physiol 300:L4–L11
14. Dumas ME, Maibaum EC, Teague C et al (2006) Assessment of analytical reproducibility of 1H NMR spectroscopy based metabonomics for large-scale epidemiological research: the INTERMAP Study. Anal Chem 78:2199–2208
15. Lenz EM, Wilson ID (2007) Analytical strategies in metabonomics. J Proteome Res 6:443–458
16. Izquierdo-Garcia JL, Nin N, Ruiz-Cabello J et al (2011) A metabolomic approach for diagnosis of experimental sepsis. Intensive Care Med 37:2023–2032
17. Shin JH, Yang JY, Jeon BY et al (2011) (1)H NMR-based metabolomic profiling in mice infected with Mycobacterium tuberculosis. J Proteome Res 10:2238–2247
18. Li Y, Hou M, Wang JG et al (2012) Changes of lymph metabolites in a rat model of sepsis induced by cecal ligation and puncture. J Trauma Acute Care Surg 73:1545–1552
19. Steelman SM, Johnson P, Jackson A, Schulze J, Chowdhary BP (2014) Serum metabolomics identifies citrulline as a predictor of adverse outcomes in an equine model of gut-derived sepsis. Physiol Genomics 46:339–347
20. Langley RJ, Tipper JL, Bruse S et al (2014) Integrative "omic" analysis of experimental bacteremia identifies a metabolic signature that distinguishes human sepsis from systemic inflammatory response syndromes. Am J Respir Crit Care Med 190:445–455
21. Antunes LC, Arena ET, Menendez A et al (2011) Impact of salmonella infection on host hormone metabolism revealed by metabolomics. Infect Immun 79:1759–1769
22. Ghosh S, Sengupta A, Sharma S, Sonawat HM (2013) Metabolic perturbations of kidney and spleen in murine cerebral malaria: (1)H NMR-based metabolomic study. PloS One 8:e73113
23. Chen L, Fan J, Li Y et al (2014) Modified Jiu Wei Qiang Huo decoction improves dysfunctional metabolomics in influenza A pneumonia-infected mice. Biomed Chromatogr 28:468–474
24. Xu PB, Lin ZY, Meng HB et al (2008) A metabonomic approach to early prognostic evaluation of experimental sepsis. J Infect 56:474–481
25. Lam CW, Law CY, To KK et al (2014) NMR-based metabolomic urinalysis: a rapid screening test for urinary tract infection. Clin Chim Acta 436:217–223

26. Lam CW, Law CY, Sze KH, To KK (2015) Quantitative metabolomics of urine for rapid etiological diagnosis of urinary tract infection: evaluation of a microbial-mammalian co-metabolite as a diagnostic biomarker. Clin Chim Acta 438:24–28

27. Gupta A, Dwivedi M, Mahdi AA, Khetrapal CL, Bhandari M (2012) Broad identification of bacterial type in urinary tract infection using (1)h NMR spectroscopy. J Proteome Res 11:1844–1854

28. Gupta A, Dwivedi M, Mahdi AA, Gowda GA, Khetrapal CL, Bhandari M (2009) 1H-nuclear magnetic resonance spectroscopy for identifying and quantifying common uropathogens: a metabolic approach to the urinary tract infection. BJU Int 104:236–244

29. Nevedomskaya E, Pacchiarotta T, Artemov A et al (2012) (1)H NMR-based metabolic profiling of urinary tract infection: combining multiple statistical models and clinical data. Metabolomics 8:1227–1235

30. Coen M, O'Sullivan M, Bubb WA, Kuchel PW, Sorrell T (2005) Proton nuclear magnetic resonance-based metabonomics for rapid diagnosis of meningitis and ventriculitis. Clin Infect Dis 41:1582–1590

31. Su L, Huang Y, Zhu Y et al (2014) Discrimination of sepsis stage metabolic profiles with an LC/MS-MS-based metabolomics approach. BMJ Open Respir Res 1:e000056

32. Langley RJ, Tsalik EL, van Velkinburgh JC et al (2013) An integrated clinico-metabolomic model improves prediction of death in sepsis. Sci Transl Med 5:195ra195

33. Mickiewicz B, Duggan GE, Winston BW, Doig C, Kubes P, Vogel HJ (2014) Metabolic profiling of serum samples by 1H nuclear magnetic resonance spectroscopy as a potential diagnostic approach for septic shock. Crit Care Med 42:1140–1149

34. Schmerler D, Neugebauer S, Ludewig K, Bremer-Streck S, Brunkhorst FM, Kiehntopf M (2012) Targeted metabolomics for discrimination of systemic inflammatory disorders in critically ill patients. J Lipid Res 53:1369–1375

35. Fanos V, Caboni P, Corsello G et al (2014) Urinary (1)H-NMR and GC-MS metabolomics predicts early and late onset neonatal sepsis. Early Hum Dev 90(Suppl 1):S78–S83

36. Mickiewicz B, Vogel HJ, Wong HR, Winston BW (2013) Metabolomics as a novel approach for early diagnosis of pediatric septic shock and its mortality. Am J Respir Crit Care Med 187:967–976

37. Dong F, Wang B, Zhang L, Tang H, Li J, Wang Y (2012) Metabolic response to Klebsiella pneumoniae infection in an experimental rat model. PloS One 7:e51060

38. Slupsky CM, Cheypesh A, Chao DV et al (2009) Streptococcus pneumoniae and Staphylococcus aureus pneumonia induce distinct metabolic responses. J Proteome Res 8:3029–3036

39. Laiakis EC, Morris GA, Fornace AJ, Howie SR (2010) Metabolomic analysis in severe childhood pneumonia in the Gambia, West Africa: findings from a pilot study. PloS One 9:5

40. Slupsky CM, Rankin KN, Fu H et al (2009) Pneumococcal pneumonia: potential for diagnosis through a urinary metabolic profile. J Proteome Res 8:5550–5558

41. Seymour CW, Yende S, Scott MJ et al (2013) Metabolomics in pneumonia and sepsis: an analysis of the GenIMS cohort study. Intensive Care Med 39:1423–1434

42. Blaise BJ, Gouel-Cheron A, Floccard B, Monneret G, Allaouchiche B (2013) Metabolic phenotyping of traumatized patients reveals a susceptibility to sepsis. Anal Chem 85:10850–10855

43. Rogers AJ, McGeachie M, Baron RM et al (2014) Metabolomic derangements are associated with mortality in critically ill adult patients. PloS One 9:e87538

44. Evans CR, Karnovsky A, Kovach MA, Standiford TJ, Burant CF, Stringer KA (2014) Untargeted LC-MS metabolomics of bronchoalveolar lavage fluid differentiates acute respiratory distress syndrome from health. J Proteome Res 13:640–649

The Rationale for Permissive Hyperglycemia in Critically Ill Patients with Diabetes

J. Mårtensson and R. Bellomo

Introduction

Avoiding extreme deviations from pre-morbid physiology is a major aim in the management of several conditions in critically ill patients. For example, vasopressors are commonly used to avoid relative hypotension in patients with chronic hypertension. Similarly, lower blood oxygen levels and higher blood carbon dioxide levels are targeted in patients with severe chronic obstructive pulmonary disease (COPD). Finally, slow correction of serum sodium is recommended in patients with chronic hyponatremia. An important exception to this logical consideration of baseline physiology and biochemistry has been blood glucose management in the intensive care unit (ICU). The most recent, and largest, randomized controlled trial on glycemic control in ICU patients, the Normoglycemia in Intensive Care Evaluation and Surviving Using Glucose Algorithm Regulation (NICE SUGAR) trial, demonstrated improved survival by targeting a blood glucose concentration of 6–10 mmol/l compared to 4–6 mmol/l [1]. Thus, since the publication of NICE SUGAR, the more 'liberal' target of 6–10 mmol/l has been recommended in international guidelines in critically ill patients and in patients undergoing cardiac surgery [2, 3]. However, several issues remain unresolved: whether uniform glycemic con-

J. Mårtensson (✉)
Department of Intensive Care, Austin Hospital
Melbourne, Australia
Department of Physiology and Pharmacology, Section of Anesthesia and Intensive Care
Medicine, Karolinska Institutet
Stockholm, Sweden
email: johan.martensson@austin.org.au

R. Bellomo
Department of Intensive Care, Austin Hospital
Melbourne, Australia
Australian and New Zealand Intensive Care Research Centre (ANZIC-RC), Department of
Epidemiology and Preventive Medicine, Monash University
Melbourne, Australia

© Springer International Publishing Switzerland 2016
J.-L. Vincent (ed.), *Annual Update in Intensive Care and Emergency Medicine 2016*,
DOI 10.1007/978-3-319-27349-5_29

trol should be used in all patients in the ICU; whether the recommended target is 'liberal' enough for patients with diabetes mellitus; and whether current practice is safe? In response to these issues, in this chapter, we introduce the novel concepts of relative hypoglycemia and permissive hyperglycemia in critically ill patients. In addition, we discuss experimental and clinical evidence that provides the rationale for applying a more liberal glycemic target in critically ill patients with diabetes in order to avoid relative hypoglycemia.

The Concept of Relative Hypoglycemia

Hypoglycemia is typically defined as a blood glucose concentration less than 3.9 mmol/l since this represents the threshold at which hormonal glucose counter-regulation is activated in individuals without diabetes [4]. Such counterregulation involves the release of epinephrine, norepinephrine, cortisol, growth hormone and, in patients with preserved pancreatic function, glucagon, which stimulates hepatic glucose production and ultimately increases blood glucose concentration toward

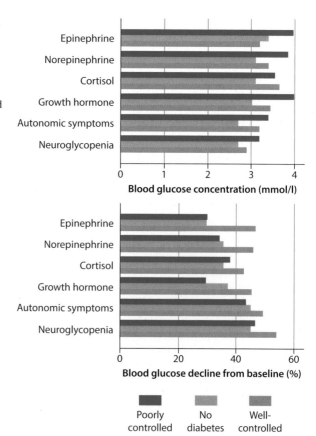

Fig. 1 Thresholds for hypoglycemia counterregulatory hormone responses and symptoms in patients with well-controlled and poorly controlled diabetes and in healthy individuals. Adapted from [4–9]

normal. In addition to this integrated hormonal response, sympathetic neural activation elicits neuroglycopenic symptoms stimulating carbohydrate ingestion.

Evidence from several experimental so-called "hypoglycemic clamp" studies in humans [4–9] suggests that counterregulatory activation occurs at higher glucose values in patients with poorly controlled diabetes than in subjects without diabetes or with well-controlled diabetes. In fact, these studies demonstrate that hypoglycemia counterregulation can occur within a normal glucose range in patients with poor glycemic control (Fig. 1), a state we would call "relative hypoglycemia". Moreover, these studies demonstrate that a 30% relative decline in blood glucose from baseline is sufficient to substantially increase circulating catecholamine levels (Fig. 1). The dangers of severe hypoglycemia are well known. Yet, the consequence of relative hypoglycemia and its contribution to mortality in critically ill patients needs to be acknowledged as well.

Effects of Relative Hypoglycemia on Cardiovascular Function

A recent episode of hypoglycemia (relative or absolutely) attenuates the humoral and symptomatic responses to subsequent episodes of hypoglycemia [10]. Such hypoglycemia-associated autonomic failure (HAAF) reduces the epinephrine response and, in conscious patients, reduces sympathetic neural response leading to hypoglycemia unawareness. In patients with insulin-dependent diabetes, strict glycemic control (meaning a glycated hemoglobin [HbA1c] of $7.1 \pm 0.7\%$), lowered the glucose level required to trigger epinephrine release during hypoglycemia [6]. Additionally, in patients without diabetes, a single episode of hypoglycemia was sufficient to impair the epinephrine and norepinephrine response to subsequent episodes of hypoglycemia [11]. Moreover, HAAF can potentially be triggered at blood glucose levels within the normal range in patients with poorly controlled diabetes [5].

In addition to an altered humoral response, activation of the carotid glomus chemoreceptors appears to contribute to cardiovascular instability during hypoglycemia (Fig. 2). In fact, emerging evidence suggests that hypoglycemia-induced chemoreceptor activation modulates hemodynamics via reduced cardiac baroreceptor sensitivity [12]. In humans without diabetes, an average reduction in blood glucose concentration from 5.4 to 3.4 mmol/l (37%) significantly increased heart rate and reduced mean arterial pressure (MAP) despite a marked increase in counterregulatory norepinephrine and epinephrine secretion [13]. Simultaneously, reduced cardiac baroreflex sensitivity (quantified by the slope of the relation between R-R interval and blood pressure) and impaired heart rate variability was observed. Furthermore, reduced baroreceptor sensitivity as well as reduced sympathetic and norepinephrine responses to nitroprusside-induced hypotension or orthostatic stress were observed approximately 16 h after correction of hypoglycemia [14]. Finally, in carotid glomus-resected patients, the baroreflex response to hypoglycemia is further blunted, supporting the role of chemoreceptor activation during hypoglycemia [15].

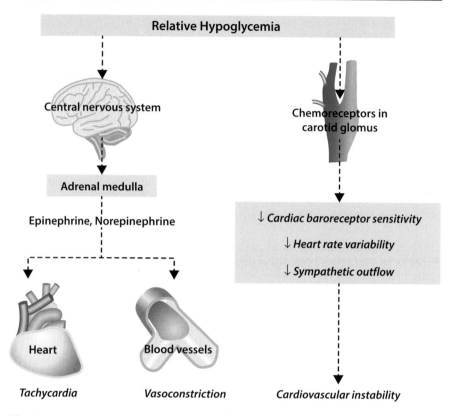

Fig. 2 Sympathoadrenal and carotid chemoreceptor responses to relative hypoglycemia

The above observations are highly relevant to critically ill patients. Firstly, a recommended blood glucose target of 6–10 mmol/l may not prevent severe hypoglycemia [1]. Secondly, applying such targets will almost certainly induce relative hypoglycemia and increase the risk of autonomic failure in patients with poorly controlled diabetes. Finally, in addition to supportive administration of vasopressors, critically ill patients depend on endogenous cardiovascular reflex mechanisms in order to maintain and recover organ function. These reflexes may well be blunted in diabetic patients. These observations suggest that "permissive hyperglycemia" may be a physiologically rational approach to glycemic control in diabetic patients.

Hyperglycemia, Hypoglycemia and Clinical Outcomes

Hyperglycemia has been suggested to contribute to mortality in critically ill patients [16, 17]. However, emerging evidence now challenges the notion that stress hyperglycemia *per se* is harmful, further justifying the rationale for "permissive hyperglycemia". Acute stress increases blood glucose concentrations via epinephrine-mediated gluconeogenesis and glycogenolysis. In addition, stress-induced hyper-lactatemia is a major source of blood glucose during physiological stress [18]. Indeed, previous studies have failed to demonstrate an independent association between stress hyperglycemia and mortality after adjusting for serum lactate [19–21], which further refutes the previous hypothesis that hyperglycemia *per se* is independently associated with increased mortality and, by association, harmful.

Yet, as hyperglycemia is a marker of illness severity, its potential causes should be sought. Importantly, cellular starvation from insulin resistance or deficiency should be excluded by measuring serum and/or urine ketones in patients with diabetes. However, to date, the epidemiology of such ketone body production during critical illness in general and during stress hyperglycemia in particular is unknown. It is possible that insulin therapy should be restricted not to patients with a particular level of glycemia but rather to patients with ketone-positive hyperglycemia. Future studies therefore need to explore whether "permissive hyperglycemia" is associated with increased ketone generation and whether premorbid glycemia together with assessment of serum ketones should be used to help guide glycemic control in critically ill patients.

Data from recent large observational studies have demonstrated lack of harm of hyperglycemia in critically ill patients with diabetes [22, 23]. In fact, Egi and co-workers found hyperglycemia to be independently associated with *lower* mortality in patients with insufficiently controlled diabetes (HbA1c > 7%, corresponding to an estimated average blood glucose concentration of > 8.5 mmol/l; see Table 1) [24]. Compared to patients with well-controlled diabetes (HbA1c ≤ 7%) and hyperglycemia in the ICU (time-weighted average glucose concentration of 12 mmol/l), patients with poor premorbid diabetes control and a similar degree of hyperglycemia in the ICU had an independent 63% lower mortality. Furthermore, time-weighted average blood glucose levels 30% below estimated pre-morbid baseline (relative hypoglycemia) were found in non-survivors whereas the difference between ICU glycemia and pre-morbid glycemia was closer to zero in survivors.

Consistent with these findings, Krinsley and coworkers found a stepwise reduction in mortality risk with increasing mean blood glucose level in the ICU in 12,880

Table 1 Relationship between glycated hemoglobin (HbA1c), estimated average glucose concentration and relative hypoglycemia

HbA1c (%)	eAG[a] (mmol/l)	Relative hypoglycemia[b] (mmol/l)
5	5.4	< 3.8
6	7.0	< 4.9
7	8.5	< 5.9
8	10.1	< 7.0
9	11.7	< 8.1
10	13.3	< 9.3

[a]eAG, estimated average glucose concentration during the last 3 months $= 1.59 \times$ HbA1c $(\%) - 2.59$ [25]
[b]Defined as a 30% decline from eAG

diabetic patients [23]. In contrast, among patients without diabetes, average blood glucose levels > 7.8 mmol/l were independently associated with increased mortality. Finally, Plummer and coworkers found a 20% increased mortality risk for every increase in blood glucose of 1 mmol/l above normoglycemia in patients without diabetes or with well-controlled diabetes [26]. However, in patients with poorly controlled diabetes, no association between acute hyperglycemia and mortality was found; not even when peak glucose levels increased > 15 mmol/l, providing further data that, during critical illness, "permissive hyperglycemia" may be a more physiologically rational approach in patients with poorly controlled pre-ICU glycemia. Consequently, although the cause of death was not reported in these studies, the observations reinforce the importance of considering pre-morbid glycemia (estimated from HbA1c) when prescribing glucose targets in critically ill patients.

In contrast to hyperglycemia, hypoglycemia is consistently associated with mortality in ICU patients irrespective of diabetic status [23, 27, 28]. Hypoglycemia-induced cardiovascular instability may explain this association. In fact, in the NICE SUGAR trial, tight glycemic control significantly increased the incidence of severe hypoglycemia as well as the risk of cardiovascular mortality [1]. Moreover, hypoglycemia occurred in 21% of patients after cardiac surgery when glucose levels between 4.4 and 7 mmol/l were targeted. In such patients, hypoglycemia was independently associated with cardiovascular instability requiring intra-aortic balloon pump insertion as well as increased mortality [29]. Finally, intensive glucose lowering therapy to achieve an HbA1c < 6% compared to more liberal control significantly increased cardiovascular mortality in ambulatory patients with poorly controlled type 2 diabetes [30].

Thus, the pursuit of strict glycemic control may decrease the degree of hyperglycemia with little or no physiological or clinical gain, while exposing patients to a greater risk of hypoglycemia, which predictably carries a real physiological and clinical cost. This effect is likely to be much greater in all diabetic patients and particularly so in those diabetic patients with poor pre-morbid glycemic control.

Detecting Relative Hypoglycemia in ICU Patients

A patient's baseline glycemic control must be known in order to monitor relative blood glucose fluctuations in the ICU. HbA1c can be measured by most laboratories and can be used to estimate the average blood glucose concentration during the 3 months prior to ICU admission. Nathan and coworkers compared blood glucose levels obtained during 3 months with HbA1c measured at the end of this period in more than 500 patients with and without diabetes [25]. They found a very close correlation ($r^2 = 0.84$) between HbA1c and the average glucose concentration. Accordingly, they developed a simple and accurate formula for conversion of HbA1c to an estimated average blood glucose concentration (eAG):

$$eAG = 1.59 \times HbA1c\ (\%) - 2.59.$$

Novel techniques to continuously monitor blood glucose concentrations [31, 32] in addition to estimated baseline premorbid glycemia will be important tools to guide blood glucose management and hence to avoid relative hypoglycemia in ICU patients (Table 1).

Conclusion

No robust evidence supports harm from hyperglycemia in critically ill patients. In fact, hyperglycemia may be beneficial in patients with poor pre-morbid glycemic control. In contrast to hyperglycemia, relative hypoglycemia, a condition previously associated with autonomic instability is particularly undesirable in critically ill patients since it may further impair cardiovascular function and hence contribute to mortality in these patients. Importantly, such relative hypoglycemia can occur at recommended blood glucose targets of 6–10 mmol/l in patients with poorly controlled diabetes. Based on these novel findings, it is time to scrutinize current practice. In particular, trials exploring the feasibility and safety of "permissive hyperglycemia" in critically ill patients with diabetes are justified.

References

1. Finfer S, Chittock DR, Su SY et al (2009) Intensive versus conventional glucose control in critically ill patients. N Engl J Med 360:1283–1297
2. Dellinger RP, Levy MM, Rhodes A et al (2013) Surviving Sepsis Campaign: international guidelines for management of severe sepsis and septic shock, 2012. Intensive Care Med 39:165–228
3. Moghissi ES, Korytkowski MT, DiNardo M et al (2009) American Association of Clinical Endocrinologists and American Diabetes Association consensus statement on inpatient glycemic control. Endocr Pract 15:353–369
4. Schwartz NS, Clutter WE, Shah SD, Cryer PE (1987) Glycemic thresholds for activation of glucose counterregulatory systems are higher than the threshold for symptoms. J Clin Invest 79:777–781
5. Korzon-Burakowska A, Hopkins D, Matyka K et al (1998) Effects of glycemic control on protective responses against hypoglycemia in type 2 diabetes. Diabetes Care 21:283–290
6. Amiel SA, Sherwin RS, Simonson DC, Tamborlane WV (1988) Effect of intensive insulin therapy on glycemic thresholds for counterregulatory hormone release. Diabetes 37:901–907
7. Boyle PJ, Schwartz NS, Shah SD, Clutter WE, Cryer PE (1988) Plasma glucose concentrations at the onset of hypoglycemic symptoms in patients with poorly controlled diabetes and in nondiabetics. N Engl J Med 318:1487–1492
8. Levy CJ, Kinsley BT, Bajaj M, Simonson DC (1998) Effect of glycemic control on glucose counterregulation during hypoglycemia in NIDDM. Diabetes Care 21:1330–1338
9. Spyer G, Hattersley AT, MacDonald IA, Amiel S, MacLeod KM (2000) Hypoglycaemic counter-regulation at normal blood glucose concentrations in patients with well controlled type-2 diabetes. Lancet 356:1970–1974
10. Cryer PE (2013) Mechanisms of hypoglycemia-associated autonomic failure in diabetes. N Engl J Med 369:362–372
11. Heller SR, Cryer PE (1991) Reduced neuroendocrine and symptomatic responses to subsequent hypoglycemia after 1 episode of hypoglycemia in nondiabetic humans. Diabetes 40:223–226

12. Conde SV, Sacramento JF, Guarino MP et al (2014) Carotid body, insulin, and metabolic diseases: unraveling the links. Front Physiol 5:418
13. Limberg JK, Taylor JL, Dube S et al (2014) Role of the carotid body chemoreceptors in baroreflex control of blood pressure during hypoglycaemia in humans. Exp Physiol 99:640–650
14. Adler GK, Bonyhay I, Failing H, Waring E, Dotson S, Freeman R (2009) Antecedent hypoglycemia impairs autonomic cardiovascular function: implications for rigorous glycemic control. Diabetes 58:360–366
15. Limberg JK, Taylor JL, Mozer MT et al (2015) Effect of bilateral carotid body resection on cardiac baroreflex control of blood pressure during hypoglycemia. Hypertension 65:1365–1371
16. Krinsley JS (2003) Association between hyperglycemia and increased hospital mortality in a heterogeneous population of critically ill patients. Mayo Clin Proc 78:1471–1478
17. Falciglia M, Freyberg RW, Almenoff PL, D'Alessio DA, Render ML (2009) Hyperglycemia-related mortality in critically ill patients varies with admission diagnosis. Crit Care Med 37:3001–3009
18. Garcia-Alvarez M, Marik P, Bellomo R (2014) Stress hyperlactataemia: present understanding and controversy. Lancet Diabetes Endocrinol 2:339–347
19. Freire AX, Bridges L, Umpierrez GE, Kuhl D, Kitabchi AE (2005) Admission hyperglycemia and other risk factors as predictors of hospital mortality in a medical ICU population. Chest 128:3109–3116
20. Kaukonen KM, Bailey M, Egi M et al (2014) Stress hyperlactatemia modifies the relationship between stress hyperglycemia and outcome: a retrospective observational study. Crit Care Med 42:1379–1385
21. Green JP, Berger T, Garg N et al (2012) Hyperlactatemia affects the association of hyperglycemia with mortality in nondiabetic adults with sepsis. Acad Emerg Med 19:1268–1275
22. Whitcomb BW, Pradhan EK, Pittas AG, Roghmann MC, Perencevich EN (2005) Impact of admission hyperglycemia on hospital mortality in various intensive care unit populations. Crit Care Med 33:2772–2777
23. Krinsley JS, Egi M, Kiss A et al (2013) Diabetic status and the relation of the three domains of glycemic control to mortality in critically ill patients: an international multicenter cohort study. Crit Care 17:R37
24. Egi M, Bellomo R, Stachowski E et al (2011) The interaction of chronic and acute glycemia with mortality in critically ill patients with diabetes. Crit Care Med 39:105–111
25. Nathan DM, Kuenen J, Borg R, Zheng H, Schoenfeld D, Heine RJ (2008) Translating the A1C assay into estimated average glucose values. Diabetes Care 31:1473–1478
26. Plummer MP, Bellomo R, Cousins CE et al (2014) Dysglycaemia in the critically ill and the interaction of chronic and acute glycaemia with mortality. Intensive Care Med 40:973–980
27. Krinsley JS, Schultz MJ, Spronk PE et al (2011) Mild hypoglycemia is independently associated with increased mortality in the critically ill. Crit Care 15:R173
28. Kalfon P, Le Manach Y, Ichai C et al (2015) Severe and multiple hypoglycemic episodes are associated with increased risk of death in ICU patients. Crit Care 19:153
29. D'Ancona G, Bertuzzi F, Sacchi L et al (2011) Iatrogenic hypoglycemia secondary to tight glucose control is an independent determinant for mortality and cardiac morbidity. Eur J Cardiothorac Surg 40:360–366
30. Gerstein HC, Miller ME, Byington RP et al (2008) Effects of intensive glucose lowering in type 2 diabetes. N Engl J Med 358:2545–2559
31. Flower OJ, Bird S, Macken L et al (2014) Continuous intra-arterial blood glucose monitoring using quenched fluorescence sensing: a product development study. Crit Care Resusc 16:54–61
32. Macken L, Flower OJ, Bird S et al (2015) Continuous intra-arterial blood glucose monitoring using quenched fluorescence sensing in intensive care patients after cardiac surgery: phase II of a product development study. Crit Care Resusc 17:190–196

Indirect Calorimetry in Critically Ill Patients: Concept, Current Use, and Future Challenges

E. De Waele, P. M. Honoré, and H. D. Spapen

Indirect Calorimetry: From Concept to Practical Use in the ICU

In the mitochondrial matrix, the Krebs cycle runs as a series of oxidation/reduction reactions that generate energy from acetate derived from carbohydrates, lipids and proteins. This process includes the electron transport chain where energy released as electrons is passed from one carrier to the next and is used to synthetize ATP from ADP and phosphate (Fig. 1). Oxygen (O_2) is consumed and water and carbon dioxide (CO_2) are released. Therefore, oxygen consumption (VO_2) and carbon dioxide production (VCO_2) are good markers of cellular, tissue and body metabolism.

The metabolic rate can be measured by analysis of inspired and expired gases. Determination of VO_2 and VCO_2 enables the respiratory quotient (RQ) and resting energy expenditure (REE) to be established [1]. Currently used indirect calorimetry techniques go back to the old principles of body heat and respiration [2]. By the end of the 18th century, the Scottish physician, Joseph Black, discovered CO_2 and accepted the fact that it was produced by the body. Lavoisier discovered that exhaled air was depleted of O_2 [3]. In 1789, he launched the term 'calorimetre' after considering heat to be a substance called 'caloric'. Since then, calorimetry has changed considerably from initial guinea pig experiments in ice calorimeters (the amount of melted ice was equivalent to the amount of produced heat!) to the portable, open-circuit, computer-based devices that are used in clinical practice today. The modified Weir equation (total kcal $= 3.941 \times l$ of O_2 used $+ 1.106 \times l$ of CO_2 produced), developed in 1949, remains the cornerstone for metabolic rate measurements. The use of a stable protein percentage of total produced calories simplifies the formula. In fact, urinary nitrogen becomes irrelevant as the error introduced by omitting it is negligible [4, 5]. For a long time, indirect calorimetry remained confined to laboratory use. Scientists considered clinicians too unexperienced to use indirect

E. De Waele · P. M. Honoré (✉) · H. D. Spapen
Department of Intensive Care, UZ Brussel-VUB University
Brussels, Belgium
email: Patrick.Honore@uzbrussel.be

© Springer International Publishing Switzerland 2016
J.-L. Vincent (ed.), *Annual Update in Intensive Care and Emergency Medicine 2016*,
DOI 10.1007/978-3-319-27349-5_30

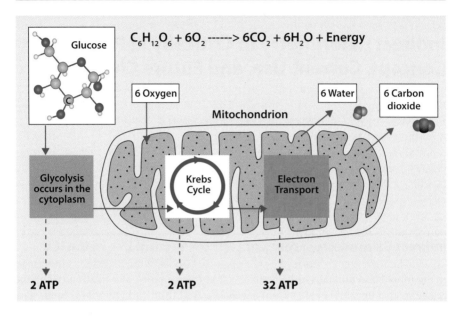

Fig. 1 Cellular respiration

calorimetry devices and the results obtained were deemed inaccurate [5]. Nevertheless, continuous progress was made by simplifying algebraic equations and developing improved technical equipment. Currently used infrared CO_2 sensors and electrochemical O_2 sensors combined with mass flow sensors make gas analysis accurate and practically feasible. Portable and less expensive devices can be used in stable patient populations [2].

Reliable instruments are imperative to permit clinical implementation of indirect calorimetry. The Deltatrac Metabolic Monitor (VIASYS Healthcare Inc, SensorMedics, Yorba Linda, CA) has been the golden standard for indirect calorimetry for almost 35 years [6] but is no longer commercialized. In studies comparing metabolic carts, the Deltatrac had the lowest coefficient of variation for comparing the validity of resting metabolic rates within subjects [7]. The technical setup of the Deltatrac is characterized by inspiratory and expiratory gas analysis without measurement of minute ventilation. In one study, it failed to deliver reliable RQ measurements [8].

Among other devices, the VmaxTM Encore 29n calorimeter is currently considered to be the most valid instrument [7] showing the least variance in measuring REE [9]. Efforts to develop a clinically useful indirect calorimeter at a reasonable cost are currently ongoing [8, 9]. Meanwhile, the VmaxTM Encore 29n calorimeter has gained a solid reputation in nutritional ICU research programs [11–13].

More than two decades ago, the American Association for Respiratory Care already published recommendations for performing metabolic cart measurements in the critical care setting [1]. However, data on feasibility and real-life practical implications are scarce. Experts disagree whether measured energy expenditure equals nutritional demands [10]. Yet, a survival benefit of indirect calorimetry-directed caloric prescription in association with adequate protein delivery was observed in mechanically ventilated, critically ill patients [14]. The length of intensive care unit (ICU) stay was substantially shortened in post-cardiac arrest patients receiving therapeutic hypothermia when the cumulative energy deficit was reduced by meeting indirect calorimetry-derived energy demands [15]. Supplementing parenteral nutrition to reach the energy target determined by indirect calorimetry significantly reduced the incidence of nosocomial infection and shortened the duration of mechanical ventilation [16]. In the Tight CAlorie balance COntrol Study (TICACOS), in which calorie intake was adapted to measured energy expenditure, hospital mortality improved despite increased ICU morbidity [17]. A large Belgian study compared early with late parenteral nutrition and found increased morbidity in the early parenteral feeding group [18]. However, caloric goals in this study were based on the somewhat 'rigid' recommendations of the American College of Chest Physicians, which are poorly correlated with measured energy expenditure. Patients at extremes of body weight especially may have been exposed to unacceptably gross under- and overfeeding [19, 20]. Ideally, indirect calorimetry should be repeated over time because repeated daily application of an upfront measured result may be inconsistent during a changing ICU course or in certain patient subgroups [21].

Indirect calorimetry has been extensively studied in critically ill children. According to the American Society of Parenteral and Enteral Nutrition guidelines, 75% of pediatric ICU patients would benefit from indirect calorimetry, in particular when aged under 2, malnourished on admission, or staying in the ICU for more than 5 days [22].

Measuring or Calculating Energy Expenditure in Critically Ill Patients?

Over the years, elaborate research has been performed on energy expenditure in different clinical settings and patient groups. Substrate and energy metabolism are sex-specific and weight-dependent [23, 24]. Adjusted REE decreases with increased body mass index (BMI): 25 kcal/kg in normal weight, 20.4 kcal/kg in obese and 16 kcal/kg in morbidly obese patients. This phenomenon relates to the principle that adipose tissue barely contributes to REE [25]. The measured REE in a cohort of underweight critically ill patients was 31 kcal/kg actual body weight [26]. Energy expenditure is also influenced by medication, as shown during barbiturate coma [26]. Energy expenditure can also vary in patients undergoing therapeutic hypothermia for severe acute cerebral injury or after successful resuscitation from cardiac arrest. A 1 °C drop in temperature causes a 6% reduction in basal metabolism [27]. An increase in REE with increasing body temperature is a constant finding [28]. During mechanical ventilation, REE did not significantly differ between medical and surgical or trauma patients. Indirect calorimetry measurements are not influenced by the ventilation mode (i.e., volume or pressure-controlled ventilation)

[29]. Infection did not alter the metabolic rate measured by indirect calorimetry in one study [30]. However, differences between REE calculated with the Harris-Benedict equation and determined by indirect calorimetry were positively correlated with C-reactive protein (CRP) in patients with sepsis, suggesting that REE in critically ill patients may increase according to inflammation [31]. Increased energy requirement for physical activity in critically ill patients was only present for active exercise and differed from that in healthy subjects [31]. Daytime variations in energy expenditure are limited and do not require continuous indirect calorimetry measurement [32].

Correct assessment of energy expenditure is a cornerstone of an adequate nutrition policy in the critically ill. Based on standardized indirect calorimetry measurements, equations have been developed that predict energy expenditure. Some formulas are called 'static' because they rely on patient height, weight, sex and age. The first described and still often used Harris-Benedict equation is based on measured energy expenditure in healthy humans. This landmark formula was initially constructed after multiple regression analysis of biometric variables, represents basal energy expenditure occurring at complete rest after an overnight fast [33], and was subsequently revised and corrected for activity and 'stress' [34]. Other equations include 'dynamic' parameters, such as body temperature, heart rate, and tidal or minute ventilation volume to account for patient variables with significant impact on REE. Finally, formulas have been developed that focus on specific subgroups of critically ill patients (e.g., the Ireton-Jones formula for trauma and burn patients [35] or the Penn State equation for obese elderly patients [36]).

Some investigators have tried to validate different equations by comparing measured energy expenditure with calculated values. Traditionally, either an 'acceptable' deviation from the true value is defined or a correlation between the values is assessed. Kross et al. compared five predictive equations with indirect calorimetry measurements in a large cohort of critically ill patients [37]. All equations failed to agree within acceptable limits with measured energy expenditure. Frankenfield et al. compared 20 equations with indirect calorimetry in 202 medico-surgical and trauma patients. From this study, the Faisy Faigon and Penn State equation emerged as the most accurate because their results deviated by less than 10% of measured values [36]. Large inconsistency between formulas and measurements rendered assessment of individual patients within certain subgroups useless. Moreover, excessive fine-tuning of formulas discriminating for age and weight status only enhances the clinical mayhem [37, 38].

Extracorporeal Techniques: A Challenge for Indirect Calorimetry

Extracorporeal treatment modalities have definitely entered modern critical care. Continuous renal replacement therapy (CRRT) is increasingly used to treat acute kidney injury (AKI) in hemodynamically unstable patients. Extracorporeal membrane oxygenation (ECMO) is a 'last stage' therapeutic option to support cardiac and/or respiratory function in patients with intractable heart failure or severe lung damage. ECMO is increasingly implemented in treatment protocols for acute respiratory distress syndrome (ARDS) [39]. With more patients exposed for longer treatment periods [40], concomitant treatment must be adjusted to extracorporeal settings. This is particularly true for antimicrobials [41] but also for enteral and parenteral nutrition.

Continuous Renal Replacement Therapy

AKI is diagnosed in 10 to 30% of patients admitted in European ICUs. Despite advances in prevention, general management, and RRT, the mortality associated with AKI remains high [42]. AKI induces metabolic and physiological disturbances that are superimposed on those produced by the initial disease. Also, AKI therapy *per se*, in particular when not carefully monitored for quality and safety, may induce harmful effects or unwarranted adverse events (i.e., the 'dialy-trauma concept') [43].

CRRT may cause substantial and incompletely quantified losses of macro- and micronutrients. Lipids or intact proteins are largely conserved during continuous hemodiafiltration [44]. However, amino acid losses may add up to 10–15 g/day because the hemodiafilter cannot discriminate between uremic toxins and nutrients [43]. Trace elements and vitamin metabolism are also thoroughly disturbed by CRRT [45]. Within 24 h of therapy, balances become negative for selenium, copper and thiamine. Despite supplementation of recommended amounts, these substances risk becoming severely depleted during prolonged CRRT. 'Apparent' losses are accompanied by more insidious heat loss [46]. CRRT indeed induces body cooling because blood circulates outside the body and interacts with cold dialysate and/or replacement fluids. A heat loss of approximately 1,000 kcal/day [47] with significant impact on energy balance has been observed [48].

During CRRT, the primary aim is to optimize nutrition whilst avoiding or reducing 'dialy-trauma'. Replenishing or compensating for the loss of macro- and micronutrients during CRRT requires higher substrate doses together with an augmented caloric and protein load [48–51].

Extracorporeal Membrane Oxygenation

ECMO provides pump-driven lung or heart-lung bypass support. Gas exchange occurs both in the native and in an artificial lung. The Extracorporeal Life Support Organization (ELSO) recently reported a 54% survival rate in 70,000 adult patients treated with extracorporeal life support in the context of respiratory, cardiac, or cardiopulmonary resuscitation [52]. Most information on REE has been retrieved from a closed-circuit indirect calorimetry technique in a neonatal ECMO setting [53]. Measurement of VO_2 and VCO_2 enabled pulmonary function to be assessed and predicted weaning from ECMO. Evaluation of energy expenditure revealed highly variable metabolic rates within and among neonates over time, which refuted the widespread belief that ECMO patients are always hypercatabolic. Protein kinetics in neonates treated with ECMO showed a negative protein balance that highly correlated with total protein turnover [54]. Increased dietary caloric intake did not improve protein catabolism but increased VCO_2, suggesting that this frail patient population needed judicious caloric supplementation. Recent work in pediatric cardiac failure reported a small increase in energy expenditure during consecutive ECMO support. Respiratory mass spectrometry proved to be feasible and obtaining information on energy expenditure and RQ enabled inadequate feeding to be avoided [55].

Data on energy requirement and nutritional consequences in adults undergoing ECMO are scant [56]. The ELSO consortium remains vague in their guidelines by merely stating "to guarantee full caloric and protein nutritional support" but without specifying how this should be accomplished [57]. A key issue in research on nutrition in ECMO is whether predictive equations are useful in this highly specific critically ill patient subgroup. For example, the observation that patients receiving ECMO had only 55% of their nutritional targets achieved could be interpreted as a failure of the stress-corrected Schofield equation that was used to estimate caloric goals in this study [58]. A recent study in adult transplant patients receiving ECMO merely recommended feeding them as any other critically ill patient [59]. Moreover, indirect calorimetry has never been studied in an adult ECMO setting mainly because of the technical challenges imposed by the presence of two simultaneously active gas exchange locations: the native and the artificial lung. Recently, De Waele et al. proposed an original method for estimating REE under ECMO conditions. According to this method, respiratory gas exchange analysis is performed separately at the ventilator and at the artificial lung. The data are then combined and introduced in the modified Weir equation to obtain the REE [60]. Preliminary clinical experience with this novel method is promising but needs prospective validation in a larger group of patients.

Conclusion

Calculating the REE in ICU patients is questionable as the discrepancy in results between the many proposed equations may merely translate into 'flipping a nutritional coin'. The 'revival' of indirect calorimetry, boosted by the commercialization of the user-friendly Vmax TM Encore 29n calorimeter, may allow more optimal fine-tuning of calorie intake in the critically ill [61]. Indirect calorimetry may also assist the clinician in handling nutrition in more complex ICU settings, such as CRRT and ECMO, but more research in this area is required.

References

1. American Association for Respiratory Care (1994) AARC clinical practice guideline. Metabolic measurement using indirect calorimetry during mechanical ventilation. Respir Care 39:1170–1175

2. Frankenfield DC (2010) On heat, respiration, and calorimetry. Nutrition 26:939–950
3. Holmes FL (1985) Lavoisier and the Chemistry Of Life. An Exploration of Scientific Creativity. University of Wisconsin Press, Madison
4. Weir JB (1949) New methods for calculating metabolic rate with special reference to protein metabolism. J Physiol 109:1–9
5. Pauling L, Wood RE, Sturdivant JH (1946) An instrument for determining the partial pressure of oxygen in a gas. Science 103:338
6. Bairiot M, Reynaert M, Roeseler J, Bachy JL (1987) Design of an automated system for assessing metabolic function in mechanically ventilated patients (Delta-Tract II & III). Acta Anaesthesiol Belg 38:45–50
7. Cooper JA, Watras AC, O'Brien MJ et al (2009) Assessing validity and reliability of resting metabolic rate in six gas analysis systems. J Am Diet Assoc 109:128–132
8. Guttormsen AB, Pichard C (2014) Determining energy requirements in the ICU. Curr Opin Clin Nutr Metab Care 17:171–176
9. Graf S, Karsegard VL, Viatte V et al (2015) Evaluation of three indirect calorimetry devices in mechanically ventilated patients: which device compares best with the Deltatrac II(®)? A prospective observational study. Clin Nutr 34:60–65
10. Preiser JC, van Zanten AR, Berger MM et al (2015) Metabolic and nutritional support of critically ill patients: consensus and controversies. Crit Care 19:35
11. De Waele E, Opsomer T, Honore PM et al (2015) Measured versus calculated resting energy expenditure in critically ill adult patients. Do mathematics match the gold standard? Minerva Anestesiol 81:272–282
12. De Waele E, Spapen H, Honoré PM et al (2012) Bedside calculation of energy expenditure does not guarantee adequate caloric prescription in long-term mechanically ventilated critically ill patients – a quality control study. ScientificWorldJournal 2012:909564
13. De Waele E, Spapen H, Honoré PM et al (2013) Introducing a new generation indirect calorimeter for estimating energy requirements in adult intensive care unit patients: Feasibility, practical considerations, and comparison with a mathematical equation. J Crit Care 28:884
14. Weijs PJ, Stapel SN, de Groot SD et al (2012) Optimal protein and energy nutrition decreases mortality in mechanically ventilated, critically ill patients: a prospective observational cohort study. JPEN J Parenter Enteral Nutr 36:60–68
15. Oshima T, Furukawa Y, Kobayashi M, Sato Y, Nihei A, Oda S (2015) Fulfilling caloric demands according to indirect calorimetry may be beneficial for post cardiac arrest patients under therapeutic hypothermia. Resuscitation 88:81–85
16. Heidegger CP, Berger MM, Graf S et al (2013) Optimisation of energy provision with supplemental parenteral nutrition in critically ill patients: a randomised controlled clinical trial. Lancet 381:385–393
17. Singer P, Anbar R, Cohen J et al (2011) The tight calorie control study (TICACOS): a prospective, randomized, controlled pilot study of nutritional support in critically ill patients. Intensive Care Med 37:601–609
18. Casaer MP, Mesotten D, Hermans G et al (2011) Early versus late parenteral nutrition in critically ill adults. N Engl J Med 365:506–517
19. Frankenfield DC, Ashcraft CM, Galvan DA (2013) Prediction of resting metabolic rate in critically ill patients at the extremes of body mass index. JPEN J Parenter Enteral Nutr 37:361–367
20. Singer P, Hiesmayr M, Biolo G et al (2014) Pragmatic approach to nutrition in the ICU: expert opinion regarding which calorie protein target. Clin Nutr 33:246–521
21. Frankenfield DC, Ashcraft CM, Galvan DA (2012) Longitudinal prediction of metabolic rate in critically ill patients. JPEN J Parenter Enteral Nutr 36:700–712
22. Kyle UG, Arriaza A, Esposito M, Coss-Bu JA (2012) Is indirect calorimetry a necessity or a luxury in the pediatric intensive care unit? JPEN J Parenter Enteral Nutr 36:177–182
23. Drolz A, Wewalka M, Horvatits T et al (2014) Gender-specific differences in energy metabolism during the initial phase of critical illness. Eur J Clin Nutr 68:707–711

24. Zauner A, Schneeweiss B, Kneidinger N, Lindner G, Zauner C (2006) Weight-adjusted resting energy expenditure is not constant in critically ill patients. Intensive Care Med 32:428–434
25. Campbell CG, Zander E, Thorland W (2005) Predicted vs measured energy expenditure in critically ill, underweight patients. Nutr Clin Pract 20:276–280
26. Ashcraft CM, Frankenfield DC (2013) Energy expenditure during barbiturate coma. Nutr Clin Pract 28:603–608
27. Saur J, Leweling H, Trinkmann F, Weissmann J, Borggrefe M, Kaden JJ (2008) Modification of the Harris-Benedict equation to predict the energy requirements of critically ill patients during mild therapeutic hypothermia. In Vivo 22:143–146
28. Oshima T, Furukawa Y, Kobayashi M, Sato Y, Nihei A, Oda S (2015) Fulfilling caloric demands according to indirect calorimetry may be beneficial for post cardiac arrest patients under therapeutic hypothermia. Resuscitation 88:81–85
29. Clapis FC, Auxiliadora-Martins M, Japur CC, Martins-Filho OA, Evora PR, Basile-Filho A (2010) Mechanical ventilation mode (volume × pressure) does not change the variables obtained by indirect calorimetry in critically ill patients. J Crit Care 25:659–716
30. Raurich JM, Ibáñez J, Marsé P, Riera M, Homar X (2007) Resting energy expenditure during mechanical ventilation and its relationship with the type of lesion. JPEN J Parenter Enteral Nutr 31:58–62
31. Hickmann CE, Roeseler J, Castanares-Zapatero D, Herrera EI, Mongodin A, Laterre PF (2014) Energy expenditure in the critically ill performing early physical therapy. Intensive Care Med 40:548–555
32. Zijlstra N, ten Dam SM, Hulshof PJ, Ram C, Hiemstra G, de Roos NM (2007) 24-hour indirect calorimetry in mechanically ventilated critically ill patients. Nutr Clin Pract 22:250–255
33. Harris JA, Benedict JA (1919) Biometric Studies of Basal Metabolism in Man. Carnegie Institute of Washington, Washington
34. Roza AM, Shizgal HM (1984) The Harris Benedict equation reevaluated: resting energy requirements and the body cell mass. Am J Clin Nutr 40:168–182
35. Ireton-Jones C, Turner W, Liepa GU, Baxter CR (1992) Equations for the estimation of energy expenditure in patients with burns with special reference to ventilatory status. J Burn Care Rehabil 13:330–333
36. Frankenfield DC, Coleman A, Alam S, Cooney RN (2009) Analysis of estimation methods for resting metabolic rate in critically ill adults. JPEN J Parenter Enteral Nutr 33:27–36
37. Kross EK, Sena M, Schmidt K, Stapleton RD (2012) A comparison of predictive equations of energy expenditure and measured energy expenditure in critically ill patients. J Crit Care 27:321
38. Faisy C, Guerot E, Diehl JL, Labrousse J, Fagon JY (2003) Assessment of resting energy expenditure in mechanically ventilated patients. Am J Clin Nutr 78:241–249
39. Schmidt M, Bailey M, Sheldrake J et al (2014) Predicting survival after extracorporeal membrane oxygenation for severe acute respiratory failure. The Respiratory Extracorporeal Membrane Oxygenation Survival Prediction (RESP) score. Am J Respir Crit Care Med 189:1374–1382
40. Schmidt M, Burrell A, Roberts L et al (2015) Predicting survival after ECMO for refractory cardiogenic shock: the survival after veno-arterial-ECMO (SAVE)-score. Eur Heart J 36:2246–2256
41. Honore PM, Jacobs R, Hendrickx I, De Waele E, Van Gorp V, Spapen HD (2015) Meropenem therapy in extracorporeal membrane oxygenation patients: an ongoing pharmacokinetic challenge. Crit Care 19:263
42. Bozfakioğlu S (2001) Nutrition in patients with acute renal failure. Nephrol Dial Transplant 16(Suppl 6):21–22
43. Maynar MJ, Honore PM, Sánchez-Izquierdo RJA, Herrera GM, Spapen HD (2012) Handling continuous renal replacement therapy-related adverse effects in intensive care unit patients: the dialytrauma concept. Blood Purif 34:177–185
44. Frankenfield DC, Reynolds HN (1995) Nutritional effect of continuous hemodiafiltration. Nutrition 11:388–393

45. Berger MM, Shenkin A, Revelly JP et al (2004) Copper, selenium, zinc, and thiamine balances during continuous venovenous hemodiafiltration in critically ill patients. Am J Clin Nutr 80:410–416
46. Yagi N, Leblanc M, Sokal K, Wright EJ, Paganini EP (1998) Cooling effect of continuous renal replacement therapy in critically ill patients. Am J Kidney Dis 32:1023–1030
47. Alvestrand A, Gutierrez A (1996) Relationship between nitrogen balance, protein, and energy intake in haemodialysis patients. Nephrol Dial Transplant 11(Suppl 2):130–133
48. Robert R, Mehaud JE, Timricht N, Goudet V, Mimoz O, Debaene B (2012) Benefits of early cooling phase in continuous renal replacement therapy for ICU patients. Ann Intensive Care 2:40
49. Honore PM, De Waele E, Jacobs R et al (2013) Nutritional and metabolic alterations during continuous renal replacement therapy. Blood Purif 35:279–284
50. Wiesen P, Van Overmeire L, Delanaye P, Dubois B, Preiser JC (2011) Nutrition disorders during acute renal failure and renal replacement therapy. JPEN J Parenter Enteral Nutr 35:217–222
51. Leverve X, Cano NJM (2010) Nutritional management in acute illness and acute kidney insuffiency. Contrib Nephrol 156:112–118
52. Extracorporeal Life Support Organization. ECLS Registry Report. Available at: https://www.elso.org/Registry/Statistics/InternationalSummary.aspx. Accessed November 2015
53. Cilley RE, Wesley JR, Zwischenberger JB, Bartlett RH (1988) Gas exchange measurements in neonates treated with extracorporeal membrane oxygenation. J Pediatr Surg 23:306–311
54. Shew SB, Keshen TH, Jahoor F, Jaksic T (1999) The determinants of protein catabolism in neonates on extracorporeal membrane oxygenation. J Pediatr Surg 34:1086–1090
55. Li X, Yu X, Cheypesh A, Li J (2015) Non-invasive measurements of energy expenditure and respiratory quotient by respiratory mass spectrometry in children on extracorporeal membrane oxygenation – a pilot study. Artif Organs 39:815–819
56. Kagan I, Singer P (2013) Nutritional imbalances during extracorporeal life support. World Rev Nutr Diet 105:154–159
57. Extracorporeal Life Support Organization. Guidelines for Extracorporeal Life Support, Version 1.3. Available at: http://www.elso.org/Portals/0/IGD/Archive/FileManager/929122ae88cusersshyerdocumentselsoguidelinesgeneralalleclsversion1.3.pdf. Accessed November 2015
58. Lukas G, Davies AR, Hilton AK, Pellegrino VA, Scheinkestel CD, Ridley E (2010) Nutritional support in adult patients receiving extracorporeal membrane oxygenation. Crit Care Resusc 12:230–234
59. Ulerich L (2014) Nutrition implications and challenges of the transplant patient undergoing extracorporeal membrane oxygenation therapy. Nutr Clin Pract 29:201–206
60. De Waele E, van Zwam K, Mattens S et al (2015) Measuring resting energy expenditure during extracorporeal membrane oxygenation: preliminary clinical experience with a proposed theoretical model. Acta Anaesthesiol Scand 59:1296–1302
61. Harvey SE, Parrott F, Harrison DA et al (2014) Trial of the route of early nutritional support in critically ill adults. N Engl J Med 371:1673–1684

Part XI
Ethical Issues

Managing Intensive Care Supply-Demand Imbalance

C. C. H. Leung, W. T. Wong, and C. D. Gomersall

Introduction

Intensive care is an expensive resource and it is common for the demand for intensive care unit (ICU) beds to exceed availability with rates of refusal of admission ranging from 17.6–42% [1–5]. Although the seven-fold difference in ICU beds per capita among different high income countries [6] makes it difficult to define the need for ICU admission and suggests that some countries may only experience a true shortfall of beds in exceptional circumstances, it is incumbent on intensive care specialists to understand the principles of managing supply-demand imbalance.

Increasing Supply

In the event of a shortage of ICU beds, physicians have an ethical obligation to try to remedy this situation by increasing the supply. This may require an increase in appropriately equipped bed spaces or simply a change in staffing ratios so that the same number of staff look after more patients. Although the latter may appear to be an attractive short-term solution, this may not be the case. Staffing ratios vary considerably from country to country indicating that there is no consensus regarding the best ratio [7]. Nevertheless, there are data indicating that lower staff-to-workload ratios are associated with increased morbidity and mortality [8]. Neuraz et al. studied patients admitted to eight ICUs in France and concluded that the risk of death was increased by 3.5 when the patient-to-nurse ratio exceeded 2.5 and was increased by 2.0 when the physician-to-patient ratio exceeded 14. Unfortunately no measures of actual workload were collected. It has been suggested that an accomplished critical care nurse should be capable of managing 40–50 Therapeutic

C. C. H. Leung · W. T. Wong · C. D. Gomersall (✉)
Department of Anaesthesia & Intensive Care, The Chinese University of Hong Kong
Shatin, Hong Kong
email: gomersall@cuhk.edu.hk

© Springer International Publishing Switzerland 2016
J.-L. Vincent (ed.), *Annual Update in Intensive Care and Emergency Medicine 2016*,
DOI 10.1007/978-3-319-27349-5_31

Intervention Scoring System (TISS-76) points [9], but this threshold has not been validated. These observations suggest that there will come a point at which increasing the number of ICU beds (without an increase in staffing) will not result in more survivors because the increased availability of beds will be offset by a reduced quality of care. This should be borne in mind when considering the appropriateness of recommendations to increase ICU bed capacity by 100–300% in a disaster [10]. There are also data suggesting that even if nursing staffing levels are maintained by employing temporary staff, an expansion in the number of beds may result in an increase in risk-adjusted mortality [11].

Elective Postoperative Admissions

In some ICUs, elective post-operative admissions constitute a significant proportion of admissions. Typically, beds are assigned to these patients before induction of anesthesia and these beds lie empty while surgery is carried out. Furthermore many of these patients require little intervention once they arrive in the ICU, but are simply monitored. This results in a highly inefficient use of beds. While there may be a benefit to this group as a whole, this benefit results entirely from those patients who develop a complication that requires urgent intervention or organ support. Those patients who do not receive any ICU-specific intervention but are only monitored, 'occupy' a bed from the time it is assigned but cannot derive benefit and may suffer harm [12]. Zimmerman and Kramer found that only 11.5% of 28,847 patients admitted to ICUs in 45 United States hospitals for monitoring received active treatment [13]. As yet, there are limited data to assist in identifying postoperative patients with a high risk of requiring intensive care intervention. 'High risk' criteria have been used to identify patients undergoing non-cardiac surgery for trials of pre-optimization [14, 15] but these criteria are poorly defined, lack an evidence base and lack specificity. We determined the 28-day mortality of 'high risk' adult surgical patients in our institution undergoing major or ultra-major general or vascular surgery lasting more than two hours. Patients were identified as being high risk based on the presence of risk factors used in previous studies of pre-optimization [14, 15]. The 28-day mortality (95% CI) was 0% for patients with no risk factors and 2.3 (0.8 to 3.7%) for patients with at least one risk factor [16]. Identifying patients at low risk may be simpler, and a fast track approach to hepatobiliary surgery that does not involve routine postoperative admission for all patients has been successfully followed in a number of centers [17, 18]. Schultz et al. reported their experience with fast track management of 100 consecutive patients undergoing hepatic resection [18]. All patients were discharged from the recovery room to a general ward except those undergoing the most advanced resections and those with an American Society of Anesthesiologists grade 3, who spent the first postoperative night in a high dependency unit. There were no deaths within 30 days of operation.

A score to identify patients likely to fail fast-track cardiac surgery has been developed and externally validated [19, 20]. By using decision curve analysis it was possible to predict how many unnecessary ICU admissions could be saved depending on the acceptable threshold risk of fast track failure. For example, if one decided that the threshold was avoidance of nine routine ICU admissions to justify the 'cost' of one unexpected admission due to fast track failure, 46% of patients could be cared for in a fast track unit rather than an ICU [20]. This approach may help individual units to determine the likely benefit from a fast track approach, depending on the demographics of patients undergoing cardiac surgery in their hospital.

ICU bed availability may also be increased by reducing the length of stay of post-operative patients. Patients randomized to short ICU stay (8 h) following cardiac surgery were found to have a similar mortality and morbidity to those randomized to conventional overnight intensive care. Not surprisingly, the cost of care was lower in the short stay group [21, 22]. In this context, reductions in duration of postoperative mechanical ventilation, which may otherwise seem trivial, become important [23]. Even a few hours difference may allow a short stay patient to be discharged during the late afternoon or early evening rather than late at night.

Delaying surgery for patients who require postoperative care is a short-term solution for a shortage of ICU beds. Superficially, this is an attractive option compared with refusing emergency admission to a critically ill patient. Delaying surgery is unlikely to have a major impact on the outcome of the patient whose operation is delayed, while refusal of emergency admission may be associated with early death. However, it is important to consider the cumulative effect of delayed surgery on those on the waiting list for surgery. For example, if each patient on a waiting list of 26 patients has their operation postponed by one week then the last patient in the queue will be delayed by the sum of those one week delays and his operation will be delayed for 26 weeks, almost 6 months. Depending on the nature of the surgery, a 6-month delay may have a significant impact on morbidity or mortality.

Emergency Admissions

The ethical principle of non-maleficence demands that prior to refusing a patient admission to intensive care on the basis of rationing, an attempt is made to transfer the patient to an ICU with an available bed. If rationing of admissions to intensive care is absolutely necessary, it may follow egalitarian or utilitarian principles. In the egalitarian approach, each patient has an equal chance of admission to ICU regardless of patient factors, including severity of illness and likelihood of benefit. In this approach, patients are generally admitted on a first-come, first-served basis with the underlying assumption that bed availability at the time of presentation is a form of natural lottery.

The utilitarian approach seeks to maximize benefit for the community. With this approach, priority is given to those patients who will achieve the greatest benefit from intensive care. When applying this approach, it is important to understand what constitutes benefit. If one considers mortality, then benefit from intensive care is not simply synonymous with the probability of survival if admitted to intensive care. Instead it is the *incremental* probability of survival if admitted to intensive care. In a similar fashion, one does not consider the benefit of a potentially life-saving drug to be the survival of those who take the drug, rather it is the difference in survival between those who take the drug and those who take a placebo [24]. Iapichino et al.'s analysis of patients admitted and refused admission to the ICU indicates that more severely ill patients derive greater benefit [25] but this is of limited help when making a triage decision for an individual patient. Thus it is important to be able to predict probability of survival if admitted to the ICU and probability of survival if refused admission. While there are extensive data addressing the predictors of survival for those admitted to the ICU, there are very limited data on the factors associated with survival of those refused admission. In the Eldicus study, age, underlying diagnosis such as cardiogenic shock and cerebrovascular accident, creatinine level, white cell and platelet counts, vasopressor requirement, Glasgow Coma Scale, Karnofsky Performance Status Scale, history of operation and presence of chronic disorder were associated with 28-day mortality in patients refused admission [5].

A few scoring systems have been proposed to aid triage decision making. These systems have been designed to identify those patients with a very high or a very low chance of death. This approach has the advantage that it is not necessary to estimate the risk of death with and without intensive care. If the risk of death is extremely high with intensive care then the incremental survival associated with intensive care must be low, even if mortality without intensive care is 100%. Similarly, if the risk of death without intensive care is very low the difference between survival with and without intensive care must be low even if mortality with intensive care is 0%. Unfortunately, so few patients referred for ICU admission fall into these categories that these scoring systems are likely to be of little practical assistance. The Eldicus prospective, observational study developed an initial rejecting score with high sensitivity for predicting mortality despite admission to ICU and a final triage score for survival even if refused. However, out of 6796 patients triaged, only 114 patients (91 for the initial score and 23 for the final score) would have been refused (1.7%) [5]. Christian et al. proposed a scoring system based on the Sequential Organ Failure Assessment (SOFA) score to triage patients in an epidemic [26]. The score was designed to exclude patients on the basis of high mortality despite admission to ICU. However, when assessed in a different environment the scoring system would have excluded patients with only moderately high mortality and when re-calibrated to exclude patients with >90% mortality would have led to the exclusion of only 0.2% of the cohort [27]. While these studies suggest that scoring systems are not currently useful for triage, this does not mean that attempts to develop appropriate scoring systems should be abandoned. One of the key components for ethical triage is justice and scoring systems should minimize the effect of bias. It may be argued that scoring systems should not be used for triage because decisions about individuals should not be based on group data. This ignores the fact that triage is a process designed to bring maximum benefit to the community not to an individual and that the whole basis of evidence-based medicine is the application of group data to individuals. Alternatively it could be argued that their discriminative ability is low and calibration poor but this pre-supposes that there is a better alternative [24]. Currently, the only alternative is clinical judgement, but the available evidence suggests that this is poor. In the Eldicus study, 25% of those refused ICU admission because they were too ill survived to hospital discharge while 12% of those considered too well died [5].

When considering benefit from intensive care, it is probably more relevant to consider survival in terms of duration rather than as an event. Thus, we should not only consider the incremental probability of survival but also the duration of survival. Conceptually, benefit could then be considered as incremental probability of survival multiplied by life expectancy. This is a logical extension of the recommendation that patients with short life expectancy should receive low priority for ICU admission [28, 29]. It also provides ethical underpinning for taking age into account when making triage decisions. Age *per se* is not the important factor but age is inversely associated with life expectancy and thus, in a utilitarian approach, older patients tend to receive a lower priority for admission.

For many, however, quality of life may be as important, if not more important, than duration of survival. Thus benefit may be considered not simply as incremental probability of survival multiplied by life expectancy but incremental probability of

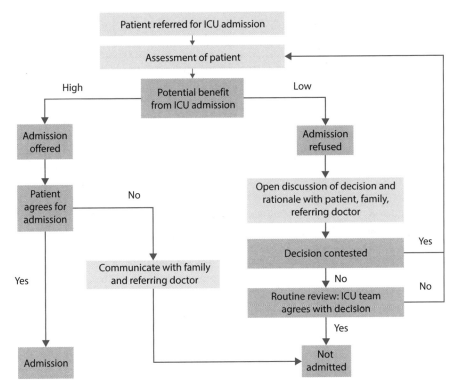

Fig. 1 The approach to triage of admissions used in our ICU. Although the process is constant, the decisions are continuously informed by discussions with referring clinicians, audit and emerging data

survival multiplied by quality-adjusted life expectancy. Although there are studies which address quality of life after intensive care, there are no data that facilitate prediction, at the time of referral, of quality of life after intensive care. However, in many patients there is no plausible mechanism by which intensive care will result in a better quality of life after discharge than before and, therefore, it may be reasonable to give a lower priority to patients with pre-existing poor quality of life. An exception are those patients with chronic disease causing poor quality of life where intensive care will give the opportunity for treatment of the chronic disease to be substantially improved.

Alternative approaches to triage are to admit patients for a limited trial of therapy or to withdraw treatment on the basis of poor likelihood of recovery. It is assumed that prognostication will be more accurate if informed by the response to a trial of therapy. Although intuitive, there are no data to support this assumption. However, perhaps more importantly, such an approach is difficult in environments in which doctors are required to obtain relatives' assent for withdrawal of treatment. Withdrawal of therapy on the basis of triage, while considered ethically equivalent to admission triage, is probably not practical and experience of this approach has not been described [29].

The approach to triage used in our ICU is illustrated in Fig. 1.

Advanced Organ Support Outside Intensive Care Units

Provision of cardiac and renal support and non-invasive ventilation (NIV) outside ICUs has been commonplace for years, however little is known about the outcome of patients receiving invasive mechanical ventilation outside the ICU or operating room. Hersch et al. described 65 patients ventilated in general wards due to a shortage of ICU beds: the mean APACHE II score was 27 and hospital mortality was 80% [30]. Lieberman et al. observed a higher mortality (68.2%) amongst patients ventilated in general wards than in the ICU but were unable to demonstrate an independent association between admission to the ICU and survival [31]. Tang et al. reported 89% mortality in 755 patients ventilated on general wards; the predicted mortality based on the Mortality Prediction Model II_0 was 75% [32]. Thus the mortality of patients ventilated in general wards appears to be high but it is unclear whether this is due to selection bias or to a lower standard of care. Nevertheless mechanical ventilation in a general ward should probably only be used as a last resort.

Conclusion

Managing supply-demand imbalance requires different approaches for elective surgical admissions and emergency admissions because of the very different consequences of refusal. Demand can potentially be reduced by identifying those elective patients who are at high risk of requiring intensive care intervention, as opposed to simple monitoring, and by shortening length of stay. For emergency admissions the focus of management is on appropriate rationing. This can be based on a first-come, first-served approach or can be based on triage designed to maximize benefit. Although triage based on benefit is recommended [28, 29, 33], its practical application is associated with considerable uncertainty [33].

References

1. Louriz M, Abidi K, Akkaoui M et al (2012) Determinants and outcomes associated with decisions to deny or to delay intensive care unit admission in Morocco. Intensive Care Med 38:830–837
2. Joynt GM, Gomersall CD, Tan P, Lee A, Cheng AY, Wong EL (2001) Prospective evaluation of patients refused admission to an intensive care unit – triage, futility and outcome. Intensive Care Med 27:1459–1465
3. Frisho-Lima P, Gurman G, Schapira A, Porath A (1994) Rationing critical care – what happens to patients who are not admitted? Theor Surg 9:208–211
4. Sprung CL, Geber D, Eidelman LA et al (1999) Evaluation of triage decisions for intensive care admission. Crit Care Med 27:1073–1079
5. Sprung CL, Baras M, Iapichino G et al (2012) The Eldicus prospective, observational study of triage decision making in European intensive care units: Part I – European Intensive Care Admission Triage Scores. Crit Care Med 40:125–131
6. Wunsch H, Angus DC, Harrison DA et al (2008) Variation in critical care services across North America and Western Europe. Crit Care Med 36:2787–2793
7. Depasse B, Pauwels D, Somers Y, Vincent JL (1998) A profile of European ICU nursing. Intensive Care Med 24:939–945
8. Neuraz A, Guérin C, Payet C et al (2015) Patient mortality is associated with staff resources and workload in the icu: a multicenter observational study. Crit Care Med 43:1587–1594
9. Keene AR, Cullen DJ (1983) Therapeutic intervention scoring system: update 1983. Crit Care Med 11:1–3
10. Sprung C, Zimmerman J, Christian M et al (2010) Recommendations for intensive care unit and hospital preparations for an influenza epidemic or mass disaster: summary report of the European Society of Intensive Care Medicine's Task Force for intensive care unit triage during an influenza epidemic or mass disaster. Intensive Care Med 36:428–443
11. Tarnow-Mordi WO, Hau C, Warden A, Shearer AJ (2000) Hospital mortality in relation to staff workload: a 4-year study in an adult intensive-care unit. Lancet 356:185–189
12. McIlroy DR, Coleman BD, Myles PS (2006) Outcomes following a shortage of high dependency unit beds for surgical patients. Anaesth Intensive Care 34:457–463
13. Zimmerman JE, Kramer AA (2010) A model for identifying patients who may not need intensive care unit admission. J Crit Care 25:205–213
14. Lobo SM, Salgado PF, Castillo VG et al (2000) Effects of maximizing oxygen delivery on morbidity and mortality in high-risk surgical patients. Crit Care Med 28:3396–3404
15. Wilson J, Woods I, Whall R, Dibb W, Morris C, McManus E (1999) Reducing the risk of major elective surgery; randomised controlled trial of preoperative optimisation of oxygen delivery. BMJ 318:1099–1103
16. Gomersall CD, Ramsay SJ, Leung P (2008) Hospital and 28-day mortality amongst 'high risk' surgical patients. A retrospective cohort study. Anaesth Intensive Care 36:20–24
17. Lee A, Chiu CH, Cho MWA et al (2014) Factors associated with failure of enhanced recovery protocol in patients undergoing major hepatobiliary and pancreatic surgery: a retrospective cohort study. BMJ Open 4:e005330
18. Schultz NA, Larsen PN, Klarskov B et al (2013) Evaluation of a fast-track programme for patients undergoing liver resection. Br J Surg 100:138–143

19. Constantinides VA, Tekkis PP, Fazil A et al (2006) Fast-track failure after cardiac surgery: Development of a prediction model. Crit Care Med 34:2875–2882
20. Lee A, Zhu F, Underwood MJ, Gomersall CD (2013) Fast-track failure after cardiac surgery: external model validation and implications to ICU bed utilization. Crit Care Med 41:1205–1213
21. van Mastrigt GAPG, Heijmans J, Severens JL et al (2006) Short-stay intensive care after coronary artery bypass surgery: Randomized clinical trial on safety and cost-effectiveness. Crit Care Med 34:1624–1634
22. van Mastrigt GA, Joore MA, Nieman FH, Severens JL, Maessen JG (2010) Health-related quality of life after fast-track treatment results from a randomized controlled clinical equivalence trial. Qual Life Res 19:631–642
23. Zhu F, Gomersall CD, Ng SK, Underwood MJ, Lee A (2015) A randomized controlled trial of adaptive support ventilation mode to wean patients after fast-track cardiac valvular surgery. Anesthesiology 122:832–840
24. Gomersall CD, Joynt GM (2011) What's the benefit in triage? Crit Care Med 39:911–912
25. Iapichino G, Corbella D, Minelli C et al (2010) Reasons for refusal of admission to intensive care and impact on mortality. Intensive Care Med 36:1772–1779
26. Christian MD, Hawryluck L, Wax RS et al (2006) Development of a triage protocol for critical care during an influenza pandemic. CMAJ 175:1377–1381
27. Shahpori R, Stelfox HT, Doig CJ, Boiteau PJE, Zygun DA (2011) Sequential organ failure assessment in H1N1 pandemic planning. Crit Care Med 39:827–832
28. Society of Critical Care Medicine ethics committee (1994) Consensus Statement on the Triage of Critically Ill Patients. JAMA 271:1200–1203
29. Christian MD, Sprung CL, King MA et al (2014) Triage: Care of the critically ill and injured during pandemics and disasters: chest consensus statement. Chest 146:e61S–e74S
30. Hersch M, Sonnenblick M, Karlic A, Einav S, Sprung CL, Izbicki G (2007) Mechanical ventilation of patients hospitalized in medical wards vs the intensive care unit – an observational, comparative study. J Crit Care 22:13–17
31. Lieberman D, Nachshon L, Miloslavsky O et al (2010) Elderly patients undergoing mechanical ventilation in and out of intensive care units: a comparative, prospective study of 579 ventilations. Crit Care 14:R48
32. Tang WM, Tong CK, Yu WC, Tong KL, Buckley TA (2012) Outcome of adult critically ill patients mechanically vertilated on general medical wards. Hong Kong Med 18:284–290
33. ATS Bioethics Task Force (1997) Fair allocation of intensive care unit resources. Am J Respir Crit Care Med 156:1282–1301

Advances in the Management of the Potential Organ Donor After Neurologic Determination of Death

A. Confalonieri, M. Smith, and G. Citerio

Introduction

Transplantation is often the only treatment for patients with end-stage organ failure, but the gap between organ availability and those awaiting a transplant remains a worldwide problem [1, 2]. A limited donor pool and low number of potentially transplantable organs retrieved from each donor are the main reasons for this ever-widening gap. Two complementary strategies for resolving this issue are:

- Increase the number and source of potential organ donors. Worldwide, the major source of deceased donor organs is from individuals in whom death has been determined by neurological criteria, i.e., donation after brain death (DBD) [3, 4]. Donation after cardiac death (DCD) is now an option that is being used in many countries to increase donation rates [5, 6], albeit one in which the number of potentially transplantable organs retrieved per donor is lower, and post-transplant graft function for some organs worse, than after DBD [7, 8]. While actions to reduce end-stage organ failure are crucial, all countries are now also encouraged to achieve self-sufficiency in organ transplantation for patients with end-

A. Confalonieri
Neurointensive Care, Department of Emergency and Intensive Care, San Gerardo Hospital
Monza, Italy

M. Smith
Department of Neurocritical Care, National Hospital for Neurology and Neurosurgery, University College London Hospitals
London, UK
National Institute for Health Research UCLH Biomedical Research Centre
London, UK

G. Citerio (✉)
School of Medicine and Surgery, University of Milan-Bicocca
Milan, Italy
Neurointensive Care, Department of Emergency and Intensive Care, San Gerardo Hospital
Monza, Italy
email: giuseppe.citerio@unimib.it

© Springer International Publishing Switzerland 2016
J.-L. Vincent (ed.), *Annual Update in Intensive Care and Emergency Medicine 2016*,
DOI 10.1007/978-3-319-27349-5_32

stage disease by increasing deceased donation rates from both DND and DCD donors [2].

- Increase the number of transplantable organs from each potential organ donor by optimizing donor maintenance and management strategies in both DBD and DCD, and by developing and implementing novel treatment and repair of donor organs using *ex vivo* techniques [9].

The intensive care unit (ICU) management of the adult brain dead potential organ donor focuses on the correction of the profound physiological derangements associated with brain death [10] in order to improve the viability of potentially transplantable organs after consent for donation [11]. Careful titration of organ support is required to maintain and maximize organ function until their retrieval [12], and intensivists and their teams are key to this process. Implementation of intensivist-led donor management protocols is associated with an increase in the number of transplantable organs retrieved from each donor [13]. Moreover, the ICU management of the brain dead donor has been informed by recent randomized controlled trials (RCTs) [14–17], and professional societies have published guidelines for the ICU management of the potential organ donor [18]. These emphasize that the same rigor that is applied to the management of living patients should also be applied to the deceased organ donor.

Physiological Changes Related to Brain Death

A rational approach to donor management is predicated on an understanding of the substantial physiological changes that accompany the onset of brain death (Fig. 1) [19]. High intracranial pressure (ICP) leads to rostral to caudal brain ischemia, which is accompanied by a massive release of catecholamines in an attempt to maintain cerebral perfusion. The classic 'Cushing's triad' of hypertension, irregular breathing (absent in ventilated patients) and bradycardia are the clinical manifestations of brainstem ischemia. In animal models of brain death, circulating catecholamine concentrations are increased by up to 800% [20]. This can result in extreme arterial hypertension, cardiac arrhythmias and left ventricular dysfunction secondary to myocardial 'stunning.' This catecholamine-related 'stress cardiomyopathy' is an acute reversible syndrome associated with typical ventricular wall motion abnormalities (apical hypokinesis/dyskinesis with sparing of the basal ventricular segment) and the development of classic myocardial histological changes, such as contraction band necrosis [21–23]. The catecholamine outpouring also causes direct injury to the lungs leading to increased pulmonary capillary permeability and pulmonary edema, as well as a profound systemic inflammatory response. Subsequently, brain herniation results in upper cord ischemia and a reduction in sympathetic tone with associated vasodilation and loss of cardiac stimulation leading to hypotension. Finally, with the onset of diencephalic ischemia there is a decrease in the levels of thyroid hormones, cortisol, antidiuretic hormone and insulin, which can exacerbate the hypotension. Central diabetes insipidus (DI), with

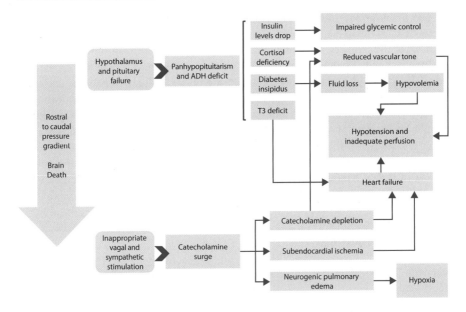

Fig. 1 The effects of brain death on systemic organ systems

its related volume depletion, further aggravates this hypotensive state. Temperature dysregulation related to hypothalamic damage is an invariable consequence of brain death, and the patient becomes poikilothermic. Thromboplastin release from ischemic brain tissue may lead to disseminated intravascular coagulation (DIC) [24].

Pathophysiological changes after brain death are exceedingly common. Hypotension occurs in 81–97% of brain dead organ donors, DI in up to 78%, DIC in 29–55%, cardiac arrhythmias in 25–32%, and pulmonary edema in 13–18% [12]. In order to maximize the chances of organ donation these profound physiological changes must be promptly identified and treated. Management of the physiologically unstable brain dead organ donor has been shown to reduce the number of donors lost during maintenance and increase the number of organs transplanted with good outcomes [25].

Deceased Organ Donation Pathways

Three deceased organ donation pathways are possible:

1. DBD following death diagnosed by neurological criteria;
2. Controlled DCD after the withdrawal of life-sustaining treatments and determination of death using cardiorespiratory criteria;
3. Uncontrolled DCD after an unexpected cardiac arrest and death, again determined using cardiorespiratory criteria.

The first two are more relevant to intensive care practice and this review will focus only on the management of the first.

In a recent series of recommendations on the management of devastating brain injuries in the ICU, the Neurocritical Care Society strongly suggests that the opportunity of organ donation should be considered and offered to patients and their families if the brain injury evolves to brain death or a decision is made to withdraw therapy [10]. Development of strategies for timely identification and triggered referral of potential donors to local organ donation services are crucial in this regard. After confirmation of brain death, the clinical team must review therapeutic goals and switch from strategies aimed at maximizing any potential for brain recovery to one of donor management in addition to discussing with family members the possibility of organ donation [26].

Donor Management

An overall donor management strategy is outlined in Fig. 2.

Hemodynamic Management

Hypotension occurs in up to 80% of potential donors, and the primary management goal is to correct low blood pressure in order to optimize perfusion for organ preservation. This is accomplished by maintaining adequate intravascular volume and cardiac output. Acceptable targets are euvolemia, mean arterial pressure (MAP) > 60 mmHg, heart rate < 100 bpm, and urine output ≥ 1 ml/kg/h.

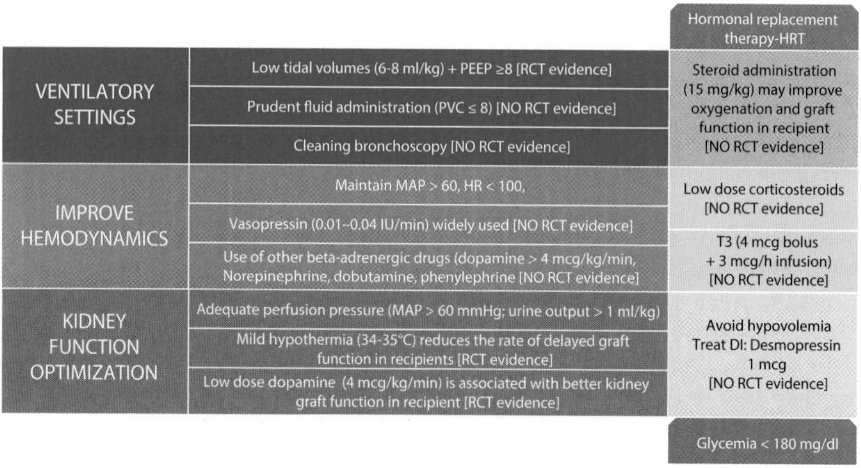

		Hormonal replacement therapy-HRT
VENTILATORY SETTINGS	Low tidal volumes (6-8 ml/kg) + PEEP ≥8 [RCT evidence]	Steroid administration (15 mg/kg) may improve oxygenation and graft function in recipient [NO RCT evidence]
	Prudent fluid administration (PVC ≤ 8) [NO RCT evidence]	
	Cleaning bronchoscopy [NO RCT evidence]	
IMPROVE HEMODYNAMICS	Maintain MAP > 60, HR < 100,	Low dose corticosteroids [NO RCT evidence]
	Vasopressin (0.01–0.04 IU/min) widely used [NO RCT evidence]	T3 (4 mcg bolus + 3 mcg/h infusion) [NO RCT evidence]
	Use of other beta-adrenergic drugs (dopamine > 4 mcg/kg/min, Norepinephrine, dobutamine, phenylephrine [NO RCT evidence]	
KIDNEY FUNCTION OPTIMIZATION	Adequate perfusion pressure (MAP > 60 mmHg; urine output > 1 ml/kg)	Avoid hypovolemia Treat DI: Desmopressin 1 mcg [NO RCT evidence]
	Mild hypothermia (34-35°C) reduces the rate of delayed graft function in recipients [RCT evidence]	
	Low dose dopamine (4 mcg/kg/min) is associated with better kidney graft function in recipient [RCT evidence]	
		Glycemia < 180 mg/dl

Fig. 2 Organ donor management. *PEEP*: positive end-expiratory pressure; *RCT*: randomized controlled trial; *MAP*: mean arterial pressure; *DI*: diabetes insipidus

Fluid Resuscitation

Brain dead patients can be volume depleted for many reasons including inadequate volume resuscitation, excessive diuresis due to DI, vasodilation secondary to loss of sympathetic tone, and the preceding use of osmotic diuretics for controlling high ICP. General principles of ICU hemodynamic management apply and, crucially, hypovolemia must be promptly identified and treated. As in other critically ill patients, invasive cardiovascular monitoring of brain dead patients is essential.

Although a central venous catheter and pulmonary artery catheter (no longer recommended) have historically been used for to guide fluid therapy, a more integrated approach is now recommended [27]. Commonly used preload measures, such as central venous pressure (CVP), have many problems and should not be used alone to guide fluid resuscitation [28]. Other methods of hemodynamic monitoring, such as bedside transthoracic echocardiogram, transpulmonary thermodilution, pulse-contour analysis and stroke volume variation, are now preferred [27, 29]. Such an integrated evaluation of volume status and volume responsiveness using dynamic variables is now relatively commonplace in the ICU, and is probably also useful in the management of brain dead organ donors [30].

A recent RCT, the Monitoring Organ Donors to Improve Transplantation Results (MOnIToR) study, assessed whether protocolized fluid therapy in brain dead donors could improve organ viability and survival in recipients [15]. In this study, brain dead patients were randomly assigned to usual care or to a protocolized volume replacement strategy in which fluids and vasopressors were titrated to pre-defined targets of cardiac index, MAP and pulse pressure variation as variables reflective of the hemodynamic status of the donor. Patients in the protocol group received more fluids compared to those in usual care group, but there was no statistically significant difference between the two groups in the number of organs retrieved per donor. A subgroup analysis of protocol fluid 'responders' demonstrated a non-statistically significant difference in the number of organs transplanted per donor, opening the possibility for future research in this area.

The recommended approach to fluid replacement in the brain dead donor is initial resuscitation with crystalloid solutions, such as 0.9% saline or lactated Ringer solution. In hypernatremic patients with DI, hyposmolar solutions (0.45% saline) in association with desmopressin (see below) can be used temporarily until sodium concentration falls below 150 mmol/l. Dextrose-containing solutions should be avoided because of resultant hyperglycemia and further osmotic diuresis, and because they extravasate into the third space. Whenever fluid replacement is required, a fluid challenge and monitored response is recommended over empirical replacement [31]. Hemodynamic support can be managed successfully with volume resuscitation and only low doses of vasopressors in 70–90% of brain dead donors [32].

In addition to the known adverse effects of hydroxyethyl starch (HES) in the critically ill generally [33], fluid replacement with HES is not recommended in potential organ donors because it can accumulate in the tissues [34] and induce renal injury and compromise renal graft function [35]. Packed red blood cells are used to maintain adequate tissue oxygenation, aiming for a hemoglobin concentration greater than 70 g/l as in the general ICU population. Other blood products may be required to manage coagulopathy.

Vasoactive Drugs

In patients who remain hypotensive despite fluid resuscitation, support with vasopressors or inotropes is required but there are insufficient data to recommend one vasopressor/inotrope over another. Dopamine, because of its inotropic and vasopressor effects, has conventionally been the first-line vasoactive agent for the management of cardiovascular collapse following brain death. It is associated with a reduced requirement for dialysis after kidney transplantation, and attenuation of the pro-inflammatory cytokine cascade. However, vasopressin (0–2.4 units/h) is now considered by many to the most appropriate first-line agent to support blood pressure, and is preferred in the presence of DI. Norepinephrine and phenylephrine should be used cautiously because of their α-receptor agonist activity, which may increase pulmonary capillary permeability and induce coronary vasoconstriction. Epinephrine may be used cautiously in primary cardiac pump dysfunction. Dobutamine may lead to undesirable hypotension and tachycardia because of its profound vasodilator effects. If hemodynamic goals are not met and/or left ventricular ejection fraction remains less than 45% with conventional hemodynamic support, hormonal replacement therapy may be considered (see below).

Ventilatory Strategy

Damage to the lungs may occur before or after brain death because of direct trauma, infection, pulmonary edema, or ventilator-induced barotrauma [36]. Lung donation proceeds in fewer than 20% of potential donors because of deterioration of lung function after brain death and highly restrictive lung donor criteria. Strategies for optimizing ventilation management to improve the quality of lungs in potential donors are urgently needed, along with extended donor criteria. The trend to protective ventilation strategies, including low tidal volume (V_T) and higher positive end-expiratory pressure (PEEP), to minimize the risk of ventilator-associated lung injury (VALI) in all critically ill patients is equally applicable to the potential brain dead organ donor. An Italian multicenter study randomized potential donors to a conventional ventilation protocol (V_T 10–12 ml/kg, 3–5 cm PEEP, open circuit for both suctioning and apnea tests) or a lung-protective protocol (V_T 6–8 ml/kg, 8–10 cm PEEP, closed circuit for suctioning, continuous positive airway pressure [CPAP] equal to previous PEEP for apnea test, and recruitment maneuvers after any disconnection from the ventilator), and found that a lung protective ventilation strategy doubled lung donation rates compared with a conventional ventilation strategy [14].

Munshi and colleagues integrated these findings into a lung preservation protocol for potential organ donors with the following recommendations [37]:

- V_T 6–8 ml/kg;
- PEEP 8–10 cmH$_2$O, with equivalent CPAP maintained during the apnea test;

- Frequent recruitment maneuvers and bronchoscopy with bronchoalveolar lavage after brain death;
- Semilateral decubitus position and recruitment maneuvers in hypoxic patients, i.e., those with PaO_2/FiO_2 fraction < 300 mmHg;
- CVP ≤ 8 mmHg and extravascular lung water < 10 ml/kg.

Implementing this intensive lung donor-treatment protocol has been shown to increase lung procurement rates in Spanish ICUs [38].

Hormonal Replacement Therapy

Given the multiple hormone dysfunction that occurs after brain death, there has been much interest in the use of hormonal replacement therapy. A standard hormonal replacement therapy regime includes 15 mg/kg of methylprednisolone, a 4.0-µg intravenous (i. v.) bolus of triiodothyronine (T3) followed by an infusion at 3 µg/h, and 0.01–0.04 IU/min of arginine vasopressin (AVP). Retrospective studies of hormonal replacement therapy have shown that it can minimize electrocardiographic changes, acid-base abnormalities and cardiovascular instability in brain dead patients, but high-quality evidence supporting its routine use in donor management is scarce. It is, therefore, prudent to reserve a standardized hormonal resuscitation package for unstable donors requiring high dose catecholamines, or those who are catecholamine unresponsive.

Vasopressin

Brain death-related AVP deficiency induces polyuria, hypovolemia, hyperosmolality and hypernatremia. The diagnosis of DI requires:

- polyuria (urine output > 2.5–3.0 ml/kg/h),
- normal/increased serum osmolality,
- diluted urine (osmolality < 200 mOsm/kg H_2O, specific gravity < 1.005) and
- hypernatremia ($Na^+ > 145$ mmol/l).

If the donor is hypotensive due to low systemic vascular resistance, a replacement dose of AVP (0.01–0.04 IU/min) is recommended in preference to other vasopressors. For DI, a starting i. v. dose of AVP of 1–4 µg, followed by additional titrated dosing (1 or 2 µg every 6 h) is recommended. However, in a recent meta-analysis of two studies, desmopressin was not associated with improved kidney graft outcomes even though it did prevent further episodes of hypotension [39].

Fluid and electrolyte balance must be monitored hourly and corrected as necessary.

Corticosteroids

A variable occurrence of corticosteroid deficiency is reported after brain death, but significant hypocortisolism is not universal. Brain death also activates a series of events leading to upregulation of pro-inflammatory and immunologic mediators.

Current guidelines recommend that administration of steroids should be considered in all donors in an attempt to minimize the effects of the inflammatory cascade on organ function following brain death [18]. However, these recommendations are based largely on observational data. A recent systematic review of the efficacy of corticosteroids in brain death donors demonstrated that 10 of the 11 RCTs included in the review yielded neutral results [40]. On the other hand, in 14 observational studies with high risks of confounding factors, the use of corticosteroids generally resulted in improved donor hemodynamics, oxygenation status, increased organ procurement, and improved recipient and graft survival. This systematic review highlights the low quality and conflicting evidence supporting the routine use of corticosteroids in the management of organ donors, and questions their generalized use. A recent multicenter study demonstrated that low-dose corticosteroids after brain death reduced the dose and duration of vasopressor use, possibly as a result of increasing cardiac and vascular sensitivity to catecholamines [41]. In the authors' opinion, administration of glucocorticoids should be considered only in patients with high catecholamine requirements and those who are catecholamine responsive.

Thyroid Hormones

Much of the evidence supporting the use of thyroid replacement therapy comes from animal studies that show significant reductions in T3 and free thyroxine (T4) levels after the onset of brain death. In humans, this reduction in T3 and T4 has not been consistently reported and, even when present, low levels of circulating thyroid hormone are not always associated with hemodynamic instability. The abnormalities in thyroid function after brain death are in fact more consistent with the disturbances in the hypothalamus-pituitary-thyroid axis frequently reported in critically ill patients generally, i.e., euthyroid sick syndrome or low T3 syndrome [42]. Rech and colleagues evaluated six RCTs estimating the effects of T3 replacement in the brain dead donor, and all had consistently negative results [39]. Even when cardiac index was used as the outcome measure, T3 replacement also turned out to be of no positive benefit in four of the RCTs. Together these findings suggest that reduced T3 and the subsequent relative hypothyroid state is not a major determinant of myocardial dysfunction after brain death, but probably an adaptive response to illness [43].

While thyroid hormone replacement therapy (4.0 µg T3 i. v. bolus followed by an infusion at 3 µg/h or 20 µg T4 i. v. bolus followed by an infusion at 10 µg/h) either alone or as part of the standardized hormonal resuscitation package is still recommended [18], the authors urge caution in its use and avoidance when possible.

Insulin

Hyperglycemia and insulin resistance may develop after brain death, and hyperglycemic deceased organ donors should be managed in a similar manner to other critically ill patients. Although debate remains regarding optimal target glucose levels [44], it is generally accepted that uncontrolled hyperglycemia should be treated with insulin. Most ICUs have adopted empirical protocols with target glucose levels < 180 mg/dl and avoidance of hypoglycemia, and this also seems a sensible approach in deceased organ donors. As noted earlier, glucose-containing fluids should be avoided.

Temperature Management

Hypothermia is the most common manifestation of hypothalamic damage after brain death, and it is current practice to warm potential donors to $\geq 35\,°C$ [12]. However, a recent RCT demonstrated that cooling to 34–35 °C was associated with a reduction in the rate of dialysis in the first week after kidney transplantation compared to normothermia, with greatest benefits in recipients of kidneys from expanded criteria donors [16]. Whether these findings will be confirmed by other studies, or are generalizable to other organs, remains to be seen.

Conclusion

The treatment of the potential brain dead organ donor is slowly changing following evidence from RCTs of the benefits of protocolized-donor management strategies in addition to the continued application of good clinical ICU practices after brain death onset. Optimal donor management focuses on treating the profound physiological derangements associated with brain death in an attempt to expand the donor pool and maximize the number of organs retrieved per donor. Nevertheless, the evidence for benefit of many of the interventions used is not strong, either for improved organ function in the donor or translation of this into increased organ utilization and transplant graft survival [45].

To radically improve organ availability, optimization strategies cannot be limited to the ICU but must be extended to DCD, and include *ex vivo* organ preservation and reconditioning strategies that are now well established in some transplant centers.

References

1. Da Silva IRF, Frontera JA (2015) Worldwide barriers to organ donation. JAMA Neurol 72:112–118
2. Rudge C, Matesanz R, Delmonico FL, Chapman J (2011) International practices of organ donation. Br J Anaesth 108:i48–i55
3. Wijdicks EFM (2001) The diagnosis of brain death. N Engl J Med 344:1215–1221
4. Shemie SD, Hornby L, Baker A et al (2014) International guideline development for the determination of death. Intensive Care Med 40:788–797

5. Gries CJ, White DB, Truog RD et al (2013) An official American Thoracic Society/International Society for Heart and Lung Transplantation/Society of Critical Care Medicine/Association of Organ and Procurement Organizations/United Network of Organ Sharing Statement: ethical and policy considerations in organ donation after circulatory determination of death. Am J Respir Crit Care Med 188:103–109

6. Algahim MF, Love RB (2015) Donation after circulatory death. Current opinion in organ transplantation 20:1–6

7. Yacoub M (2015) Cardiac donation after circulatory death: a time to reflect. The Lancet 385:2554–2556

8. Wall SP, Plunkett C, Caplan A (2015) A potential solution to the shortage of solid organs for transplantation. JAMA 313:2321–2322

9. Reeb J, Keshavjee S, Cypel M (2015) Expanding the lung donor pool: advancements and emerging pathways. Curr Opin Organ Transplant 20:498–505

10. Souter MJ, Blissitt PA, Blosser S et al (2015) Recommendations for the critical care management of devastating brain injury: prognostication, psychosocial, and ethical management. Neurocrit Care 23:4–13

11. Domínguez-Gil B, Murphy P, Procaccio F (2015) Ten changes that could improve organ donation in the intensive care unit. Intensive Care Med (in press)

12. McKeown DW, Bonser RS, Kellum JA (2011) Management of the heartbeating brain-dead organ donor. Br J Anaesth 108:i96–i107

13. Singbartl K, Murugan R, Kaynar AM et al (2011) Intensivist-led management of brain-dead donors is associated with an increase in organ recovery for transplantation. Am J Transplant 11:1517–1521

14. Mascia L, Pasero D, Slutsky AS et al (2010) Effect of a lung protective strategy for organ donors on eligibility and availability of lungs for transplantation: a randomized controlled trial. JAMA 304:2620–2627

15. Al-Khafaji A, Elder M, Lebovitz DJ et al (2015) Protocolized fluid therapy in brain-dead donors: the multicenter randomized MOnIToR trial. Intensive Care Med 41:418–426

16. Niemann CU, Feiner J, Swain S et al (2015) Therapeutic hypothermia in deceased organ donors and kidney-graft function. N Engl J Med 373:405–414

17. Dikdan GS, Mora-Esteves C, Koneru B (2012) Review of randomized clinical trials of donor management and organ preservation in deceased donors. Transplantation 94:425–441

18. Kotloff RM, Blosser S, Fulda GJ et al (2015) Management of the potential organ donor in the ICU: Society of Critical Care Medicine/American College of Chest Physicians/Association of Organ Procurement Organizations Consensus Statement. Crit Care Med 43:1291–1325

19. Smith M (2004) Physiologic changes during brain stem death – lessons for management of the organ donor. J Heart Lung Transplant 23:S217–S222

20. Chen EP, Bittner HB, Kendall SW, Van Trigt P (1996) Hormonal and hemodynamic changes in a validated animal model of brain death. Crit Care Med 24:1352–1359

21. Lee VH, Oh JK, Mulvagh SL, Wijdicks EFM (2006) Mechanisms in neurogenic stress cardiomyopathy after aneurysmal subarachnoid hemorrhage. Neurocrit Care 5:243–249

22. Hollenberg SM (2015) Understanding stress cardiomyopathy. Intensive Care Med (in press)

23. Templin C, Ghadri JR, Diekmann J et al (2015) Clinical features and outcomes of Takotsubo (stress) cardiomyopathy. N Engl J Med 373:929–938

24. Lisman T, Leuvenink HGD, Porte RJ, Ploeg RJ (2011) Activation of hemostasis in brain dead organ donors: an observational study. J Thromb Haemost 9:1959–1965

25. Wood K, Becker B, McCartney J et al (2004) Care of the potential organ donor. N Engl J Med 351:2730

26. McKeown DW, Ball J (2014) Treating the donor. Curr Opin Organ Transplant 19:85–91

27. Cecconi M, De Backer D, Antonelli M et al (2014) Consensus on circulatory shock and hemo-dynamic monitoring. Task force of the European Society of Intensive Care Medicine. Intensive Care Med 40:1795–1815
28. Marik PE, Cavallazzi R (2013) Does the central venous pressure predict fluid responsiveness? An updated meta-analysis and a plea for some common sense. Crit Care Med 41:1774–1781
29. Downs EA, Isbell JM (2014) Impact of hemodynamic monitoring on clinical outcomes. Best Pract Res Clin Anaesthesiol 28:463–476
30. Marik PE, Cavallazzi R, Vasu T, Hirani A (2009) Dynamic changes in arterial waveform derived variables and fluid responsiveness in mechanically ventilated patients: a systematic review of the literature. Crit Care Med 37:2642–2647
31. Cecconi M, Parsons AK, Rhodes A (2011) What is a fluid challenge? Curr Opin Crit Care 17:290–295
32. Dare AJ, Bartlett AS, Fraser JF (2012) Critical care of the potential organ donor. Curr Neurol Neurosci Rep 12:456–465
33. Bion J, Bellomo R, Myburgh J et al (2014) Hydroxyethyl starch: putting patient safety first. Intensive Care Med 40:256–259
34. Wiedermann CJ, Joannidis M (2013) Accumulation of hydroxyethyl starch in human and ani-mal tissues: a systematic review. Intensive Care Med 40:160–170
35. Cittanova ML, Leblanc I, Legendre C et al (1996) Effect of hydroxyethylstarch in brain-dead kidney donors on renal function in kidney-transplant recipients. The Lancet 348:1620–1622
36. Mascia L (2009) Acute lung injury in patients with severe brain injury: A double hit model. Neurocrit Care 11:417–426
37. Munshi L, Keshavjee S, Cypel M (2013) Donor management and lung preservation for lung transplantation. Lancet Respir Med 1:318–328
38. Miñambres E, Pérez-Villares JM, Chico-Fernández M et al (2015) Lung donor treatment pro-tocol in brain dead-donors: A multicenter study. J Heart Lung Transplant 34:773–780
39. Rech TH, Moraes RB, Crispim D et al (2013) Management of the brain-dead organ donor: a systematic review and meta-analysis. Transplantation 95:966–974
40. Dupuis S, Amiel J-A, Desgroseilliers M et al (2014) Corticosteroids in the management of brain-dead potential organ donors: a systematic review. Br J Anaesth 113:346–359
41. Pinsard M, Ragot S, Mertes PM et al (2014) Interest of low-dose hydrocortisone therapy during brain-dead organ donor resuscitation: the CORTICOME study. Crit Care 18:R158
42. Mebis L, Van den Berghe G (2009) The hypothalamus-pituitary-thyroid axis in critical illness. Neth J Med 67:332–340
43. Boonen E, Van den Berghe G (2014) Endocrine responses to critical illness: novel insights and therapeutic implications. J Clin Endocrinol Metab 99:1569–1582
44. Van den Berghe G (2013) What's new in glucose control in the ICU? Intensive Care Med 39:823–825
45. Dhanani S, Shemie SD (2015) Advancing the science of organ donor management. Crit Care 18:1–3

Humanizing Intensive Care: Theory, Evidence, and Possibilities

S. M. Brown, S. J. Beesley, and R. O. Hopkins

Introduction

Intensive care units (ICUs) are showcases for many of the most stunning techno-logical advances in medicine. Survival from once routinely fatal diseases is rapidly increasing [1]. Unfortunately, the severity of illness and the invasiveness of inten-sive therapies can make the ICU a brutal place for all involved [2, 3]. Patients report violations of their dignity and most survivors and family members experi-ence symptoms of anxiety, depression, or posttraumatic stress disorder (PTSD) [4]. For patients who die in or shortly after the ICU stay, many of the deaths will have been deformed by an overemphasis on medical technology [5]. ICU admission may threaten the individual's sense of self, both from the threat of annihilation through death and the dehumanization attendant to critical illness, its treatments, and clin-ician behaviors [2]. The sometimes brutal realities of contemporary ICU care are generating appropriate debates about how to humanize the ICU. Several possible solutions have been proposed [6], but the topic has often been associated with a lack of clear thinking, particularly in the ICU.

The dehumanization of the ICU has persisted for many reasons, including struc-tural/organizational problems and defense mechanisms and cognitive errors on the part of clinicians. These cognitive errors are understandable, even predictable. The ICU is stressful and disorienting enough that all participants – clinicians, patients,

S. M. Brown (✉) · S. J. Beesley
Center for Humanizing Critical Care, Intermountain Medical Center
Murray, USA
Pulmonary and Critical Care Medicine, University of Utah School of Medicine
Salt Lake City, USA
email: Samuel.Brown@imail.org

R. O. Hopkins
Center for Humanizing Critical Care, Intermountain Medical Center
Murray, USA
Psychology and Neuroscience Center, Brigham Young University
Provo, USA

© Springer International Publishing Switzerland 2016
J.-L. Vincent (ed.), *Annual Update in Intensive Care and Emergency Medicine 2016*,
DOI 10.1007/978-3-319-27349-5_33

405

and families – are prone to misperceive the situation in ways that contribute to dehumanization. While clinician diagnostic errors have been well described by cognitive psychologists in recent decades [7], the risks of misapprehension and cognitive errors related to human aspects of the ICU experience are also endemic and merit consideration. Increasingly sophisticated work in cognitive psychology and judgment and decision making may shed considerable light on the problems of dehumanization in the ICU. In this chapter, we consider theory, evidence, and early solutions with an eye toward clarifying the cognitive errors and blind spots that often interfere with humanization in the ICU.

Theory

Contemporary Western bioethics (and indeed much of political philosophy) is based on individual rights and autonomy, a political, economic, and philosophical system that dates to the European Enlightenment, with acceleration in the last half-century in Europe and USA [8]. In this understanding, the primary locus of meaning and authority is the individual and his self-determination. This cultural understanding has led to great social and cultural changes and has been associated with substantial protections of the rights of minorities and improvements in the status of women and people of color. In this modern cultural understanding, the self is something that is constituted by acts of self-determination, and the primary role of government in Western democracies (and other communal structures such as the medical system) is to facilitate individual self-determination as much as possible. On this view, what is human is the individual who can consciously choose a path for himself; the process of choosing must be supported wherever possible.

Within the medical system, this modern cultural consensus has led to the steady erosion of 'paternalistic' ideas about the relationships between clinicians and patients [9]. In place of paternalism has come what some term the 'consumerist' model of medicine, in which patients are independent consumers and clinicians are 'providers' of healthcare, which may be the case in elective, low-risk procedures and routine health screening. Some have complained that the consumerist model is not true to how people process serious threats to their health and make decisions during such crises [10]. The assumptions of the consumerist model of healthcare may be less applicable in critical care environments, in which people are bewildered, life is threatened, and treatments are often uncomfortable. In such times of crisis, many patients (and their families) want to be considered more than merely 'customers' and may resist the burden of making difficult decisions under tragic circumstances.

Within the modern cultural context, humanization has tended to refer to two ideas, perhaps at the opposite ends of the spectrum. One view is that the individual matters, in all his/her particularity. To be treated as a human being means to be treated as if your individuality were important, even paramount. The other view is an expression of solidarity. To be treated as a human being is to be treated as if the individuals interacting with you (e.g., clinicians) see you as a peer. This view need not mean that power is equal but that any power difference is morally neutral. Whereas in pre-Enlightenment Europe rigid hierarchies were the norm, such hierarchies are much less pervasive now, even if unwelcome remnants persist. What people mean by their humanity is often, perhaps ironically, the ways in which they *differ* from other human beings. Often that individuality is favored over the commonality, although both matter. Both specificity and generality are relevant in the humanization of critical care. In parallel with these philosophical considerations, social psychologists discuss dehumanization as a failure to attribute human-defining or human-unique attributes to others (in the former case, the dehumanized individual is viewed as an inanimate object; in the latter case the dehumanized individual is seen as a non-human animal). Psychologists (and others) have long observed that people as a general rule treat others as less human, especially when these other individuals are part of an 'outgroup'. While such dehumanization is perhaps most familiar from political or social violence, subtle but important patterns are also observed in modern Western medicine [11].

Box 1. Elements of Humanization and Barriers to it

Elements of Humanization
- Self-awareness
- Self-determination
- Sense of being respected
- Attention to individuality in support and decision making
- Feeling known by clinicians
- Therapeutic alliance
- Attention to modesty
- Ownership of personal space in the ICU room
- Attention to needs of family/loved ones

Barriers to Humanization
- Altered consciousness
- Inability to exercise choice
- Fear of death
- Discomfort
- Invasive procedures
- Immodest medical clothing
- Sedation
- Loss of individuality
- Clinician burnout and blindspots
- Physical exclusion of family from ICU rooms

The modern focus on autonomy and self-determination can be difficult to apply in the ICU because so many patients lack the intact consciousness required to exercise that autonomy. The close tie between self determination and autonomy can inadvertently compound dehumanization, as ICU patients lack those markers of full humanity by token of their illness and associated disruptions of consciousness [11]. A kind of inertia can develop in the presence of altered consciousness, which heightens the risk of the dehumanization inherent to critical illness. This is of course only one of many threats to humanization. In Box 1 we display both key elements of and threats to humanization of patients in the ICU.

The individualistic focus of contemporary political philosophy has led to blind spots, especially when it comes to the people who accompany ICU patients during their illness. ICU family members (sometimes called 'caregivers' or 'surrogates') have often been seen as passive conduits for patients' self-determination rather than people with legitimate concerns in their own right, although some theoretical work has laid the groundwork for incorporation of families into ethical reasoning in healthcare [12]. The inattention to families has perhaps contributed to the strikingly high rates of post-intensive care syndrome among family members, a syndrome marked by substantial psychological distress, including anxiety, depression, and PTSD [13].

'Respect' and 'dignity' are often used to describe the opposite of dehumanization. While these terms originally referred to a person's status in a hierarchy (people higher in the hierarchy were more dignified and thereby more deserving of respect), part of the cultural changes that leveled hierarchy suggested that all people, regardless of their social status, merited respect for their dignity. While the precise meaning of the terms are debated, investigators have proposed that 'respect' describes actions that preserve an individual's 'dignity' inherent to them as human beings. To borrow a useable, if somewhat circular definition, dignity is "the intrinsic, unconditional value of all human beings that makes them worthy of respect" [14]. Alternatively, dignity means that a person does not need to do anything to merit "unconditional positive regard" [15]. Where hierarchies still exist, such as in medical encounters, risks to respect and dignity may be accentuated.

Beyond general philosophical considerations, another matter looms large in the contemporary ICU: the inherent, ineluctable uncertainty about life-and-death outcomes. This uncertainty can contribute substantially to blind spots in contemporary ICU environments.

The Nature of Uncertainty

In the high-stakes setting of the ICU, many participants and observers see patients as belonging in one of two groups. They are either going to die, in which case they merit palliative care focused on the end of life, or they are going to survive, in which case technological imperatives focused on prolonging life predominate. Unfortunately, by the time patients aggregate into such categories – if in fact they ever actually do, which has not been true when prognosis is ascertained for in-hospital deaths [16] – much of the psychological damage of ICU dehumanization has already occurred.

If predictions were entirely reliable, uncertainty would not be a problem. Statistical prediction models do exist, in multiple iterations. While these scores usefully adjust for severity of illness for hospital benchmarking, their utility for individual prediction is tenuous at best. While most models are judged by their discrimination – how often survivors' scores are lower than non-survivors' scores – patients and families are more likely to care about calibration – how close predicted and observed mortality are to each other – which is most relevant to their own general prospects for recovery. Unfortunately, the regression equations used to predict ICU mortality are best calibrated in the middle ranges, where the most supporting data exist. But if prognosis is crucial for a given person, their actual decision thresholds will be relevant. We suspect that few people, if they are not already in their final phase of life, would reject a 10% chance of recovery. But prediction models are poorly calibrated in that range. For example, the mortality in the highest decile of APACHE IV-predicted mortality is only 63%. When patients' decisional thresholds reside outside the well-calibrated ranges of prediction scores, a raw prognostic estimate is unlikely to change decisions meaningfully.

Clinician predictions may be favored over statistical models by both clinicians and patients, even if families tend to discount prognostic estimates in general [17]. However, the evidence that clinician prognoses are superior to statistical models is mixed at best [18]. In fact, clinician moral distress may contribute to undue pessimism regarding prognosis; in some studies, nurses, the clinicians closest to the indignities of critical illness, make the most pessimistic predictions of outcome [19].

To put it simply, current prognostication is not accurate enough to eliminate uncertainty. Since uncertainty is unavoidable, solutions intended to humanize the ICU experience will need to come to terms with that uncertainty.

Clinicians and families may rush to collapse patients into specific categories as a way to resolve the tension associated with prognostic uncertainty. Anthropologists describe 'liminal' entities which sit on the threshold between established categories, states, or conditions [20]. Such liminal entities are difficult to accommodate in clinical care, as in the rest of life. Sick patients in the ICU are often liminal in precisely that sense, and clinicians and families may want the patients to fit into one of the established categories 'going to survive' or 'dying'. The reality is that nature is continuous, and so are the probabilities of recovery. Careful communication that seeks to understand and honor the individual's values, goals, and priorities is likely crucial to dealing with ICU existence between life and death. Where clinicians push for premature certainty about outcome, families may bear substantial burdens of guilt, even when the patient survives (if, e.g., a family member wanted to stop treatment in response to a dire prognostication by a clinician).

Potential Barriers to a More Human ICU

The provision of intensive care is demanding, exhausting work and it requires being in the presence of patients' terribly disfigured bodies that often lack the conscious-ness that makes people familiar as people. ICU clinicians experience high rates of burnout, 'vicarious traumatization' and 'compassion fatigue', with attendant men-tal illness and reduced quality of life [21]. Dehumanization may be adaptive for clinicians in the ICU: thinking too often about the humanity of patients could hy-pothetically increase the risk of burnout [22]. Notably, though, burnout tends to be associated with moral distress, emotional depletion, toxic communication environ-ments, and feelings of helplessness, which need not be inevitable in the ICU. It is possible that increased humanization, especially through the practice of empathy, in the ICU could decrease the risks of burnout [23]. Whatever the specific relationship between humanization and clinician burnout, a human ICU will need to be healthful for clinicians as well as patients and families.

Intense time demands on ICU clinicians may also prevent humanization. Clini-cians may worry that it will take more time to honor the humanity of a patient since such efforts may add to the time required for the technical medical components of care. On the contrary, it may be that improved communication and humanization decreases the amount of time spent resolving conflicts. These are open empirical questions that merit careful research.

The residual effects of medical paternalism may also interfere with humaniza-tion [2]. Specifically, some clinicians may be tempted to treat patients as children. While paternalism may be born of excellent motives – a desire to protect vulnerable individuals from unwanted stress – in addition to less worthy motives – a desire to maintain physician power – treating patients as children when their sense of self is already under attack may both demoralize and interfere with communication. In contemporary society, people expect to be treated as independently worthy indi-viduals; paternalism directly counteracts that assumption. However inadvertently, paternalism contributes to dehumanization. The balancing act of full, meaningful collaboration between clinicians and patients that is necessary for humanization will be hard to achieve, but clinicians will need to bring their expertise and commitment to bear in a way that treats patients and families as partners rather than dependents.

Practical Solutions

In Box 2, we display the attributes of a traditional ICU model vs. a humanized model of the ICU. In the following sections we consider several of the questions relevant to humanizing the ICU.

> **Box 2. Attributes of Traditional Versus Humanized ICUs**
>
> **Traditional ICU**
> - Patients sedated and immobilized
> - Personality defined by clinicians
> - Social network excluded
> - Patients dependent/passive
> - Lost sense of self
> - Activities defined by clinicians
> - No ownership of space or body
> - Patients unable to communicate
> - Patients not addressed by name
> - Decisions often don't reflect values and priorities of patients
> - Policies decided exclusively by clinicians
> - Communication haphazard, with limited training
>
> **Humanized ICU**
> - Sedation minimized
> - Mobilization maximized
> - Personal history known to clinicians
> - Families are full partners in care
> - Patients and families participate in care
> - Activities defined in part by patient/families
> - Adaptive communication technologies used
> - Clinicians knock before entering and ask permission to touch patient
> - Clinicians address patient by name
> - Decisions reflect values and priorities of patients
> - Policies decided in collaboration with patients and families
> - May involve communication facilitators

Engagement

"Patient and family engagement" is a current emphasis in healthcare [24, 25]. While definitions of engagement vary somewhat, they all focus on inclusion and active partnership among clinicians, patients, and families. Engagement in the ICU differs from outpatient models of engagement for chronic disease management [26], but despite such differences, engagement should help address the high prevalence of learned helplessness in the ICU [27]. While patients, families, and clinicians may in fact be powerless in the face of a relentless critical illness, engagement may help ease the burden of critical illness by decreasing the sense of isolation or helplessness and allowing families to contribute to ultimate recovery.

Let Them In

A crucial barrier to engagement and humanization more broadly is a traditional exclusion of patients' loved ones from the ICU bedside. People's social networks (people we call 'family' as a shorthand for those whom a patient would want involved in his/her medical care [26]) are crucial to their identity, especially during health crises. Families are caregivers, both before and after the ICU admission, but they also represent the individual in ways that would otherwise be inaccessible to clinicians. Historically, families have been excluded from the ICU despite their importance to patients for emotional and social support.

It is time to stop excluding families from the ICU. Sufficient data already exist to support generally open visitation policies [28]. Accumulating experience suggests that families should be involved in ICU rounds [29]. Small studies suggest that all benefit from families participating in certain bedside care activities [30]. Early evidence from cardiopulmonary resuscitation (CPR) [31] suggests that families should even be allowed to be present during procedures within the ICU. Such openness to physical presence is in keeping with the wishes of patients and family members, who have for decades advocated for access to ICUs and partnership with the medical team [28, 29]. It is time the medical system honored those wishes.

Improving the Exercise of Respect

While humanization may sound nebulous, the practice of respect may be easier to grasp. Patients and families clearly and consistently want to be treated with respect [32]. Considering 'respect and dignity' as important outcomes may be a useful entry into solutions that enhance patient and family engagement and humanize the ICU experience. One group has begun defining violations of respect as preventable harms requiring root-cause analysis [33]. Relatively simple interventions may go a long way towards improving respect. Learning patient and family names, knocking before entering the room, asking permission before touching the patient, addressing even unconscious patients as if they merited social engagement, emphasizing the coordination of communication and many other practices basic to respect could dramatically improve humanization.

Central to treatment with respect is the need to tailor medical treatments to the values and priorities of the individual patients in ways that honor them in their entire humanity. Thus far, solutions to that problem have been of low quality [34]. We propose in their place a new paradigm that emphasizes real-time personalization of medical care during serious illness, tailored to the individual and the expected trajectory of illness.

Personalized Care During Serious Illness

While historical paternalism has been appropriately criticized, some have swung to the opposite extreme, a thoughtless application of autonomism [34]. Without care, extreme autonomism may inadvertently dehumanize participants by placing ill-equipped individuals into decision-making environments where they are likely to fail. Patients and families often founder in an overly legalistic environment at a time of crisis. Importantly, many uses of advance directives remain prone to clinician bias by diverting attention from patient-oriented considerations to clinician-oriented questions, such as whether to perform CPR [2, 34].

As a cautionary tale, a substantial proportion of patients listed as do-not-resuscitate/do-not intubate (DNR/DNI) were merely trying to communicate that they did not want to persist in a vegetative state [35]. When proclamations rejecting certain extreme states are misinterpreted, they may lead to unnecessary premature death. A patient with early cancer, for example, may have requested DNR/DNI only to avoid treatments when all hope is lost, but his statement could be misconstrued as a refusal of mechanical ventilation even for pneumonia, despite excellent prospects of recovery to several more years of quality life. Without substantial assistance, many individuals might inadvertently communicate something they did not intend.

A hybrid approach, rather than either extreme of paternalism or autonomism, is indicated in our view. We believe it is important to strike a balance that honors the person as an individual while not forcing a view of the problem on them that is alien to their desires and experience or in conflict with their values and priorities [2]. We advocate "personalized care during serious illness" (PCSI, outlined in contrast to the traditional model in Table 1) as a model for using more patient-centered approaches to replace traditional advance directives. Within the PCSI framework, we advocate close collaboration and personalized guidance as a path to solutions that best align treatments with patients' values and priorities and honor the patient as a person. The older advance directive model has focused on specific procedures to refuse in a hypothetical future, exemplified by questions we have heard physician trainees ask patients, such as, "should we pound on your chest if your heart stops?". The PCSI model advocates a focus on understanding the individual, coming to understand what phase of life they understand themselves to be in, and discussing likely upcoming medical events. Rather than focusing on stigmatized procedures like CPR, the focus in PCSI is on the patient, his/her hopes, values, and priorities, and the concrete medical situations in which those values and priorities will be brought to bear. PCSI begins by asking, "who are you [or your loved one] as a person?" and "what phase of life are you [or your loved one] in?" and proceeds from there to develop individualized plans of care, specific to the person as an individual and the likely course of disease.

Recent work, focused on patients dying in the ICU, has taken a pragmatic approach to identification of individual patient's priorities, using the framing of 'wishes' for the end of life [32]. By helping patients and families focus on final tasks that can be performed before death, including mechanisms to summarize and honor the meaning of a life, clinicians can help create meaning as life is near its

Table 1 Comparison of traditional advance directives and personalized care during serious illness (PCSI)

Attribute	Advance Directives	PCSI
Focus of efforts	Procedures to be refused, such as mechanical ventilation	Experience and goals; likely trajectories of illness and recovery
Sources of insight	Patient and a legal document	Patient and family
Relevance of post-intensive care syndrome	Used to justify refusal of treatment	Incorporates individualized treatment and rehabilitation plans
Bias	Toward the clinicians who perform procedures	Toward the patient and family who experience and will remember the procedure
Relation to uncertainty	Assumes that certainty exists	Embraces uncertainty and seeks collaborative path through it
Paradigm	Consumer autonomy	Respect, collaboration, and desired guidance
Timing	Long before needed; generally when illness is still theoretical	Just-in-time, tied to expected disease trajectories
View of living will documents	Authoritative legal instruction	Element of communication about serious illness

close. Strenuous efforts in support of humanization should be undertaken for those who ultimately die and those who ultimately survive.

The main thrust of the PCSI model is to create concordance between the treatments provided, the ways they are provided and patients' actual values, goals, and priorities. Such efforts to improve the match between medical treatments provided and the patients' values, goals, and priorities will depend on conscientious, effective communication.

Learning to Communicate

Improved communication skills appear to help in high-stakes clinical encounters. Communication training and a bereavement pamphlet helped in France [36]. ICU clinicians have proved trainable in terms of basic communication skills [37]. However, a large randomized trial raised the possibility that brief simulation-based communication training may not lead to better outcomes for patients, a crucial problem [38]. Studies of communication will need to demonstrate improvements in patient-centered outcomes rather than just intermediate outcomes.

Despite these caveats, some general observations appear valid. Families prefer family meetings when they are allowed to speak more [39]. Training in sympathetic communication combined with a bereavement brochure decreased PTSD among families of ICU patients near death [36]. Families are more satisfied when they have more information [40], likely due to the empowerment that comes from understanding the generally unfamiliar ICU environment and a loved one's condition. An intensive communication strategy decreased ICU length-of-stay without affecting the mortality rate [41]. Substantially more work remains to be done to define optimal methods of both communication and training for clinicians. Ultimately it is likely that optimal communication methods will need to be tailored to the specific individuals involved.

Confronting Our Blindspots: The Practice of Situational Awareness

Psychologists have extensively documented the fact that experts are just as susceptible to predictable cognitive errors as laypeople. Certain industries (e.g., military, aviation) employ explicit techniques to foster 'situational awareness'. These methods help participants step out of automatic thinking into more deliberate modes of reasoning. Such explicit techniques may decrease errors [7]. In intensive care, procedures and the medical treatment of dynamic patients require situational awareness. But situational awareness is also important in interactions with patients and families at a human level. We suspect that most of the dehumanization in the ICU occurs unconsciously, driven in large parts by factors that escape participants' awareness.

In Box 3 we display some of the risks to situational awareness for all participants in the complex environment of the ICU.

Box 3. Vulnerabilities and Sources of Blindspots of ICU Participants

Clinician
- Personal fear of death
- Personal religious convictions (including atheism)
- Experiences with other patients
- Chronic workplace stress
- Guilt
- Difficult work conditions
- Intra-team conflict
- Inexperience
- Stress at home
- Burnout
- Power structures
- Historical medical culture

Patient
- Personal fear of death
- Personal religious convictions (including atheism)
- Pain

- Altered consciousness
- Acute stress reaction
- Unfamiliarity with the ICU
- Dyspnea
- Sleep disruption
- Limited self-efficacy
- Poor coping skills
- Limited resilience
- Immobility
- Low health literacy

Family
- Personal fear of death
- Personal religious convictions (including atheism)
- Sleeplessness
- Anxiety
- Unfamiliarity with the ICU
- Acute stress reaction
- Learned helplessness
- Relationship with patient
- Prior caregiving burden
- Anticipated caregiving burden
- Low health literacy

Turnbull et al. have shown that intensivists may rely on unconscious biases in their recommendations regarding life support decisions in ways that do not accurately honor patients' values and priorities [42]. Those findings are likely the tip of an iceberg. While decision aids might improve the quality of decisions [43], it is nevertheless important to be careful to apply such aids in ways that do not amplify clinician bias. The risk of clinician bias is particularly severe when biased 'nudges' are employed, e.g., videos designed to decrease the rate of 'full code' designations among patients [44].

Maintenance of Mental Health During the ICU Experience

Crucial to humanizing the ICU is recognizing the needs participants have for psychological health after the ICU experience. Relatively little work has been done on how best to prevent later psychological distress in the ICU, although Davidson et al. have suggested that involvement in bedside care helps families [30], and Cox et al. have begun work on early coping interventions for ICU families [45]. Empirically, ICU diaries decrease post-traumatic stress by helping families to support survivors in the consolidation of true memories in place of delusional memories associated with critical illness encephalopathy [46]. Additional research is urgently required to decrease psychological distress for patients and families after the ICU admission. It may be that recruiting additional experts into the ICU milieu may improve situational awareness and psychological outcomes among participants in the ICU.

New Experts

Peers and Doulas

It is common when bias is a substantial risk to introduce a third party whose blind spots do not overlap with those of the principals. This is probably true in medical encounters as well as in more general problem solving. Such a third party may well have a specific role to play in the ICU. In labor and delivery, a 'doula' exists to mediate between prospective parents and their clinicians. Such an individual may have a similar role to play in the ICU. Two large randomized, controlled studies are evaluating similar individuals as communication facilitators [47, 48]. Social workers or chaplains may fill such a role. Others are pursuing the question of whether veterans of the ICU experience could serve in such a role, as part of a much larger effort to encourage peer support among ICU patients and families [49]. Such activities make intuitive sense but are not yet evidence-based. Research on their optimal structure and efficacy is urgently indicated. Independent of specific ICU admissions, non-clinician experts may have an important role to play in shaping the structure and function of the medical system.

Patient-Family Advisory Councils (PFACs)

PFACs began in the USA in pediatric hospitals [50]. Currently about a third of US hospitals report having a PFAC, at least at the hospital level [25]. Anecdotally, these councils work well at providing layperson insights into the experience of intensive care, although how best to integrate PFACs into hospital operations is not yet firmly known and may be an appropriate topic for additional research. In our institution, members of the ICU PFAC have written manuscripts with us, performed in-service training with clinicians, revised our unit orientation process, created streamlined methods for visitor authentication, performed content validation of survey materials, and guided development of study protocols. Some such improvements should be considered straightforward operational improvements, while other aspects should be subjected to rigorous study.

Conclusion

The medical technology in the ICU is by and large familiar and robust enough that we can safely focus effort on rehumanizing the ICU. Some aspects of humanization should begin immediately. We can already say that ICU visitation should be open and that ICU diaries should be made available. Careful attention to communication for patients at very high risk of death is supported by multiple studies. Other interventions will require careful multidisciplinary research before a sufficient evidence base exists to support them. How best to nurture peer support and how to optimize the personalization is still largely unknown. How to deal with clinician burnout is also important, as rehumanization strategies that worsen clinician distress and burnout are unlikely to be ultimately successful. Opportunities for meaningful research and patient-centered reform should be embraced.

References

1. Zimmerman JE, Kramer AA, Knaus WA (2013) Changes in hospital mortality for United States intensive care unit admissions from 1988 to 2012. Crit Care 17:R81
2. Brown SM (2016) Through the Valley of Shadows: Living Wills, Intensive Care, and Making Medicine Human. Oxford University Press, New York
3. Alonso-Ovies A, Heras La Calle G (2016) ICU: a branch of hell? Intensive Care Med (in press)
4. Needham DM, Davidson J, Cohen H et al (2012) Improving long-term outcomes after discharge from intensive care unit: report from a stakeholders' conference. Crit Care Med 40:502–509
5. Callahan D (1993) The Troubled Dream of Life: in Search of Peaceful Death. Simon and Schuster, New York
6. Haque OS, Waytz A (2012) Dehumanization in medicine: causes, solutions, and functions. Perspect Psychol Sci 7:176–186
7. Singh H, Petersen LA, Thomas EJ (2006) Understanding diagnostic errors in medicine: a lesson from aviation. Qual Saf Health Care 15:159–164
8. Taylor C (2007) A Secular Age. Harvard University Press, Cambridge
9. Katz J (1984) The Silent World of Doctor and Patient. Free Press, New York
10. Rosenbaum L (2015) The paternalism preference – choosing unshared decision making. N Engl J Med 373:589–592
11. Haslam N (2006) Dehumanization: an integrative review. Pers Soc Psychol Rev 10:252–264
12. Nelson H, Nelson J (1995) The Patient in the Family: An Ethics of Medicine and Families. Routledge, New York
13. Netzer G, Sullivan DR (2014) Recognizing, naming, and measuring a family intensive care unit syndrome. Ann Am Thorac Soc 11:435–441
14. Aboumatar H, Forbes L, Branyon E et al (2015) Understanding treatment with respect and dignity in the intensive care unit. Narrat Inq Bioeth 5:55A–67A
15. Frosch DL, Tai-Seale M (2014) R-E-S-P-E-C-T – what it means to patients. J Gen Intern Med 29:427–428
16. Lynn J, Harrell F Jr, Cohn F, Wagner D, Connors AF Jr (1997) Prognoses of seriously ill hospitalized patients on the days before death: implications for patient care and public policy. New Horiz 5:56–61
17. Zier LS, Sottile, Hong SY, Weissfield LA, White DB (2012) Surrogate decision makers' interpretation of prognostic information: a mixed-methods study. Ann Intern Med 156:360–366
18. Keegan MT, Gajic O, Afessa B (2011) Severity of illness scoring systems in the intensive care unit. Crit Care Med 39:163–169
19. Rocker G, Cook D, Sjokvist P et al (2004) Clinician predictions of intensive care unit mortality. Crit Care Med 32:1149–1154
20. Turner VW (1964) Betwixt and between: the liminal period in rites de passage. The Proceedings of the American Ethnological Society 1964:4–20
21. Embriaco N, Papazian L, Kentish-Barnes N, Pochard F, Azoulay E (2007) Burnout syndrome among critical care healthcare workers. Curr Opin Crit Care 13:482–488

22. Vaes J, Muratore M (2013) Defensive dehumanization in the medical practice: a cross-sectional study from a health care worker's perspective. Br J Soc Psychol 52:180–190

23. Haslam N (2007) Humanizing medical practice: the role of empathy. Med J Aust 187:381–382

24. Carman KL, Dardess P, Maurer M et al (2013) Patient and family engagement: a framework for understanding the elements and developing interventions and policies. Health Aff (Millwood) 32:223–231

25. Herrin J, Harris KG, Kenward K, Hines S, Joshi MS, Frosch DL (2016) Patient and family engagement: a survey of US hospital practices. BMJ Qual Saf (in press)

26. Brown SM, Rozenblum R, Aboumatar H et al (2015) Defining patient and family engagement in the intensive care unit. Am J Respir Crit Care Med 191:358–360

27. Sullivan DR, Liu X, Corwin DS et al (2012) Learned helplessness among families and surrogate decision-makers of patients admitted to medical, surgical, and trauma ICUs. Chest 142:1440–1446

28. Brown SM (2015) We still lack patient centered visitation in intensive care units. BMJ 350:h792

29. Davidson JE, Powers K, Hedayat KM et al (2007) Clinical practice guidelines for support of the family in the patient-centered intensive care unit: American College of Critical Care Medicine Task Force 2004–2005. Crit Care Med 35:605–622

30. Davidson JE, Daly BJ, Agan D, Brady NR, Higgins PA (2010) Facilitated sensemaking: a feasibility study for the provision of a family support program in the intensive care unit. Crit Care Nurs Q 33:177–189

31. Jabre P, Tazarourte K, Azoulay E et al (2014) Offering the opportunity for family to be present during cardiopulmonary resuscitation: 1-year assessment. Intensive Care Med 40:981–987

32. Cook D, Swinton M, Toledo F et al (2015) Personalizing death in the intensive care unit: the 3 wishes project: a mixed-methods study. Ann Intern Med 163:271–279

33. Sokol-Hessner L, Folcarelli PH, Sands KE (2015) Emotional harm from disrespect: the neglected preventable harm. BMJ Qual Saf 24:550–553

34. Schneider CE (1998) The Practice of Autonomy: Patients, Doctors, and Medical Decisions. Oxford University Press, New York

35. Jesus JE, Allen MB, Michael GE et al (2013) Preferences for resuscitation and intubation among patients with do-not-resuscitate/do-not-intubate orders. Mayo Clin Proc 88:658–665

36. Lautrette A, Darmon M, Megarbane B et al (2007) A communication strategy and brochure for relatives of patients dying in the ICU. N Engl J Med 356:469–478

37. Shaw DJ, Davidson JE, Smilde RI, Sondoozi T, Agan D (2014) Multidisciplinary team training to enhance family communication in the ICU. Crit Care Med 42:265–271

38. Curtis JR, Back AL, Ford DW et al (2013) Effect of communication skills training for residents and nurse practitioners on quality of communication with patients with serious illness: a randomized trial. JAMA 310:2271–2281

39. McDonagh JR, Elliott TB, Engelberg RA et al (2004) Family satisfaction with family conferences about end-of-life care in the intensive care unit: increased proportion of family speech is associated with increased satisfaction. Crit Care Med 32:1484–1488

40. Azoulay E, Pochard F, Chevret S et al (2002) Impact of a family information leaflet on effectiveness of information provided to family members of intensive care unit patients: a multicenter, prospective, randomized, controlled trial. Am J Respir Crit Care Med 165:438–442

41. Lilly CM, De Meo DL, Sonna LA et al (2000) An intensive communication intervention for the critically ill. Am J Med 109:469–475

42. Turnbull AE, Krall JR, Ruhl AP et al (2014) A scenario-based, randomized trial of patient values and functional prognosis on intensivist intent to discuss withdrawing life support. Crit Care Med 42:1455–1462

43. Cox CE, White DB, Abernethy AP (2014) A universal decision support system. Addressing the decision-making needs of patients, families, and clinicians in the setting of critical illness. Am J Respir Crit Care Med 190:366–373

44. Billings JA (2012) The need for safeguards in advance care planning. J Gen Intern Med 27:595–600
45. Cox CE, Porter LS, Hough CL et al (2012) Development and preliminary evaluation of a telephone-based coping skills training intervention for survivors of acute lung injury and their informal caregivers. Intensive Care Med 38:1289–1297
46. Garrouste-Orgeas M, Coquet I, Perier A et al (2012) Impact of an intensive care unit diary on psychological distress in patients and relatives. Crit Care Med 40:2033–2040
47. Curtis JR, Ciechanowski PS, Downey L et al (2012) Development and evaluation of an inter-professional communication intervention to improve family outcomes in the ICU. Contemp Clin Trials 33:1245–1254
48. White DB, Cua SM, Walk R et al (2012) Nurse-led intervention to improve surrogate decision making for patients with advanced critical illness. Am J Crit Care 21:396–409
49. Mikkelsen ME, Iwashyna TJ, Thompson C (2015) Why ICU clinicians need to care about post-intensive care syndrome. SCCM Critical Connections Aug 4
50. Webster P, Johnson B (2000) Developing and Sustaining a Patient and Family Advisory Council. Institute for Family-Centered Care, Bethesda

Part XII
Applying New Technology

Ultrasound Simulation Education for Intensive Care and Emergency Medicine

F. Clau-Terré, A. Vegas, and N. Fletcher

Introduction

The widespread uptake of ultrasound in intensive care, anesthesiology and emergency medicine has been greatly commented on and is recognized to be a key growth area for the next generation of clinicians. In addition to point-of-care diagnosis, ultrasound can guide procedures and interventions and is complementary to many monitors that are used in such environments. The size, portability, ease of use and high quality imaging now available in affordable ultrasound platforms has removed many barriers to its routine use. Herein lies a problem – ultrasound is a technical skill with a significant learning curve, particularly for cardiac ultrasound or echocardiography. Instructors in intensive care and emergency medicine are trying to determine how to best educate current and future trainees to achieve clinical competence in ultrasound within a time limited and constantly expanding medical curriculum. The manpower, expense and time required for supervision and training cannot be underestimated. The use of simulation-based ultrasound learning to accelerate and enhance traditional clinical teaching is therefore very attractive [1]. In this chapter, we discuss the evidence and recent advances, whilst suggesting

F. Clau-Terré (✉)
Department of Critical Care, Consorci Sanitari Terrassa
Barcelona, Spain
Department of Anesthesia, Vall d'Hebron Research Institute
Barcelona, Spain
email: fclau_terre@yahoo.es

A. Vegas
Department of Anesthesia and Pain Management, Toronto General Hospital
Toronto, Canada

N. Fletcher
Department of Critical Care, St Georges University Hospital
London, UK
Department of Anaesthesia, University of London
London, UK

© Springer International Publishing Switzerland 2016
J.-L. Vincent (ed.), *Annual Update in Intensive Care and Emergency Medicine 2016*,
DOI 10.1007/978-3-319-27349-5_34

how ultrasound simulation may be best incorporated into teaching programs, with a particular focus on echocardiography.

Current Practice

Echocardiography

Echocardiography has been used as a diagnostic modality for a long time in critical care and emergency medicine, but was mostly delivered by cardiologists and trained ultrasonography technicians. Recent emphasis has been on critical care and emergency room clinicians delivering this service. Training has been broadly defined as either basic or advanced. Basic competence encompasses mostly a limited set of 2D imaging planes using a transthoracic (TTE) or transesophageal (TEE) approach to diagnose severe and potentially life-threatening pathology. Advanced practice uses the full range of anatomical and Doppler imaging to their full potential to diagnose subtle pathologies and monitor hemodynamic interventions.

Lung Ultrasound

Lung ultrasound has been widely adopted as an immediate point-of-care diagnostic technique. The experienced practitioner can differentiate pneumothorax, pleural effusion, consolidation and pulmonary edema with increasing levels of expertise. There are the advantages of portability over X-rays and computed tomography (CT) scanning, as well as intra-procedural guidance for the insertion of chest drains. Lung ultrasound is incorporated into a number of bedside ultrasound protocols (Table 1).

Abdominal Ultrasound

Point-of-care abdominal ultrasound for trauma has become popularized in the emergency room (Table 1). Rapid diagnosis of free fluid is essential in the triage of such cases. Critical care clinicians are increasingly using ultrasound to visualize various viscera in particular the kidneys, great vessels and bladder.

Vascular Ultrasound

Vascular ultrasound has revolutionized the safer insertion of venous and arterial cannulae. Many professional guidelines now stipulate that procedural ultrasound should be an integral part of any central line insertion.

Table 1 Overview of the commonly used introductory focused surface ultrasound protocols

Name, year	Echocardiography views	Context	Other content	Number of scans required for certification
Basic FATE, 1989	Parasternal long axis, parasternal short axis, apical 4 chamber, subcostal 4 chamber, pleura	Postoperative cardiac surgery, ICU	M-mode Pleural views for effusion	Not applicable
FAST, 1999	Parasternal long axis, subcostal 4 chamber	Trauma, EM	Pleural views Abdominal views	
Advanced FATE	As FATE plus apical 2 chamber, apical 5 chamber, subcostal inferior vena cava	Same as for basic FATE	As above plus more quantification	Not applicable
HEART.scan®, 2008	Parasternal long axis, parasternal short axis, apical 4 chamber, apical 2 chamber, apical 3 chamber, apical 5 chamber, subcostal 4 chamber, subcostal inferior vena cava, RV inflow	Hemodynamic state and valvular assessment	Quantification	Approximately 30 scans
FEEL, 2009	Parasternal long axis, parasternal short axis, apical 4 chamber, subcostal 4 chamber	Resuscitation	No	50 supervised scans
FICE, 2012	Parasternal long axis, parasternal short axis, apical 4 chamber, subcostal 4 chamber, subcostal inferior vena cava 2D only	ICU, EM	Pleural views for effusion	50 supervised scans

HEART: Hemodynamic Echocardiography Assessment in Real Time; *FEEL*: Focused Echocardiography in Emergency Life-support; *FATE*: Focused Assessed Transthoracic Echocardiography; *FICE*: Focused Intensive Care Echocardiography; *RV*: right ventricular; *ICU*: intensive care unit; *EM*: emergency medicine

Ultrasound Protocols

Many protocols have been developed in different geographic regions encompassing diverse areas of practice. Most are focused applications of echocardiography, with the addition of lung or abdominal ultrasound depending on the context (Table 1). The general principle of these protocols is an initial limited scan searching for obvious pathology that needs immediate intervention. Further assessment by experts should take place once the patient is more stable. These protocols are specifically designed with the trainee in mind and some have an embedded curriculum, supervision, educational content and a competency sign off.

Simulation

The use of simulation in medicine has a long tradition as an educational tool. Diverse situations are tested repeatedly to achieve success in actual patient management. This has allowed the repetition of different scenarios, high risk in some cases, rare and infrequent in others, to improve performance at the clinical sharp end [2]. Simulation can also be used to enhance performance of procedures requiring skill and precision. In recent years, with the evolution of high-fidelity technology, simulator models have emerged for the development of these skills. Surgeons have benefitted from shortened learning times, improved outcomes, and reduced complication rates. Currently, simulation is included within a broader context combining manual dexterity with actions, decisions, knowledge and leadership to improve real outcome in situations that are difficult to recreate in the clinical sphere.

Simulation itself is not a simple process and occurs in different forms. Three styles of simulation are commonly described: live, virtual and constructive. Live simulation involves activity with humans and/or equipment in a setting where they would operate for real. Virtual simulation entails using humans and/or equipment in a computer-controlled setting. Time is less relevant, allowing users to concentrate on the crucial details. Constructive simulation does not engage humans or equipment as participants. This is driven more by the proper sequencing of events, rather than by time. All three types of simulation are applicable to ultrasound training.

Ultrasound Simulation Technology

A significant recent development in ultrasound training has been the emergence of ultrasound simulators. These have expanded the opportunities for acquisition of relevant knowledge and technical skills. An appreciation of sonographic anatomy is the key first step to an understanding of ultrasound images, which are often initially challenging to interpret. The ultrasound platform merely displays a two dimensional grayscale representation of anatomy. The three dimensional reconstruction we make is a cognitive process that cannot easily be achieved from clinical teaching. A simulator is an elegant method of relating ultrasonic anatomy and imaging planes to topographical anatomy and probe position. We will discuss some of the simulators available with their advantages and disadvantages.

Web-Based Ultrasound Simulators
Web-based ultrasound simulation is an example of a low-fidelity system that is inexpensive yet highly accessible and thus may be used to train large numbers of people.

Table 2 An overview of currently available echocardiography mannequin simulators

	Developer	Initial studies	Image acquisition and display	Dummy Probe	Mmode Doppler included	E-learning package
Heart-Works	Inventive Medical, UK, 2008	Bose et al. [15]	Virtual reality; computer digital reconstruction (grayscale images) from a beating heart model	TEE, TTE	Yes	Yes
Vimedix	CAE Healthcare, Canada, 2009	Platts et al. [22]	Virtual reality; computer-based digital reconstruction (grayscale images) from a beating heart model	TEE, TTE Lung Abdomen	Yes	Yes
EchoCom	Leipzig University Germany, 2007	Weidenbach et al. [34]	Augmented reality; real-time 2D image derivation from a beating heart model and 3D TTE dataset	TTE TEE	Yes	Yes
Schallware	Schallware, Berlin, Germany	Weidenbach et al. [33]	Virtual reality; 3D image dataset. Multiple scanning modes	TTE Abdomen	Yes	Yes

TTE: transthoracic echocardiography; *TEE*: transesophageal echocardiography

These are interactive tools that the user can manipulate to varying degrees. An attached educational package offers the potential for self-directed learning. These types of simulators can be accessed for free or at minimal cost on the internet. Examples include CT2TEE [3], Toronto Virtual TEE and TTE [4] and SonoSim [5], which includes a dummy TTE probe. Applications are available for tablets and smartphones enabling users to bring the simulation to the clinical interface. The web-based simulators permit distance learning, but do not allow the supervision of physical manipulation skills that is vital to competence.

Phantom Simulators

Phantoms are simulation devices that mimic anatomical features to aid the development of ultrasound-guided procedural skills. The procedures of most interest here are central venous cannulation, thoracocentesis and paracentesis. There is no computerized interface; instead a real ultrasound probe is placed on the mannequin surface/phantom generating an ultrasound image similar to that obtained from a patient. To add to the fidelity of the situation, mock blood or fluids can be tapped from rechargeable containers within the model.

Probe and Mannequin-Based High-Fidelity Ultrasound Simulators

These simulators have a mannequin and replica ultrasound probe connected to a computer and high resolution monitor (Table 2). A haptic interface locates the probe on the mannequin and displays a dynamic 3D heart model with the corresponding acquired grayscale ultrasound plane. A considerable body of anatomical and animation expertise has contributed to these models. EchoCom (Leipzig, Germany), Schallware (Berlin, Germany), Heartworks (Inventive Medical, London UK) and Vimedix (CAE Healthcare, Quebec, Canada) offer these simulators on a commercial basis. All provide both TTE and TEE probes except the Schallware which offers only TTE. The Vimedix and Heartworks systems contain the most features and are the most widely used and researched. Heartworks has a very realistic computer heart model, whereas the Vimedix provides lung and abdominal scanning with metrics feedback functionality. Both contain pathological echocardiographic findings, which can be selected in addition to M-mode and all the fluid Doppler modes. The simulator can provide an environment for dedicated teaching away from the stress of clinical interaction. Trainees can practice image acquisition with expert supervision or after some initial tuition use the enabled e-learning packages for self-directed learning. These systems are expensive, limiting availability and require the student to be co-located.

Evidence of Benefit from Ultrasound Simulation Education

There is now a considerable body of evidence to support the positive impact of simulation in medical education [6, 7]. The increasing availability of high-fidelity ultrasound simulators and trainers and the pressure to develop competent point of care ultrasound physician practitioners has resulted in an increasing evidence base for their adoption (Table 3). All critical care program directors in a recent survey in the US considered simulation to be an essential part of an ultrasound teaching program [8]. Most of the evidence for echocardiography simulation comes from research in cardiac anesthesia TEE teaching programs. This relates to the fact that TEE is more invasive and also already well established in cardiac anesthesia. In contrast there is less research for TTE simulation use in critical care, possibly because it can be adequately demonstrated with real human models. Most studies are randomized but underpowered and involve trainees at an early point in the learning curve. Nevertheless, the consistent finding of a benefit of simulation is impressive and it is possible to translate this into general critical care echocardiography training as critical care overlaps with cardiac anesthesia. High-fidelity simulator software development has also been so rapid that evidence inevitably has a significant lag time. However, certain guiding principles have been established, which have implications for critical care and emergency medicine practice.

Table 3 An overview of the key evidence supporting echocardiography simulators

Author (year)	Participants (n)	Study type	Modality studied	Conclusion
Weidenbach et al. (2007) [34]	56 (25 experts and 31 novice users)	Questionnaire-based survey	EchoCom TEE	Experts rated the simulator as realistic and novice users felt that it supported spatial orientation
Bose et al. (2011) [15]	14	Prospective randomized; benefit assessed using pre- and post-test	HeartWorks TEE simulator	Simulator-based teaching is better than conventional methods of TEE teaching
Jerath et al. (2011) [35]	10	Prospective observational; benefit assessed using pre- and post-tests	Virtual TEE website; standard views module	Significant improvement in knowledge of cardiac anatomy on TEE following review of the website
Vegas et al. (2012) [10]	10	Prospective observational; benefit assessed using pre- and post-tests	Virtual TEE website; simulation module	Use of simulation module significantly improves knowledge of navigating 20 standard TEE views
Platts et al. (2012) [22]	82 (42 trainees and 42 attendees at TEE workshop)	Prospective observational; assessed using questionnaire-based survey	VIMEDIX TTE and TOE simulator	Simulation provides a realistic method of image acquisition and improves spatial relationship
Neelankavil et al. (2012) [36]	61	Prospective randomized; effect assessed using pre- and post-tests and TTE scan on volunteers	HeartWorks TTE simulator	Simulation-based teaching significantly improves TTE image acquisition and anatomy identification as compared to lecture-based methods
Sharma et al. (2013) [13]	28	Prospective randomized; benefit assessed using pre- and post-tests	Virtual TEE website and HeartWorks TEE simulator	Internet and simulation-based teaching significantly improves TEE knowledge compared with traditional methods
Jelacic et al. (2013) [31]	37	Prospective observational; benefit assessed using pre- and post-tests	Heartworks TEE simulator	Significant improvement in knowledge of normal echocardiography anatomy after simulation-based teaching session

TEE: transesophageal echocardiography; *TTE*: transthoracic echocardiography

Simulation vs Conventional Teaching

Traditional learning of ultrasound is based on reading, study of DVDs and online educational material and attending lecture-based teaching along with point-of-care instruction on patients. It has been shown that only 12% of the concepts taught in an oral session of an ultrasound course are retained within two weeks [9].

The application of virtual reality is a superior method of enabling trainees to recognize ultrasound planes and images when compared with the conventional teaching methods described above. Using the pre-intervention and post-intervention testing method, researchers demonstrated better image recognition in those groups that had learned anatomical and spatial concepts with virtual reality simulation [10–13]

Hands-on teaching of ultrasound techniques with patients will always remain the principal route to clinical competence [14]. Manipulation of the ultrasound probe is a fundamental skill. Acquisition of probe manipulation skills using TEE is more difficult than TTE due to the potential for harm and the lack of willing volunteer models! High-fidelity simulator mannequins with replica TTE and TEE probes permit safe practice in a less stressful environment. They have been shown to be effective in the acquisition of theoretical knowledge [15, 16], but importantly also in the necessary psychomotor skills for probe manipulation [17, 18]. A new system of metrics in the Vimedix platform enables the operator to receive graded feedback on task performance [19, 20]. Evidence for an educational benefit of TTE simulation comes from educational interventions with anesthesiology residents and sonographers in two studies [21, 22]. Continuous innovation in simulator platforms has made select pathologies and clinical situations available for goal-directed scanning [23–25].

Simulation vs Clinical Teaching

A recent study directly compared simulation teaching with clinical teaching in the cardiac operating room in echo-naïve subjects [26]. The simulation group outperformed the control group on post-intervention testing of their recognition of imaging planes. The confounding effect of protected teaching time away from the stress of cardiac surgery cannot be excluded from this study, yet this is a 'real world' finding in support of simulation.

Significance for Educational Programs

The concept of competence is now widely entrenched in medical education. Education with simulation has a structured number of elements that make it a consistent and effective process. An effective simulation based curriculum for ultrasound training must incorporate key elements for physician skill teaching (Box 1).

Box 1. Simulation-Based Ultrasound Curriculum

- Clear goals and carefully structured objectives
- Conveniently accessed, graduated, longitudinal instruction
- A protected and optimal learning environment
- Repetition of concepts and technical skills
- Progressive expectations for understanding and skill development
- Introduction of abnormalities after understanding normal anatomy and probe manipulation
- Live learning sessions that are customizable to meet learner needs and individualized proctoring in skill sessions

---

Professional bodies should design and oversee the minimum content of curricula, which incorporates a curriculum of knowledge and skills, defined methods of assessment and a sign off. The process is overseen by a supervisor with the necessary qualifications and experience to assume the role. Discussion still remains whether this should be time-based or caseload-based. Trainee feedback is vital in ensuring the process continually evolves. Many international curricula in critical care and emergency medicine now have embedded ultrasound-guided vascular access. The same cannot be observed for echocardiography as the learning curve is longer and competence is more difficult to achieve. Most echocardiography curricula remain an additional competence that the motivated trainee may choose to acquire. This state of affairs is rapidly evolving with different solutions around the world [27, 28]. Most accreditators have adopted a caseload-based logbook with a variation in the numbers required. The learning curve appears to flatten for Focused Abdominal Sonogram for Trauma (FAST) anywhere between 30 to 100 studies [29]. Hemodynamic critical care TEE requires 30 supervised studies to achieve clinical competence [30]. Basic accreditation seems to cluster around a caseload of 50 in 6 months, with more advanced accreditation requiring up to 250 cases over 2 years. There is always a tendency to require a larger number of cases to protect both the individual and the accrediting body. The question we need to ask here is – would the inclusion of high-fidelity simulation into the cardiac ultrasound curriculum help to shorten the learning curve? The accumulated evidence above suggests that it would, albeit when introduced at an early stage. If an early appreciation of cardiac sonoanatomy can be gained during initial training, trainees will have a solid basis on which to develop the accompanying manual skills essential for competence during subsequent training.

What do the trainees themselves want? The incorporation of a TEE simulation-based teaching session into the cardiothoracic anesthesia rotation curriculum was strongly endorsed by senior anesthesia residents according to one study [31]. Simulation is incorporated in leading international postgraduate teaching courses, with a high degree of participant satisfaction scoring. It is vital that we listen to the trainee voice – the educational experiences of the next generation may be very different to those of their senior colleagues who are their trainers. Clearly it is also essential not to oversell simulation as a panacea to a pressing global educational need. Expert clinical supervision and mentorship are by far the more important assets along with courses, books, and e-learning applications. The concept of blended learning is an important one – there have never been so many options for a young doctor who is driven to learn the various forms of ultrasound [32].

Future Developments

So far, we have discussed virtual and constructive simulation. We have focused on the acquisition of technical skills and knowledge from a calm interaction between learner, simulator and supervisor. The next step is the introduction of ultrasound into live team simulation. Just as the operating room or emergency room can be reconstructed in the simulation center so can the critical care unit. The most important outcome is for appropriate treatment of the critically ill and unstable patient. The ability to rapidly perform ultrasound can lead to coherent interventions and communication with the rest of the critical care team. Rare events, such as acute massive pulmonary embolus, trauma, cardiac tamponade, pneumothorax and cardiac arrest, can only be practiced and deconstructed in the setting of simulation.

Inevitably simulator manufacturers will enhance the fidelity of the platforms. The interface will more accurately resemble the actual ultrasound machine with applications and controls to match. Larger pathology libraries will be assimilated and streamlined with education bundles that follow the various accreditations and protocols. The simulator companies are moving in the direction of more mobile technology whereby an ultrasound 'skin' (TTE mobile, Heartworks) with a haptic interface can be placed over a mannequin or human, placing ultrasound-based decision-making at the center of the scenario.

Conclusion

Many forms of ultrasound have been adopted into intensive care and emergency medical practice. From simple central venous access to sophisticated hemodynamic assessment with TEE, the clinicians in these areas are increasingly delivering this service. There is a challenge to educate the next generation of doctors, particularly in echocardiography which is a complex technical skill with a significant learning curve. There is a growing evidence base in anesthesia educational research that high-fidelity ultrasound simulators can enhance anatomical understanding of echocardiographic planes, assist in the appreciation of probe manipulation and shorten this learning curve. This has yet to be translated to research in the intensive care unit and emergency room context. Incorporation of high-fidelity echocardiography simulation should be considered by those organizing curricula and courses, particularly during the initial phase of learning.

References

1. Clau-Terre F, Sharma V, Cholley B et al (2014) Can simulation help to answer the demand for echocardiography education? Anesthesiology 120:32–41
2. Owen H (2012) Early use of simulation in medical education. Simul Healthc 7:102–116
3. CT2TEE: on-line TEE simulator based on CT. http://www.ct2tee.agh.edu.pl. Accessed November 2015
4. Toronto University Virtual Echocardiography Simulator. http://pie.med.utoronto.ca. Accessed November 2015
5. Sonosim® Virtual Simulator. http://sonosim.com. Accessed November 2015
6. Zendejas B, Brydges R, Wang A, Cook DA (2013) Patient outcomes in simulation-based medical education: A Systematic Review. J Gen Intern Med 28:1078–1089
7. Cook DA, Hatala R, Brydges R (2011) Technology-enhanced simulation for health professions education: a systematic review and meta-analysis. JAMA 305:978–988
8. Mosier JM, Malo J, Stolz LA (2014) Critical care ultrasound training: a survey of US fellowship directors. J Crit Care 29:645–649
9. Hempel D, Stenger T, Campo Dell' Orto M et al (2014) Analysis of trainees' memory after classroom presentations of didactical ultrasound courses. Crit Ultrasound J 6:10
10. Vegas A, Meineri M, Jerath A, Corrin M, Silversides C, Tait G (2013) Impact of online transesophageal echocardiographic simulation on learning to navigate the 20 standard views. J Cardiothorac Vasc Anesth 27:531–535
11. Kempny A, Piórkowski A (2010) CT2TEE – a novel, internet-based simulator of transoesophageal echocardiography in congenital heart disease. Kardiol Pol 68:374–379
12. Zhu D, Fang DF, Zhou L et al (2013) Preliminary report on use of 3-dimensional computed tomographic images in a disease-based transesophageal echocardiographic simulation system. Tex Heart Inst J 40:250–255
13. Sharma V, Chamos C, Valencia O, Meineri M, Fletcher SN (2013) The impact of internet and simulation-based training on transoesophageal echocardiography learning in anaesthetic trainees: a prospective randomised study. Anaesthesia 68:621–627
14. Maus TM (2011) Simulation: the importance of "hands-on" learning. J Cardiothorac Vasc Anesth 25:209–211
15. Bose RR, Matyal R, Warraich HJ et al (2011) Utility of a transesophageal echocardiographic simulator as a teaching tool. J Cardiothorac Vasc Anesth 25:212–215
16. Ferrero NA, Bortsov AV, Arora H et al (2014) Simulator training enhances resident performance in transesophageal echocardiography. Anesthesiology 120:149–159
17. Bick JS, Demaria S Jr, Kennedy JD et al (2013) Comparison of expert and novice performance of a simulated transesophageal echocardiography examination. Simul Healthc 8:329–334
18. Sohmer B, Hudson C, Hudson J, Posner GD, Naik V (2014) Transesophageal echocardiography simulation is an effective tool in teaching psychomotor skills to novice echocardiographers. Can J Anaesth 61:235–241
19. Shakil O, Mahmood B, Matyal R, Jainandunsing JS, Mitchell J, Mahmood F (2013) Simulation training in echocardiography: the evolution of metrics. J Cardiothorac Vasc Anesth 27:1034–1040
20. Matyal R, Mitchell JD, Hess PE (2014) Simulator-based transesophageal echocardiographic training with motion analysis: a curriculum-based approach. Anesthesiology 121:389–399
21. Neelankavil J, Howard-Quijano K, Hsieh TC (2012) Transthoracic echocardiography simulation is an efficient method to train anesthesiologists in basic transthoracic echocardiography skills. Anesth Analg 115:1042–1051
22. Platts DG, Humphries J, Burstow DJ, Anderson B, Forshaw T, Scalia GM (2012) The use of computerised simulators for training of transthoracic and transoesophageal echocardiography. The future of echocardiographic training? Heart Lung Circ 21:267–274
23. Wagner R, Razek V, Gräfe F et al (2013) Effectiveness of simulator-based echocardiography training of noncardiologists in congenital heart diseases. Echocardiography 30:693–698

24. Zhu D, Fang DF, Zhou L et al (2013) Preliminary report on use of 3-dimensional computed tomographic images in a disease-based transesophageal echocardiographic simulation system. Tex Heart Inst J 40:250–255

25. Damp J, Anthony R, Davidson MA, Mendes L (2013) Effects of transesophageal echocardiography simulator training on learning and performance in cardiovascular medicine fellows. J Am Soc Echocardiogr 26:1450–1456

26. Ogilvie E, Vlachou A, Edsell M et al (2015) Simulation-based teaching is more effective than point-of-care teaching to assist trainees to identify basic transoesophageal echocardiography views: a prospective randomised study. Anaesthesia 70:330–335

27. Fletcher SN, Grounds RM (2012) Critical care echocardiography: cleared for take up. Br J Anaesth 109:490–92

28. Expert Round Table on Echocardiography in ICU (2014) International consensus statement on training standards for advanced critical care echocardiography. Intensive Care Med 40:654–666

29. Gracias VH, Frankel HL, Gupta R et al (2001) Defining the learning curve for the Focused Abdominal Sonogram for Trauma (FAST) examination: implications for credentialing. American Surg 4:364–368

30. Charron C, Vignon P, Prat G et al (2013) Number of supervised studies required to reach competence in advanced critical care transesophageal echocardiography. Intensive Care Med 39:1019–1024

31. Jelacic S, Bowdle A, Togashi K, VonHomeyer P (2013) The use of TEE simulation in teaching basic echocardiography skills to senior anesthesiology residents. J Cardiothorac Vasc Anesth 27:670–675

32. Lewiss RE, Hoffmann B, Beaulieu Y, Phelan MB (2013) Point-of-care ultrasound education: the increasing role of simulation and multimedia resources. J Ultrasound Med 33:27–32

33. Weidenbach M, Drachsler H, Wild F et al (2007) EchoComTEE – a simulator for transoesophageal echocardiography. Anaesthesia 62:347–353

34. Weidenbach M, Wild F, Scheer K et al (2005) Computer-based training in two-dimensional echocardiography using an echocardiography simulator. J Am Soc Echocardiogr 18:362–366

35. Jerath A, Vegas A, Meineri M et al (2011) An interactive online 3D model of the heart assists in learning standard transesophageal echocardiography views. Can J Anaesth 58:14–21

36. Neelankavil J, Howard-Quijano K, Hsieh TC et al (2012) Transthoracic echocardiography simulation is an efficient method to train anesthesiologists in basic transthoracic echocardiography skills. Anesth Analg 115:1042–1051

Virtual Patients and Virtual Cohorts: A New Way to Think About the Design and Implementation of Personalized ICU Treatments

J. G. Chase, T. Desaive, and J.-C. Preiser

Introduction

Intensive care unit (ICU) patients exhibit complex and highly variable behavior, making them very difficult to manage efficiently and safely. More pragmatically, the cost of intensive care in healthcare systems has dramatically risen over the last decades mostly because of patient ageing. The next generation and challenge for ICU care is thus to personalize and improve care to manage inter- and intra-patient variability and improve cost and productivity. Defeating 'one size fits all' protocolized approaches and moving to a 'one method fits all' personalized approach could provide the big step forward required to handle the demographic tsunami and rising costs.

Computer models offer one powerful opportunity to personalize care by using clinical data and system identification methods to create a so-called 'virtual patient' representing the patient in a particular state. This approach relies on identifying patient-specific parameters that are time varying, capture inter- and intra-patient variability, and are not a function of the therapeutic inputs. Such 'sensitivities' are the key to unlocking virtual patients and model-based care. Thus, the approach predefines the type of deterministic physiological models used. These models have a long history in physiological studies, but a much shorter one in clinical studies. However, over the last 10 years, the successful design and implementation of

J. G. Chase (✉)
Department of Mechanical Engineering, University of Canterbury
Christchurch, New Zealand
email: geoff.chase@canterbury.ac.nz

T. Desaive
GIGA – Cardiovascular Sciences, University of Liège
Liège, Belgium

J.-C. Preiser
Department of Intensive Care, Erasme University Hospital, Université libre de Bruxelles
Brussels, Belgium

© Springer International Publishing Switzerland 2016
J.-L. Vincent (ed.), *Annual Update in Intensive Care and Emergency Medicine 2016*,
DOI 10.1007/978-3-319-27349-5_35

model-based sensors or decision support systems [1, 2] has demonstrated the potential of this approach to provide personalized solutions for ICU patients.

Moreover, there is further power to be obtained by using clinical data to create virtual patients. These virtual patients would represent real patients based on their data, but, when simulated could be used to test different approaches to care than what was actually used. Hence, the underlying models can provide not only a means of controlling individual patients, but a means of safely and rapidly prototyping and optimizing treatment protocols *in silico* in virtual randomized trials.

In addition to speed and safety, virtual cohorts offer the opportunity to improve on the difficulties encountered in evidence-based randomized controlled trials (RCTs) in the ICU, which are often confounded by lack of generality across broader cohorts and/or the interaction of a wide variety of related conditions that serve to confound care of a particular dysfunction [3]. Thus, virtual cohorts and trials offer the opportunity to develop optimal solutions that directly account for inter- and intra-patient variability in response to care, as well as in condition; the latter is difficult to control in a RCT, but can be easily created in a broad enough virtual cohort. Thus, one can ensure that a protocol is safe and robust to both forms of variability. In effect permitting a series of single patient clinical trials to be performed *in silico*.

Finally, a validated *in silico* virtual trials platform with appropriate virtual cohorts offers significant opportunities to reduce the number of phase II/III human trials, or even to replace them. There is the possibility, already partly realized, that they could be used to replace or augment human trials as an alternative, accepted form of evidence in regulatory submissions [4], thus better linking device design and clinical utilization [1]. Finally, they could be used directly by clinicians and medical device companies in concert to design novel devices that best suit optimized delivery protocols.

In this chapter, we examine the necessary modeling and computational methods required to create virtual patients. In particular, we talk about the types of model required, the data required for such models, and how the resulting virtual patients and trials should be validated to ensure a quality result. In each section, we explore the results to date in each area, with a particular focus on glycemic control, for which there is a long history of metabolic modeling that has crossed over to the ICU.

Model Types and Requirements

A mathematical model is a mathematical description of reality. In physiology, such a model underlies a certain number of assumptions about the physical, chemical and biological processes involved. These mathematical models may vary significantly in their complexity and their objectives. They can range from relatively simple lumped-compartment models (e.g., [5, 6]) to very complex network representations and finite element models of several million degrees of freedom (e.g., [7, 8]). A virtual patient model must be able to meet the following requirements:

- Physiologically relevant,
- Clinically relevant,
- Defined by an identifiable treatment sensitivity,
- Identifiable from the data available or presumed to be available at the bedside.

The first requirement (physiological relevance) means that the model has a fixed structure that contains the relevant physiological dynamics that impact care. At one level, no model can capture all complexity. However, any model for use must be able to capture the observed or measured physiological dynamics seen in critical care patients. In addition, its inputs and outputs must be related by known physiological dynamics in the model structure, and inputs should appear at rates observed in physiological studies. This requirement thus ensures the model captures fundamental physiology and also sets a lower limit on model complexity.

The second requirement (clinical relevance) focuses on models that can be simulated in clinical real-time, which is the time between measurements and/or decisions. It should have all the same inputs that one sees clinically in treating the specific dysfunctions associated with the physiological system. It should deliver an output model response that is a measured variable used to titrate care, or a close surrogate of one. Thus, it should have inputs and outputs that are used to guide care so it is directly clinically relevant, and these inputs and outputs should be connected by known clinical input-output responses. This requirement serves to further define the model structure so that all inputs and outputs are known.

The third requirement (identifiable treatment sensitivity) is the key element in creating a virtual patient or using a model to guide care. Ideally, all care is guided by a measured response to patient treatment inputs. Specifically, the model outputs in response to the model inputs, as defined above. The 'rate of exchange' between the input and the output is the sensitivity of the output to the input parameter(s). Thus, for example, insulin sensitivity reflects the 'rate of exchange' between insulin and nutrition inputs, and glycemic response, and lung elastance reflects the independent output pressure (volume) response to a controlled mechanical ventilation volume (pressure) input [9]. While these sensitivities are some examples, they are of course not the only possibilities, and the only limitation in creating such models is the need to maintain physiological relevance within the modeled dynamics.

However, sensitivities are the clinical key to capturing inter- and intra-patient variability in response to care and thus to guiding therapy, and are regularly measured clinically in assessing response to care. In particular, highly sensitive patients with all relevant inputs accounted for need less treatment input and *vice versa*. Thus, a physiologically relevant sensitivity metric that captures the transfer of input to output response to care is a critical element as response to care is guided by physiology and patient condition. Overall, this requirement further defines the model structure and organization.

The fourth requirement (identifiable from the data available) is used to ensure that the model can be made patient-specific. For guiding care, this requirement means that a clinically relevant set of data obtained in a clinically relevant time frame can be used to identify the model. For creating virtual patients, it must be possible to identify the necessary sensitivity, and any other relevant parameters, with the data available. These data requirements should be the same, and the identified sensitivity value must capture the inter- and intra-patient variability over time and/or inputs so that it represents the patient at any given time and, over time, it

Dextrose Absorption

$$P(t) = \min(d_2 P_2, P_{max})$$
$$\dot{P}_2 = -\min(d_2 P_2, P_{max}) + d_1 P_1$$
$$\dot{P}_1 = -d_1 P_1 + D(t)$$

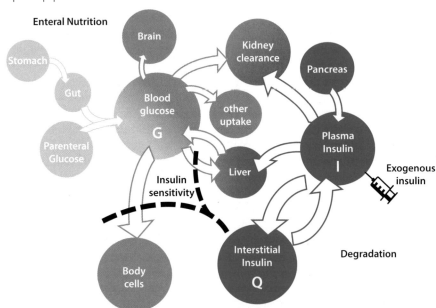

$$\dot{G} = -p_G G(t) - S_I G(t) \frac{Q(t)}{1 + \alpha_G Q(t)} + \frac{\min(d_2 P_2, P_{max}) + EGP_b - CNS + PN(t)}{V_G}$$

$$\dot{Q} = n_I(I(t) - Q(t)) - n_c \frac{Q(t)}{1 + \alpha_G Q(t)}$$

$$\dot{I} = -\frac{n_L I(t)}{1 + \alpha_I I(t)} - n_K I(t) - n_I(I(t) - Q(t)) + \frac{u_{ex}(t)}{V_I} + (1 - x_L)\frac{u_{en}(G)}{V_I}$$

Fig. 1 Glucose-insulin pharmacokinetic and pharmacodynamics model used for virtual patients. See [10] for abbreviations

captures the evolution in patient state as verified by other external clinical observations or knowledge. Pragmatically, with limited data, only limited parameters can be identified in clinically relevant timeframes, thus this requirement puts an upper limit on model complexity.

In summary, a model must have all necessary physiology to guide treatment, the model structure must include inputs and outputs that are clinically relevant, as well as a sensitivity parameter relating the throughput or rate of exchange of the output response to that input. Identified from clinical data over time these sensitivity profiles can capture inter-patient variability, as well as the patient's evolution over time of their response to care, which is the intra-patient variability. In summary, these requirements allow you to create models that can be used to create virtual patients and personalize care.

Figure 1 shows a metabolic model designed for creating virtual patients and designing glycemic protocols [10] and the series of equations used to capture it. The inputs are the parenteral [PN(t)] and enteral [P(t)] nutritional carbohydrate inputs, with appropriate appearance dynamics, along with the exogenous intravenous insulin input [$u_{ex}(t)$]. The model structure includes all relevant insulin kinetics and nutrition dynamics to ensure appropriate times of appearance. The pharmacodynamics equation for glycemia [G(t)] is then defined by the combination of these inputs to deliver a glycemic response as a function of the insulin sensitivity [$S_I(t)$]. This sensitivity can be identified hourly or more frequently depending on data density and has been shown to capture patient specific dynamics and their evolution [11, 12].

Data Required for Virtual Patients

Virtual patients are created directly from clinical data using a model as defined in the previous section and shown schematically in Fig. 2. To identify sensitivities one must have data for all the clinically relevant inputs, such as insulin and all forms of nutrition for glycemic control and pressure/volume for ventilation, as well as the clinically relevant and modeled output, such as glucose or volume/pressure for the examples noted. From this input-output data, model-based sensitivity can be identified via any number of means [11] between any set of one or more input-output data. Captured over time, it captures the patient-specific evolution of this sensitivity to care, which can then be used to simulate how new forms of care would lead to new, possibly improved, output variables.

The key to virtual patients is ensuring one captures the relevant physiological and clinically observed dynamics. If patient evolution with a condition is slow, then these parameters or sensitivities need only be identified at a similarly slow or slightly faster rate. Equally, if clinical interventions will only vary slowly or can only vary slowly due to limited or highly invasive measurements, then these parameters need only be identified at a similar rate. In contrast, typical ICU patient dysfunction is often characterized by rapidly changing dynamics [13], requiring rapid response. Thus, the data must be obtained frequently enough to be able

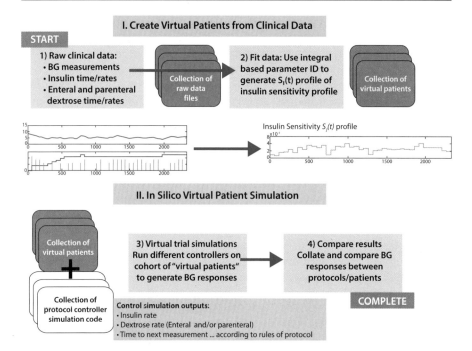

Fig. 2 Virtual patient and cohort creation (*top*) and virtual trials process (*bottom*). *BG*: blood glucose

to identify these rates of evolution [11, 14–16], subject to a trade-off on nursing workload if the data must be manually, rather than electronically and automatically, collected.

Thus, the data must be obtained at a rate suitable for safely and successfully capturing these dynamics. Too infrequent, and the model will not be able to capture patient evolution. Fortunately, most clinical sensors at this time provide far more data than necessary, such as that found from cardiovascular catheters providing pressures every few seconds, or breathing inputs sampled at 100–400 times per breath. In addition, increasing numbers of sensors used in the ICU are electronically accessible and can thus be sampled automatically using standard data acquisition systems at very high rates, such as obtaining pressure data from a catheter or glucose data from a continuous glucose monitor [17], reducing the workload required to obtain the data [18]. Hence, it is only necessary to ensure that the data sampled and models used can provide accurate estimates of the sensitivity to care that captures the clinically observed dynamics.

Virtual Patients, Cohorts and their Validation

Virtual Patients

Virtual patients can thus be created as defined in Fig. 2. These trajectories of sensitivities offer significant insight in and of themselves. It is critical to note that a virtual patient represent that patient's specific responses as defined by the model. Thus, if the model is representative, the outputs will represent and capture that condition and its evolution. One could then use these trajectories to compare across different conditions, such as sepsis vs non-sepsis patients for diagnostics, improved resolution or other insight [1]. However, while, to date, such approaches have been limited, there is a growing explosion of use as data becomes ever easier to obtain electronically from medical devices.

In the metabolic domain, insulin sensitivity trajectories have been used to identify the impact of other drug therapies [19, 20], to provide insight into patient condition evolution over time and thus how treatment should best proceed [21–23], and to diagnose the absence of sepsis [24]. In pulmonary mechanics, elastance has been used to identify the impact and effect of recruitment maneuvers and how they decline or wear-off over time [15, 16, 25], as well as the impact of different breathing modes [9, 15, 26, 27].

More directly, virtual patients form a platform for defining and optimizing new protocols and approaches to care. Several protocols have been optimized in this way for metabolic control [28–35], and some have gone on to show the close results of their clinical use to that simulated [32, 36]. This approach can thus aid protocol development and offer a patient-specific approach that allows direct management of the intra- and inter-patient variability that has been shown, particularly in the glycemic control space, to be a major contributor to the failure of large clinical trials using fixed protocols [13].

However, virtual patients can also be used to analyze a given protocol as well. Simulation possibilities are numerous but can include testing protocol variations, such as timing, sensor errors, errors in dosing, and patient variability [13, 37, 38]. Equally, they can be used to test the impact of fixed, physiological model parameters that cannot be identified. Thus, they can be used to test the impact of model parameters and variations in expected or unexpected physiology.

Finally, it is important to note that all of these modeling elements that create virtual patients are built from a long history of physiological modeling used in identifying physiological parameters [5, 6]. The concept of virtual patients, first introduced to the best of the authors' knowledge for use in designing a protocol for use as a standard of care [34], has thus extended these early works to the patient simulators and models now in use. A recent analysis of how ICU research can proceed and its current critical failures, noted that we too often study syndromes and specific cohorts that do not generalize and that perhaps the time of the "single patient trial" was approaching [3, 39]. Virtual patients can offer these single patient trials *in silico*, which can, once safe, be extended for use in model-based personalized care protocols that does the same for each patient in a 'one method fits all approach'.

Virtual Cohorts

Virtual cohorts are collections of virtual patients. Thus, any group of relevant and useful patient data can be used to create virtual patients and thus cohorts, which must be representative of the intended treatment cohort.

This requirement states that a given cohort of data should represent the study cohort or treatment cohort as broadly and completely as possible. It is critical that all reasonably expected patient dynamics that might be observed when the protocol is in use should be present in the virtual cohort. A glycemic control virtual cohort with no sudden, or gradual, rises in insulin sensitivity that can lead to hypoglycemia and its attendant risks in control, would not be representative. It is the authors' experience that, in fact, it is better to slightly over represent these more outlying cases to ensure protocol robustness and safety.

Thus, a virtual cohort should capture all relevant cohort dynamics just as a model and data should capture all relevant patient dynamics. Failure to be representative means that any protocol design is skewed by the missing dynamics and thus poses a risk to either safety or performance in use. These episodes and cohorts should thus be large enough to be representative of all dynamics, particularly outlying effects, as well as representative of what would be encountered in practice, so that virtual trial simulations of virtual cohorts yield results that would be expected in practice.

Similarly, the recent analysis of how ICU research can proceed and its current critical failures, noted that narrow cohort clinical trials often do not generalize [39]. Virtual cohorts offer the opportunity to design protocols for whole cohorts that are general and typical; a 'one method fits all' form of care that can translate to all patients, thus offering the ability to safely and robustly perform clinical trials and studies on all patients in a way that represents the real clinical situation, and thus ensures greater potential generalizability of the results.

Validation: How to Ensure the Model Is Good

Virtual patients and cohorts can be created, but the key question with any modeling is how does one know if the model is representative and captures the observed dynamics? The ability to fit a model to data does not ensure that the sensitivity parameters, and any others, identified to make the model patient-specific will capture the response to treatment accurately. The only way to test this value is to see whether, once identified, the model captures the outcome of a new input. The question is thus, how can such virtual patients and models be validated?

There are three forms of validation that can ensure a model and virtual patient cohort are valid and will be clinically useful:

- Patient level: Using clinical data, a patient can be identified at a given moment in time and then the inputs simulated. The output predictions can then be compared to the measured data. This tests the model's predictive behavior where it is assumed that accurate prediction results from accurate identification of underlying system dynamics and patient-specific sensitivity. It thus provides validation of the model dynamics within the range of intra-patient variability.

- Cohort level before-after: A virtual cohort can be simulated with a protocol, and then compared to later clinical use of the protocol. Overall cohort results and per-patient median performance can offer the ability to see if cohort level median and variability data are captured, and that all individual patients in that cohort have reasonable response. It provides validation of the method, the virtual patients in general over an episode or stay, and the overall design approach, but not of the specific patients since they are different.

- Cohort level cross validation: This approach requires clinical data from two or more clinically matched cohorts. Virtual patients are created and the original protocols can be tested. The cross validation occurs when the virtual patients of Cohort A treated with Protocol A, are tested on the remaining protocols (Protocols B, C ...) and compared to Clinical Data B, C, ... The quality of the match of all possible cross validations compared to clinical data validates the independence of the sensitivities identified to create virtual patients, as well as their ability to capture the underlying patient dynamics well enough that when treated with another protocol the expected clinical results occur.

These validations serve together to validate the model, the sensitivity parameters, and the ability to accurate design for both patient and cohort levels.

Examples of the first validation are seen in [10] and have been used in a number of model studies [35, 40, 41]. The comparison to clinical data is a gold standard. However, this validation tests not the fit of model to data, but the ability to predict clinical outcomes. Other ways of doing this form of validation can occur in pilot trials where clinical data are collected using a model and protocol prospectively (e.g., [42, 43]). These predictions can only be as accurate as the ability of the patient to vary in condition over the prediction time interval, as assessed for example by stochastic models used in control to capture intra-patient variability [13, 14]. However, most intra-patient variations are smaller, and it is thus a fundamental first validation of the model and sensitivity identified, as the ability to predict outcomes to clinical inputs is the key element.

The second form of validation has only been performed, to the best of the authors' knowledge, twice [32, 36]. These results are shown in Fig. 3 and clearly show that, for the metabolic model of Fig. 1, it is able to predict cohort level median and variability, first and second order statistics that are crucial to understanding performance and risk. Equally, these studies both captured percentage glucose within safety (blood glucose < 4.0 mmol/l, hypoglycemic events) and performance (blood glucose in the 4.0–7.0 or 4.0–8.0 mmol/l range or similar) very well, yielding further validation and confidence in the model and methods. These before-after validations also show how protocols can be designed with virtual patients and cohorts and still accurately capture the cohort and thus the outcomes of the protocols – well in advance of clinical use, and far faster and safer. Thus, these results show how virtual patients and cohorts may be validated as well as their potential power to design effective new treatments.

Fig. 3 Cohort-level before-after validation of virtual trials designed glycemic control cohorts for *SPRINT* (Specialized Relative Insulin Nutrition Tables) versus other protocols used for comparison in design (Panel **a**); and SPRINT's successor, *STAR* (Stochastic TARgeted), compared to SPRINT (Panel **b**)

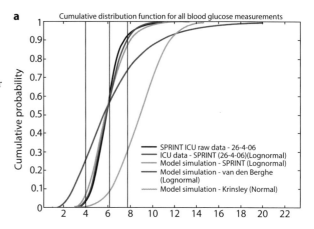

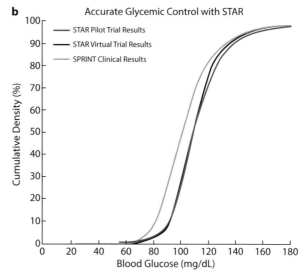

The final form of validation has also been performed twice ([12, 44]), using two and three cohorts, respectively. In each case, as shown in Fig. 4, the cross validation comparisons to clinical data were very good. These results show the validation of the underlying assumptions that the identified insulin sensitivity parameter in these studies was truly representative of patient condition, patient evolution across a virtual patient, and the underlying patient state in general.

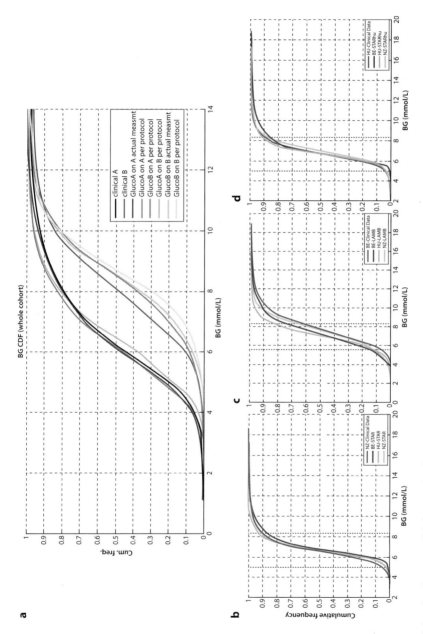

Fig. 4 Cohort-level cross validation results for Glucontrol A and B cohorts from [45] (**a**); and three matched cohorts using different forms of glycemic control data in New Zealand (**b**), Belgium (**c**) and Hungary (**d**) are shown. *BG*: blood glucose

Conclusion

The fields of engineering modeling and computation and intensive care medicine are converging rapidly. Increasing access to data and its use increase the ability to use computation to enable clinical professionals to provide better care, as well as to design better protocols. The virtual patients and cohort methods reviewed here are a nascent tip of an emerging iceberg.

Clinical data can increasingly be merged with engineering modeling to create virtual patients and, together, virtual cohorts. Properly validated, these models and resulting virtual trials can be used to analyze and optimize existing care, ensure the safety of existing care, test the impact of new sensors or delivery devices, develop new optimal protocols, and test the safety and performance of potential protocols in a specific ICU cohort – all before testing on patients, thus directly saving time and reducing risk. As a result, they offer a host of new avenues for understanding and improving care, not the least of which is the potential to develop and implement personalized protocols and care.

Personalized care is widely seen as the next major step in care. The transition from 'one size fits all' protocols with little or no adaptation to inter- and intra-patient variability and evolution to personalized, time-varying 'one method fits all' approaches offers the chance to achieve far better care and outcomes than the current non-computerized approach. The key to these therapies is the use of virtual patient models and methods.

In future, virtual patient cohorts could be collected and curated for use by all in the design and analysis of new treatment methods. These cohorts could be created by accessing data from central electronic data management services. What is the next biggest hurdle for this next-generation approach, whether for virtual cohorts or use in model-based decision support at the bedside? Obtaining direct, free and open access to patient treatment data from medical sensors and treatment devices – but this is an argument for another day.

References

1. Chase JG, Le Compte AJ, Preiser JC, Shaw GM, Penning S, Desaive T (2011) Physiological modeling, tight glycemic control, and the ICU clinician: what are models and how can they affect practice? Ann Intensive Care 1:11
2. Dong Y, Chbat NW, Gupta A, Hadzikadic M, Gajic O (2012) Systems modeling and simulation applications for critical care medicine. Ann Intensive Care 2:18
3. Vincent JL (2010) We should abandon randomized controlled trials in the intensive care unit. Crit Care Med 38(10 Suppl):S534–S538
4. Kovatchev BP, Breton M, Man CD, Cobelli C (2009) In silico preclinical trials: a proof of concept in closed-loop control of type 1 diabetes. J Diabetes Sci Technol 3:44–55
5. Carson ER, Cobelli C (2001) Modelling Methodology For Physiology And Medicine. Elsevier, Amsterdam
6. Keener JP, Sneyd J (1998) Mathematical Physiology. Springer, New York
7. Hunter P, Coveney PV, de Bono B et al (2010) A vision and strategy for the virtual physiological human in 2010 and beyond. Philos Transact A Math Phys Eng Sci 368:2595–2614

8. Tawhai MH, Burrowes KS, Hoffman EA (2006) Computational models of structure-function relationships in the pulmonary circulation and their validation. Exp Physiol 91:285–293

9. Chiew YS, Pretty C, Docherty PD et al (2015) Time-varying respiratory system elastance: a physiological model for patients who are spontaneously breathing. PLoS One 10:e0114847

10. Lin J, Razak NN, Pretty CG et al (2011) A physiological Intensive Control Insulin-Nutrition-Glucose (ICING) model validated in critically ill patients. Comput Methods Programs Biomed 102:192–205

11. Hann CE, Chase JG, Lin J, Lotz T, Doran CV, Shaw GM (2005) Integral-based parameter identification for long-term dynamic verification of a glucose-insulin system model. Comput Methods Programs Biomed 77:259–270

12. Chase JG, Suhaimi F, Penning S et al (2010) Validation of a model-based virtual trials method for tight glycemic control in intensive care. Biomed Eng Online 9:84

13. Chase JG, Le Compte AJ, Suhaimi F et al (2011) Tight glycemic control in critical care. The leading role of insulin sensitivity and patient variability: A review and model-based analysis. Comput Methods Programs Biomed 102:156–171

14. Lin J, Lee D, Chase JG et al (2008) Stochastic modelling of insulin sensitivity and adaptive glycemic control for critical care. Comput Methods Programs Biomed 89:141–152

15. van Drunen VE, Chiew YS, Zhao Z et al (2013) Visualisation of time-variant respiratory system elastance in ARDS models. Biomed Tech (Berl) 58(Suppl 1):4328

16. Chiew YS, Chase JG, Shaw GM, Sundaresan A, Desaive T (2011) Model-based PEEP optimisation in mechanical ventilation. Biomed Eng Online 10:111

17. Wernerman J, Desaive T, Finfer S et al (2014) Continuous glucose control in the ICU: report of a 2013 round table meeting. Crit Care 18:226

18. Aragon D (2006) Evaluation of nursing work effort and perceptions about blood glucose testing in tight glycemic control. Am J Crit Care 15:370–377

19. Pretty C, Chase JG, Lin J et al (2011) Impact of glucocorticoids on insulin resistance in the critically ill. Comput Methods Programs Biomed 102:172–180

20. Pretty C, Chase JG, Le Compte A, Lin J, Shaw G (2011) Impact of metoprolol on insulin sensitivity in the ICU. Trauma 4:4

21. Pretty CG, Le Compte AJ, Chase JG et al (2012) Variability of insulin sensitivity during the first 4 days of critical illness: implications for tight glycemic control. Ann Intensive Care 2:17

22. Sah PA, Chase JG, Pretty CG et al (2014) Evolution of insulin sensitivity and its variability in out-of-hospital cardiac arrest (OHCA) patients treated with hypothermia. Crit Care 18:586

23. Ferenci T, Benyo B, Kovacs L, Fisk L, Shaw GM, Chase JG (2013) Daily evolution of insulin sensitivity variability with respect to diagnosis in the critically ill. PloS one 8:e57119

24. Lin J, Parente JD, Chase JG et al (2011) Development of a model-based clinical sepsis biomarker for critically ill patients. Comp Methods Programs Biomed 102:149–155

25. van Drunen EJ, Chase JG, Chiew YS, Shaw GM, Desaive T (2013) Analysis of different model-based approaches for estimating dFRC for real-time application. Biomed Eng Online 12:9

26. Chiew YS, Chase JG, Lambermont B et al (2013) Effects of neurally adjusted ventilatory assist (NAVA) levels in non-invasive ventilated patients: titrating NAVA levels with electric diaphragmatic activity and tidal volume matching. Biomed Eng Online 12:61

27. van Drunen EJ, Chiew YS, Chase JG et al (2013) Expiratory model-based method to monitor ARDS disease state. Biomed Eng Online 12:57

28. Pielmeier U, Andreassen S, Juliussen B, Chase JG, Nielsen BS, Haure P (2010) The Glucosafe system for tight glycemic control in critical care: a pilot evaluation study. J Crit Care 25:97–104

29. Plank J, Blaha J, Cordingley J et al (2006) Multicentric, randomized, controlled trial to evaluate blood glucose control by the model predictive control algorithm versus routine glucose management protocols in intensive care unit patients. Diabetes Care 29:271–276

30. Van Herpe T, Mesotten D, Wouters PJ et al (2013) LOGIC-insulin algorithm-guided versus nurse-directed blood glucose control during critical illness: The LOGIC-1 single-center randomized, controlled clinical trial. Diabetes Care 36:189–194
31. Evans A, Le Compte A, Tan CS et al (2012) Stochastic targeted (STAR) Glycemic control: design, safety, and performance. J Diabetes Sci Technol 6:102–115
32. Fisk L, Lecompte A, Penning S, Desaive T, Shaw G, Chase G (2012) STAR Development and Protocol Comparison. IEEE Trans Biomed Eng 59:3357–3364
33. Le Compte AJ, Chase JG, Lynn A, Hann CE, Shaw GM, Lin J (2011) Development of blood glucose control for extremely premature infants. Comput Methods Programs Biomed 102:181–191
34. Lonergan T, LeCompte A, Willacy M et al (2006) A simple insulin-nutrition protocol for tight glycemic control in critical illness: development and protocol comparison. Diabetes Technol Ther 8:191–206
35. Wilinska ME, Chassin L, Hovorka R (2008) In silico testing – impact on the progress of the closed loop insulin infusion for critically ill patients project. J Diabetes Sci Technol 2:417–423
36. Chase JG, Shaw GM, Lotz T et al (2007) Model-based insulin and nutrition administration for tight glycaemic control in critical care. Curr Drug Deliv 4:283–296
37. Le Compte AJ, Pretty CG, Lin J, Shaw GM, Lynn A, Chase JG (2011) Impact of variation in patient response on model-based control of glycaemia in critically ill patients. Comput Methods Programs Biomed 109:211–219
38. Pretty CG, Signal M, Fisk L et al (2014) Impact of sensor and measurement timing errors on model-based insulin sensitivity. Comput Methods Programs Biomed 114:e79–e86
39. Vincent JL, Hall JB, Slutsky AS (2015) Ten big mistakes in intensive care medicine. Intensive Care Med 41:505–507
40. Van Herpe T, Pluymers B, Espinoza M, Van den Berghe G, De Moor B (2006) A minimal model for glycemia control in critically ill patients. Conf Proc IEEE Eng Med Biol Soc 1:5432–5435
41. Hovorka R, Chassin LJ, Ellmerer M, Plank J, Wilinska ME (2008) A simulation model of glucose regulation in the critically ill. Physiol Meas 29:959–978
42. Evans A, Shaw GM, Le Compte A et al (2011) Pilot proof of concept clinical trials of Stochastic Targeted (STAR) glycemic control. Ann Intensive Care 1:38
43. Lonergan T, Compte AL, Willacy M et al (2006) A pilot study of the SPRINT protocol for tight glycemic control in critically Ill patients. Diabetes Technol Ther 8:449–462
44. Pretty CG (2012) Analysis, classification and management of insulin sensitivity variability in a glucose-insulin system model for critical illness. http://ir.canterbury.ac.nz/bitstream/handle/10092/6580/thesis_fulltext.pdf?sequence=1. Accessed November 2015
45. Preiser JC, Devos P, Ruiz-Santana S et al (2009) A prospective randomised multi-centre controlled trial on tight glucose control by intensive insulin therapy in adult intensive care units: the Glucontrol study. Intensive Care Med 35:1738–1748

Part XIII

Intensive Care Unit Trajectories: The Bigger Picture

Predicting Cardiorespiratory Instability

M. R. Pinsky, G. Clermont, and M. Hravnak

Introduction

Identification of patients with overt cardiorespiratory insufficiency or at high risk of impending cardiorespiratory insufficiency is often difficult outside the venue of directly observed patients in highly staffed areas of the hospital, such as the operating room, intensive care unit (ICU) or emergency department. And even in these care locations, identification of cardiorespiratory insufficiency early or predicting its development beforehand is often challenging. The clinical literature has historically prized early recognition of cardiorespiratory insufficiency and its prompt correction as being valuable at minimizing patient morbidity and mortality while simultaneously reducing healthcare costs. Recent data support the statement that integrated monitoring systems that create derived fused parameters of stability or instability using machine learning algorithms, accurately identify cardiorespiratory insufficiency and can predict their occurrence. In this overview, we describe integrated monitoring systems based on established machine learning analysis using various established tools, including artificial neural networks, k-nearest neighbor, support vector machine, random forest classifier and others on routinely acquired non-invasive and invasive hemodynamic measures to identify cardiorespiratory insufficiency and display them in real-time with a high degree of precision.

M. R. Pinsky (✉)
Department of Critical Care Medicine, University of Pittsburgh
Pittsburgh, USA
Department of Anesthesiology, University of California, San Diego
La Jolla, USA
email: pinsky@pitt.edu

G. Clermont
Department of Critical Care Medicine, University of Pittsburgh
Pittsburgh, USA

M. Hravnak
Department of Tertiary Care Nursing, University of Pittsburgh
Pittsburgh, USA

© Springer International Publishing Switzerland 2016   451
J.-L. Vincent (ed.), *Annual Update in Intensive Care and Emergency Medicine 2016*,
DOI 10.1007/978-3-319-27349-5_36

The implications of these approaches for all healthcare monitoring across the spectrum of in-patient to chronic care is clear, even though the need may appear more pressing for the acute care setting to those of us whose daily life is centered there. The underlying assumption of these approaches is that measured changes in easily acquired physiologic variables reflect complex patient-specific interactions amongst multiple regulatory autonomic, hormonal and metabolic systems. Accordingly, simple algorithm approaches to such interactions, like the use of the existing severity scoring systems or computer-based treatment protocols, are unlikely to improve outcomes other than by standardizing therapies. Potentially, by using functional hemodynamic monitoring principles, previously described and validated, we can predict with a high degree of accuracy volume responsiveness and central arterial tone in all patients. But one needs to identify who is unstable or going to be unstable before applying these functional hemodynamic monitoring approaches.

Integrated Monitoring Systems Improve Diagnosis of Cardiorespiratory Insufficiency and Treatment Effectiveness

Current resuscitation decisions are typically made in response to a falling blood pressure (BP), persistently high heart rate (HR) or arterial desaturation [1]. Individual vital signs (BP, HR, respiratory rate, pulse oximeter oxygen saturation [SpO_2], and end-tidal CO_2) are usually assessed as mean values and interpreted independently. These point estimates may not reach an actionable level until the patient has already progressed to late (or decompensated) cardiorespiratory insufficiency. Alternatively, an integrated monitoring system can use fused data, collected and synthesized to identify physiologic patterns, which are predictive of instability in real-time and before overt clinical deterioration [2]. To see whether such an integrated monitoring system could identify overt cardiorespiratory insufficiency earlier in its course and reduce overall patient instability, we used a Food and Drug Administration (FDA)-approved Visensia™ monitor (OBS Medical, Carmel, IN) that amalgamates non-invasive vital signs (BP, HR, respiratory rate, SpO_2) and derives a calculated index score (vital signs index [VSI]) between zero and ten using an artificial neuronet approach [3]. Using our 600 step-down unit (SDU) patient cohort as a calibration set, we recalibrated the VSI algorithm to fit our cohort, wherein VSI values of >3.2 correlated significantly with independently estimated instability based on clinical assessment (r = 0.815) [4]. An example of one patient who progressively deteriorated over a 6 h period is shown in Fig. 1. Note that deterioration is not steady but phasic (blue arrows) with periods of failed recovery ending in collapse (black arrow). Furthermore, when the VSI alert was coupled with an effector arm of direct immediate nursing bedside activation and protocolized treatment, overall instability decreased by 150% and the progression from mild to severe instability was reduced by 300% [5, 6]. Importantly, the VSI alert occurred before clinically-apparent instability in 80% of cases, with an advance time of 9.4 ± 9.2 min. Thus, such bedside-displayed VSI data can often detect the onset of cardiorespiratory in-

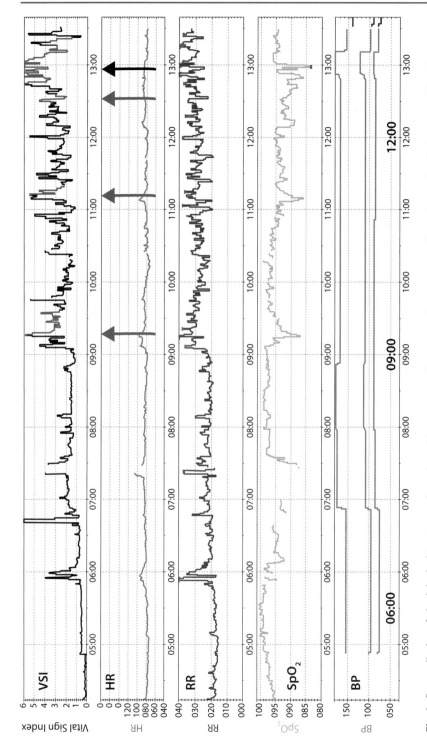

Fig. 1 Screen display of physiologic data stream of a patient with progressive decompensation to overt cardiorespiratory insufficiency over 6 h. *Blue arrows* mark times when the fused instability index (*vital signs index* [VSI]) exceeds "normal" and the *black arrow*, the time when medical emergency response team activation occurred. *HR*: heart rate; *RR*: respiratory rate; *SpO₂*: pulse oximeter oxygen saturation; *BP*: blood pressure

sufficiency before overt symptoms are present and when coupled to appropriate immediate treatment plans markedly reduces patient instability.

Demographic and clinical characteristics are useful in predicting mortality for groups of patients using static snapshot models such as APACHE III [7] or IV [8], and also help to predict mortality when added to intermittent vital sign amalgamation. Smith et al. [9] determined that adding age to a single-parameter instability-concern model (RR < 5 or > 36/min, HR < 40 or > 140/min, systolic BP < 90 mmHg, sudden fall in level of consciousness) or the intermittently determined Modified Early Warning System (MEWS) improved mortality prediction. Patients ≥ 80 years of age with a RR of 24–25 per minute had 4 times the mortality of patients 40–64 years of age, and those ≥ 80 years of age with a systolic BP of 90–94 mmHg had 10 times the mortality of those aged 40–64 years of age. Higher age also increased mortality prediction as MEWS score increased. We subsequently validated this improved predictive index in our SDU cohort, wherein adding low frequency data (demographics) markedly improved the predictive value of the VSI alerts in SDU patients [10].

Advanced Signal Processing Improves Predictive Value of HR for Identifying Impending Instability

Batchinsky et al. showed that advanced signal processing R-R intervals could be used to predict trauma survivorship [11]. They then showed clear differences in HR complexity in 31 pre-hospital trauma patients during their helicopter transport to a level 1 trauma center who survived (20 survived) or died (11 died) after admission. Although mean HR was not different between groups (117 ± 9 vs. 100 ± 4/min, non-survivors vs. survivors), their HR variability, quantified by the instantaneous R-R interval changes on a beat-to-beat basis were clearly different. They quantified HR variability by assessing approximate entropy (ApEn), sample entropy (SampEn) and similarity of distributions. Traditionally, heart rate variability, estimated, as the standard deviation of the R-R interval, requires at least 800 beats to derive robust values. However, these authors showed that by using these derived parameters of variability, SampEn not only displayed clear separation of values between survivors and non-survivors, but the strength of the discrimination persisted even when the datasets were reduced from 800 to 100 R-R intervals [11]. Furthermore, these electrocardiographic (EKG)-derived signal differences were also associated with the need for life-saving interventions in these same trauma patients [12]. Finally, they verified the above findings in a mixed cohort of prehospital trauma patients [13]. Thus, readily available vital sign data can be used to derive clinically-relevant prediction parameters with precision and a markedly reduced lead time.

Advanced Signal Processing of Physiologic Variable Time Series Identifies Those SDU Patients Who Will Become Unstable From Those Who Will Not

Using the above SDU patient data series [5, 6], we analyzed HR variability parameters similar to those described by Batchinsky et al. [11–13]. We created a HR variability index based on HR autocorrelation, standard deviation, high frequency power of HR frequency spectrum and ApEn. The resulting fused parameter was significantly different for the 80 patients in the 307 patient cohort who experienced at least one cardiorespiratory insufficiency episode. Importantly, when displayed as 5 min epochs moving backward from the instability event or discharge in the two groups, HR variability discriminated between the two groups > 48 h before these events (Fig. 2) [14]. Thus, advanced signal processing of clinical data can identify instability before it becomes clinically apparent, often with many hours of lead time.

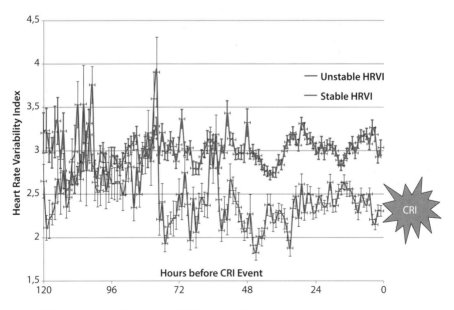

Fig. 2 Heart rate variability index (*HRVI*) of step-down unit patients who were never unstable (*blue*) and those who would become unstable (*gray*) at time zero. Times are displayed preceding instability events for the patients wo would become unstable and a similar time frame but at random to hospital stay for a matched cohort of stable step-down unit patients. *CRI*: cardiorespiratory instability

Advanced Monitoring-Derived Comprehensive Libraries

It is not enough to use existing data streams to predict instability. One must also create physiological libraries of complex and dynamic states, such as hemorrhage, sepsis, pump failure, or evolving acute lung injury (ALI). Normal physiological reflexes aggressively support blood flow to the heart and brain and thus may well obfuscate bedside assessment. We used highly instrumented animal models to define high fidelity physiologic patterns of individual animal response to disease. We studied these patterns of response in compensated trauma/hemorrhagic shock, both during the progression to cardiovascular collapse and its response to resuscitation therapies. As with the above vital sign analysis, we note not only the absolute values of measured hemodynamic variables ascertained from non-invasive and minimally invasive biosensors, but also their dynamic response to prescribed physiological challenges. Compensation, exhaustion and response to therapy reflect the three primary processes studied.

The experimental hemorrhage protocol is designed to simulate a dynamically changing clinical situation by modifying a Wigger's model using several discrete bleeding episodes based on the animal's physiologic response. Lightly anesthetized swine followed an arterial pressure-driven experimental hemorrhage protocol to a mean arterial pressure (MAP) of 30 mmHg, held there for a maximum of 90 min then resuscitated. The porcine trauma/hemorrhagic shock model plays into the unique nature of each test animal by having the level of bleed defined by the subsequent MAP and not by the amount of blood shed. This allowing us to examine the specific compensating mechanisms, unique measures of decompensation and tissue viability and response to therapy [15]. High fidelity (256 Hz) hemodynamic waveform collection and low frequency endocrine, metabolic and immunologic parameters can also be recorded throughout the experiment. Instrumentation with additional biosensors to assess tissue O_2 saturation (StO_2), tissue CO_2 and pH, capillary blood flow and mucosal $NADH_2$ levels were also performed as well as dynamic stress tests described below. The partial list of 'non-traditional' biosensors we have used in this model and that can be used clinically going forward is given in Table 1.

The cause of cardiovascular collapse from compensated trauma/hemorrhagic shock appears to be related to failure of compensatory response mechanisms rooted in autonomic balance. Trauma/hemorrhagic shock acts as a trigger for a cascade of post-traumatic events involving hemodynamic, neuro-endocrine and inflammatory systems interactions, among others. Such varied multifactorial interactions lend themselves to complexity modeling because analyses performed to identify the onset of cardiovascular collapse reflect variable interactions rather than single parameter changes. Thus, the intrinsic variability of response among subjects that makes linear analysis of trauma/hemorrhagic shock difficult is actually a desired quality to build a predictive complexity model. The normal interaction between measured variables will be altered by responses to pathological insults. For example, failure of sympathetic drive and related endocrine response to trauma/hemorrhagic shock account for refractoriness to conventional resuscitation [16–21]. Failure of sympathetic/endocrine coupling effectors (e.g., epinephrine) and vascular endothelial-

Table 1 FDA-approved non-invasive non-traditional biosensors available and previously used by us

Sensor Name	Parameters measured	Manufacturer
Trendcare Multiparameter	Tissue PCO_2, PO_2, pH	Diametrics Medical
CritiView CRV3	Mitochondrial function ($NADH_2$ fluorescence), microcirculatory blood flow, volume and oxygenation	CritiSence Inc.
InSpectra	Tissue O_2 saturation	Hutchinson Industry
CV InSight	Vascular tone	iNTELOMED
Microscan	Microcirculatory flow	Microvision Medical
Cytoscan	Microcirculatory flow	Cytometrics
Clearsight finger plethysmograph	Blood pressure and cardiac output	Edwards Lifesciences
CNAP finger plethysmograph	Blood pressure and cardiac output	cnsystems
NICOM	Cardiac output, stroke volume variation, thoracic fluid	Cheetah Medical
Navigator-1	Mean systemic pressure, cardiac power	Applied Physiology

smooth muscle coupling may explain cardiovascular refractoriness and cardiovascular collapse in trauma/hemorrhagic shock [22]. Cellular energetic failure through impaired mitochondrial oxidative phosphorylation may further explain the vasodilatation seen in late stages of hemorrhagic shock similar to that reported in septic shock [23, 24]. Elevated $NADH_2$ levels mirror hypotension but often persist for several minutes during resuscitation despite restoration of MAP [25].

Extending Biosensor Utility Using Functional Hemodynamic Monitoring for Prediction

Fully half of all hemodynamically unstable ICU patients are not volume-responsive [26]. Estimates of preload (e.g., right [RV] or left [LV] ventricular volumes, intrathoracic blood volume or ventricular filling pressures) do not predict volume-responsiveness. Functional hemodynamic monitoring overcomes this limitation of traditional hemodynamic monitoring [27, 28]. In this case, functional hemodynamic monitoring uses a small volume loading challenge to perturb the cardiovascular autoregulatory function. Examples of preload challenges validated in multiple clinical trials include small rapid bolus volume infusions (i.e., fluid challenge), positive-pressure breathing [29] and passive leg-raising (PLR) to 30° [30]. If LV stroke volume increases transiently with these maneuvers, then cardiac output will also increase with subsequent fluid infusion. The degree of increase is quantified as the ratio of the maximal change in pulse pressure or stroke volume over 4–5 breaths or with PLR to the mean pulse pressure or stroke volume, referred to as pulse pressure variation (PPV) or stroke volume variation (SVV), respectively. The disadvantages of a traditional fluid challenge are that it takes time, often is given too slowly, thus masking volume responders, and is irreversible. Functional hemodynamic monitoring techniques give reliable predictions of preload response immediately and do not require fluid infusions to make this prediction. Both positive-pressure ventilation by physically decreasing venous return with inspiration and leg-raising by transiently increasing venous return fulfill these criteria [29, 30]. PPV and SVV can be easily monitored using several FDA-approved minimally invasive monitoring devices. Thus, in patients receiving positive-pressure breathing, simple inspection of the arterial PPV will continuously define volume responsiveness. The magnitude of PPV and SVV during ventilation will also be a function of the size of the tidal breath [31], thus this approach is only useful during controlled mechanical ventilation at a fixed tidal volume, which is not the case in spontaneously breathing patients. Furthermore, PPV and SVV do not reflect volume responsiveness in patients with atrial fibrillation where R-R intervals vary widely. However, a PLR maneuver with leg elevation to 30° displays the same predictive information in all patients [30]. We and others have extensively documented that a PPV > 13% or a SVV > 10% at a tidal volume of 7 ml/kg or a maximal increase in mean cardiac output > 10% during a PLR maneuver are predictive of preload responsiveness (> 90% sensitivity and specificity) [32]. Several minimally-invasive devices report cardiac output, PPV and SVV during positive-pressure breathing or change in cardiac output with PLR using arterial waveform analysis (e.g., PiCCO plus™ [Pulsion Medical Systems], LiDCO plus™ and LiDCO rapid™ [LiDCO Group Plc] and FloTrac™ [Edwards Lifesciences]). We have previously defined the operating characteristics and reliability of all these devices [33, 34]. Finally, the PPV/SVV ratio reflects central arterial elastance and can be used to monitor changes in vasomotor tone [12].

Importantly, FDA-approved non-invasive surrogate estimates of arterial pulse pressure and stroke volume exist, including pulse oximetry signal, bioreactance (NICOM, Cheetah) and transthoracic ultrasound (USCom) techniques. Pulse oximetry density profiles derived from the unprocessed pulse oximetry plethysmographic waveform amplitude (Nonin, Nelcor and Massimo), and pressure-sensitive optical sensors (BMEYE, Edwards Lifesciences) can be featurized to estimate pulse pressure, stroke volume and changing vasomotor tone [35]. The BMEYE pressure-sensitive, high fidelity, rapid-response optic sensor has the ability to track the arterial pressure profile to measure instantaneous cardiac output [36] and, along with the pulse oximetry plethysmographic profile, reflect two real-time waveform signals that we can use to extract predictive features of the cardiovascular system. Importantly, these non-invasive waveform data can be analyzed independent of their mean values and expand the utility of these analyses and predictive modeling beyond invasive monitoring to less invasive monitoring environments, markedly increasing generalizability of this featurized approach.

Non-Invasive Measures of Oxygen Sufficiency

An unanswered question in shock resuscitation is the relationship between tissue perfusion and wellness. Neither MAP, cardiac output or mixed venous oxygen

Fig. 3 Graphic display of the thenar tissue oxygen saturation (StO_2) at baseline and in response to a total vascular occlusion to a minimal StO_2 then release, referred to as a vascular occlusion test. Deoxygenation post-occlusion (DeO_2) and reoxygenation upon release (ReO_2)

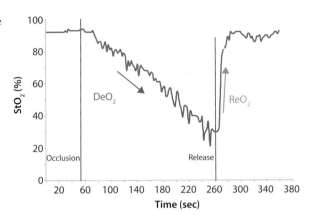

saturation (SvO_2) define tissue oxygenation. Near infra-red spectroscopy (NIRS) permits continuous, non-invasive measurement of StO_2. Although StO_2 values do not decrease until tissue perfusion is very low, StO_2 becomes more sensitive and specific when monitoring its change in response to a vascular occlusion test (VOT) (Fig. 3). If the StO_2 probe is placed on the thenar eminence and a downstream arm blood pressure cuff is inflated to a pressure higher than systolic arterial pressure and held there, total ischemia occurs. The occlusion is sustained until StO_2 decreases to $<40\%$ and then the cuff rapidly deflated. The StO_2 down slope is dependent on local metabolic rate and blood flow distribution. The StO_2 recovery rate assesses cardiovascular reserve, as we validated in trauma and septic patients compared to normal volunteers [37].

Predicting the Need for Life-Saving Interventions In Stat Medevac Air Transport

We assessed the predictive value of the VOT StO_2 and spot lactate levels in trauma patients during emergency air transport from an accident site. All patients were monitored using 3-lead EKG, non-invasive BP, HR, SpO_2, and when intubated, end-tidal CO_2 capnography. These single vital signs are not sensitive at identifying shock until advanced [38]. Protocol-based algorithms typically rely on individual vital signs or clinical parameters (e.g., cyanosis, altered mental status) to identify the need for life-saving interventions [39, 40] and subjective measures (mental status changes) are difficult to standardize [41]. We hypothesized that in-flight measures of VOT StO_2 and lactate would identify shock trauma subjects in need of life-saving interventions [42, 43]. We studied 400 transported trauma patients with lactate sampling and 194 patients also with VOT StO_2. Patients with pre-hospital lactate levels $>4\,mmol/l$ had greater need for emergent operation, intubation, and vasopressor (p = 0.02). This association persisted after adjustment for age, Glasgow Coma Scale (GCS) score and initial vital signs. The VOT StO_2 deoxygenation slopes were predictive of the need for life-saving interventions (p = 0.007), while a delayed reoxygenation slope was predictive of mortality (p = 0.006) [44]. These data collectively document that the measurement of readily available physiological variables when coupled to functional hemodynamic monitoring principles (PLR and VOT) can predict clinically relevant physiological states and the subsequent need for life-saving interventions.

Using Machine Learning Principles to Define Health and Disease

One never truly sees hypovolemia, sepsis, heart failure or ALI in the critically ill patients under our care, one sees the phenotypic physiological response of the host to these pathological processes. Thus, a fundamental aspect of both traditional monitoring and any novel approach is to identify normal biological variability and separate it out from adaptive/reflexive responses and pathological sequelae of these primary processes. For identification and predictive purposes this is very useful because most pathological process presenting as circulatory shock and respiratory insufficiency evolve over time. For example, hypovolemia in the setting of active intravascular volume loss starts with no measurable changes because the volume loss is so small. However, with progressive volume loss by any mechanism (hemorrhage, 3rd space loss, diarrhea), adaptive processes and hemodynamic phenotypic signatures evolve which may not be easily identified early on using primary mean hemodynamic values. However, derived parameters, based on validated machine learning approaches, such as the artificial neuronet of interacting variables or SampEn of time series single source data, can markedly improve the early identification of critical illness. Thus, we hypothesize that by advanced analysis of existing biological data series, one can detect adaptive and maladaptive processes earlier than we presently do such that definitive therapy can be started to reverse these processes before they become severe, induce remote organ injury or become irreversible. For example, an acute asthma attack can often be easily reversible with simple inhalational bronchodilators, whereas if the same process is left untreated until severe status asthmaticus, much more aggressive therapies need to be given to reverse the same process. And this disease and those required therapies (e.g., steroids) markedly increase morbidity and mortality.

Thus, the process of creating accurate sensitive and specific alerts and decision support systems is both iterative and based on creating libraries of 'normal' and 'not-normal' physiological interactions or 'behaviors', and to have a deeper understanding of the fuzziness of the boundary of normality for each of these behaviors. For example, one could use the previously described baseline porcine data prior to trauma/hemorrhagic shock to 'train' the model as to normal biological variability. We will then use the bleeding time, changes in endotoxin infusion, burn or smoke inhalation as time-dependent pathological stressors to calibrate the 'not-normal' states, as described below. We then use these relatively pure pathological insults to define process-specific signatures of disease to identify both the pathological process and its severity. Inherent in this analysis is that if therapy reverses these pathological processes, the derived measure of disease also decreases.

Three major barriers arise when iterating clinical data based on animal experimental data. First, our patient cohorts are often not previously healthy and then subjected to a defined relatively pure insult. They arrive in varying states of illness, preexisting co-morbidities and ongoing therapies. Using a young trauma cohort for initial model development may minimize this effect. Second, human data are typically not as rich in terms of frequency and number of variables collected given field conditions and other pragmatic reasons. Patients get disconnected from monitoring devices for various reasons (e.g., X-rays, turning), EKG electrodes and pulse oximeter probes fall off and primary signals can be inaccurate (clotted catheter). Thus, an initial data processing aspect of any model building needs to review these data streams and identify gaps in data flow and artifacts. Finally, one cannot truly define 'normal' in our critically ill patients, only normal behavior. For example, an animal in hemorrhagic shock may appear to be normal based on measured variables and derived parameters if they are also getting vasopressor therapy. Thus, the best we can do across all pathophysiological domains is to report not-normal and stability, both of which must be interpreted within the context of therapy.

Within these constraints, one must first determine the minimal data set (independent monitored signal, sampling frequency and lead time) required to identify not-normal with an acceptable level of false alerts and long enough lead time to overt disease expression as to be clinically relevant. We refer to this approach as "hemodynamic monitoring parsimony". Intuitively, one expects tradeoffs between parsimony, lead time and accuracy. Initially, a 15 min advanced warning may be the minimal lead time for cardiorespiratory instability to be clinically relevant. Once an alert of not-normal is made, one may sequentially insert additional measures to determine their ability to improve sensitivity and specificity of these alerts in defining specific disease processes so as to guide therapy. The concept of monitoring parsimony extends beyond hemodynamic monitoring. As the ability to merge hemodynamic data with other clinically relevant data streams, it is expected that a parsimonious set of clinical features useful to cardiorespiratory instability detection and prediction will include non-hemodynamic data as well.

How do we put all of this together? At the mathematical level there are two main problems. The first is how to predict the occurrence of events in data rich scenarios, such as in our porcine data, and the second is how to do the same in humans, which usually will involve only a few biomarkers. In addition, why do we need animal models to predict human behavior? Cannot this analysis be done completely on the human data using only a few biomarkers such as BP, HR, respiratory, SpO_2 and minimally invasive measures? Our preliminary analysis of the porcine dataset, which involves many biomarkers, and VSI human data involving the four physiological variables mentioned above [4–6] suggest that our insight can be improved tremendously by using the animal data. It is possible that the variables we use now from the animal trauma/hemorrhagic shock model are not the best for human instability prediction. For example, the grouping and its variation over time is not apparent in the small human dataset we collected of trauma SDU patients [6]. The animal models that are very close to human disease will allow us to gain a much better understanding of the dynamic features and which of these are the important players at different stages of stress, compensation, resuscitation, recovery and death. These animal analyses may also suggest which variables can be omitted in certain cases, and what omission implies about disease level and adaptation, etc. We hypothesize that data-driven prediction modeling approaches will enable healthcare professionals both at the bedside and in remote settings to predict those patients most likely to develop future instability. We also hypothesize that dynamic systems modeling will further improve prediction, including the provision of various signatures for instability subtype. This is and will continue to be an amazing and informative journey.

Acknowledgement

This work was supported in part by NIH grant NR013912.

References

1. Goodrich C (2006) Endpoints of resuscitation: what should we be monitoring? AACN Adv Crit Care 17:306–316
2. Hravnak M, DeVita M, Edwards L, Clontz A, Valenta C, Pinsky MR (2008) Cardiorespiratory instability before and after implementing an integrated monitoring system. Am J Respir Crit Care Med 177:A842 (abst)
3. Tarassenko L, Hann A, Young D (2006) Integrated monitoring and analysis for early warning of patient deterioration. Br J Anaesth 97:64–68
4. Hravnak M, Edwards L, Clontz A, Valenta C, DeVita M, Pinsky MR (2008) Defining the incidence of cardio-respiratory instability in step-down unit patients using an electronic integrated monitoring system. Arch Intern Med 168:1300–1308
5. Hravnak M, Edwards L, Foster-Heasley M et al (2007) Electronic integrated monitoring of medical emergency team calls to a step down unit. Circulation 116(II):939 (abst)
6. Hravnak M, DeVita MA, Clontz A, Edwards L, Valenta C, Pinsky MR (2011) Cardiorespiratory Instability Before and After Implementing an Integrated Monitoring System. Crit Care Med 39:65–72
7. Knaus WA, Wagner DP, Draper EA et al (1991) The APACHE III prognostic system. Risk prediction of hospital mortality for critically ill hospitalized adults. Chest 100:1619–1636
8. Zimmerman JE, Kramer AA, McNair DS, Malila FM (2006) Acute Physiology and Chronic Health Evaluation (APACHE) IVL hospital mortality assessment for today's critically ill patients. Crit Care Med 34:1297–1310
9. Smith GB, Prytherch DR, Schmidt PE et al (2008) Should age be included as a component of track and trigger systems used to identify sick adult patients? Resuscitation 78:109–115
10. Yousef K, Pinsky MR, DeVita MA, Sereika S, Hravnak M (2012) Demographic and clinical predictors of cardiorespiratory instability in a step-down unit: pilot study. Am J Crit Care 21:344–350
11. Batchinsky AI, Salina J, Kuusela T, Necsoiu C, Jones J, Cancio LC (2009) Rapid prediction of trauma patients survival by analysis of heart rate complexity: impact of reducing data set size. Shock 32:565–571
12. Cancio LC, Batchinsky AI, Salinas J et al (2008) Heart-rate complexity for prediction of prehospital lifesaving interventions in trauma patients. J Trauma 65:813–819
13.

Batchinsky AI, Salinas J, Jones JA, Necsoiu C, Cancio LC (2009) Predicting the need to perform life-saving interventions in trauma patients using new vital signs and artificial neural networks. Lecture Notes in Computer Science. Springer, Berlin

14. Ogundele O, Clermont G, Sileanu F, Pinsky MR (2013) Use of derived physiologic variable to predict individual patients' probability of hemodynamic instability. Am J Respir Crit Care Med 187:A5067 (abst)

15. Zenker S, Polanco PM, Kim HK et al (2007) Threshold area over the curve of spectrometric tissue oxygen saturation as an indicator of volume resuscitability in an acute porcine model of hemorrhagic shock. J Trauma 63:573–580

16. Gannon TA, Britt RC, Weireter LJ, Cole FJ, Collins JN, Britt LD (2006) Adrenal insufficiency in the critically III trauma population. Am Surg 72:373–376

17. Porter MH, Cutchins A, Fine JB, Bai Y, DiGirolamo M (2002) Effects of TNF-alpha on glucose metabolism and lipolysis in adipose tissue and isolated fat-cell preparations. J Lab Clin Med 139:140–146

18. Helling TS (2005) The liver and hemorrhagic shock. J Am Coll Surg 201:774–783

19. Evans DA, Jacobs DO, Wilmore DW (1989) Tumor necrosis factor enhances glucose uptake by peripheral tissues. Am J Physiol 257:R1182–R1189

20. Chang CG, Van Way CW 3rd, Dhar A, Helling T Jr, Hahn Y (2000) The use of insulin and glucose during resuscitation from hemorrhagic shock increases hepatic ATP. J Surg Res 92:171–176

21. Carey LC, Curtin R, Sapira JD (1976) Influence of hemorrhage on adrenal secretion, blood glucose and serum insulin in the awake pig. Ann Surg 183:185–192

22. Landry DW, Oliver JA (2001) The pathogenesis of vasodilatory shock. N Engl J Med 345:588–595

23. Singer M (2007) Mitochondrial function in sepsis: acute phase versus multiple organ failure. Crit Care Med 35:441–448

24. Leverve XM (2007) Mitochondrial function and substrate availability. Crit Care Med 35:S454–S460

25. Clavijo-Alvarez JA, Sims CA, Soller B, Pinsky MR, Puyana JC (2005) Monitoring skeletal muscle and subcutaneous tissue acid-base status and oxygenation during hemorrhagic shock and resuscitation. Shock 24:270–275

26. Michard F, Teboul JL (2002) Predicting fluid responsiveness in ICU patients: A critical analysis of the evidence. Chest 212:2000–2008

27. Pinsky MR (2007) Hemodynamic evaluation and monitoring in the ICU. Chest 123:2020–2029

28. Pinsky MR (2009) Functional hemodynamic monitoring: use of derived variable to diagnose and manage the critically ill. Acta Anaesthesiol Scand 53(suppl 119):9–11

29. Michard F, Chemla D, Richard C et al (1999) Clinical use of respiratory changes in arterial pulse pressure to monitor the hemodynamic effects of PEEP. Am J Respir Crit Care Med 159:935–939

30. Monnet X, Rienzo M, Osman D et al (2006) Response to leg raising predicts fluid responsiveness in critically ill. Crit Care Med 34:1402–1407

31. Kim HK, Pinsky MR (2008) Effect of tidal volume, sampling duration and cardiac contractility on pulse pressure and stroke volume variation during positive-pressure ventilation. Crit Care Med 36:2858–2862

32. Pinsky MR (2009) Functional hemodynamic monitoring: A personal perspective. In: Vincent JL (ed) Yearbook of Emergency and Intensive Care Medicine. Springer-Verlag, Berlin, pp 306–310

33. Marquez J, McCurry K, Severyn DA, Pinsky MR (2008) Ability of pulse power, esophageal Doppler and arterial pressure to estimate rapid changes in stroke volume in humans. Crit Care Med 36:3001–3007

34. Hadian M, Kim HK, Severyn D, Pinsky MR (2010) Cross-comparison of continuous cardiac output trending accuracy of LiDCO, PiCCO, FloTrac and pulmonary artery catheters. Crit Care 14:R212

35. Cannesson M, Besnard C, Durand PG, Bohé J, Jacques D (2005) Relation between respiratory variations in pulse oximetry plethysmographic waveform amplitude and arterial pulse pressure in ventilated patients. Crit Care 9:R562–R568

36. Benomar B, Quattara A, Estagnasie P, Brusset A, Squara P (2010) Fluid responsiveness predicted by non-invasive bioreactance-based passive leg raise test. Intensive Care Med 36:1875–1881

37. Gomez H, Torres A, Zenker S et al (2008) Use of non-invasive NIRS during vascular occlusion test to assess dynamic tissue O2 saturation response. Intensive Care Med 34:1600–1607

38. Wo CCJ, Shoemaker WC, Appel PL et al (1993) Unreliability of blood pressure and heart rate to evaluate cardiac output in emergency resuscitation and critical illness. Crit Care Med 21:218–223

39. Holcomb JB, Niles SE, Miller CC, Hinds D, Duke JH, Moore FA (2005) Prehospital physiologic data and lifesaving interventions in trauma patients. Mil Med 170:7–13

40. Holcomb JB, Salinas J, McManus JJ, Miller CC, Cooke WH, Convertino VA (2005) Manual vital signs reliably predict need for life-saving interventions in trauma patients. J Trauma 59:821–829

41. Porter JM, Ivatury RR (1998) In search of the optimal end points of resuscitation in trauma patients: a review. J Trauma 44:908–914

42. Guyette FX, Suffoletto BP, Castillio JL, Puyana JC (2009) Identification of occult shock using out-of-hospital lactate. Ann Emerg Med 54:S142 (abst)

43. Castillio JL, Guyette FX, Suffoletto BP, Peitzman AB, Puyana JC (2009) The role of prehospital lactate as a predictor of outcomes in trauma patients. J Trauma 63:S138 (abst)

44. Guyette F, Gomez H, Suffoletto B et al (2009) Prehospital dynamic tissue O2 saturation response predicts in-hospital mortality in trauma patients. Crit Care Med 37(12 Suppl):A28 (abst)

Long-Term Outcomes After Critical Illness Relevant to Randomized Clinical Trials

C. L. Hodgson, N. R. Watts, and T. J. Iwashyna

Introduction

The traditional goal of intensive care has been to prevent death. Intensive care units (ICUs) are getting better at this with data from several sources suggesting that mortality rates are declining [1]. Many survivors have long-term, sometimes permanent, impairment of one or more aspects of physical, psychological or cognitive function [2–5]. Declining mortality rates may be producing a new and as yet unmet health care need: an increasing number of patients who have survived treatment in an ICU but with incomplete functional recovery leading to poor long-term outcomes [2, 6, 7].

In this context, there is an urgent need to accurately describe the longer term outcomes of ICU survivors to gain a more complete understanding of physical function, cognitive ability and other attributes. Specific tools may be already available or may need to be developed to meet the needs of the varied stakeholders involved – clinicians, researchers, patients, health care service providers and industry.

On behalf of the Australian and New Zealand Intensive Care Society Clinical Trials Group Working Party on Long-Term Outcomes

C. L. Hodgson
Australian and New Zealand Intensive Care Research Center, Monash University
Melbourne, Australia
Physiotherapy Department, The Alfred Hospital
Melbourne, Australia

N. R. Watts
Division of Critical Care and Trauma, The George Institute for Global Health
Sydney, Australia

T. J. Iwashyna (✉)
Department of Internal Medicine, University of Michigan
Ann Arbor, USA
Center for Clinical Management Research, VA Ann Arbor Health System
Ann Arbor, USA
email: tiwashyn@umich.edu

© Springer International Publishing Switzerland 2016
J.-L. Vincent (ed.), *Annual Update in Intensive Care and Emergency Medicine 2016*,
DOI 10.1007/978-3-319-27349-5_37

In this chapter, we highlight the need to be able to describe the long-term outcomes of patients who survive critical illness and highlight some early international initiatives to develop a standardized approach to this for clinical trials.

Short-Term Physiological Outcomes and Mortality Versus Long-Term Functional Assessment

The decompressive craniectomy in diffuse traumatic brain injury (TBI) trial (DE-CRA) randomized 155 patients to early decompressive craniectomy (intervention) or non-surgical standard care (control) [8]. The intervention was associated with a substantial immediate reduction in intracranial pressure (ICP), fewer days of mechanical ventilation and shorter length of stay, with no difference in mortality. If this trial had used these endpoints, it could have been suggested that decompressive craniectomy was safe and effective for this patient population.

However, the results for the designated primary outcome for the study, the extended Glasgow Outcome Scale (GOS-E) at 6 months, a measure of functional recovery, provided a very different conclusion: patients who underwent craniectomy were much more likely to survive with severe disability or in a vegetative state than those who did not have craniectomy (70% vs 51%, p = 0.02) indicating that early decompressive craniectomy was harmful (Fig. 1). This example illustrates the importance of considering the impact of treatments on long-term patient-centered outcomes, rather than focusing on short-term effects on physiology and mortality.

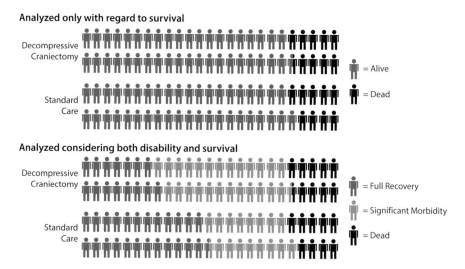

Fig. 1 Two analyses of the same trial highlight the need to consider long-term outcomes other than mortality. Data from DECRA [8]

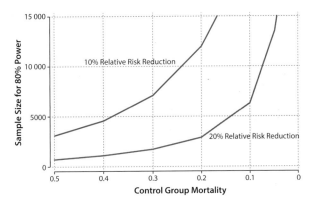

Fig. 2 Sample size calculations for mortality in ICU trials with mortality as the endpoint

Declining Mortality Rates Mean That Clinical Trials Using Mortality May Be Unfeasible

Survival rates have improved across many patient groups admitted to the ICU, including severe sepsis [1], TBI [9] and patients mechanically ventilated for greater than 12 h [10]. This may be due to many factors, including improved quality of ICU care [11], earlier recognition of deterioration (for example the use of medical emergency teams [12]) or improved health systems [13]. The improved survival rates for ICU patients have had a substantial effect on sample size calculations for clinical trials that have mortality as a primary endpoint. With declining mortality in the ICU, the size of clinical trials required to detect feasible relative risk reductions is increasing substantially. For example, if control group mortality is 20% and you power a study for a 20% relative risk reduction, the sample size required is 2,894. However, if testing a therapy with the same relative risk reduction but in a population with control group mortality of 10%, the sample size required is 6426 patients. The increase in sample size is exponential thereafter, and even steeper for interventions with a more modest 10% relative risk reduction (Fig. 2). It is therefore likely that relying on mortality as a primary endpoint will become impractical, and alternative outcome measures will need to be considered.

Prior Approaches to Describing Long-Term Outcome in Australia and New Zealand

Clinical trials have traditionally focused on mortality as the primary outcome and have rarely used long-term (non-mortality) outcomes as the primary endpoint. We conducted a review of all past or current randomized clinical trials that were endorsed by the Australia and New Zealand Clinical Trials Group (ANZICS-CTG) and that measured any patient-reported outcome at a minimum of six months after intensive care admission. We identified 21 randomized clinical trials and one observational study. In these 22 studies, 16 different long-term outcomes measures were

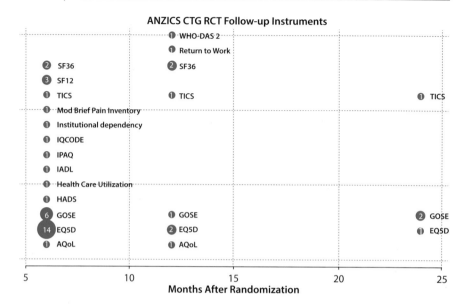

Fig. 3 Instruments used by the Australia and New Zealand Clinical Trials Group (*ANZICS-CTG*) in intensive care unit (*ICU*) clinical trials to measure long-term follow-up over the past decade. Not shown: 48-month dialysis use, SF-12 and EQ5D from POST-RENAL. *SF*: Short Form; *GOS*: Glasgow Outcome Scale; *HADS*: Hospital Anxiety and Depression Scale; *IADL*: Instrumental Activities of Daily Living; *IPAQ*: International Physical Activity Questionnaire; *IQCODE*: Informant Questionnaire on Cognitive Decline in the Elderly

used. The majority (14 of 22, 64%) of studies measured health-related quality of life as a secondary outcome using the EQ-5D at 6 months, with TBI trials measuring the GOS-E (Fig. 3). Four studies used the Short Form 12 (SF-12) and four the Short Form 36 (SF-36).

International Collaboration and Consensus on Measuring Long-Term Outcomes

Over a decade ago, at the Brussels Round Table on surviving ICU [6], key questions included whether treatments in the ICU would change if their effects on long-term outcomes were known. Recommendations from this Round Table were that clinical trials include measures of long-term follow-up of health-related quality of life, functional status and costs of care. A decade later, the Society of Critical Care Medicine Stakeholders' Conference on improving long-term outcomes after discharge from the ICU [4] reported ongoing research gaps related to mechanisms and epidemiology of post-ICU impairments, design of post-ICU interventions and links between physical function, cognition and mental health. A new Round Table meeting is being convened in 2016.

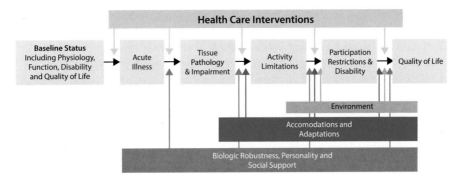

Fig. 4 Measuring long-term outcomes, including impairment, activity limitations, disability and health-related quality of life. Potential interventions and uncontrolled effect modifiers are shown as *vertical arrows*. Reproduced from [23]

The default for measuring long-term outcome in clinical trials in the past has been a measure of health-related quality of life [6]. It has been argued that health-related quality of life is patient-centered, can measure long-term health and well-being and has the additional benefit of allowing health economic evaluation [14]. However, health-related quality of life does not include important information about organ impairment, cognitive impairment, activity limitation, disability and other aspects of the recovery included in the international classification of function (Fig. 4) [15]. Additionally, generic measures (e.g., SF-36, EQ-5D) are not particularly sensitive in disease-specific groups [16].

Pros and Cons of Standardizing Outcomes Assessment

With growing numbers of trials in Australia, New Zealand and around the world collecting outcomes at 6 months and later, there are movements to standardize the measures they collect. The goal of such standardization is to ensure that all future clinical trials include the same reproducible outcome measures to allow comparability between studies. There are strong benefits of standardizing core outcome sets across clinical trials including: (1) improved signal detection in systematic reviews; (2) preventing selective reporting; and (3) enhanced comparability across trials [17]. Standardization facilitates comparison across trials, including the potential for individual patient meta-analysis, with the ability to conduct secondary analyses to explore subgroup response to interventions.

Standardizing core outcome sets may solve the problem of comparability between studies for trials focused on long-term outcomes, but careful consideration and testing of the outcome measures is needed. Clinical trials are the foundation of evidence-based practice and, as such, it is crucial that the data generated is rigorous. This is achieved through appropriate selection and definition of primary and secondary outcome measures. However, investigators conducting similar trials may not measure the same trial outcomes and, where similar outcomes are measured, they are not measured consistently [17]. The need to pick one and only one primary randomized clinical trial endpoint for sample size calculations also highlights the dangers of premature standardization. If a therapy has targeted benefits, then standardization to an endpoint that imperfectly measures the specific domain of benefit would increase measurement error and decreases the power of an randomized trial to detect a real effect. That is, standardization may encourage investigators (or funding bodies) to use outcomes for clinical trials that may not be able to detect an effect that is truly beneficial or harmful.

International Efforts to Standardize Outcomes or International Consensus Process

In 2008, the International Forum for Acute Care Trialists (InFACT) was launched as a network of investigator-led clinical research groups and academic institutions whose focus is the optimal care of acutely ill patients. Its vision is "to improve the care of acutely ill patients around the world by promoting high quality clinical research into the causes, prevention, and optimal management of acute, life-threatening illness" [18]. Members include over 20 organizations from around the world, including the ANZICS-CTG. InFACT believes the globalization of critical care trials requires consensus on core outcomes, with strong regional input required for agreement on both definitions and outcomes.

Complementing InFACT's efforts and coordinated with them, Prof Dale Needham, Director of the Outcomes After Critical Illness and Surgery (OACIS) Group at Johns Hopkins University School of Medicine, leads a systematic effort to define the psychometric properties of existing measures; develop a website for dissemination [19]; and broadly engage representatives in a Delphi process on selecting core outcome measures for acute respiratory failure. Similarly, Bronagh Blackwood and the COVenT study group are working to develop a core outcome set for trials aiming to reduce lung injury from or duration of mechanical ventilation [20].

These are examples of international work examining core outcomes for trials in acutely and critically ill patients with the aim of standardizing core outcome measures and instruments for randomized clinical trials.

ANZICS-CTG Long-Term Outcomes Program

The ANZICS-CTG have recently convened a Working Party on long-term outcomes after critical illness. The Working Party's goals are to make recommendations for a standardized set of long-term outcomes that should be incorporated into all ANZICS-CTG trials, to recommend a single scale for a non-mortality primary endpoint (if local consensus is possible), and to achieve this in an expedited fashion, given that several major CTG randomized clinical trials are in a late planning stage.

Based on our existing review of the literature, we do not believe that there are sufficient data to unequivocally recommend one primary outcome measure as most appropriate for all patient groups. We have therefore initiated a multi-pronged research agenda to provide a more robust evidence base for outcome selection within ANZCIS-CTG trials, and to contribute to international efforts to standardize outcome measures. A few tenets guide this program:

- Outcome scales should measure things valued by patients.
- Outcome scales should be persuasive to clinicians.
- Outcome measures should exhibit reliability, validity and responsiveness.
- In-person assessments that require return to hospital may not be feasible for many in Australia and New Zealand and carry risk of an unacceptable number of patients being lost to follow up.
- Costs are an essential aspect of feasibility.
- Linkages to existing registries that already collect outcome measure (for example, death or readmission to hospital) should be investigated and optimized.

Projects initiated through the program are outlined below.

Patient-Centered Outcomes

Outcome scales should measure things valued by patients, and it is unclear from our existing health-related quality of life scales whether the current domains reflect those that are most valued by patients. In particular, it is important to determine whether there are domains missing from the existing scales that patients value highly and should be included in future research. To this end, we are conducting qualitative studies of ICU survivors to determine patients' values, preferences, and needs. This will inform future work on patient-centered long-term outcomes and will contribute to similar work being conducted internationally, adding to the existing body of knowledge in this area.

Additionally, we are considering a range of patient-centered outcomes including days alive and out of hospital (including rehabilitation/nursing home), an outcome measure that encompasses death, hospital stay, need for ongoing rehabilitation, and re-admission. It reflects personal, social and economic benefits. We are also testing various measures of disability, including the World Health Organization's Disability Assessment Scale which has a direct link to the International Classification of Function [21].

Clinician Opinion

The ANZICS-CTG have worked in collaboration with Prof Dale Needham and colleagues at Johns Hopkins, to solicit clinician and researcher input on the domains that should be included in a core outcome set for research on long-term outcomes following acute respiratory failure. This work has included a structured deliberation process that occurred this year in both the USA and Australia and that will result in an international comparative list of domains considered important for future research in studies of long-term outcomes for patients following respiratory failure. This preliminary work will inform a future Delphi process led by Prof Needham and lead to further investigation of clinicians' opinions across Australian and New Zealand stakeholder groups (e.g., rehabilitation clinicians, psychologists, general practitioners).

Remote Monitoring

In-person assessments that require return to the hospital are not feasible in Australian and New Zealand CTG studies because of the long distance many people live from the treating hospital. One solution to this problem may be to use remote monitoring devices. A recent study found that many smartphone applications and wearable devices produced accurate results when compared with direct observation of step counts, a metric which has been successfully used in interventions to improve clinical outcomes [22]. This study was conducted in healthy American college students, and the accuracy of these applications and devices in other populations, such as post-intensive care, is unknown. However, this may be an important area of future research, particularly in large multicenter trials that limit face-to-face follow-up. We plan to test remote monitoring devices in the ICU population to determine reliability, feasibility and validity against other standard measures of step count and walking.

Registry Linkage

Evaluating hospital outcomes and risk prediction is an integral part of the reporting and benchmarking achieved by the ANZICS Centre for Outcome and Resource Evaluation (CORE). We plan to expand the data recorded within the CORE database to include hospital readmissions, long-term mortality and disability, in order to capture long-term outcomes and associated costs beyond hospital discharge. This will be facilitated by linkage with large national registries, for example the Australian Rehabilitation Outcome Registry.

Conclusion

The increased numbers of survivors of critical illness has resulted in international interest in the quality of survival. Mortality rates in clinical trials may need to be qualified by an understanding of the recovery profile of survivors to measure the true effectiveness of ICU interventions. Measures of quality of survival need to be patient-centered, reliable, valid and responsive. While patient preferences should be paramount, they also need to be persuasive to multidisciplinary clinicians. The application of such measures may eventually facilitate decision-making in clinical practice, assist in the translation of research findings, and also help with the planning of health care resource use.

Acknowledgements

This manuscript was written on behalf of the ANZICS-CTG Long-Term Outcome Working Party, including Rinaldo Bellomo, Jamie Cooper, Simon Finfer, Lisa Higgins, Imogen Mitchell, Lynne Murray, Neil Orford, David Pilcher, Manoj Saxena and Paul Young. This work was supported by the National Health and Medical Research Council of Australia as part of a Fellowship scheme (CH). We appreciate the assistance of Madeline Page Cenedese in conducting the review of ANZICS-CTG randomized clinical trials.

References

1. Kaukonen KM, Bailey M, Suzuki S, Pilcher D, Bellomo R (2014) Mortality related to severe sepsis and septic shock among critically ill patients in Australia and New Zealand, 2000–2012. JAMA 311:1308–1316
2. Herridge MS, Tansey CM, Matte A et al (2011) Functional disability 5 years after acute respiratory distress syndrome. N Engl J Med 364:1293–1304
3. Pandharipande PP, Girard TD, Jackson JC et al (2013) Long-term cognitive impairment after critical illness. N Engl J Med 369:1306–1316
4. Needham DM, Davidson J, Cohen H et al (2012) Improving long-term outcomes after discharge from intensive care unit: report from a stakeholders' conference. Crit Care Med 40:502–509
5. The TEAM Study Investigators (2015) Early mobilization and recovery in mechanically ventilated patients in the ICU: a bi-national, multi-centre, prospective cohort study. Crit Care 19:81
6. Angus DC, Carlet J (2003) Surviving intensive care: a report from the 2002 Brussels Roundtable. Intensive Care Med 29:368–377
7. Cuthbertson BH, Roughton S, Jenkinson D, Maclennan G, Vale L (2010) Quality of life in the five years after intensive care: a cohort study. Crit Care 14:R6
8. Cooper DJ, Rosenfeld JV, Murray L et al (2011) Decompressive craniectomy in diffuse traumatic brain injury. N Engl J Med 364:1493–1502
9. Gabbe BJ, Simpson PM, Sutherland AM et al (2012) Improved functional outcomes for major trauma patients in a regionalized, inclusive trauma system. Ann Surg 255:1009–1015
10. Esteban A, Frutos-Vivar F, Muriel A et al (2013) Evolution of mortality over time in patients receiving mechanical ventilation. Am J Respir Crit Care Med 88:220–230
11. Berenholtz SM, Dorman T, Ngo K, Pronovost PJ (2002) Qualitative review of intensive care unit quality indicators. J Crit Care 17:1–12
12. Jones D, Egi M, Bellomo R, Goldsmith D (2007) Effect of the medical emergency team on long-term mortality following major surgery. Crit Care 11:R12
13. Cameron PA, Gabbe BJ, Cooper DJ, Walker T, Judson R, McNeil J (2008) A statewide system of trauma care in Victoria: effect on patient survival. Med J Aust 189:546–550
14. Angus DC, Musthafa AA, Clermont G et al (2001) Quality-adjusted survival in the first year after the acute respiratory distress syndrome. Am J Respir Crit Care Med 163:1389–1394
15. Iwashyna TJ (2012) Trajectories of recovery and dysfunction after acute illness, with implications for clinical trial design. Am J Respir Crit Care Med 86:302–304
16. Wiebe S, Guyatt G, Weaver B, Matijevic S, Sidwell C (2003) Comparative responsiveness of generic and specific quality-of-life instruments. J Clin Epidemiol 56:52–60
17. Blackwood B, Clarke M, McAuley DF, McGuigan PJ, Marshall JC, Rose L (2014) How outcomes are defined in clinical trials of mechanically ventilated adults and children. Am J Respir Crit Care Med 89:886–893
18. International Forum for Acute Care Trialists. http://www.infactglobal.org

19. Improving Long-Term Outcomes Research for Acute Respiratory Failure. http://www.infactglobal.org
20. Blackwood B, Ringrow S, Clarke M et al (2015) Core Outcomes in Ventilation Trials (COVenT): protocol for a core outcome set using a Delphi survey with a nested randomised trial and observational cohort study. Trials 16:368
21. Von Korff M, Crane PK, Alonso J et al (2008) Modified WHODAS-II provides valid measure of global disability but filter items increased skewness. J Clin Epidemiol 61:1132–1143
22. Case MA, Burwick HA, Volpp KG, Patel MS (2015) Accuracy of smartphone applications and wearable devices for tracking physical activity data. JAMA 313:625–626
23. Iwashyna TJ, Odden AJ (2013) Sepsis after Scotland: enough with the averages, show us the effect modifiers. Crit Care 17:148

Long-Term Consequences of Acute Inflammation in the Surgical Patient: New Findings and Perspectives

P. Forget

Introduction

Perioperative inflammation is now considered not only as a therapeutic target but is also included in new screening strategies, patient stratification, preoperative optimization, especially in cancer, and also in the frail patient at risk of infectious and ischemic complications.

Acute Inflammation in Cancer Surgery

Acute inflammation is clearly associated with the natural history of cancer [1]. At least for solid tumors, surgery can be curative. Unfortunately, rapid recurrences can occur after surgery with, sometimes, evidence of accelerated growth of metastases, probably linked to the perioperative, acute inflammatory reaction [2]. More than 10 years ago, a bimodal pattern of postoperative cancer relapse was suggested. This was shown in breast cancer patients treated only by mastectomy by different teams [3–6]. Analysis of these databases showed an early peak of relapses during the first two years. Most of the relapses (50–80%) occurred during this early peak. The time of occurrence of early relapses seemed to be chronologically related to surgery. Is this surprising? Probably not so much if we remember that surgery induces some pro-inflammatory pathways that are not only associated with the necessary mechanisms of wound healing but are also typically described as part of the cancer pathophysiology [7] (Fig. 1).

P. Forget (✉)
Department of Anesthesiology, Cliniques Universitaires Saint-Luc
Brussels, Belgium
Institute of Neuroscience, Université Catholique de Louvain
Brussels, Belgium
email: forgetpatrice@yahoo.fr

© Springer International Publishing Switzerland 2016
J.-L. Vincent (ed.), *Annual Update in Intensive Care and Emergency Medicine 2016*,
DOI 10.1007/978-3-319-27349-5_38

VASCULAR DISEASE

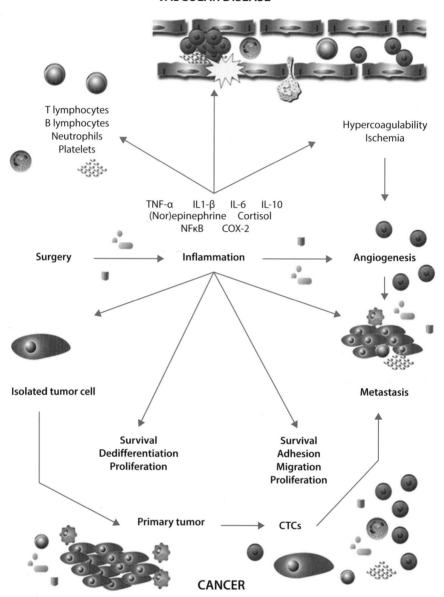

T lymphocytes
B lymphocytes
Neutrophils
Platelets

Hypercoagulability
Ischemia

TNF-α   IL1-β   IL-6   IL-10
(Nor)epinephrine   Cortisol
NFκB   COX-2

Surgery ⟶ Inflammation ⟶ Angiogenesis

Isolated tumor cell

Metastasis

Survival
Dedifferentiation
Proliferation

Survival
Adhesion
Migration
Proliferation

Primary tumor ⟶ CTCs

CANCER

Fig. 1 Surgery and inflammation are closely associated, and linked to mechanisms promoting tumor growth, such as atherothrombotic complications. At the time of the extirpation of the tumor, the incidence of circulating tumor cells (*CTCs*) depends on several mechanisms, including the inflammatory environment around the tumor itself. Inflammation promotes escape into the bloodstream, but also growth of metastases. Platelets can be involved in this dissemination process, by adhesion mechanisms and/or by the synthesis of mediators. Immune cells could participate in the elimination of cancer cells (B and T lymphocytes, neutrophils) and in the suppression of the immune response (neutrophils). Cyclooxygenase (*COX*)-2 is overexpressed in tumor cells and in immune suppressor cells, like macrophages. Prostaglandin E2 (*PGE2*) can promote growth of the tumor directly and indirectly, via suppression of cellular-mediated immunity. The cytokines interleukin (*IL*)-1β, IL-6 and tumor necrosis factor (*TNF*)-α can also directly suppress the activity of immune cells and promote the number and the activation of suppressor cells. All these factors have also been implicated in hypercoagulability, ischemia, and atherothrombotic complications after surgery, suggesting common mechanisms. *NF-kB*: nuclear factor-kappa B. Adapted from [7] with permission

Acute Inflammation in Non-Cancer Surgery

In non-cancer surgery, a dysregulated inflammatory reaction is also associated with worse outcome. Early mortality is probably due to the combination of surgical insult (in major surgery), concurrent medical problems and a low physiological reserve, all of which can worsen immune reactivity. As identifying which patients are at greatest risk of developing complications and which types of complications are life-threatening is essential, could we propose inflammation as an early therapeutic target to improve outcome? Two phenomena, not mutually exclusive, could explain worse outcomes in patients with persisting inflammation. The first is the cumulative effect of a persistent acute inflammatory response. The second is a later response, more toxic and different in nature. Indeed, the acute inflammatory response can be observed minutes after a vascular lesion or an acute ischemic event [8]. This response is characterized by increases in interleukin (IL)-1β and IL-6 secretion, at least partially by activated neutrophils (Fig. 1). Cross-talk between neutrophils and platelets permits platelet activation. This cross-talk occurs rapidly and participates in the destabilization of atherosclerotic plaques, enhances coagulation and perpetuates thrombus formation. Neutrophils then induce secretion of growth factors, reactive-oxygen species (ROS), prostaglandins, tumor necrosis factor (TNF)-α and enzymes, which induce further vascular damage.

This suggestion is supported by observations in elderly patients after hip fracture. The main causes of death at 3 months after hip fracture are cardiovascular complications and chest infection [9]. Indeed, many recent studies have highlighted the neutrophil-to-lymphocyte ratio (NLR) as a 'new cardiovascular risk factor', which may improve patient screening. A recent observational study including diabetic patients with a follow-up of four years showed that the NLR was an independent predictor of major cardiac events [10]. In this cohort, patients with an NLR > 2.4 had a significantly worse survival rate (21.4% vs 5.3%) than those with an NLR < 1.6. This attractive role of a high NLR to predict cardiovascular outcome and early postoperative mortality has been confirmed by others [11–15].

The Vision

The Neutrophil-to-Lymphocyte Ratio Emerges as a Screening and a Stratification Tool

Various inflammatory markers have been proposed for use in cancer and non-cancer patients, including C-reactive protein (CRP) level, white blood cell (WBC) count, NLR, platelet-to-lymphocyte ratio, the modified Glasgow prognostic score (mGPS), the prognostic index, and the prognostic nutritional index (PNI) [16].

In perioperative settings, the NLR may be an interesting parameter, at least for breast, lung, and kidney cancer patients undergoing surgical resection of their primary tumor. In non-cancer patients, the NLR has been proposed as an objective risk factor for mortality, cardiovascular morbidity and infections in the early and late postoperative period, if not normalized five days after surgery [3].

However, although inflammatory biomarkers and scores are modified after surgery, the lack of concordance between the inflammatory scores shows that they are not interchangeable during the perioperative period and should not be interpreted as such. Indeed, performances of the NLR and CRP seem to be different, following different kinetics after surgery. Interest in these scores is increasing during and after surgery despite limited data and the presence of limitations (small series, monocenter studies, not all types of surgery). To select the best score to be used during the perioperative period, description of evolution over time is an important step.

Why introduce the NLR, rather than simply using CRP? We already know that before surgery these parameters do not necessarily reflect the same phenomenon, since they arise, at least in part, from different mechanisms. After surgery, these differences are evident as the evolutions of the NLR and CRP are not parallel. An analysis of a cohort of patients undergoing major abdominal surgery showed that the correlation between the NLR and CRP was moderate before surgery and on postoperative day 7 ($R^2 = 0.40$ and 0.38, respectively, $p < 0.05$). In contrast, although statistically significant, correlation was poor on postoperative days 1 and 2 ($R^2 = 0.06$ and 0.10, respectively, $p < 0.05$) [17]. Interestingly, on postoperative day 7, an increased NLR was the only parameter independently associated with complications ($p < 0.001$). In other words, complications are associated with a greater inflammatory response to abdominal surgery, which is better reflected by a higher NLR 7 days after the surgery than by the CRP level. Indeed, the NLR remained elevated in patients developing postoperative complications compared with patients who had no complications. In a multivariable analysis, the NLR value on postoperative day 7 was the only factor associated with postoperative complications. CRP levels had delayed kinetics compared to the NLR, increasing on postoperative day 2 and not normalizing by day 7 whether or not there were complications. This confirms previous observations by Vaughan-Shaw et al. and Cook et al. [18, 19]. A persistently high NLR value after one week has been associated not only with short term morbidity (cardiovascular and septic) but also with higher long-term mortality after lung cancer surgery and orthopedic surgery for hip fracture.

In brief, inflammatory biomarkers are not interchangeable, may be insufficient in some situations (e.g., immunonutrition programs), and more sensitive and rapid markers, such as NLR, should be introduced [20].

The Options

To Control the Inflammatory Reaction

There is a strong rationale for perioperative testing of interventions that could be associated with optimal control of the inflammatory reaction to prevent the perioperative disequilibrium in cancer patients that can lead to postoperative accelerated tumor growth and early relapse [21]. Even if persistence of the inflammatory process is a consequence rather than a cause, investigation of this phenomenon may be interesting. In other words, are there pathophysiological mechanisms linking a persisting high NLR value with a worse outcome? And could we propose an early therapeutic intervention to improve outcome?

Non-Steroidal Anti-Inflammatory Drugs
Among the possible interventions used by anesthesiologists, one has attracted most attention: non-steroidal anti-inflammatory drugs (NSAIDs). NSAIDs have been shown to impair the growth of tumors at all the steps described above. Indeed, in addition to their opiate-sparing effect, NSAIDs present a promising anticancer profile with respect to the pathophysiological steps of tumor proliferation and dissemination [22]. These therapeutic effects of chronic NSAIDs in cancer have been described for various carcinomas, with considerable concordance between studies. While the role of NSAIDS in cancer prevention remains unclear, this is not related to a lack of data on their anticancer effect but, rather, to adverse effects associated with chronic administration [23, 24]. In animal surgical models, concordant data have been published, suggesting a direct specific effect of NSAIDs on perioperative protumoral events that lead circulating tumors cells and/or micrometastases to survive and proliferate [25, 26]. Unfortunately, in human studies focusing on perioperative interventions to influence postoperative cancer outcome, methodological pitfalls including endpoint selection and unreported NSAID use preclude any definitive conclusions [27]. Consequently, additional studies have been conducted, using existing prospective patient lists and high quality databases, in breast, prostate, lung and kidney cancer surgery [28].

Endothelial Function: Statins and Clonidine
Well-known/validated in the chronic treatment of inflammatory vascular atherosclerotic disease, statins and/or aspirin may find a place in high-risk population cancer and non-cancer surgery. Statins may help reduce the acute phase of the inflammatory response, endothelial dysfunction and the procoagulant profile as well as the toxic cross-talk existing between platelets and neutrophils that occurs days after the first event [29]. Clonidine, an α_2-agonist used in the perioperative period

as a co-analgesic and anti-hypertensive drug, may also be associated with cardiovascular protection via its anti-inflammatory properties and protection of post-ischemic endothelial function. Aspirin, acting on the cardiovascular profile by various mechanisms, including neutrophil-platelet adhesion, could also be an important therapeutic intervention. Unfortunately, in heterogeneous series of moderate risk patients, neither aspirin nor clonidine has proven their utility to prevent major vascular events [30, 31]. Therefore, it appears that a paradigm shift is necessary if we want to improve the efficiency of our research. We propose that retrospective analyses are of prime importance to convert observations to theories and to identify potential therapeutic targets. This approach can be used to select biomarkers, to analyze the influence of our interventions and/or to improve comprehension of long-term outcomes, in non-cancer and in cancer research [1, 32].

Time for a Paradigm Shift

Subgroup identification can be important to understand the effects of our interventions; it has helped us in understanding of the effect of NSAIDs in breast and prostate cancer patients. Other examples exist in which development of drug candidates was stopped when it may have been successful in some subgroups. One condition of a successful test is to focus on patients most likely to benefit from the drug. The incorporation of biomarkers is, at least partially, a response to try and identify these patients. In our work, incorporation of the NLR led to a better understanding and documentation of the biology. This approach may prevent failure of clinical trials testing drug candidates. Another example is the high incidence of early relapse observed after breast cancer surgery in triple-negative histological type patients. A selection of patients based on this prognostic biomarker has been proposed to test the influence of ketorolac. This approach could reduce the high attrition rate and minimize futile exposure of patients to ineffective investigational therapies. In the same direction, we can also propose to use the data from large available series, e.g., the PeriOperative Ischemic Evaluation-2 Trial (POISE-2). This is an example of a large database (10,000 patients) that could be used to monitor the effects of aspirin on cancer recurrence, even if it was not designed for this goal.

Additionally, and as detailed above, a potential role of high NLR to identify high-risk patients has been proposed in cancer and in non-cancer settings. NLR values could be assessed in the preoperative period and followed after surgery. We propose that the NLR should be used to screen patients and to monitor response to cancer and to surgery. This monitoring could be used in clinical practice from diagnosis to the end of the postoperative recovery. NLR values could also be used as an inclusion criterion in clinical trials.

Conclusion

Inflammation is a major prognostic factor after major cancer and non-cancer surgery, as well as in non-surgical settings. Biomarkers like the NLR can reflect this process and can be used in clinical practice and integrated into clinical research. Biomarkers are now proposed not only in cancer surgery, but also to identify high-risk subgroups in non-cancer surgery to potentially prevent morbidity and mortality, or at least to treat preventable risk factors. We have possible pharmacological interventions, such as NSAIDs, statins and clonidine, for use in the perioperative period of major surgery. We suggest how the NLR could be incorporated into prospective trials. Database analyses and incorporation of biomarkers into clinical research will probably play a major role in the future.

References

1. Forget P, De Kock M (2014) Perspectives in anaesthesia for cancer surgery. J Cancer Res Clin Oncol 140:353–359
2. Demicheli R, Retsky MW, Hrushesky WJM, Baum M (2007) Tumor dormancy and surgery-driven dormancy interruption in breast cancer: learning from failures. Nature Clin Pract Oncol 4:699–710
3. Retsky MW, Demicheli R, Hrushesky WJ, Baum M, Gukas ID (2008) Dormancy and surgery-driven escape from dormancy help explain some clinical features of breast cancer. APMIS 116:730–741
4. Jatoi I, Tsimelzon A, Weiss H, Clark GM, Hilsenbeck SG (2005) Hazard rates of recurrence following diagnosis of primary breast cancer. Breast Cancer Res Treat 89:173–178
5. Hilsenbeck SG, Ravdin PM, de Moor CA, Chamness GC, Osborne CK, Clark GM (1998) Time-dependence of hazard ratios for prognostic factors in primary breast cancer. Breast Cancer Res Treat 52:227–237
6. Baum M, Demicheli R, Hrushesky W, Retsky M (2005) Does surgery unfavourably perturb the "natural history" of early breast cancer by accelerating the appearance of distant metastases? Eur J Cancer 41:508–515
7. Forget P, Coulie PG, Retsky M, Demicheli R, Machiels JP, De Kock M (2013) Is there a rationale for an anesthesiologist's role against cancer recurrence? Acta Anaesthesiol Belg 64:15–24
8. Gourdin M, Dubois P, Mullier F et al (2012) The effect of clonidine, an alpha-2 adrenergic receptor agonist, on inflammatory response and postischaemic endothelium function during early reperfusion in healthy volunteers. J Cardiovas Pharmacol 60:553–560
9. Roche JJ, Wenn RT, Sahota O, Moran CG (2005) Effect of comorbidities and postoperative complications on mortality after hip fracture in elderly people: prospective observational cohort study. BMJ 331:1374
10. Azab B, Chainani V, Shah N, Mc GJT (2012) Neutrophil-Lymphocyte ratio as a predictor of major adverse cardiac events among diabetic population: a 4-year follow-up study. Angiology 64:456–465
11. Forget P, Moreau N, Engel H et al (2015) The neutrophil-to-lymphocyte ratio (NLR) after surgery for hip fracture (HF). Arch Gerontol Geriatr 60:366–371
12. Lee GK, Lee LC, Chong E et al (2012) The long-term predictive value of the neutrophil-to-lymphocyte ratio in type 2 diabetic patients presenting with acute myocardial infarction. QJM 105:1075–1082
13.

Duffy BK, Gurm HS, Rajagopal V, Gupta R, Ellis SG, Bhaatt DL (2006) Usefulness of an elevated neutrophil to lymphocyte ratio in predicting long-term mortality after percutaneous coronary intervention. Am J Cardiol 97:993–996

14. Tamhane UU, Aneja S, Montgomery D, Rogers E-K, Eagle KA, Gurm HS (2008) Association between admission neutrophil to lymphocyte ratio and outcomes in patients with acute coronary syndrome. Am J Cardiol 102:653–657

15. Nunez J, Nunez E, Bodi V et al (2008) Usefulness of the neutrophil to lymphocyte ratio in predicting long-term mortality in ST segment elevation myocardial infarction". Am J Cardiol 101:747–752

16. Forget P, Rengger N, Berliere M, De Kock M (2014) Inflammatory scores are not interchangeable during the perioperative period of breast cancer surgery. Int J Surg 12:1360–1362

17. Forget P, Dinant V, De Kock M (2015) Is the Neutrophil-to-Lymphocyte Ratio more correlated than C-reactive protein with postoperative complications after major abdominal surgery? PeerJ 3:e713

18. Vaughan-Shaw PG, Rees JR, King AT (2012) Neutrophil lymphocyte ratio in outcome prediction after emergency abdominal surgery in the elderly. Int J Surg 10:157–162

19. Cook EJ, Walsh SR, Faroog N, Alberts JC, Justin TA, Keeling NJ (2007) Post-operative Neutrophil-lymphocyte ratio predicts complications following colorectal surgery. Int J Surg 5:27–30

20. Forget P, Echeverria G, Giglioli S et al (2015) Biomarkers in immunonutrition programme, is there still a need for new ones? A brief review. Ecancermedicalscience 9:546

21. Forget P, Simonet O, De Kock M (2013) Cancer surgery induces inflammation, immunosuppression and neo-angiogenesis, but is it influenced by analgesics? F1000Res 2:102

22. Forget P (2014) A single dose of ketorolac during surgery may suppress cancer relapse: something for nothing? Proc Belg Royal Acad Med 3:53–60

23. Holmes MD, Chen WY, Li L, Hertzmark E, Spiegelman D, Hankinson SE (2010) Aspirin intake and survival after breast cancer. J Clin Oncol 28:1467–1472

24. Burn J, Gerdes AM, Macrae F et al (2012) Long-term effect of aspirin on cancer risk in carriers of hereditary colorectal cancer: an analysis from the CAPP2 randomised controlled trial. Lancet 378:2081–2087

25. Forget P, Collet V, Lavand'homme P, De Kock M (2010) Does analgesia and condition influence immunity after surgery? Effects of fentanyl, ketamine and clonidine on natural killer activity at different ages. Eur J Anaesthesiol 27:233–240

26. Forget P, De Kock M (2009) Could anaesthesia, analgesia and sympathetic modulation affect neoplasic recurrence after surgery? A systematic review centred over the modulation of natural killer cells activity. Ann Fr Anesth Reanim 28:751–768

27. Forget P, Leonard D, Kartheuser A, De Kock M (2011) Choice of Endpoint and Not Reporting All the Analgesics Used May Render Inconclusive Studies on Oncological Outcome. Anesthesiology 114:717

28. Forget P, Machiels JP, Coulie PG et al (2013) Neutrophil:lymphocyte ratio and intraoperative use of ketorolac or diclofenac are prognostic factors in different cohorts of patients undergoing breast, lung and kidney cancer surgery. Ann Surg Oncol 20(suppl 3):S650–S660

29. Manfredi AA, Rovere-Querini P, Maugeri N (2010) Dangerous connections: neutrophils and the phagocytic clearance of activated platelets. Curr Opin Hematol 17:3–8

30. POISE-2 Investigators (2014) Aspirin in patients undergoing noncardiac surgery. N Engl J Med 370:1494–1503

31. POISE-2 Investigators (2014) Clonidine in patients undergoing noncardiac surgery. N Engl J Med 370:1504–1513

32. Lacombe D, Burock S, Meunier F (2012) Academia-Industry Partnerships: Are we ready for new models of partnership?: The point of view of the EORTC, an academic clinical cancer research organisation. Eur J Cancer 49:1–7

Kairotropy: Discovering Critical Illness Trajectories Using Clinical Phenotypes with Big Data

G. E. Weissman and S. D. Halpern

Introduction

In 1967, Alvan Feinstein defined "iatrotropic stimulus" as "the particular reason why a person decided to seek medical attention at a particular time" [1]. His purpose was to draw the attention of clinicians and researchers to the fact that the medical system becomes aware of a disease only at the moment a patient decides to arrive into the healthcare system, and not necessarily at the time that the disease begins. This concept is powerful in that it encourages the clinician as well as the epidemiologist to see the broader picture of a patient's experience and understand the contextual drivers behind utilization patterns. The primary care setting is often the first point of catchment for iatrotropy, suggesting that "health problems are presented to healthcare workers for the first time because they are not solvable by patients and their social networks without professional medical help" [2]. Given the unique causes, costs, and sequelae of critical illness, a particular kind of health problem, here we introduce the term "kairotropic stimulus" to signify "the particular reason why a person is in need of critical care services at a particular time".

Consider a patient presenting in respiratory failure to the intensive care unit (ICU). This patient may present with a chief complaint of dyspnea and be given a diagnosis of 'chronic obstructive pulmonary disease (COPD) exacerbation'. To the bedside clinician, these are good explanations for the patient's need for critical care.

G. E. Weissman
Pulmonary, Allergy, and Critical Care Division, Hospital of the University of Pennsylvania
Philadelphia, USA
Leonard Davis Institute of Health Economics, University of Pennsylvania
Philadelphia, USA

S. D. Halpern (✉)
Pulmonary, Allergy, and Critical Care Division, Hospital of the University of Pennsylvania
Philadelphia, USA
Department of Medicine, University of Pennsylvania
Philadelphia, USA
email: shalpern@exchange.upenn.edu

© Springer International Publishing Switzerland 2016
J.-L. Vincent (ed.), *Annual Update in Intensive Care and Emergency Medicine 2016*,
DOI 10.1007/978-3-319-27349-5_39

A deeper look, however, may reveal that the kairotropic stimulus was actually the loss of employment, resulting in loss of insurance coverage for chronic medications, such as inhalers, thus leading to decompensated respiratory failure. An outpatient consult with a social worker to re-enroll the patient in a low-cost insurance plan, or access to free medications through a public clinic might have prevented this ICU stay.

Next consider a patient with known stage IV pancreatic cancer who presents to the ICU with hemorrhagic shock. Emergent endoscopy reveals that the tumor has invaded the duodenum. Again, the first-line clinician may reasonably conclude that the cancer caused the bleed, which caused the shock. However, a more holistic perspective may suggest that the kairotropic stimulus was not the invasive tumor, but rather the unmet need for palliative and hospice services that might have prevented a costly and potentially unwanted ICU admission.

Identifying the specific reasons that lead to critical care utilization has broad consequences. The societal burden of critical illness continues to rise as the population ages and healthcare technologies expand, driving both an expansion in ICU beds and greater strain on ICU capacities to provide high-quality care [3–6]. Further, ICU survivorship is increasing, leading to more survivors of critical illness living with psychiatric, cognitive, functional [7, 8] and economic [9] burdens years following discharge from the ICU. For these and other reasons, there are strong incentives to prevent critical illness when possible, or to provide timely alternatives to ICU admission when appropriate.

The ICU provides significant benefits for properly selected patients [10]. In other populations, however, ICU care may represent a low-value distribution of health system resources. In one study, for example, 15% of ICU admissions were for ambulatory care sensitive conditions [11], suggesting that timely and appropriate primary care may have achieved similar or improved outcomes at lower cost. Similarly, a large proportion of healthcare costs occur at the end of life, often in people with known advanced, chronic disease [12]. This suggests an unmet need for palliative care services and advance care planning that may have both improved provision of care consistent with patient preferences, and reduced costly ICU and other hospital care.

The longitudinal trajectory of critical illness begins long before physiological derangements occur, often continues through a grueling and uncertain ICU stay, and, if the patient survives, frequently culminates in a state that has been termed the post-intensive care syndrome [8], with increased debility and risk for readmission. Each segment of this trajectory includes its own risks, challenges for patients, families, providers, and researchers, and opportunities for meaningful intervention to align care with patient preferences and improve the value of delivered health care.

In this chapter, we offer a new approach for understanding the contextual roots of critical illness with an emphasis on the earliest segment of this longitudinal trajectory. The framework of kairotropy challenges the nosologic habits of critical care practitioners to consider social, demographic, and other extra-medical factors as potential root causes of critical illness. We further describe how analyses of aggregated, population-level electronic health information (EHI) can elucidate opportunities for interventions that may improve realization of patient preferences and increase the value of critical care delivery. In sum, we describe how analyzing Big Data can elucidate kairotropic phenotypes to provide clinically and socially actionable knowledge.

The Kairotropic Stimulus

The ancient Greek word kairos ($\kappa\alpha\iota\rho\delta\varsigma$) refers to a "critical time, season, or opportunity" or a "vital" part of the body [13] – apt references to the time-sensitive and vital threats faced by the contemporary critically ill patient. The term has been described as "a passing instant when an opening appears which must be driven through with force if success is to be achieved" [14] – appropriate both for students of classical rhetoric and for ICU clinicians. Finally, in the New Testament, the word kairos represents critical times or events on a divine scale (Matthew 26:18). And -tropy, derived from the Greek word tropos ($\tau\rho\sigma\pi\sigma\varsigma$) meaning 'turning', has been used in combination with Greek terms to form combined words "denoting types of spatial orientation or directional movement or growth in response to a stimulus" [15]. Therefore, kairotropy intends the moving towards a state of critical illness.

This view of critical illness alters the scope of work of front-line providers. In seeking to identify the kairotropic stimulus, the history of present illness must be expanded to include contextual questions about social, cultural, demographic, and personal information. This line of questioning illuminates opportunities for a range of interventions, such as outpatient care coordination, home safety evaluation, hospice referral, and others, which may prevent future ICU admissions. Such knowledge would frame the strategy for anticipatory guidance and high-value interventions for patients and families that provide patient-centered care.

One limitation of the kairotropic stimulus framework may be that, in some ways, the ICU is merely a place in a larger healthcare system, the use of which is guided, in part, by idiosyncratic decision-making processes and other factors external to the patient. Thus, our definition purposefully includes patients 'in need of' the life support and close monitoring that characterize critical care, rather than those who are actually admitted to an ICU. Many hospitalized patients do not receive the appropriate level of care required by their illness at the correct time. Some potential reasons for unrealized kairotropy include lack of beds, inefficiencies in triage, lack of regional referral networks, or misrecognition of disease severity.

Although defining kairotropic stimuli among patients in need of critical care is conceptually sound, this definition may be difficult to achieve practically. Patients must at least arrive in the hospital and present to an emergency room or ICU, to be counted. A homeless patient who suffers from hypothermia, trauma, or sepsis in the community may indeed have a kairotropic stimulus, but it never reaches its apotheosis, the actual receipt of timely and appropriate critical care. These patients, unfortunately, often fly below the epidemiologic and Big Data radars.

Globally, kairotropy will look different in different countries where the resources that are accessible outside the ICU differ. In lower-resourced settings, kairotropy

Table 1 Potentially preventable forms of kairotropy and associated interventions

Kairotropic Phenotype	Kairotropic Stimulus	Upstream Intervention
Ambulatory care sensitive condition	– Lack of timely access to care provider (e.g., primary care, behavioral health, etc.) – Lack of health insurance, or under-insurance – Lack of transportation to pharmacy, dialysis center, or other health service	– Health system 'navigator', coach, social worker, or community health worker depending on specific need – Enrollment in low-cost health insurance plan on insurance exchange – Pre-arrange transportation services
Unmet need for palliative care	– Lack of advanced care planning in patient at high risk for critical illness	– Early outpatient referral to palliative and/or hospice services
Frailty	– Mechanical fall – Medication error – Aspiration event	– Home safety evaluation with installation of support bars and rails, and removal of trip-risks – Outpatient pharmacist consult with visiting nurse and medication teaching – Swallow evaluation with follow up therapy, including family education
Unstable social situations	– Lack of or unstable housing – Lack of or unstable social support network – Exposure to domestic violence and trauma	– Social worker or other social services case worker – Peer groups, counseling, housing services – Child care

will be more strongly correlated with mortality because the requisite resources to provide critical care will be less available. In such settings, the impetus for prospective identification and early intervention, where possible, will be correspondingly greater.

Finally, not all kairotropy will be preventable. A person undergoing lung transplantation, for example, will inexorably arrive in the ICU postoperatively. Such predictable and appropriate uses of the ICU fall outside our current consideration. Instead, our focus is on the common phenotypic trajectories for which there may be a reasonable likelihood of preventing critical illness or an unwanted ICU stay. Table 1 summarizes these phenotypes and associated interventions.

Data Signatures and Phenotypes of Kairotropy

In this section, we propose several potentially common phenotypes of kairotropy that may be important for critical care clinicians, population health researchers, leaders of healthcare delivery systems, and payers. We selected these phenotypes based on our clinical experience caring for patients in a medical ICU, and on published literature regarding known risks for critical illness and hospital admission. Before describing the selected phenotypes, several caveats are in order.

First, there certainly exist many other kairotropic phenotypes not mentioned here. We focus on those that are most likely to be preventable, and acknowledge that research is needed to refine these phenotypes and to uncover new ones. Second, we note that the designation of phenotypes as preventable depends on the interventions available in a given setting. If, for example, a community does not have a local palliative care clinic or service, then predicting unmet needs for palliative care will not immediately alter care for patients. However, such prediction could be used to motivate local investment in palliative resources. Third, some patients will exhibit combinations of multiple phenotypes, rather than fitting neatly into only one category. In such cases, multiple actions may be needed to prevent the manifestation of critical illness. Finally, we emphasize an approach to characterizing kairotropy that includes an *a priori* specification of phenotypes, rather than a hypothetical approach that seeks to allow the data to independently determine the kairotropic stimulus. Although both approaches are viable, and may indeed be used complementarily, specifying patterns of interest may promote the chances that actionable interventions emerge from the predictive models.

In the sections below we present a number of kairotropic stimuli that merit future investigation, and summarize these in Fig. 1.

Location-Dependent

Some preventable kairotropic phenotypes are particular to a location. It is the clinical, demographic and social milieu of that location which drives a patient toward critical illness. In this section, we present some examples of location-dependent, preventable kairotropy. The location is important because embedded in it are the risks for critical illness as well as the site and means of intervention.

Ambulatory Kairotropy

Known types of preventable kairotropy among community-dwelling populations are centered around lack of access to appropriate and timely care. In one ICU, for example, a review of admissions revealed that 15% were for ambulatory care-sensitive conditions [11], suggesting that timely access to a primary care provider could have prevented the ICU admission.

It is also likely that timely and appropriate outpatient referral to palliative and/or hospice services may prevent low-value ICU admissions. One in five Americans dies receiving ICU services, and an estimated 43,100 people with metastatic malignancy die in the ICU each year in the USA [16]. One in three Medicare beneficiaries are admitted to the ICU in the last month of their lives [17].

Our first phenotype represents patients with unmet needs for palliative care. Such patients likely have diagnostic codes in claims and encounter notes relating to advanced stage malignancy, or an array of non-malignant disorders, such as end-stage renal disease or advanced COPD or heart failure [18]. They may also have sufficient codes to suggest the presence of frailty [19, 20]. However, these patients will lack claims for palliative care consultation or for prescriptions for indicated palliative

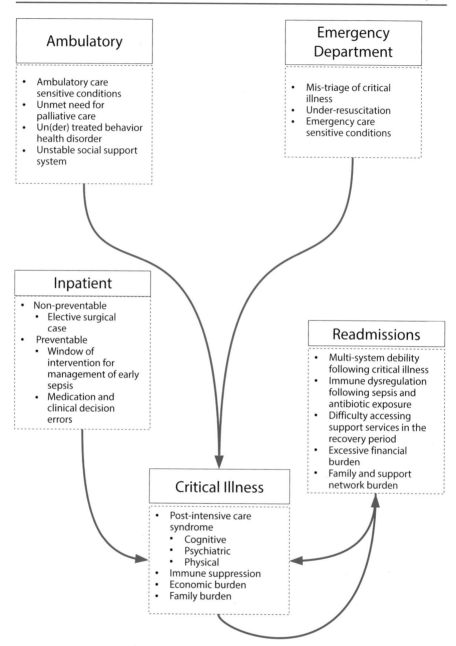

Fig. 1 Kairotropic phenotypes and their causes

medications. Frequent address changes in administrative databases, likely a marker of social instability, are associated with higher rates of hospital admission [21].

A phenotype of frailty is common among patients prior to development of critical illness [19]. Numerous models exist to identify frailty [19, 22, 23] and burden of morbidity [24, 25] from clinical and administrative data, and might be used to target interventions aimed at advance care planning. Some of these interventions may actually prevent critical illness, where others may instead offer care more closely aligned with patient preferences when critical illness does occur. Prospective identification of patients with frailty, paired with a targeted, multidisciplinary intervention can reduce costs and hospital admissions [22].

It has also been observed that low health literacy [26], unstable housing, drug use, history of a missed clinic visit and history of depression or anxiety [21] are risk factors for hospital admissions from the community. Such factors might also contribute specifically to ICU admission risk. However, it is unclear how many ICU admissions for common indications, such as respiratory failure, sepsis, and hemorrhage [27], manifest from trajectories of preventable kairotropic phenotypes.

Early identification of patients with the above risks would allow for care providers or administrators to schedule timely interventions in the community setting to community health workers, social workers, behavioral health specialists, or provide transportation or literacy support where needed. It is very likely that if these interventions were successful in preventing an ICU admission, then any such outpatient intervention would be highly cost-effective and perhaps cost-saving.

Emergency Department Kairotropy

The emergency department (ED) represents a common catchment for patients who are unable to sufficiently manage health problems with outpatient resources. Once triaged, patients presenting to the ED may be discharged home, observed, or admitted to the hospital for further management. Of those sick enough to be admitted, some go to a ward bed, others to an ICU, and still others to care units with intermediate nurse:patient ratios and monitoring capacities. The choice between these locations is not always clear. In this section we explore risks for critical illness and ICU transfer among those patients presenting to the ED.

Unplanned transfer to the ICU within 24 h of admission to the hospital is associated with increased mortality [28]. Among community hospitals, risks for such transfers include lower hospital volume and increased burdens of acute and chronic diseases, while the availability of a step-down or telemetry unit was associated with reduced ICU admissions [29]. Physiologic derangements measured by abnormal vital signs and laboratory tests have been used to predict admission to the ICU from the ED [30].

'Emergency care sensitive conditions' are those "for which rapid diagnosis and early intervention in acute illness or acutely decompensated chronic illness improve patient outcomes" [31]. Failure to provide appropriate early diagnosis and intervention, such as early resuscitation for sepsis, could lead to progression to critical illness.

Inpatient Kairotropy

Kairotropy among patients already admitted to a hospital is common, but prospective identification of preventable, clinical decompensation is an elusive target [32]. In a single-center study, the use of a rapid response team was associated with reduced rates of out-of-ICU cardiac arrest, increased ICU admissions, and equivocal effects on mortality [33]. Such services may also reduce ICU admission among patients too sick to benefit from critical care by providing timely discussions about goals of care. Fewer available ICU beds at the time of sudden clinical deterioration among hospitalized patients is associated with fewer ICU admissions and increased rates of change of care goals to no-resuscitation or to comfort measures [34]. This finding suggests that ICU-bed scarcity may help to reduce inpatient kairotropy by prompting previously unmet need for discussion of care goals [35]. Other specialized services may also reduce inpatient kairotropy. For example, early consultation with infectious disease specialists has been associated with decreased mortality, ICU length of stay, and readmission rates, although the proportion of patients requiring ICU care was not reported [36].

Location-Independent

Readmissions Kairotropy

Hospital readmissions have become a topic of national interest such that Centers for Medicare & Medicaid Services (CMS) will reduce reimbursement to hospitals that underperform relative to expected readmissions rates generated from a CMS model [37]. However, the observations that almost 35% of ICU readmissions occur more than 120 h following ICU discharge [38], and that readmissions are more closely associated with patient factors rather than ICU care [39], suggest that disease trajectories may be a potential target for intervention.

Patients with severe sepsis have higher health care utilization in the year following their admission, more alive days spent in a facility compared to patients with non-sepsis hospitalization [40], and have an increased rate of hospital admissions for ambulatory care sensitive conditions [41]. Survivors of hospitalizations that promote dysbiosis (primarily infection with associated antibiotic exposure) are also at higher risk of subsequent severe sepsis [42].

Prior work suggests that some low cost interventions, such as community health workers, may reduce readmission rates for those patients with social and material needs that compete with the need for medical care [43]. Interventions that prevent readmissions for disease-specific phenotypes have shown, for example, reduced admission rates in patients with COPD who receive transitional care management programs [44] and timely post-discharge follow-visit with a pulmonologist [45]. Identification of those patients likely to benefit from such low-cost interventions remains a goal of reducing readmissions kairotropy.

Why ICU Admissions Are Unique

Hospital utilization and readmissions have become topics of national concern for health care policy-makers and in public discourse [37, 46]. Given that the ICU is merely a place within a hospital designed to provide specialized care that commonly includes life support, is it important to distinguish ICU admissions and readmissions from those to non-ICU inpatient services?

There are clear economic motives for doing so. In 2011, the mean charge for a non-ICU hospitalization was \$25,200, compared with \$61,800 for those hospitalizations that included an ICU stay [47]. Thus, interventions that prevent ICU admissions might be significantly more cost-effective than those that prevent hospital admissions without ICU care.

Given the distinct intensity of ICU admissions both for patients and for families, who can also suffer from the family variant of post-intensive care syndrome [8], outpatient discussions with caregivers about patient and family preferences for hospital admission may vary based on the probability of an ICU stay compared to a non-ICU admission.

Finally, the ICU admission itself may present a distinct opportunity for gathering information and intervening to alter a patient's future trajectory. ICU admissions may be viewed as sentinel events in a patient's disease courses, during which frank discussions with patients and families are common. This allows clinicians to gather contextual information that may help reveal a kairotropic stimulus, which could lead to personalized interventions during an ICU stay.

Breaking down 'Big Data'

Asch et al. [48] observed that patients spend only a few hours each year in contact with the healthcare system, and more than 5000 h awake and doing everything else. This fact makes it difficult for health care providers to monitor patients and know who will get sick and when. Despite the promise of 'Big Data' to improve healthcare delivery, it is not clear exactly how this trend may augment understanding of patients' trajectories through the healthcare system.

At a practical level, Big Data means aggregating large amounts of information from multiple sources so as to strategically improve patient health. Although physicians spend little time with patients, patients do emit a sort of Global Positioning System (GPS) signal each time they come into contact with a billable healthcare service. This signal, while intermittent, may include information about laboratory results, pharmacy utilization, outpatient care and other services, and may prove sufficient to generate an accurate prediction of patients' future clinical trajectories. Appropriately used, such aggregated data from multiple types of patient encounters with the healthcare system provides unique opportunities to observe patients at risk for and following critical illness as traversing a longitudinal path, rather than merely appearing and disappearing in episodic ICU encounters. Thus, studying patients' arrays of interactions with the healthcare system may reveal 'signatures' in utilization patterns that correspond to clinical phenotypes.

But for Big Data to fulfill its promise in this regard, it must produce timely, clinically relevant, and actionable knowledge for the healthcare provider, patient, administrator, or researcher. For example, building a predictive model to identify people at risk for ICU admission in the next 30 days might serve as a useful harbinger of upcoming capacity strain or staffing needs. The reasons for ICU admission are myriad and complex, and so it would also be helpful to know why a person is going to be admitted. In this regard, the advent of supervised learning methods [49] may enable accurate assessments of the attributable risks conferred by each potential predictor variable. However, to be clinically actionable, such information must be translatable into a specific, appropriate intervention for patients.

Building predictive models using supervised learning methods with an *a priori* phenotype in mind may increase the probability that the ensuing model will illuminate opportunities for direct action. There is also value, however, in using *un*supervised learning methods [49] to segment the population and identify utilization signatures and kairotropic risk not previously characterized. Identification of such phenotypes and risk factors may prompt further investigations (both qualitative and quantitative), but may not immediately evince an actionable intervention.

Areas for Future Investigation

The framework of kairotropy suggests many new areas of investigation. First, previously developed predictive models of hospital admission from the community do not specifically account for those admissions requiring ICU services. It is unclear whether a severity adjustment alone will enable existing models to stratify ICU and non-ICU admissions, or if distinct risk factors among community-dwelling populations will emerge.

Other important unknowns in studying kairotropy are the optimal time horizons for data gathering and making predictions. The answers to these questions are also likely to be phenotype-specific, and depend on which interventions are available in a given region. Upon enrollment into an insurance plan, a patient identified as 100 years old on an administrative form should prompt inquiry into needs for advanced care planning. A patient with an unstable social support network, however, may take many months to build an electronic signature in clinical and administrative records demonstrating repeated low-value utilization patterns. Table 2 provides a summary of these and other areas of future investigation in the study of kairotropy.

Table 2 Areas for future investigation in the study of kairotropy

Unknown	Research questions
Risk factors for ICU admission among community-dwelling population	– Do existing models of admission risk appropriately identify ICU admission risk factors? – Is the difference between an ICU and non-ICU admission only a matter of "dose" of severity or risk? – Are there distinct risk factors for ICU admission that vary based on the kairotropic phenotype?
Time horizons of information and prediction	– What is the optimal time period over which to gather clinical, administrative, and demographic data to optimize the test characteristics of a predictive model for ICU admission? – What is the optimal time period over which to predict ICU admission? Does this vary by available intervention, kairotropic phenotype, or patient preference?
Preventive interventions	– Can interventions such as community health workers, advance care planning teams, and social workers that are known to prevent hospital admissions and readmissions, also address preventable kairotropy? – How does the cost-effectiveness of preventing ICU admissions change the scope of beneficial interventions? – Does the ICU itself offer new opportunities for location-specific interventions to prevent readmissions kairotropy?
Patient-centered data use	– What aspects of an ICU admission would be important to a patient if it could be predicted in advance? – Are there probability thresholds that would or would not change the way a patient would want to discuss potential future ICU admissions? – How do predictive models built on massive data sets best account for heterogeneity and provide accurate information for individual patients?

Conclusion

Prospective identification of kairotropy in the general population may provide opportunities for early intervention that can improve quality of life, align care with patient preferences, reduce costs, and increase the value of care. Leveraging Big Data trends of aggregated patient information across multiple types and locations, combined with statistical learning methods and clinical insight, can transform large amounts of information into clinically relevant, actionable knowledge.

This framework is relevant for clinical providers, population health researchers, health system leaders, and all risk-bearing entities. Ongoing data collection and information sharing between these stakeholders in the future will allow for increased predictive power of models that rely on a combination of clinical, administrative, and demographic information. Given the unique burdens and costs of critical illness, prevention of critical illness or provision of higher-value care in its place, is likely to yield significant benefits to patients, families, and health systems.

Acknowledgements

Gary Weissman is supported by an NIH training grant (T32-HL098054) and is grateful to Kabeera Weissman for reviewing this chapter and providing helpful comments and insights.

References

1. Feinstein AR (1967) Clinical Judgment. Williams & Wilkins, Baltimore
2. Knottnerus JA (2002) Between iatrotropic stimulus and interiatric referral: the domain of primary care research. J Clin Epidemiol 55:1201–1206
3. Carson SS (2003) The epidemiology of critical illness in the elderly. Crit Care Clin 19:605–617
4. Milbrandt EB, Kersten A, Rahim MT et al (2008) Growth of intensive care unit resource use and its estimated cost in Medicare. Crit Care Med 36:2504–2510
5. Halpern SD (2011) ICU capacity strain and the quality and allocation of critical care. Curr Opin Crit Care 17:648–657
6. Wallace DJ, Angus DC, Seymour CW, Barnato AE, Kahn JM (2014) Critical care bed growth in the United States: A comparison of regional and national trends. Am J Respir Crit Care Med 191:410–416
7. Herridge MS, Tansey CM, Matté A et al (2011) Functional disability 5 years after acute respiratory distress syndrome. N Engl J Med 364:1293–1304
8. Elliott D, Davidson JE, Harvey MA et al (2014) Exploring the scope of post-intensive care syndrome therapy and care: engagement of non-critical care providers and survivors in a second stakeholders meeting. Crit Care Med 42:2518–2526
9. Griffiths J, Hatch RA, Bishop J et al (2013) An exploration of social and economic outcome and associated health-related quality of life after critical illness in general intensive care unit survivors: A 12-month follow-up study. Crit Care 17:R100
10. Shmueli A, Sprung CL (2005) Assessing the in-hospital survival benefits of intensive care. Int J Technol Assess Health Care 21:66–72
11. Burr J, Sherman G, Prentice D, Hill C, Fraser V, Kollef MH (2003) Ambulatory care-sensitive conditions: Clinical outcomes and impact on intensive care unit resource use. South Med J 96:172–178
12. Hogan C, Lunney J, Gable J, Lynne J (2001) Medicare beneficiaries' costs of care in the last year of life. Health Affairs 20:188–195
13. Liddell HG, Scott R, Jones SHS, McKenzie R (1940) A Greek-English Lexicon: A New Edition Revised and Augmented Throughout by Sir Henry Stuart Jones, with the Assistance of Roderick McKenzie. Clarendon Press, Oxford (2 Vols)
14. White EC (1987) Kaironomia: On the Will-to-Invent. Cornell University Press, London
15. OED online (2015) -tropy, comb. form. Available at http://www.oed.com/view/Entry/236528. Accessed September 2015
16. Angus DC, Barnato AE, Linde-Zwirble WT et al (2004) Use of intensive care at the end of life in the United States: An epidemiologic study. Crit Care Med 32:638–643
17. Teno JM, Gozalo PL, Bynum JP et al (2013) Change in end-of-life care for Medicare beneficiaries: Site of death, place of care, and health care transitions in 2000, 2005, and 2009. JAMA 309:470–477
18. Weissman DE, Meier DE (2011) Identifying patients in need of a palliative care assessment in the hospital setting: A consensus report from the center to advance palliative care. J Palliat Med 14:17–23
19. Hope AA, Gong MN, Guerra C, Wunsch H (2015) Frailty before critical illness and mortality for elderly medicare beneficiaries. J Am Geriatr Soc 63:1121–1128

20. Ensrud KE, Ewing SK, Taylor BC et al (2008) Comparison of 2 frailty indexes for prediction of falls, disability, fractures, and death in older women. Arch Intern Med 168:382–389

21. Amarasingham R, Moore BJ, Tabak YP et al (2010) An automated model to identify heart failure patients at risk for 30-day readmission or death using electronic medical record data. Med Care 48:981–988

22. Baker A, Leak P, Ritchie LD, Lee AJ, Fielding S (2012) Anticipatory care planning and integration: A primary care pilot study aimed at reducing unplanned hospitalisation. Br J Gen Pract 62:e113–e120

23. Baldwin MR, Reid MC, Westlake AA et al (2014) The feasibility of measuring frailty to predict disability and mortality in older medical intensive care unit survivors. J Crit Care 29:401–408

24. Charlson ME, Charlson RE, Peterson JC, Marinopoulos SS, Briggs WM, Hollenberg JP (2008) The Charlson comorbidity index is adapted to predict costs of chronic disease in primary care patients. J Clin Epidemiol 61:1234–1240

25. Huntley AL, Johnson R, Purdy S, Valderas JM, Salisbury C (2012) Measures of multimorbidity and morbidity burden for use in primary care and community settings: A systematic review and guide. Ann Fam Med 10:134–141

26. Baker DW, Gazmararian JA, Williams MV et al (2002) Functional health literacy and the risk of hospital admission among medicare managed care enrollees. Am J Public Health 92:1278–1283

27. Lilly CM, Zuckerman IH, Badawi O, Riker RR (2011) Benchmark data from more than 240,000 adults that reflect the current practice of critical care in the United States. Chest 140:1232–1242

28. Liu V, Kipnis P, Rizk NW, Escobar GJ (2012) Adverse outcomes associated with delayed intensive care unit transfers in an integrated healthcare system. J Hosp Med 7:224–230

29. Delgado MK, Liu V, Pines JM, Kipnis P, Gardner MN, Escobar GJ (2013) Risk factors for unplanned transfer to intensive care within 24 hours of admission from the emergency department in an integrated healthcare system. J Hosp Med 8:13–19

30. Labarere J, Schuetz P, Renaud B, Claessens YE, Albrich W, Mueller B (2012) Validation of a clinical prediction model for early admission to the intensive care unit of patients with pneumonia. Acad Emerg Med 19:993–1003

31. Carr BG, Conway PH, Meisel ZF, Steiner CA, Clancy C (2010) Defining the emergency care sensitive condition: A health policy research agenda in emergency medicine. Ann Emerg Med 56:49–51

32. Umscheid CA, Betesh J, VanZandbergen C et al (2015) Development, implementation, and impact of an automated early warning and response system for sepsis. J Hosp Med 10:26–31

33. Karpman C, Keegan MT, Jensen JB, Bauer PR, Brown DR, Afessa B (2013) The impact of rapid response team on outcome of patients transferred from the ward to the ICU: A single-center study. Crit Care Med 41:2284–2291

34. Stelfox HT, Hemmelgarn BR, Bagshaw SM et al (2012) Intensive care unit bed availability and outcomes for hospitalized patients with sudden clinical deterioration. Arch Intern Med 172:467–474

35. Wagner J, Halpern SD (2012) Deferred admission to the intensive care unit: Rationing critical care or expediting care transitions?: Comment on "Intensive care unit bed availability and outcomes for hospitalized patients with sudden clinical deterioration". Arch Intern Med 172:474–476

36. Schmitt S, McQuillen DP, Nahass R et al (2014) Infectious diseases specialty intervention is associated with decreased mortality and lower healthcare costs. Clin Infect Dis 58:22–28

37. Joynt KE, Jha AK (2013) Characteristics of hospitals receiving penalties under the hospital readmissions reduction program. JAMA 309:342–343

38. Brown SES, Ratcliffe SJ, Kahn JM, Halpern SD (2012) The epidemiology of intensive care unit readmissions in the United States. Am J Respir Crit Care Med 185:955–964

39. Brown SE, Ratcliffe SJ, Halpern SD (2014) An empirical comparison of key statistical attributes among potential ICU quality indicators. Crit Care Med 42(8):1821–1831

40. Prescott HC, Langa KM, Liu V, Escobar GJ, Iwashyna TJ (2014) Increased 1-year healthcare use in survivors of severe sepsis. Am J Respir Crit Care Med 190:62–69
41. Prescott HC, Langa KM, Iwashyna TJ (2015) Readmission diagnoses after hospitalization for severe sepsis and other acute medical conditions. JAMA 313:1055–1057
42. Prescott HC, Dickson RP, Rogers MAM, Langa KM, Iwashyna TJ (2015) Hospitalization type and subsequent severe sepsis. Am J Respir Crit Care Med 192(5):581–588
43. Kangovi S, Long JA, Emanuel E (2012) Community health workers combat readmission. Arch Int Med 172:1756–1757
44. Kangovi S, Grande D (2014) Transitional care management reimbursement to reduce COPD readmission. Chest 145:149–155
45. Gavish R, Levy A, Dekel OK, Karp E, Maimon N (2015) The association between hospital readmission and pulmonologist follow-up visits in patients with COPD. Chest 148:375–381
46. Gawande A (2011) The Hot Spotters. New Yorker Jan 24, 2011. http://www.newyorker.com/magazine/2011/01/24/the-hot-spotters. Accessed November 2015
47. Barrett M, Smith M, Elixhauser A, Honigman L, Pines J (2014) HCUP Statistical Brief #185: Utilization of Intensive Care Services. Agency for Healthcare Research and Quality. http://www.hcup-us.ahrq.gov/reports/statbriefs/sb185-Hospital-Intensive-Care-Units-2011.pdf. Accessed September 2015
48. Asch DA, Muller RW, Volpp KG (2012) Automated hovering in health care – watching over the 5000 hours. N Engl J Med 367:1–3
49. Hastie TJ, Tibshirani RJ, Friedman JH (2009) The Elements of Statistical Learning: Data Mining, Inference, and Prediction. Springer-Verlag, New York

Index

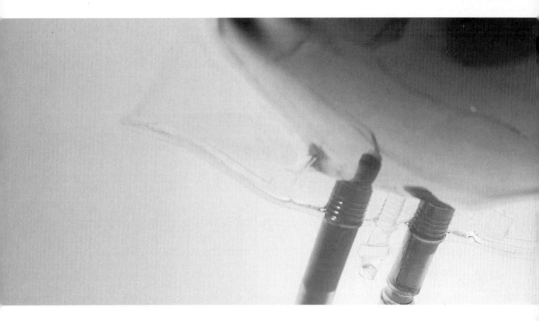
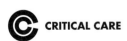
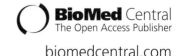

Printing and Binding: PHOENIX PRINT GmbH, Würzburg